Pearls and Pitfalls in
# HEAD AND NECK AND
# NEUROIMAGING
## Variants and Other
## Difficult Diagnoses

# Pearls and Pitfalls in
# HEAD AND NECK AND NEUROIMAGING

## Variants and Other Difficult Diagnoses

### Nafi Aygun

Associate Professor of Radiology and Director of the Neuroradiology
Fellowship Program, Johns Hopkins University, Baltimore, MD, USA

### Gaurang Shah

Associate Professor of Radiology, University of Michigan Health
System, Ann Arbor, MI, USA

### Dheeraj Gandhi

Professor of Radiology, Neurology and Neurosurgery at the
University of Maryland School of Medicine, Baltimore, MD, USA

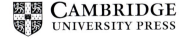
CAMBRIDGE
UNIVERSITY PRESS

# CAMBRIDGE
## UNIVERSITY PRESS

University Printing House, Cambridge CB2 8BS, United Kingdom

Published in the United States of America by Cambridge University Press, New York

Cambridge University Press is part of the University of Cambridge.

It furthers the University's mission by disseminating knowledge in the pursuit of education, learning and research at the highest international levels of excellence.

www.cambridge.org
Information on this title: www.cambridge.org/9781107026643

First published 2013

Printed in Spain by Grafos SA, Arte sobre papel

*A catalog record for this publication is available from the British Library*

*Library of Congress Cataloging in Publication data*
Aygun, Nafi.
Pearls and pitfalls in head and neck and neuroimaging / Nafi Aygun, Gaurang Shah, Dheeraj Gandhi.
    p. ; cm.
Includes bibliographical references.
ISBN 978-1-107-02664-3 (Hardback)
I. Shah, Gaurang.   II. Gandhi, Dheeraj.   III. Title.
[DNLM: 1. Neuroimaging–methods.   2. Central Nervous System Diseases–diagnosis.
3. Diagnosis, Differential.   4. Otorhinolaryngologic Diseases–diagnosis.   WL 141.5.N47]
RC349.D52
616.8′04754–dc23   2013010572

ISBN 978-1-107-02664-3 Hardback

To my parents, Vrindavan and Vinu Shah, for their love and support;
my wife Kinnari, for taking the journey with me; and my sons Sharvil and Sahil,
for bringing joy into our lives.

Gaurang Shah

To Bobby, my best friend and life partner and for Shreya and Diya,
my beautiful daughters and the love of my life.

Dheeraj Gandhi

# Contents

*Preface*   ix

## Section 1   Cerebrovascular diseases

Case 1   Dense basilar artery sign   1
Case 2   Global anoxic brain injury   4
Case 3   Acute infarction   8
Case 4   Vertebral artery dissection   10
Case 5   Subacute infarct   13
Case 6   Subarachnoid hemorrhage   17
Case 7   Intracranial aneurysms   21
Case 8   Giant aneurysms   23
Case 9   Acute intracerebral hematoma   26
Case 10   Cerebral amyloid angiopathy   30
Case 11   Primary CNS vasculitis   34
Case 12   Reversible cerebral vasoconstriction
          syndrome   37
Case 13   Moyamoya disease/syndrome   40
Case 14   Cortical venous thrombosis   43
Case 15   Developmental venous anomalies   46
Case 16   Dural arteriovenous fistula   49
Case 17   Cavernous malformation   52

## Section 2   Demyelinating and inflammatory diseases

Case 18   Tumefactive demyelinating lesion   55
Case 19   Acute disseminated encephalomyelitis   58
Case 20   Progressive multifocal
          leukoencephalopathy   62
Case 21   Osmotic myelinolysis   65
Case 22   Neurosarcoidosis   72

## Section 3   Tumors

Case 23   Posterior fossa masses in children   80
Case 24   Low-grade glioma   92
Case 25   Diffuse intrinsic pontine glioma   105
Case 26   Pseudoprogression of GBM   109
Case 27   Pseudoresponse in treatment of GBM   112
Case 28   Low-grade oligodendroglioma   114
Case 29   Primary CNS lymphoma   116
Case 30   Pineal region tumors   125
Case 31   Intraventricular masses   140
Case 32   Colloid cyst   153
Case 33   Primary intraosseous meningioma   161
Case 34   Suprasellar meningioma   171
Case 35   Pituitary macroadenoma   180

## Section 4   Infectious diseases

Case 36   Brain abscess   191
Case 37   Neurocysticercosis   194
Case 38   Tuberculosis   198
Case 39   Creutzfeldt–Jakob disease   207
Case 40   Herpes encephalitis   210

## Section 5   Metabolic and neurodegenerative conditions

Case 41   Wernicke's encephalopathy   213
Case 42   Hypertrophic olivary degeneration   217
Case 43   Adrenoleukodystrophy   219

## Section 6   Trauma

Case 44   Mild traumatic brain injury   224
Case 45   Isodense subdural hematoma   227

## Section 7   Miscellaneous

Case 46   Posterior reversible encephalopathy syndrome   229
Case 47   Late-onset adult hydrocephalus secondary to
          aqueductal stenosis   232
Case 48   Intracranial hypotension   234
Case 49   Idiopathic intracranial hypertension   238
Case 50   Rathke's cleft cyst   240

## Section 8   Artifacts and anatomic variations

Case 51   FLAIR sulcal hyperintensity secondary to general
          anesthesia   245
Case 52   Virchow–Robin spaces   250
Case 53   Arachnoid granulations   255
Case 54   Benign external hydrocephalus   257
Case 55   Pitfalls in CTA   260
Case 56   Asymmetric pneumatization of the anterior
          clinoid process   264

## Section 9   Skull base

Case 57   Fibrous dysplasia of skull base   267
Case 58   Sphenoid bone pseudolesion   271
Case 59   Clival lesions   276
Case 60   Perineural spread   282

## Section 10  Temporal bone

Case 61  Cochlear dysplasia   285
Case 62  Labyrinthitis ossificans   289
Case 63  Superior semicircular canal dehiscence   292
Case 64  Fluid entrapment in the petrous apex cells   294
Case 65  Acquired cholesteatoma   299
Case 66  Malignant otitis externa   304
Case 67  Temporal bone fractures   307

## Section 11  Paranasal sinuses

Case 68  Allergic fungal sinusitis   310
Case 69  Invasive fungal sinusitis   316
Case 70  Spontaneous CSF leaks and sphenoid
         cephaloceles   324
Case 71  Juvenile nasal angiofibroma   328

## Section 12  Orbits

Case 72  Idiopathic orbital pseudotumor   331
Case 73  Optic neuritis   336

## Section 13  Salivary glands

Case 74  Intraparotid lymph nodes   342
Case 75  Benign mixed tumor   344
Case 76  First branchial cleft cyst   350

## Section 14  Neck

Case 77  Nasopharyngeal cysts   354
Case 78  Cystic nodal metastasis   357
Case 79  Low-flow vascular malformations   360
Case 80  Parapharyngeal masses   364

## Section 15  Thyroid and parathyroid

Case 81  Third branchial apparatus anomaly   370
Case 82  Parathyroid adenoma   372
Case 83  String sign   378

## Section 16  Vessels

Case 84  Carotid artery dissection   381
Case 85  Traumatic arterial injury   384

## Section 17  Spinal column

Case 86  Craniovertebral junction injuries   387
Case 87  Odontoid fractures   390
Case 88  Vertebral compression fractures   398
Case 89  Sacral insufficiency fracture   401
Case 90  Paget's disease of the spine   405
Case 91  Renal osteodystrophy   409
Case 92  Calcific tendinitis of the longus colli   414

## Section 18  Intervertebral discs

Case 93  T2 hyperintense disc herniation   419
Case 94  Disc herniation and cord compression   424
Case 95  Postoperative disc herniation versus postsurgical
         scarring   427
Case 96  Degenerative endplate alterations   430

## Section 19  Spinal canal contents

Case 97   Spinal dysraphism   434
Case 98   Tethered spinal cord   445
Case 99   Chiari I malformation   449
Case 100  Spinal vascular malformations   455
Case 101  Cord compression   458
Case 102  Demyelinating/inflammatory spinal
          cord lesion   466
Case 103  Subacute combined degeneration   469
Case 104  Intradural cyst   471
Case 105  Spinal CSF leaks   475
Case 106  Leptomeningeal drop metastases   478

*Index*   486

# Preface

*"A teacher is one who makes himself progressively unnecessary."*
– *Thomas Carruthers*

It is with a great sense of pride that we introduce our endeavor entitled *Pearls and Pitfalls in Head and Neck and Neuroimaging*. We hope that this book will be fun to read and foster the understanding of difficult diagnoses and common pitfalls in Neuroimaging.

We have different backgrounds and sub-specialty Neuroimaging expertise, but have one thing in common – the love and passion for teaching the residents and fellows. This has resulted in accumulation of thousands of teaching files in our respective libraries. Years spent with the trainees in the reading room in wonderful academic institutions have given us an understanding of diagnoses that are commonly missed and imaging findings that are likely to be misinterpreted.

While a number of excellent books exist on the subject and practice of Neuroradiology, a book like this is unique. It aims to cover the lacunae that commonly exist in the knowledge of Neuroimaging and gives clarity to diagnoses that are difficult to make with certainty.

After deciding to proceed with this project, the three of us brainstormed and came up with 106 topics that we wanted to cover. These topics were divided into 19 sections.

Each chapter is concise, yet gives a comprehensive overview of the subject matter.

We understand that time is precious and therefore wanted to create a resource that is precise and trustworthy. It is our hope that this treatise is easy to follow, unpretentious, and helpful.

We would like to thank all the Cambridge University Press staff who helped us tremendously every step of the way. In particular, we express our gratitude to Nisha Doshi and Beata Mako. Gaurang would also like to express his gratitude to Suresh Mukherji, Mark Shiroishi, Sanjay Jain, Prasan Rao, Jayant Narang and Mohammad Arabi for sharing their images and wisdom.

Our sincere thanks to the clinicians working with us for providing ever so important clinical feedback and learning that comes with it. Last but not the least, we thank our families for their unconditional support and patience during the writing of this project.

We hope that the readers will enjoy reading this book. We are open to any suggestions or criticism that the readers may have for its improvement and look forward to hearing from you.

**Nafi, Gaurang, and Dheeraj**

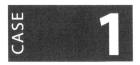

# Dense basilar artery sign

## Imaging description

Intravascular clot can be seen on unenhanced CT as a focal hyperattenuation and may be the only sign of acute ischemia (Fig. 1.1). A thrombosed vessel has a higher CT attenuation value than a normal vessel, because clot contains more protein and less serum than blood due to the deposition of fibrinogen and other clotting proteins and extraction of serum during the process of thrombus formation. When CT shows a focal hyperattenuation in the middle cerebral artery (MCA) this is known as the dense MCA sign. This provides not only a diagnosis of MCA territory infarct but also some prognostic information, because stroke patients who demonstrate a dense MCA sign on their initial CT do relatively poorly compared to those who do not have this sign (Fig 1.2) [1]. Clot in the basilar artery is not as common as MCA thrombus, but the same principles that lead to the dense MCA sign apply to basilar artery thrombosis (Fig. 1.1) [2]. Similarly, thrombosis of the other intracranial vessels, including the veins and dural sinuses, can be diagnosed on the basis of dense clot present within the vessel (Figs. 1.3, 1.4).

## Importance

Unenhanced CT is the first imaging study performed in most acute neurologic presentations. Diagnosing a vascular occlusion early has great prognostic significance. Early initiation of treatment is the most important factor in achieving improved outcomes in the setting of basilar occlusion [3].

## Typical clinical scenario

MCA territory infarcts are relatively easy to diagnose clinically, as patients present with focal neurologic deficits and consciousness is usually not altered. Basilar artery territory infarcts, on the other hand, may lack localizing features and are associated with varying degrees of alteration in consciousness that require a broader clinical differential diagnosis than anterior circulation infarcts.

## Differential diagnosis

Increased attenuation in a vessel can result from increased attenuation of the blood or the vessel wall in addition to intraluminal clot formation. Atherosclerosis results in focally increased attenuation in vessel wall that can mimic thrombus. Increased hematocrit due to hemoconcentration or systemic disorders such as chronic obstructive lung diseases may cause diffusely hyperdense vessels that can potentially mimic the dense artery sign. Partial volume averaging, vessel tortuosity, or ectasia may also make a portion of the vessel appear denser than the other parts. Most of these possibilities can be eliminated by using thinner slices and comparing the vessel segment in question to other vessels of similar size on the same CT [4]. Of course, it is crucial to have appropriate clinical correlation. Contrast-enhanced CT/CTA or MRI/MRA can be used as a problem solver in ambiguous cases. It should be also kept in mind that the sensitivity of the dense vessel sign is relatively low. In other words, absence of dense artery sign does not exclude vessel occlusion or brain infarct.

## Teaching points

The dense basilar artery sign indicates basilar artery thrombosis, basilar artery territory infarcts, and a poor outcome. In the appropriate clinical setting, the specificity of this finding is high although sensitivity is only moderate. Using thinner slices, comparing the density of the vessel in question to that of other vessels of similar size, helps to differentiate intraluminal clot from mimickers such as atherosclerosis, hemoconcentration, and vessel tortuosity. To confirm the presence of vessel occlusion, contrast-enhanced CT may be employed as a quick problem solving tool, although CTA, MRI/MRA, and sometimes digital subtraction angiography (DSA) are necessary to better characterize the extent of vessel occlusion, collateral vessels, and infarcted areas.

REFERENCES

1. Zorzon M, Masè G, Pozzi-Mucelli F, et al. Increased density in the middle cerebral artery by nonenhanced computed tomography: prognostic value in acute cerebral infarction. Eur Neurol 1993; 33: 256–9.
2. Goldmakher GV, Camargo EC, Furie KL, et al. Hyperdense basilar artery sign on unenhanced CT predicts thrombus and outcome in acute posterior circulation stroke. Stroke 2009; 40: 134–9.
3. Eckert B, Kucinski T, Pfeiffer G, Groden C, Zeumer H. Endovascular therapy of acute vertebrobasilar occlusion: early treatment onset as the most important factor. Cerebrovasc Dis 2002; 14: 42–50.
4. Gadda D, Vannucchi L, Niccolai F, et al. Multidetector computed tomography of the head in acute stroke: predictive value of different patterns of the dense artery sign revealed by maximum intensity projection reformations for location and extent of the infarcted area. Eur Radiol 2005; 15: 2387–95.

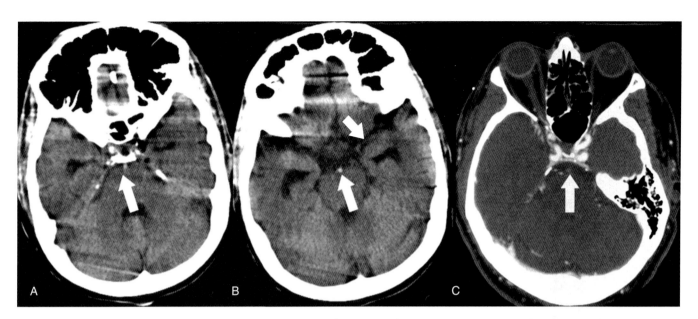

**Figure 1.1** Acute basilar artery thrombosis. (**A, B**) Axial unenhanced CT images show increased attenuation in the basilar artery (arrows) as compared to the left middle cerebral artery (short arrow), indicating basilar artery thrombosis, in this patient with acute deterioration of neurologic status and alertness. (**C**) Axial image from a CTA performed shortly after shows lack of contrast filling of the basilar artery (arrow) compared to the carotids.

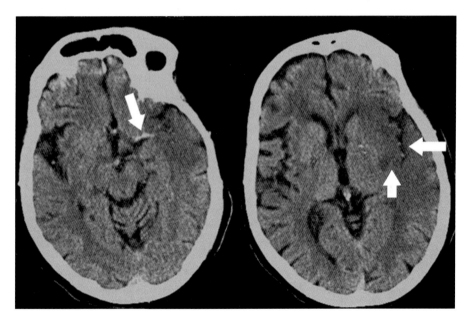

**Figure 1.2** Axial CT images show increased attenuation associated with the left MCA and its branches (arrows) compatible with thrombosis. Decreased gray/white differentiation in the left insular ribbon and putamen (short arrow) is compatible with acute infarct.

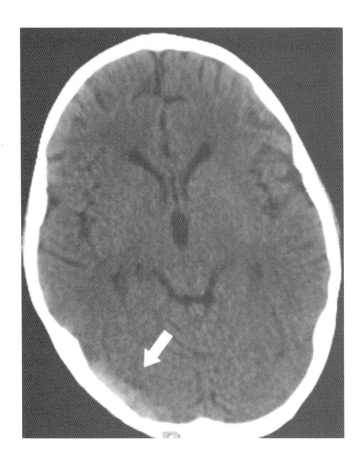

**Figure 1.3** Axial CT shows a marked hyperattenuation in the right transverse sinus, which was confirmed to represent acute thrombosis.

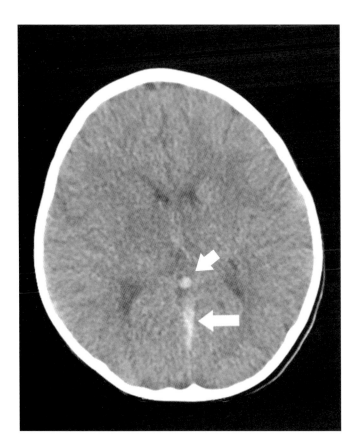

**Figure 1.4** Axial CT shows thrombosis of the straight sinus (arrow) and the vein of Galen (short arrow) with associated hypoattenuation in the bilateral thalami.

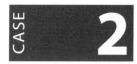

# Global anoxic brain injury

## Imaging description

Anoxic–ischemic injury to the brain as a result of cardiorespiratory insufficiency, such as seen in cardiac arrest, respiratory arrest, prolonged hypotension, and asphyxia, is difficult to diagnose because of the subtlety and symmetry of abnormalities seen on MRI and CT scans. These scans are frequently misinterpreted, particularly when radiologists are not aware of the clinical circumstances. CT scans show diffuse decrease in gray/white differentiation and mild edema in the early stages. On MRI, diffuse increase in the cortical signal is seen on FLAIR/T2-weighted images as well as diffusion-weighted images (DWI) in most cases (Figs. 2.1, 2.2), although different patterns are occasionally encountered, including signal changes in the deep gray matter structures only, in both gray and white matter, and in the white matter only [1].

The underlying pathophysiologic processes leading to differences in pattern are not clearly understood, although essentially all types of global anoxic–ischemic injury portend a very poor prognosis. DWI sequence is the most sensitive imaging modality. DWI shows a much increased contrast difference between the diffusely abnormal cortex and relatively preserved white matter, creating a more "eye-pleasing" appearance compared to a normal DWI scan, which shows only a mild difference between gray and white matter (Fig. 2.3). However, there are differences in the normal contrast present between the cortex and white matter in different MRI scanners and different DWI sequences, and radiologists should become familiar with the normal appearance of the DWI images in their practice settings. High-b-value DWI may increase sensitivity [2].

## Importance

Anoxic–ischemic injury, particularly when it is severe, often results in brain death, which has enormous implications for cessation of life support, family counseling, and organ harvesting.

## Typical clinical scenario

Patients are typically comatose following cardiorespiratory arrest, prolonged hypotensive episode, asphyxia, drowning, etc.

## Differential diagnosis

In the proper clinical setting there is no differential diagnosis. In strict radiological terms the differential diagnosis is between a normal scan and a severely abnormal scan, as missing this injury will result in generation of a normal MRI or CT report. One important clue is the difference in attenuation/signal of the supratentorial brain and cerebellum. Because the supratentorial structures are preferentially affected there is usually a stark difference between cerebellum and brain. When only the deep gray matter is involved (Fig. 2.4) the differential diagnosis may include Creutzfeldt–Jakob disease (CJD) and metabolic toxic injury, although the clinical features should be helpful in differentiating these. Only white matter involvement may be confused with leukoencephalopathies radiologically (Fig. 2.5).

> ### Teaching points
> Global hypoxic injury results in symmetric and subtle changes on MRI and CT scans that are easily missed. Radiologists should be familiar with the normal contrast present between the gray and white matter on their DWI sequences and look for changes in that contrast in comatose patients.

REFERENCES

1. Kim E, Sohn CH, Chang KH, Chang HW, Lee DH. Patterns of accentuated grey-white differentiation on diffusion-weighted imaging or the apparent diffusion coefficient maps in comatose survivors after global brain injury. *Clin Radiol* 2011; **66**: 440–8.

2. Tha KK, Terae S, Yamamoto T, *et al.* Early detection of global cerebral anoxia: improved accuracy by high-b-value diffusion-weighted imaging with long echo time. *AJNR Am J Neuroradiol* 2005; **26**: 1487–97.

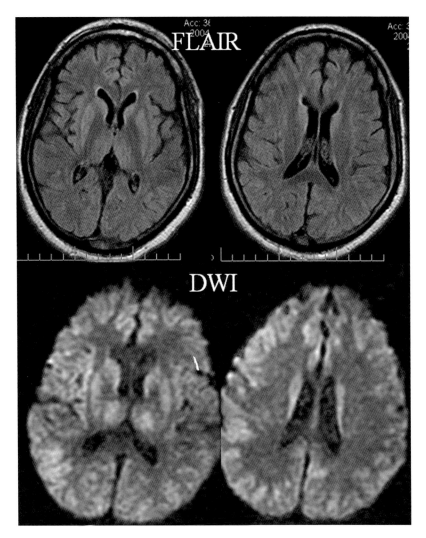

**Figure 2.1** Axial FLAIR and DWI images show diffusely and symmetrically increased signal in the cortex and deep gray matter structures compatible with global anoxic injury. The patient had a cardiac arrest and was declared brain-dead shortly after the MRI.

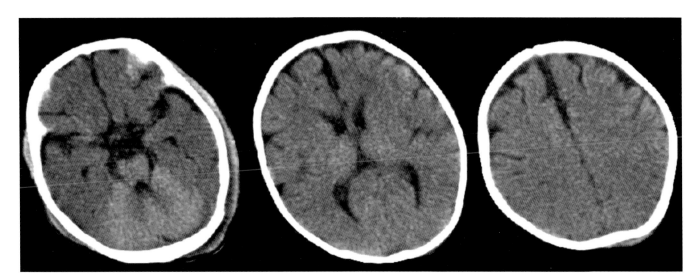

**Figure 2.2** Axial CT images show diffuse loss of gray/white differentiation throughout the supratentorial brain compatible with global anoxic injury. Note the attenuation of the cerebellum, which appears prominent relative to diffusely decreased attenuation of the brain. This is the "white cerebellum sign." Similar differences are observed on MRI, in particular in DWI images.

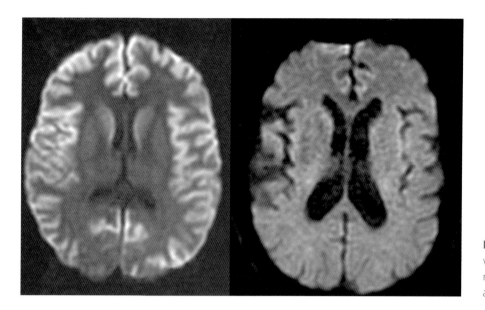

**Figure 2.3** Axial DWI images of a patient with global anoxic injury (left) and of a normal individual (right) highlight the abnormality more clearly.

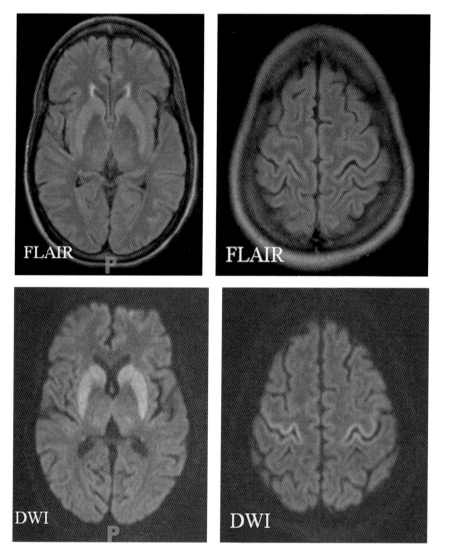

**Figure 2.4** A less common pattern of global anoxic injury. Axial FLAIR and DWI images show preferential involvement of the deep gray matter with preservation of the cortex except in the perirolandic area.

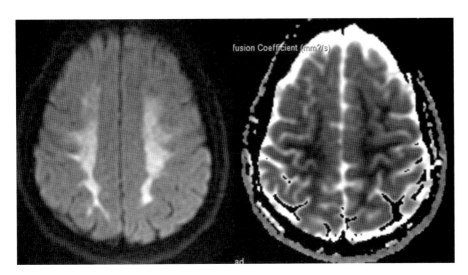

**Figure 2.5** A much rarer form of global anoxic injury. White matter is involved and the cortex is spared, although quantitative apparent diffusion coefficient (ADC) evaluation showed some cortical abnormality as well.

## Imaging description

CT has an unparalleled track record in the detection of intracranial hemorrhage and therefore is the first imaging study obtained in this setting. In addition to excluding intracranial hemorrhage, CT may help demonstrate early signs of acute ischemic stroke (AIS), such as insular ribbon sign, hyperdense cerebral artery sign, sulcal effacement, and development of acute parenchymal low attenuation (Fig. 3.1). Patients who have advanced signs of infarction involving more than one-third of the middle cerebral artery (MCA) territory are generally excluded from intravenous tissue plasminogen activator (tPA) therapy because of a higher risk for hemorrhagic conversion.

Advanced imaging as a triage tool for selecting patients for intravenous (IV) or intra-arterial (IA) stroke therapies beyond 3 hours is a focus of evaluation of many ongoing clinical trials [1]. Central to the idea of advanced imaging is to obtain a precise measure of the area of ischemic core versus ischemic but still viable tissue that is at risk for infarction in the absence of early recanalization (penumbra). It can be argued that patients can only benefit from recanalization if there is a relatively modest area of already infarcted tissue and significant (ideally >20% of area of core infarction) ischemic tissue that can be potentially salvaged.

Ideally, imaging would provide an assessment (or confirmation) of occlusion of a major cerebral artery, a precise measure of the area of irreversible infarction, and assessment of the surrounding perfusion abnormality. MRI, using diffusion-weighted imaging (DWI), has become the gold standard to demonstrate the area of irreversible infarction. This tissue demonstrates high signal on DWI images and corresponding reduction in apparent diffusion coefficient (ADC) values. Salvageable penumbra can be operationally defined as a mismatch between the perfusion MR volume and the DW MR volume, where the perfusion MR volume indicates presumably ischemic, hypoperfused penumbral tissue and the DW MR volume represents irreversibly ischemic infarct core (Fig. 3.2).

CT imaging has its proponents, and they rely on a combination of CT angiography (CTA) (to demonstrate the vascular occlusion/cut-off) and CT perfusion (CTP). The area of irreversible infarction on CTP should demonstrate decrease in cerebral blood volume (CBV), and it can serve as a surrogate for DWI imaging. Similar to DWI–PWI mismatch,

investigators have used cerebral blood flow (CBF)–CBV mismatch or mean transit time (MTT)–CBV mismatch to assess the penumbral tissue on CTP, although the latter maps may be optimal (Fig. 3.3). However, CT has disadvantages of radiation exposure and, in institutions lacking 256- or 320-slice CTs, entire brain coverage is not possible. Post-processing is relatively more cumbersome, and thresholds vary based on post-processing techniques.

## Importance

Radiologists must be familiar with early signs of stroke on CT as well as assessment of perfusion abnormalities in the setting of stroke.

## Typical clinical scenario

Stroke is characterized by a sudden, acute neurologic deficit that is referable to the involved vascular territory. Common presentations include hemiparesis, facial droop, aphasia, and loss of consciousness, although a myriad of possible combinations of neurologic signs and symptoms are possible.

## Differential diagnosis

With proper clinical correlation, imaging diagnosis of stroke is easily accomplished, especially on MRI. However, one must be alert to the possibility that there are numerous causes of restricted diffusion on DWI studies that need to be differentiated from acute stroke. Common causes of diffusion abnormalities other than stroke include encephalitis, traumatic lesions, acute demyelination, brain abscess, and highly cellular neoplasms.

> ## Teaching points
>
> Revascularization may be futile if there is no significant salvageable penumbral tissue (DWI–PWI mismatch). Moreover, such recanalization is potentially harmful, since it would restore blood flow to an already infarcted area.

REFERENCES

1. Köhrmann M, Schellinger PD. Acute stroke triage to intravenous thrombolysis and other therapies with advanced CT or MR imaging: pro MR imaging. *Radiology* 2009; **251**: 627–33.

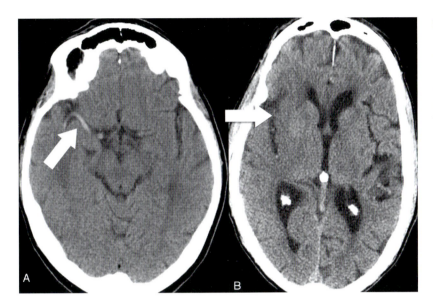

**Figure 3.1** (**A**) Hyperdense middle cerebral artery (MCA) sign in a patient with acute left hemiparesis (arrow). (**B**) In another patient with acute stroke, the insular ribbon sign is noted (arrow). Additionally, the right-sided sulci are effaced and there is early parenchymal hypoattenuation, in comparison with the normal left side.

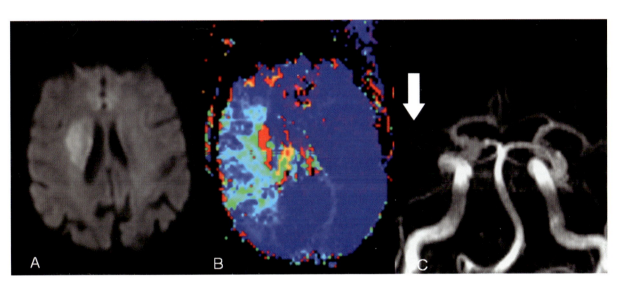

**Figure 3.2** Utility of MRI as a trial tool for IA thrombolysis. (**A**) DWI, (**B**) PWI (MTT map), and (**C**) 3D time-of-flight (TOF) MRA are demonstrated in a patient with acute right MCA occlusion. Note a very small ischemic core on DWI, relatively large PWI defect, and occlusion of right M1 segment (arrow). This was successfully recanalized with IA thrombolysis, and neurologic deficits markedly improved.

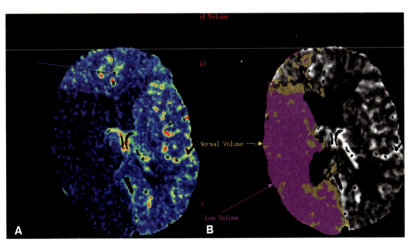

**Figure 3.3** MCA ischemia of 90 minutes duration. (**A**) CBV map reveals an essentially completely infarcted right MCA and PCA territory. (**B**) A "penumbra" map. The purple area corresponds to CBV reduction and yellow areas highlight "penumbral tissue (MTT–CBV)." It would be futile to intervene in this patient because of lack of salvageable tissue.

## Imaging description

Vertebral artery dissections (VADs) result from intimal injury, laceration of the arterial wall, or spontaneous hemorrhage of the vasa vasorum causing a subintimal or intramural hematoma. Spontaneous dissections are presumably related to an inherent arteriopathy due to genetic factors and connective tissue disorders such as Ehlers–Danlos syndrome type IV, Marfan syndrome, and fibromuscular dysplasia. Traumatic and iatrogenic dissections are predominantly due to blunt/penetrating injuries, chiropractic manipulation, or catheter angiography.

The imaging findings of VAD are similar to carotid artery dissection (CAD, see Case 84) with characteristic MR imaging findings of wall thickening or hematoma, crescentric high signal in subacute phase, and narrowing of the flow void (Fig. 4.1). In some cases, however, the lumen many be enlarged due to development of dissecting aneurysm. MRA and CTA are both utilized in the diagnosis of VAD, although CTA may be superior in identifying subtle signs of VAD (Fig. 4.2) such as small dissection flaps and dissecting aneurysms [1]. Lum *et al.* have described a "suboccipital rind sign" in VADs that involve the V3 segment [2]. They argue that in some cases of V3 dissections, the only imaging abnormality is the vertebral artery wall thickening, and the lumen appears normal in caliber.

The V1 and V3 segments of the vertebral artery at the points of entry (C6–C7) and exit (C1–C2 loops) from the foramen transversarium are common locations for VADs (Fig. 4.3). The V1 segment dissections are most common. Ischemic findings are common in VADs and generally embolic in nature. Embolic infarcts from VADs are most frequently observed in the distribution of the affected posterior inferior cerebellar artery although other presentations include basilar artery thrombosis or ischemia in the posterior cerebral artery.

The distal, V3 segment dissections can migrate intracranially and result in dissecting aneurysms and subarachnoid hemorrhage (SAH) (Fig. 4.4). SAH is a particularly feared complication of distal V3 dissections since this complication carries a high risk of morbidity and mortality.

## Importance

VADs are an important cause of stroke in the posterior circulation, particularly in young patients. Imaging signs are generally more subtle than in CAD because of the smaller size of vertebral arteries.

## Typical clinical scenario

VADs are often associated with posterior neck pain and brainstem or cerebellar ischemia. Ischemia from VADs is most frequently observed in the distribution of the affected posterior inferior cerebellar artery and commonly presents with lateral medullary (Wallenberg) syndrome. Nearly 10% of vertebral artery dissections extend intracranially, with the potential to form dissecting aneurysms, thereby presenting with subarachnoid hemorrhage.

## Differential diagnosis

Proximal VADs need to be distinguished from atherosclerotic steno-occlusive disease. One should remember that VAD generally occurs slightly distal to the origin of the vertebral artery, and the origin is relatively spared. In contrast, atherosclerotic disease has a predilection for the vertebral artery origin.

### Teaching points

The junction of the V1 and V2 segments is the most common location of VAD. Proximal VADs typically spare the origin of the vertebral artery. Intradural extension of distal VADs is a feared complication, with associated risk of SAH. The intradural VA is more susceptible to rupture than the extradural VA because it has a much thinner adventitia layer.

REFERENCES

1. Vertinsky AT, Schwartz NE, Fishbein NJ, *et al.* Comparison of multidetector CT angiography and MR imaging of cervical artery dissection. *AJNR Am J Neuroradiol* 2008; **29**: 1753–60.
2. Lum C, Chakraborty S, Schlossmacher M, *et al.* Vertebral artery dissection with a normal-appearing lumen at multisection CT angiography: the importance of identifying wall hematoma. *AJNR Am J Neuroradiol* 2009; **30**: 787–92.

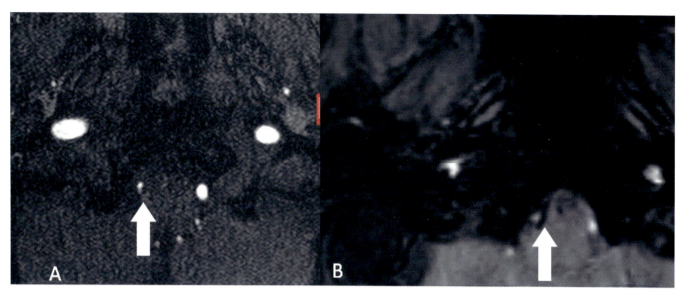

**Figure 4.1** (**A**) MRA source image and (**B**) susceptibility-weighted image (SWI) in a patient with right-sided lateral medullary syndrome. The source image shows narrowing of the vertebral artery (arrow). There is a small intramural hematoma that is well appreciated on SWI as a rim of hypointensity (arrow).

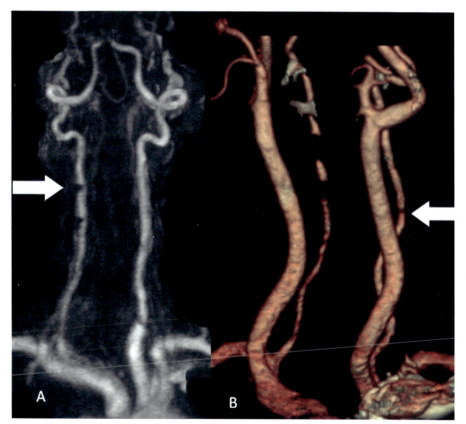

**Figure 4.2** (**A**) Contrast-enhanced MRA and (**B**) CTA reconstructions in a patient with MVA. The MRA reveals possible dissection of right vertebral artery but it is difficult to be certain that this is not an artifact (arrow). CTA is complementary and clearly shows severe narrowing of the right vertebral artery. CTA also additionally demonstrates a small left vertebral artery dissection.

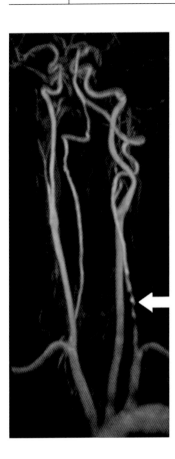

**Figure 4.3** VAD involving the V1 segment, where the vertebral artery enters the foramen transversarium (arrow). Note that the vertebral origin is spared, differentiating it from atherosclerotic disease.

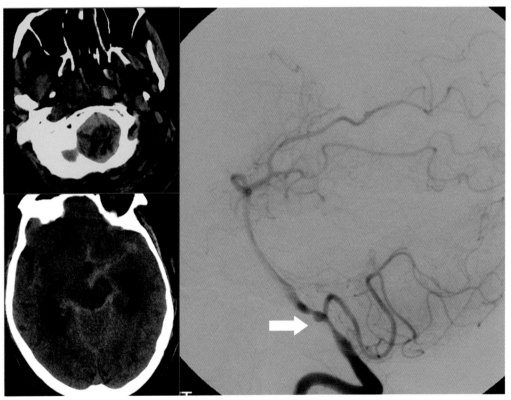

**Figure 4.4** Subarachnoid hemorrhage from dissection of the right vertebral artery. Non-contrast CT images reveal extensive subarachnoid hemorrhage. The DSA image is a lateral view of the right vertebral artery. Note the focal narrowing of vertebral artery and an associated small dissecting aneurysm (arrow).

## Imaging description

Brain infarcts in the subacute stage demonstrate enhancement and may mimic enhancing tumors or infectious processes (Fig. 5.1). Enhancement of the infarcted brain parenchyma is different than "luxury perfusion," which involves enhancement of the vessels around the infarct in the acute phase. Infarcted tissue enhancement usually starts approximately 4–5 days after the insult and may increase in the following week [1]. Edema associated with infarcts peaks around the fourth day and starts dissipating afterwards, although some level of swelling of the infarcted tissue is usually present for approximately 2 weeks. Diffusion-weighted imaging (DWI) signal increase (apparent diffusion coefficient [ADC] signal decrease) is seen shortly after the infarct, peaks around the second day and gradually diminishes afterwards, with ADC normalization occurring around day 10. Brain MRI performed 5–14 days after the infarct may show an enhancing lesion with swelling and relative lack or absence of ADC signal decrease that might lead to an erroneous diagnosis.

## Importance

Enhancing mass-like lesions of the brain usually require extensive work-up that frequently involves invasive procedures which may be harmful. Misdiagnosing an infarct leads not only to unnecessary work-up but also to delay in identifying and treating the underlying cause of the infarct for secondary stroke prevention.

## Typical clinical scenario

Most infarcts, particularly of the anterior circulation, present with acute symptoms that are easily recognized by the patient and healthcare personnel. MRI performed at the early stages of infarcts is very sensitive and specific for acute infarcts, and no significant diagnostic difficulty is encountered in this phase. Infarcts that lack motor or sensory deficits, however, may be relatively asymptomatic or have symptoms that are nonspecific, which may lead to delayed clinical presentations and delayed imaging. Posterior cerebral artery (PCA) territory infarcts may potentially present late because the visual field cut caused by the infarct may not be noticed by the patient [2]. Likewise, patients with multiple small infarcts occasionally present late, as they may not have any significant neurologic deficits. The non-specific symptoms they have, such as headache, dizziness, drowsiness, and weakness, may be attributable to other underlying conditions.

## Differential diagnosis

Most infarcts have specific clinical and radiologic features and therefore require no differential diagnosis. The enhancing subacute infarcts can be recognized by their distinctive shape and location that conform to a vascular territory, most commonly the PCA territory. A gyral pattern of enhancement is seen in subacute infarcts, with a greater degree of enhancement of the cortex compared to white matter (Fig. 5.2). Multiple small infarcts in the subacute phase may mimic metastases or other enhancing lesions (Fig. 5.3). The distribution within a vascular territory or in the watershed zones is helpful in differential diagnosis. Short-term follow-up imaging may be very helpful in problem cases, as evolving infarcts show significant changes and often improve over a short interval, in contrast to mass lesions.

---

### Teaching points

PCA territory infarcts and small embolic infarcts may come to clinical attention late and present with non-specific symptoms. Subacute infarcts show parenchymal enhancement and mass effect on MRI, which when coupled with lack of clinical suspicion and restricted diffusion mimic masses, metastases, and other enhancing lesions.

---

REFERENCES

1. Elster AD. Magnetic resonance contrast enhancement in cerebral infarction. *Neuroimaging Clin N Am* 1994; **4**: 89–100.
2. Finelli PF. Neuroimaging in acute posterior cerebral artery infarction. *Neurologist* 2008; **14**: 170–80.

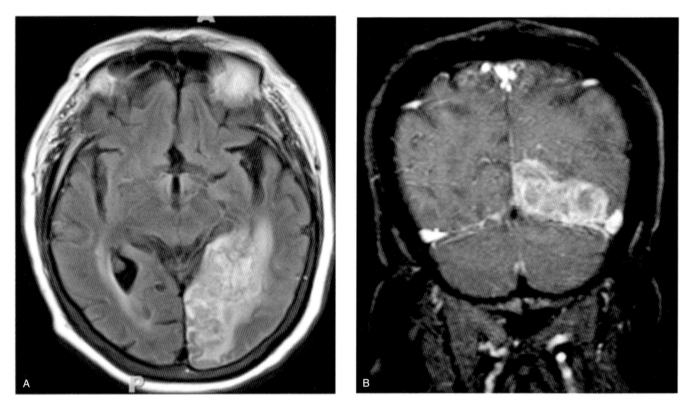

**Figure 5.1** (**A**) Axial FLAIR and (**B**) post-contrast coronal T1-weighted images show a large area of abnormal signal and enhancement in the left temporo-occipital region within the PCA territory with associated swelling. Accompanying DWI did not show significant signal abnormality. This was the first imaging study performed on this patient with subacute infarct.

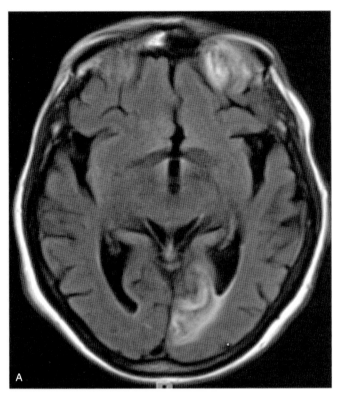

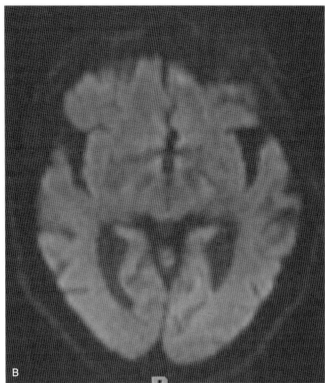

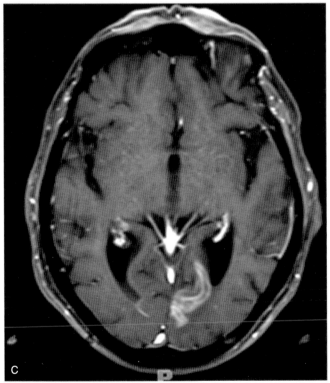

**Figure 5.2** (**A**) Axial FLAIR image shows an area of hyperintensity in the left mesial occipital lobe with no significant mass effect or volume loss. (**B**) DWI showed no signal increase, and a gyral pattern of enhancement is seen on (**C**) post-contrast T1-weighted image. This patient presented with a 7-day history of headache and drowsiness.

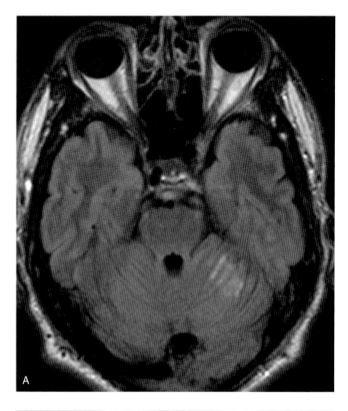

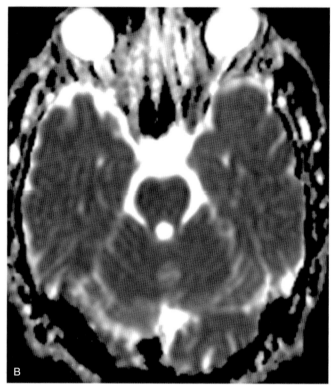

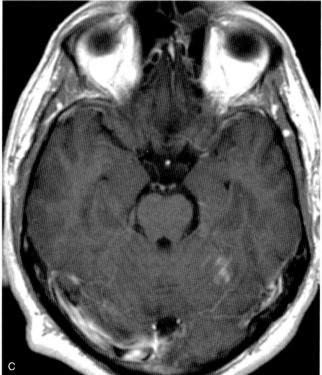

**Figure 5.3** (**A**) Axial FLAIR through the posterior fossa shows a cortical signal abnormality in the left cerebellum with (**B**) normal ADC map and (**C**) patchy enhancement on post-contrast T1-weighted image in a patient with pancreatic cancer and no recent symptoms. This was initially interpreted as possible metastasis but later confirmed to be a subacute infarct.

## Imaging description

Acute hemorrhage in the subarachnoid space appears as areas of hyperdensity in the basal cisterns, cerebral sulci, and/or the ventricles. There are several imaging findings that can help locate the site of a ruptured aneurysm. The distribution of blood in the subarachnoid space and thickness of a localized clot can often help with such localization. Additionally, the presence of a parenchymal hematoma is one of the most significant predictors for evaluating the location of the ruptured aneurysm (Fig. 6.1).

CTA is increasingly gaining popularity as the procedure of choice for initial, and in a majority of cases definitive, evaluation (Fig. 6.2). The advantages of CTA include its near-uniform availability, safety profile, high spatial resolution, and limited time required to perform the test. Additionally, it can be obtained at the same sitting when the patient gets the non-contrast CT. CTA has the ability to demonstrate the precise relationship between bony structures of the skull and the aneurysm. CTA may also help demonstrate other characteristics of the aneurysm that are less well studied on digital subtraction angiography (DSA) – for example, presence of endoluminal thrombus as well as calcification of the aneurysm wall. Preoperative knowledge of these aneurysm characteristics significantly aids in therapeutic decisions. The reported overall sensitivity of CTA exceeds 90% when compared with DSA in most recent publications [1]. However, if there is any doubt regarding the findings on CTA, one should have a low threshold for recommending further evaluation with a DSA.

DSA still remains the gold-standard imaging study for evaluation of intracranial aneurysms, with highest reported sensitivity. The advantages include its very high spatial resolution and its ability to demonstrate small vessels and their relationship with the neck of the aneurysm, as well as yielding information for planning endovascular repair (Fig. 6.1). However, it is not uniformly available and has an associated risk of ischemic complications due to its invasive nature. "Diagnostic" cerebral angiography is therefore being increasingly replaced by CTA, although it still retains its place as a prelude to endovascular intervention and also as a definitive means of evaluation if initial CTA is negative.

## Importance

Aneurysmal subarachnoid hemorrhage (SAH) is a medical emergency with a very high rate of morbidity and mortality. Patients should receive a prompt work-up and timely intervention to prevent the secondary mortality from aneurysm rebleeding.

## Typical clinical scenario

Most patients experience a sudden, worst headache of their life. However, higher-grade patients may experience altered level of consciousness or focal neurological deficits, or become comatose. Nearly 40–50% of patients may die within the first week after the hemorrhage.

## Differential diagnosis

Perimesencephalic hemorrhage may have an imaging appearance that can be confused with aneurysmal SAH. A location centered around the anterior aspect of the midbrain, absence of large amounts of intraventricular blood, and potential extension to the posterior interhemispheric fissure are characteristic imaging features of this condition (Fig. 6.3). There is lack of parenchymal hematoma and a 4-vessel angiogram is negative for aneurysm.

One of the most common causes of false positive detection of aneurysm on CTA is infundibular dilatation at the origin of posterior communicating (Fig. 6.4) or anterior choroidal arteries [1]. The infundibulum is typically conical in shape, measures 3 mm or smaller, and has a vessel that arises from its apex. Also, venous contamination may result in false positive diagnosis of aneurysm when venous structures abut the arterial bifurcation (Fig. 6.5).

### Teaching points

CTA is gaining widespread popularity as the initial, and in many cases definitive, evaluation for aneurysmal SAH. However, potential possible pitfalls of CTA should be kept in mind.

REFERENCES

1. Marshall SA, Kathuria S, Nyquist P, Gandhi D. Noninvasive imaging techniques in the diagnosis and management of aneurysmal subarachnoid hemorrhage. *Neurosurg Clin N Am* 2010; **21**: 305–23.

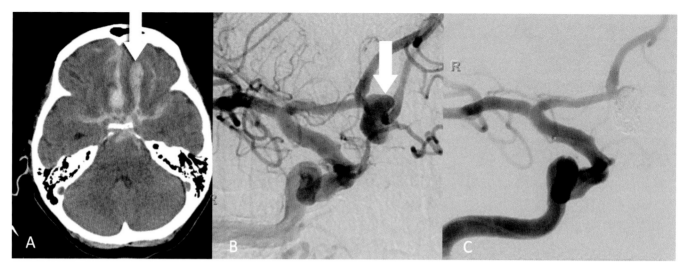

**Figure 6.1** (**A**) CT reveals diffuse SAH and a left-sided gyrus rectus hematoma, predictive of ruptured anterior communicating artery (Acom) aneurysm. (**B**) An irregular Acom aneurysm is confirmed (arrow) on DSA of right ICA. (C) The aneurysm was embolized at the same sitting.

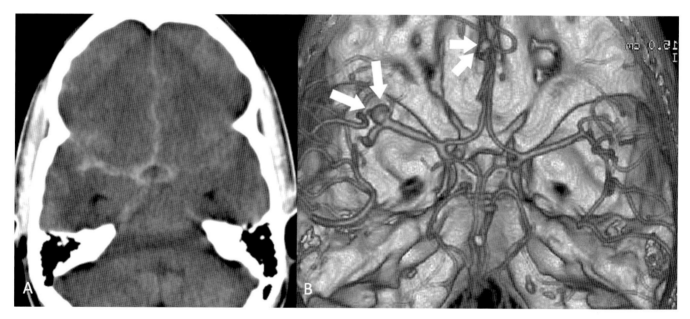

**Figure 6.2** (**A**) SAH with slightly thicker hematoma along the right MCA, suggesting the possibility of right MCA aneurysm. (**B**) CTA reveals a right MCA (arrows) as well as a pericallosal aneurysm (short arrows). Right MCA aneurysm was the source of the SAH, confirmed at surgery.

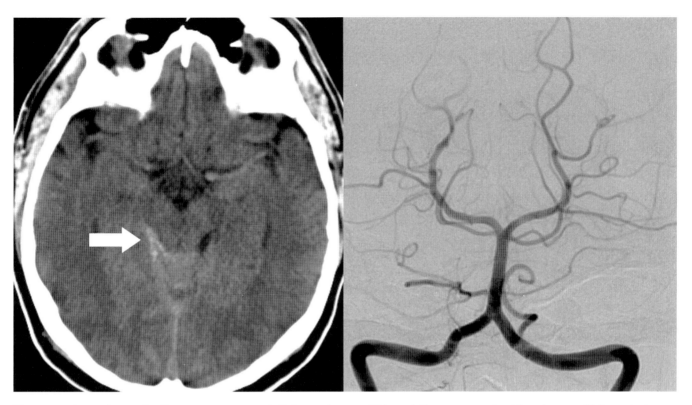

**Figure 6.3** A typical example of benign perimesencephalic hemorrhage on CT (arrow). The accompanying AP angiogram of left vertebral artery is unremarkable for an aneurysm in the posterior fossa.

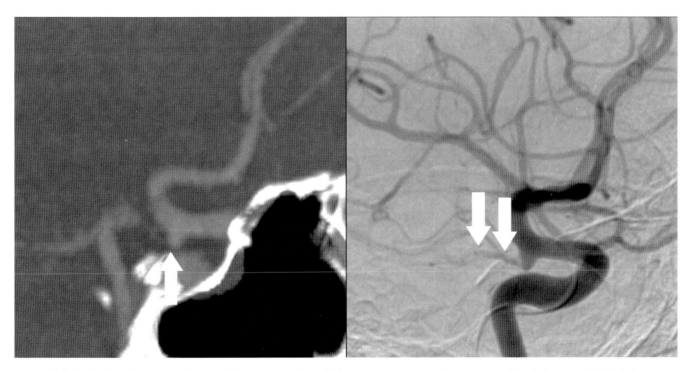

**Figure 6.4** Sagittal MIP image reveals a possible aneurysm (arrow) along the communicating segment of the ICA, although it is difficult to exclude an infundibulum. A DSA clearly demonstrates a small vessel (Pcom: double arrow) arising from the apex, confirming this to be an infundibulum.

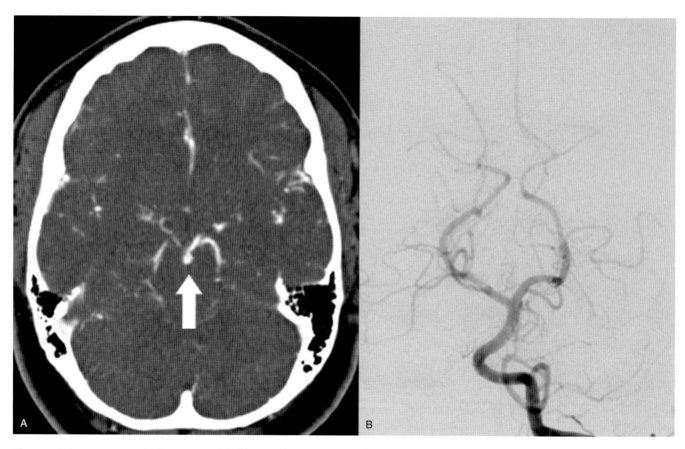

**Figure 6.5** Venous contamination can result in false positive appearance of an aneurysm. (**A**) In this patient with SAH, a basilar tip aneurysm (arrow) was diagnosed on CTA, contaminated by venous filling. (**B**) The DSA shows the basilar tip to be unremarkable.

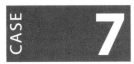

# CASE 7 Intracranial aneurysms

## Imaging description

Intracranial saccular (berry) aneurysms are common intracranial vascular lesions with an estimated prevalence in the general population ranging from 2% to 6% [1]. Digital subtraction angiography (DSA) has the highest spatial resolution of all vascular imaging studies and remains a gold-standard technique. However, while DSA is the most sensitive for such detection and characterization of aneurysms, it is not practical as a screening tool because of its invasive nature and a small risk of neurologic complications.

The sensitivity of CTA has continued to increase, with some studies reporting it to be even comparable to that of DSA [1]. Images are generally reconstructed in 2D maximum intensity projection (MIP) or 3D volume rendering (VR) (Fig. 7.1). The sensitivity and specificity are reported to be as high as 90%, but depend on the size of the aneurysm. According to Villablanca et al., CTA has >90% sensitivity for aneurysms of the middle cerebral artery, regardless of the size of the aneurysm [2]. However, CTA may not clearly identify small aneurysms in the area of the carotid siphon and paraclinoid region.

Magnetic resonance angiography (MRA) is an excellent screening diagnostic method in asymptomatic patients with risk of harboring an intracranial aneurysm. The advantages include its non-invasive nature, the lack of radiation exposure, and the high sensitivity. Multiple overlapping thin-slice acquisition (MOTSA) combines the advantages of 2D and 3D time-of-flight (TOF) techniques (Fig. 7.2) and is widely utilized for the circle of Willis MRA. In a systematic review comparing MRA with DSA, MRA had a sensitivity of 87%, a specificity of 95%, a positive predictive value of 97% per aneurysm [3]. MRA is often a preferred screening technique for unruptured aneurysms.

## Importance

Rupture of intracranial aneurysm results in subarachnoid hemorrhage, a condition with significant morbidity and mortality. Therefore, the screening techniques used for detection of unruptured aneurysms should have very high sensitivity as well as specificity to be useful.

## Typical clinical scenario

There is no evidence to support screening the general population for intracranial aneurysms. Nevertheless, specific patient populations present an increased risk for formation of intracranial aneurysms. These include patients with polycystic kidney disease, Marfan syndrome, coarctation of the aorta, fibromuscular dysplasia, family history of intracranial aneurysms, and Ehlers–Danlos syndrome. These patients should receive screening with a highly sensitive and specific technique.

## Differential diagnosis

Infundibular dilatation at the vessel origins may simulate an aneurysm on CTA or MRA (Fig. 7.3). The characteristic features of infundibula that separate these from aneurysms are their conical shape, diameter less than 3 mm, and a vessel arising from the apex. Occasionally, a vessel loop may simulate an aneurysm on MIP projections. However, careful review of source images or generation of multiplanar reconstruction (MPR) images in different planes will generally resolve one from the other. Occasionally, a venous structure in close proximity to the artery may simulate an aneurysm on CTA (see Fig. 6.5).

---

### Teaching points

Multi-slice CTA and MRA, especially at 3T strength, are excellent techniques for the detection of intracranial aneurysms. MRA has a slight advantage, since there is lack of ionizing radiation and it can be obtained without the need to inject contrast agent.

---

REFERENCES
1. Pozzi-Mucelli F, Bruni S, Doddi M, et al. Detection of intracranial aneurysms with 64 channel multidetector row computed tomography: comparison with digital subtraction angiography. *Eur J Radiol* 2007; **64**: 15–26.
2. Villablanca JP, Hooshi P, Martin N et al. Three-dimensional helical computerized tomography angiography in the diagnosis, characterization, and management of middle cerebral artery aneurysms: comparison with conventional angiography and intraoperative findings. *Journal of Neurosurgery*, 2002; **97**: 1322–32.
3. White PM, Wardlaw JM, Easton V. Can noninvasive imaging accurately depict intracranial aneurysms? A systematic review. *Radiology* 2000; **217**: 361–70.

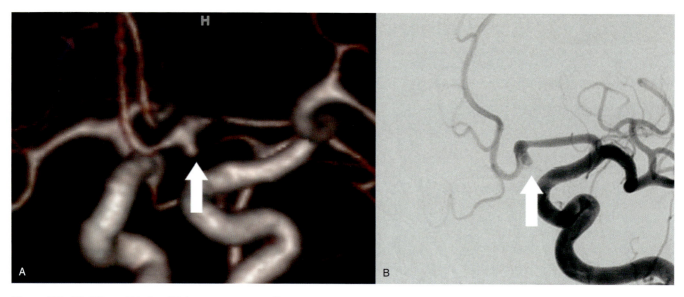

**Figure 7.1** (**A**) CTA on 320 slice CT demonstrating excellent automated bone subtraction and a tiny, 2 mm left anterior cerebral artery aneurysm (arrow). (**B**) This aneurysm is confirmed on DSA (arrow).

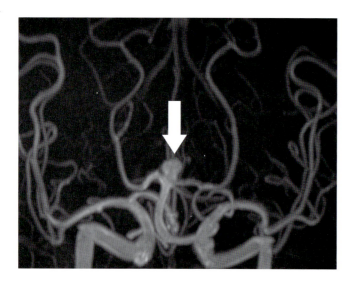

**Figure 7.2** 3D MOTSA TOF MRA was performed as a screening test in a 38-year-old female with polycystic kidney disease. Note a 5 mm basilar tip aneurysm (arrow).

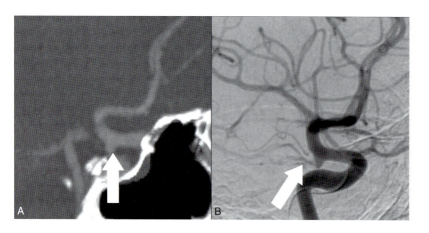

**Figure 7.3** (**A**) Lower resolution of CTA and MRA (compared to DSA) may result in false positive diagnosis of aneurysm (arrow, in this case on CTA). (**B**) DSA is able to display a conical shape of the abnormality and small posterior communicating artery arising from the apex of this lesion (arrow), confirming this to be an infundibulum.

## Imaging description

Giant intracranial aneurysms present unique challenges in diagnosis, characterization, and management. By definition, aneurysms that exceed 25 mm in greatest diameter are termed giant aneurysms. Giant aneurysms may be either saccular or fusiform in morphology.

In terms of location, these lesions are most commonly identified in the extradural internal carotid artery (ICA), more specifically in the cavernous segment. Other locations that are involved with some frequency include the middle cerebral artery (MCA) and the vertebral-basilar system. CT is generally the first imaging study obtained, especially in the patients where the initial presentation is with subarachnoid hemorrhage (SAH) or ischemic symptoms. Giant aneurysms are appreciated as round or oval masses that are slightly hyperdense compared to the gray matter (Fig. 8.1). Calcification is a frequent occurrence and can be seen either in the periphery in an "egg shell" fashion or scattered within the thrombosed portion of the lumen. Administration of contrast allows the identification of the patent lumen of the aneurysm.

Cerebral digital subtraction angiography (DSA) is frequently needed, and is helpful both in delineating the branch vessels and for planning therapy. However, as a sole imaging study, it is insufficient in precise characterization of these complex aneurysms. Because it only demonstrates the patent lumen, it may sometimes grossly underestimate the size or the extent of the aneurysm (Fig. 8.2). DSA must always be complemented with cross-sectional studies for evaluating these complex lesions.

MRI is a very useful tool for the evaluation of giant aneurysms, but it can be confusing to interpret. Partially thrombosed giant aneurysms appear as extra-axial masses that consist of areas of mixed signal intensities representing clot of varying ages [1]. An eccentric or central patent lumen may be seen as an area of flow void (Figs. 8.1, 8.3). The pulsations of the aneurysm or vessel wall create unique ghosting artifacts on MR, propagating in the phase-encoding direction (Fig. 8.1). This artifact is quite helpful in making a specific diagnosis of giant aneurysm. MRA is complementary to MRI in depicting the patent portion of the lumen. A standard 3D MRA may occasionally be misleading and fail to demonstrate the aneurysm if there is very slow flow in the sac of the aneurysm. Contrast-enhanced 3D time-of-flight (TOF) MRA and dynamic contrast-enhanced MRA may be able to provide better detail of the lumen.

## Importance

Giant aneurysms are rare but very difficult lesions in terms of their characterization on imaging, as well as management. Care should be taken not to confuse these with other intracranial masses.

## Typical clinical scenario

Giant aneurysms most often present with symptoms of mass effect on adjacent structures, although SAH may also be the initial presentation in some patients. Cavernous ICA aneurysms may exert mass effect on the nerves coursing through the cavernous sinus, resulting in compressive neuropathies of 3rd, 4th and/or 6th cranial nerves. Giant aneurysms may also result in ischemic symptoms, due to embolic phenomenon occurring from intraluminal thrombus that these lesions frequently harbor.

## Differential diagnosis

Differential considerations include other intracranial masses. For example, the aneurysms in the cavernous ICA frequently project into the pituitary sella and suprasellar cistern and may be misdiagnosed as hemorrhagic pituitary macroadenomas. Clues to the correct recognition include demonstrating the continuity of the mass with the carotid artery, identification of a flow void, and pulsatility artifacts. Hemorrhagic primary neoplasms and large cavernous malformations can simulate giant aneurysm on account of blood products of varying ages (Fig. 8.4). However, these lesions are intra-axial, whereas giant aneurysms are located in the subarachnoid space.

### Teaching points

Giant aneurysms should always be entertained in the differential diagnosis of large extra-axial masses, especially those that are hyperdense on CT and/or demonstrate blood products on MRI.

REFERENCES
1. Atlas SW, Grossman RI, Goldberg HI, *et al.* Partially thrombosed giant intracranial aneurysms: correlation of MR and pathologic findings. *Radiology* 1987; **162**: 111–14.

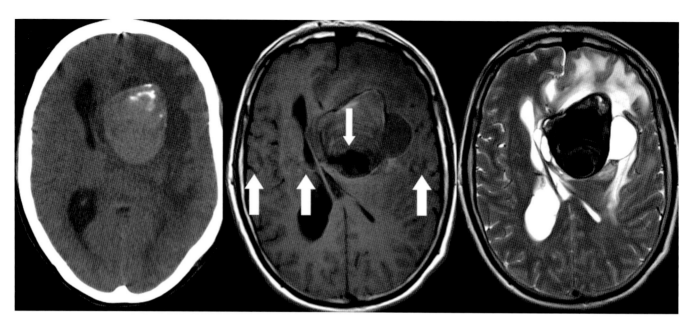

**Figure 8.1** Giant ICA terminus aneurysm. CT demonstrates a high-density mass with speckled peripheral calcification. The aneurysm has variegated thrombus that is better seen on T1-weighted image and a smaller, patent lumen seen as a flow void (thin arrow). The clue to recognize this as aneurysm is pulsatility artifact in the phase-encoding direction (thick arrows).

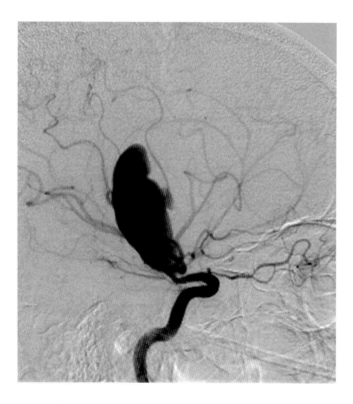

**Figure 8.2** Lateral view of left ICA on DSA of the same patient as in Fig. 8.1 reveals a saccular, carotid terminus aneurysm. Note that DSA significantly underestimates the actual size of the aneurysm, as it shows only the patent lumen.

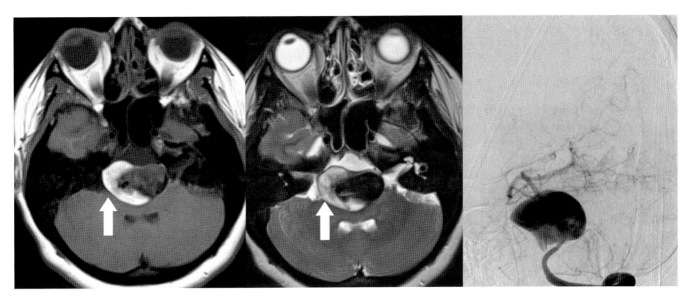

**Figure 8.3** Giant vertebral-basilar (fusiform) aneurysm with subacute peripheral thrombus on the right (arrow) and a patent lumen on the left seen as a flow void. Note the subarachnoid location and marked mass effect on the pons.

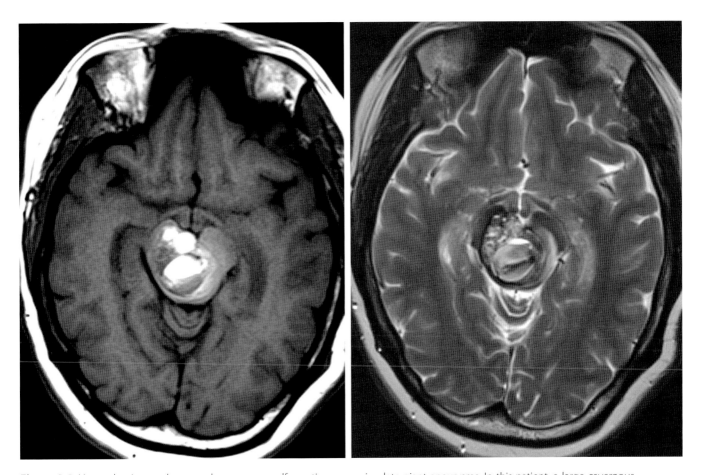

**Figure 8.4** Hemorrhagic neoplasms and cavernous malformations may simulate giant aneurysms. In this patient, a large cavernous malformation is present in the midbrain. The key to correct diagnosis is recognition of its intra-axial location.

# Acute intracerebral hematoma

## Imaging description

Acute intracerebral hematoma (ICH) accounts for 10–15% of all strokes and is associated with a higher mortality rate than both ischemic stroke and subarachnoid hemorrhage (SAH). Common causes include hypertension, amyloid angiopathy, trauma, coagulopathy, vascular anomalies including cavernomas and arteriovenous malformations (AVMs), tumors, and various drugs. Hypertension remains the single greatest modifiable risk factor for ICH.

Although clinical information is invaluable in helping to distill a reasonably short differential for acute ICH, there are many features on imaging that can be quite helpful. Amongst the features to be analyzed include location, multiplicity, symmetry, mass effect, and presence of enhancement within the hematoma. CT has a high sensitivity and the modality of choice in detecting ICH. However, MRI is very helpful to evaluate for possible underlying lesions.

Hypertensive hemorrhages most commonly occur within the basal ganglia, thalamus, and cerebellum (Fig. 9.1). However, primary brainstem and lobar bleeds can also occur in a smaller number of patients. These locations correspond to the location of microscopic changes of hyalinization, necrosis, tortuosity, and microaneurysm formation in the perforating vessels. Large lesions may extend into the ventricular system, or less commonly into the subarachnoid space. CT angiography is being increasingly utilized in the work-up of ICH. Presence of "spot sign" on CTA may be indicative of future hematoma expansion (Fig. 9.2). It is defined as spot-like and/or serpiginous foci of enhancement, within the margin of a parenchymal hematoma without obvious connection to outside vessels [1].

Amyloid angiopathy (AA) (see Case 10) results in lobar hemorrhages, often of differing ages. AA spares the basal ganglia and most commonly involves the parieto-occipital region. Microbleeds in the cortex or subcortical white matter suggest an underlying AA. Post-traumatic hemorrhages occur at characteristic locations, i.e., basal frontal and temporal lobes, gray–white junctions, corpus callosum, and upper dorsal brainstem (see Case 10).

ICH may occur from a variety of coagulopathies including blood dyscrasias, anticoagulant and antiplatelet drugs, and liver failure. The coagulopathic hemorrhages favor intraparenchymal and subdural locations. Presence of heterogeneity, areas of low attenuation suggesting active extravasation, fluid-fluid levels, and satellite sites of hemorrhage may all point to coagulopathy, although these are not specific to this etiology (Fig. 9.3).

Hemorrhage from vascular abnormalities such as AVM or dural AV fistula (dAVF) may occur in any area of the brain. The presence of linear or speckled calcifications favors an underlying AVM (Fig. 9.4).

On occasion, acute intratumoral hemorrhage may be an event that brings a tumor to clinical attention. Differentiation from bland hemorrhage may be difficult on CT, but MRI may help with this distinction (Fig. 9.5). The hemorrhage within a tumor frequently has a heterogeneous appearance and consists of an admixture of various stages. There may be foci within the hematoma that enhance with contrast, and thereby point towards the correct etiology.

## Importance

ICH is associated with morbidity and mortality that exceeds that of SAH and ischemic stroke. Moreover, spontaneous ICH occurs in relatively younger patients. Careful analysis of the imaging pattern is helpful in determining the exact etiology of ICH.

## Typical clinical scenario

The clinical presentation depends on the location and size of the ICH. Large hematomas may be fatal due to acutely developing mass effect and herniation. Smaller hematomas may present with acute neurologic deficits referable to the location of the bleed.

## Differential diagnosis

See *Imaging description*, above.

---

## Teaching points

Location, multiplicity, and MR characteristics of hematoma, coupled with clinical history, allow a precise diagnosis of etiology of intracerebral bleed in a vast majority of cases. Hypertensive hemorrhage is the most common type of spontaneous ICH, recognized by its location, association with microbleeds in the basal ganglia, and clinical history of long-standing hypertension.

---

REFERENCES

1. Thompson AL, Kosior JC, Gladstone DJ, *et al.*; PREDICTS/ Sunnybrook ICH CTA Study Group. Defining the CT angiography 'spot sign' in primary intracerebral hemorrhage. *Can J Neurol Sci* 2009; **36**: 456–61.

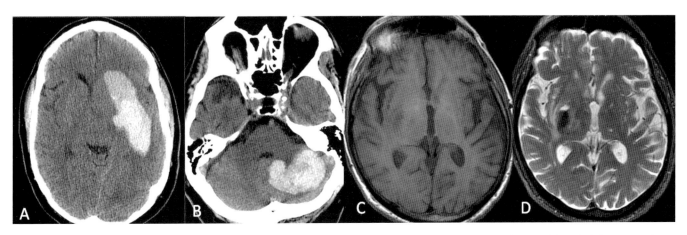

**Figure 9.1** Typical locations of hypertensive bleeds with involvement of (**A**) lenticular nucleus, (**B**) cerebellum, and (**C, D**) thalamocapsular region. MRI is invaluable in assessing the age of the bleed (for example, acute stage, C, D) and establishing the etiology.

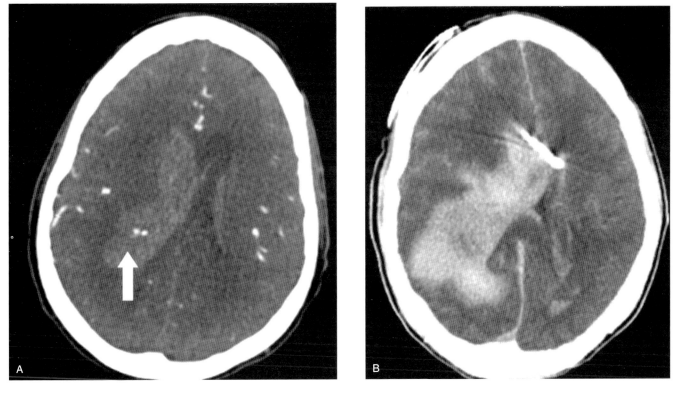

**Figure 9.2** (**A**) Acute parenchymal hematoma with intraventricular extension. Note two small enhancing foci (arrow) which are not related to a visible vessel, i.e., "spot sign." (**B**) Follow-up CT showed marked hematoma expansion.

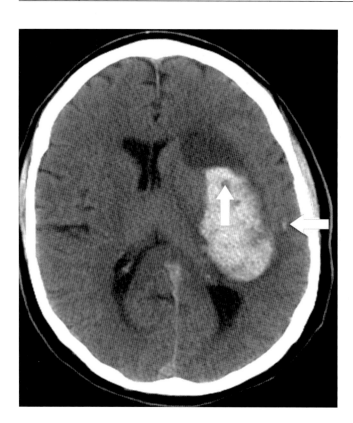

**Figure 9.3** Large basal ganglia hemorrhage in a coagulopathic patient. Presence of fluid levels (vertical arrow) and satellite areas of bleed (horizontal arrow) are suggestive but not specific to this etiology.

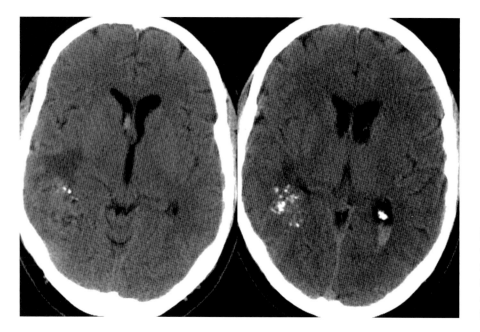

**Figure 9.4** Acute hemorrhage in a patient with temporo-occipital AVM. Note the speckled calcifications of the nidus and edema in right peritrigonal white matter. A small amount of blood is noted in right frontal horn and left ventricular trigone.

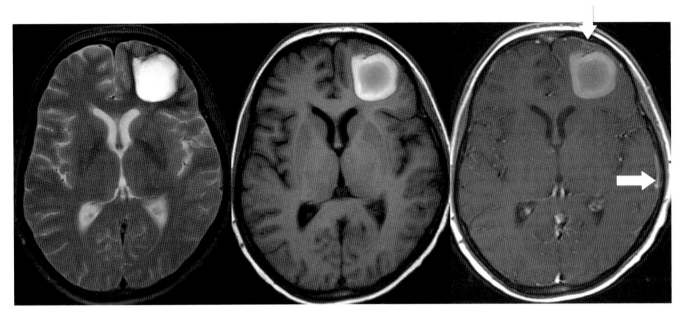

**Figure 9.5** Melanoma metastasis masquerading as a subacute hematoma. The only hints to the neoplastic etiology are nodular areas of enhancement in the parenchyma (vertical arrow) and areas of leptomeningeal enhancement (horizontal arrow).

# 10 Cerebral amyloid angiopathy

## Imaging description

Cerebral amyloid angiopathy (CAA) is a heterogeneous group of biochemically and genetically diverse disorders that is characterized by the deposition of β-amyloid protein in the media and adventitia of small and medium-sized vessels of the cerebral cortex, subcortex, and leptomeninges. The deposition of amyloid results in weakening of blood vessels, leading to both asymptomatic microbleeds and symptomatic lobar intracerebral hemorrhage (ICH). CAA is a common cause of lobar hemorrhage in normotensive elderly patients [1].

On non-contrast CT, hematomas are easily identified and are typically noted in the cortex or subcortical region. Deep white matter, basal ganglia, and brainstem are generally spared. Other neuroimaging features that support a diagnosis of CAA include multiplicity and recurrent nature of lobar hematomas. The hematomas may be accompanied by subarachnoid, intraventricular, or subdural extension, especially when large. When a diagnosis of CAA is entertained, MRI should be performed with the addition of gradient echo (GRE) or susceptibility-weighted imaging (SWI). These sequences are sensitive to local magnetic field inhomogeneity and readily demonstrate small petechial hemorrhages in the cortical–subcortical regions associated with CAA (Figs. 10.1, 10.2). The petechial hemorrhages are typically less than 5 mm in diameter and can sometimes be quite extensive (Fig. 10.2). Identification of these microbleeds lends specificity to a diagnosis of CAA in a patient with acute ICH. More recently, positron emission tomography (PET) imaging with the β-amyloid-binding Pittsburgh Compound B has been proposed as a potential non-invasive method for CAA detection in living subjects [1]. Other non-specific findings are frequently noted in patients with CAA, including leukoariosis and generalized brain volume loss (atrophy).

## Importance

CAA is a common disorder that is frequently asymptomatic, and its prevalence increases with advancing age [1]. Accurate diagnosis is heavily dependent on imaging characteristics, thereby resulting in proper treatment and avoidance of unnecessary further work-up.

## Typical clinical scenario

CAA is typically diagnosed in elderly patients (>55 years) who present with focal neurologic symptoms related to acute ICH or dementia. The Boston criteria serve as a tool to improve and standardize the diagnosis of CAA [2].

## Differential diagnosis

CAA-related hemorrhages must be differentiated from other common causes of ICH including hypertension, trauma, coagulopathy, vascular malformations, tumors, and illicit drug use [2]. The clinical history, coupled with specific features on imaging studies, is helpful in making a correct diagnosis. For example, in contrast to CAA, the hypertensive hemorrhages occur most commonly in the basal ganglia, thalami, or the brainstem. Although microbleeds can be seen in hypertensive patients, these are typically confined to deep gray matter as well and spare the cortex and subcortical regions.

Conditions that result in multiple areas of susceptibility on GRE or SWI sequences may mimic CAA. These include diffuse axonal injury (DAI), multiple cavernous malformations, and hemorrhagic metastases (Fig. 10.3). Factors such as clinical history, the age of the patient, and the size (<5 mm) and distribution of microbleeds in cortical–subcortical regions help differentiate CAA from other disorders. For example, the areas typically involved by petechial hemorrhages in DAI include the gray–white matter junction, splenium of the corpus callosum, and dorsolateral brainstem (Fig. 10.4), and a history of trauma is usually forthcoming.

## Teaching points

ICH from CAA is an important but underdiagnosed cause of morbidity and mortality in normotensive elderly patients. Findings on neuroimaging studies are often characteristic of CAA.

REFERENCES

1. Greenberg SM, Biffi A. Cerebral amyloid angiopathy: a systematic review. *J Clin Neurol* 2011; **7**: 1–9.
2. Knudsen KA, Rosand J, Karluk D, Greenberg SM. Clinical diagnosis of cerebral amyloid angiopathy: validation of the Boston criteria. *Neurology* 2001; **56**: 537–9.

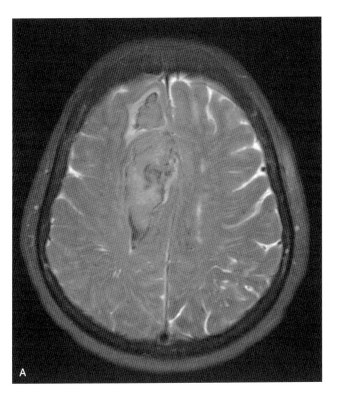
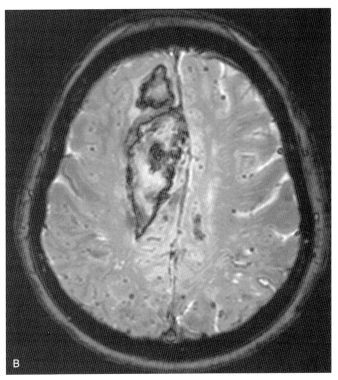

**Figure 10.1** (**A**) A lobar, right frontal hematoma in an elderly patient is noted on T2-weighted sequence. Although CAA can be suspected based on the location of the bleed and the age of the patient, the diagnosis can be more confidently made with the addition of sequences that highlight the magnetic field inhomogeneity. (**B**) The GRE sequence at the same level demonstrates multiple cortical and subcortical foci of microbleeds, highly suggestive of CAA.

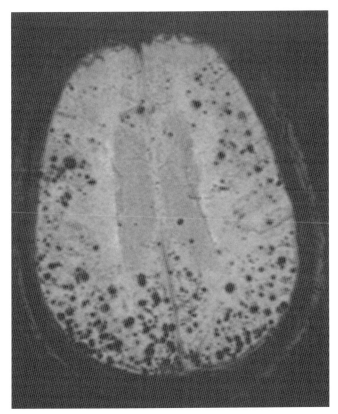

**Figure 10.2** SWI sequence offers the highest sensitivity for detection of cerebral petechial hemorrhages (microbleeds). The microbleeds are very extensive in this case. Note the relative sparing of deep white matter and periventricular regions.

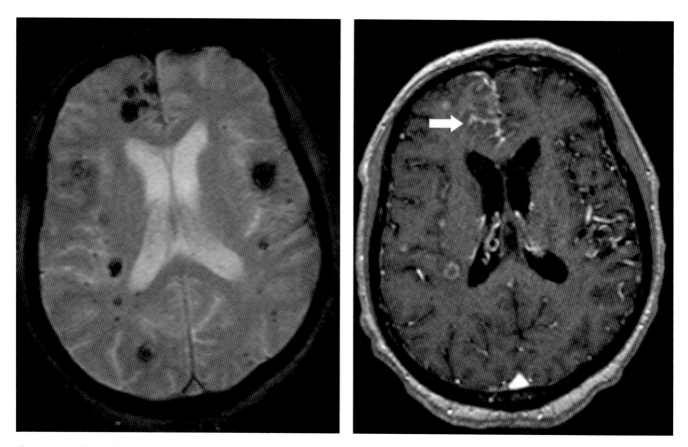

**Figure 10.3** Hemorrhagic metastasis from lung carcinoma simulating CAA on GRE images. Several of these lesions enhance with contrast, thereby favoring metastatic disease. Also note the presence of leptomeningeal metastatic disease (arrow).

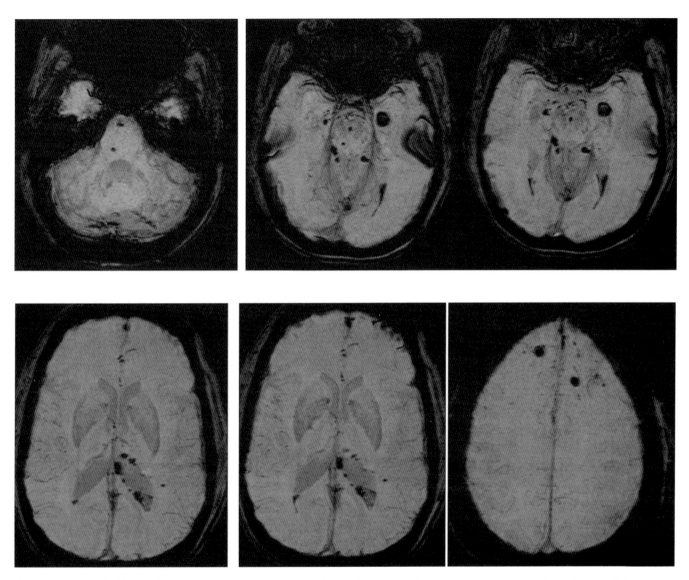

**Figure 10.4** Petechial hemorrhages in DAI have a characteristic distribution and involve gray–white matter junction, splenium of the corpus callosum, and dorsolateral brainstem.

# Primary CNS vasculitis

## Imaging description

Primary CNS vasculitis (PCNSV) is a relatively uncommon disease that is limited to the brain and spinal cord. The imaging manifestations are varied and non-specific, but help make the diagnosis in the setting of an appropriate clinical scenario. An MRI of the brain is almost always abnormal, although the observed abnormalities are non-specific. Findings on MRI include cortical or subcortical infarcts (Figs. 11.1, 11.2), often of varied ages. Abnormal enhancement can be seen involving the parenchyma as well as leptomeninges. Scattered, non-specific alterations are frequently present in the white matter. Intracranial hemorrhage is a less common but well-recognized manifestation of PCNSV. Fewer than 5% of patients demonstrate tumor-like mass lesions [1,2]. Advanced MRI techniques may in future be able to better characterize the vessel wall abnormalities and demonstrate mural enhancement that may suggest a diagnosis of vasculitis (Fig. 11.3) [2].

Non-invasive vascular studies such as MRA and CTA may demonstrate areas of focal and segmental narrowing, irregularity, and beading, which is suggestive of vasculitis, but may be completely normal if the predominant involvement is of distal vessels. Cerebral digital subtraction angiography (DSA) has been considered a gold-standard test for cerebral vascular imaging but is not without limitations. DSA can reveal classic changes of alternate areas of narrowing and dilatation, irregularity, beading (Fig. 11.2), vessel cut-off, or sometimes even microaneurysm formation. The sensitivity of this study varies from 40% to 90%, and the specificity can be as low as 30% [2]. Therefore, angiographic changes should always be interpreted in the light of clinical presentation and supportive laboratory data.

## Importance

A prompt diagnosis of CNS vasculitis is important, because timely institution of steroid or immunosuppressive agents can halt the progress and result in clinical improvement. On the other hand, it is very important to distinguish PCNSV from other causes of vascular abnormalities such as reversible cerebral vasoconstriction syndrome (RCVS: see Case 12) and infectious abnormalities, where treatment with steroids and immunosuppressants may result in serious morbidity.

## Typical clinical scenario

Several subsets of CNS vasculitis have been identified which differ in their degree of severity and prognosis. PCNSV can have either a progressive or a relapsing course with transient or fixed neurologic deficits, headaches, and decreased cognition. The serologic markers are generally negative but cerebrospinal fluid (CSF) demonstrates evidence of inflammatory process. Definitive diagnosis requires brain and meningeal biopsy, but presumptive diagnosis can be made based on a combination of supportive clinical, laboratory, neuroimaging, and angiographic findings.

## Differential diagnosis

Correct diagnosis of PCNSV may be difficult, since a number of disease entities can demonstrate similar imaging characteristics (Table 11.1, Fig. 11.4). Careful assessment of clinical, laboratory, and imaging data may help formulate a presumptive diagnosis of PCNSV. However, brain biopsy may be needed to establish a correct diagnosis. In general, biopsies targeting abnormal areas (lesions) in the brain are more likely to result in a positive result [1].

**Table 11.1** Differential diagnosis of PCNSV (adapted from [2]).

| **Diseases that mimic angiographic findings of PCNSV** |
| --- |
| Reversible cerebral vasoconstriction syndrome (RCVS) |
| Radiation vasculopathy |
| Intravascular lymphoma |
| Atherosclerosis |
| Vasospasm |
| **Diseases that mimic MRI findings of PCNSV** |
| Demyelinating diseases (multiple sclerosis, progressive multifocal leukoencephalopathy) |
| Posterior reversible leukoencephalopathy |
| Neoplasms (intravascular lymphoma, gliomatosis) |
| **Systemic diseases** |
| Rheumatologic diseases (scleroderma, polyarteritis nodosa, SLE) |
| Infections (herpes, chronic bacterial infections such as tuberculosis and syphilis, fungal infections) |

## Teaching points

PCNSV is the most common form of vasculitis affecting the CNS. A presumptive diagnosis can be established on the basis of clinical, laboratory, and neuroimaging data, but biopsy may still be necessary for accurate diagnosis. One of the commonest conditions that can be confused with PCNSV is RCVS (see Case 12). In contrast to RCVS, PCNSV has generally insidious onset with less severe intensity of headaches and a more progressive course of neurologic deterioration.

REFERENCES

1. Salvarani C, Brown RD, Hunder GG. Adult primary central nervous system vasculitis: an update. *Curr Opin Rheumatol* 2012; **24**: 46–52.
2. Hajj-Ali RA, Singhal AB, Benseler S, Molloy E, Calabrese LH. Primary angiitis of the CNS. *Lancet Neurol* 2011; **10**: 561–72.

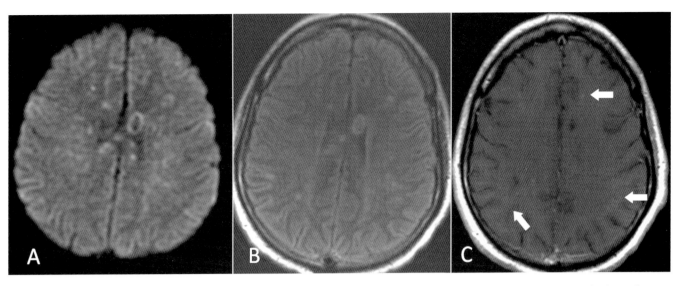

**Figure 11.1** MRI in a patient with proven PCNSV. (**A**) DWI and (**B**) FLAIR images reveal infarcts of various ages including multiple small acute subcortical infarcts. (**C**) There are scattered areas of parenchymal enhancement on T1-weighted enhanced sequence (arrows), some along the distribution of periventricular spaces.

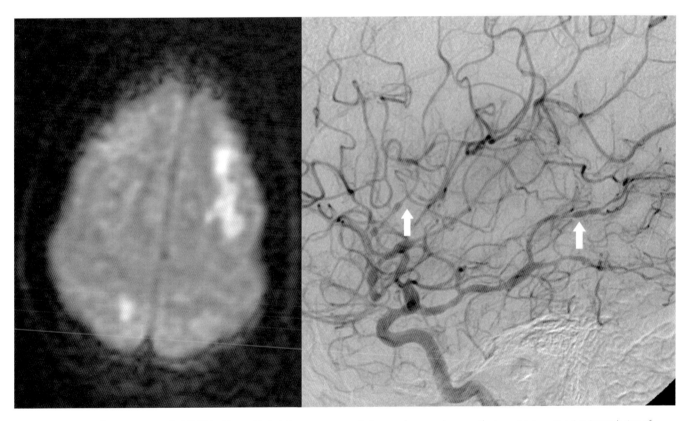

**Figure 11.2** Another patient with PCNSV with multiple infarcts at presentation and an angiogram that suggests extensive irregularity of the cortical vessels and multifocal beading (arrows). It should be remembered, however, that these changes may be identified in other types of vasculopathies as well.

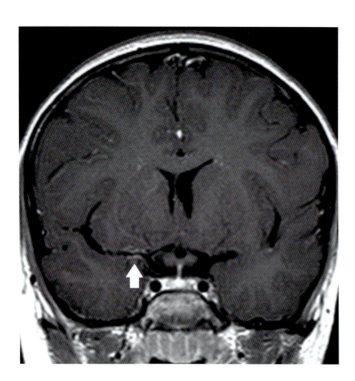

**Figure 11.3** A child with varicella vasculitis presented with sudden-onset left hemiparesis. Note the intramural enhancement of the right MCA, suggesting inflammation of vessel wall.

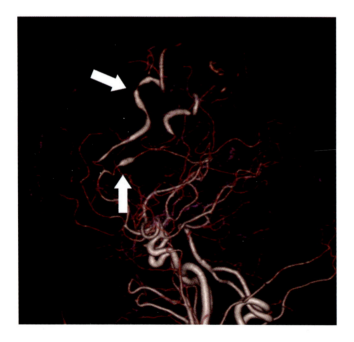

**Figure 11.4** CTA demonstrating extensive changes of vasculitis with vessel irregularity and beading (arrows). The etiology for these vascular alterations in this case was radiation arteritis.

# Reversible cerebral vasoconstriction syndrome

## Imaging description

Reversible cerebral vasoconstriction syndromes (RCVS) represent a heterogeneous group of cerebrovascular disorders that share similar clinical and imaging features. These disorders are associated with thunderclap headache, with or without neurologic symptoms and transient segmental narrowing of the distal intracranial arteries [1,2]. The neuroimaging features are variable, but the presence of unilateral or bilateral cortical subarachnoid hemorrhage (SAH) is very suggestive, in the appropriate clinical scenario. The amount of blood is generally small and may manifest as hyperdensity of cortical sulci on CT (Fig. 12.1) or hyperintense signal in sulci on FLAIR sequence. Areas of infarction may be identified as areas of restricted diffusion and can be seen in as many as 7–54% of patients. The least common finding is parenchymal hematomas (Fig. 12.2).

An imaging hallmark of this disease is the presence of multifocal areas of segmental vascular narrowing (Figs. 12.1, 12.2, 12.3). Typically, more than one vascular distribution is involved and the vessels demonstrate a beaded appearance. These changes may be seen on CTA, MRA, or digital subtraction angiography (DSA). In some instances only second- and third-order vessels are involved, and therefore CTA and MRA may be false negative and DSA is required to establish the diagnosis. Of note, vascular imaging studies generally demonstrate an absence of ruptured aneurysm or a vascular malformation. The vascular changes of RCVS resolve on follow-up studies, within a period of 3 months (Fig. 12.3).

## Importance

An accurate diagnosis of this condition is very important, since it can prevent unnecessary and often invasive further work-up. RCVS is often mistaken for primary angiitis of CNS (PACNS) / primary CNS vasculitis (PCNSV), and thus patients may be subjected to unnecessary brain biopsy and/or long-term treatment with high-dose steroids and/or cytotoxic agents that may have harmful side effects [1]. On the other hand, misdiagnosis of this condition as SAH-associated vasospasm may initiate triple-H therapy (hypervolemia, hypertension, hemodilution) or unnecessary and potentially dangerous angioplasty.

## Typical clinical scenario

The most common clinical presentation is sudden, severe (thunderclap) headache. The severity of headache generally results in a work-up for aneurysmal SAH, with CT of the brain and, in many cases, lumbar puncture. There is female preponderance. A small number of patients present with acute neurologic symptoms related to ischemic or hemorrhagic brain lesions. Although considered idiopathic, RCVS has been associated with a multitude of factors, including vasoactive substances, medications, postpartum state, and headache disorders. The implicated substances have included alcohol, amphetamines, cannabis, cocaine, methylendioxymethamphetamine ("ecstasy"), bromocriptine, ergotamine, pseudophedrine, sympathomimetics, SSRIs, interferon, nicotine patches, and triptans.

## Differential diagnosis

There have been numerous reports of various types of reversible vasoconstriction syndromes within the literature under a multitude of nosologies including, but not limited to, benign isolated arteritis of the CNS, benign angiopathy of the CNS, migrainous vasospasm, postpartum cerebral angiopathy, thunderclap headache with vasospasm, and drug-induced vasospasm, which can now be unified under the diagnosis of RCVS.

On vascular studies, this condition can be mistaken for PCNSV or SAH-associated vasospasm (Fig. 12.4). RCVS-associated SAH may be distinguished from SAH-related vasospasm based on the absence of ruptured aneurysm on vascular imaging and diffuse distribution and disproportionate extent of vasoconstriction relative to the focal cortical subarachnoid blood. While second- and third-order vessels are involved by RCVS, SAH-induced vasospasm generally causes smooth, long-segment narrowing of the proximal cisternal vessels (A1, M1, P1 segments) correlating with the location and amount of subarachnoid blood.

In addition to short-term reversibility of vascular changes on follow-up angiography, the distinction between RCVS and PCNSV is aided by diligent clinical assessment and CSF analysis. PCNSV usually has an insidious course of progressive neurologic deterioration, whereas RCVS occurs acutely and has a self-limited course (see Case 11). CSF analysis may be helpful and is often near normal in patients with RCVS, with occasional mild protein or white blood cell elevation [3]. In contrast, patients with PCNSV typically demonstrate abnormal CSF values with elevated protein levels >100mg/dL and leukocytosis in excess of 5–10 cells/mm$^3$ [4].

## Teaching points

RCVS is an underdiagnosed and often misdiagnosed entity. A knowledge of typical clinical and imaging characteristics along with reversible segmental vasoconstriction demonstrated on vascular studies can help establish the correct diagnosis and avoid unnecessary and invasive investigations.

REFERENCES

1. Ansari SA, Rath T, Gandhi D. Reversible cerebral vasoconstriction syndromes presenting with subarachnoid hemorrhage: a case series. *Journal of Neurointerv Surg* 2011; **3**: 272–8.

2. Ducros A, Boukobza M, Porcher R, *et al.* The clinical and radiological spectrum of reversible cerebral vasoconstriction syndrome. a prospective series of 67 patients. *Brain* 2007; **130**: 3091.

3. Hajj-Ali RA, Furlan A, Abou-Chebel A, *et al.* Benign angiopathy of the central nervous system: cohort of 16 patients with clinical course and long-term follow-up. *Arthritis Rheum* 2002; **47**: 662–9.

4. Duna GF, Calabrese LH. Limitations of invasive modalities in the diagnosis of primary angiitis of the central nervous system. *J Rheumatol* 1995; **22**: 662–7.

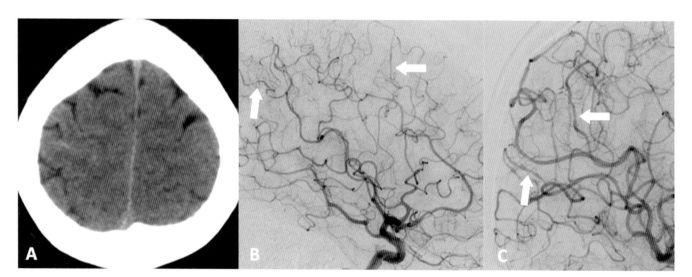

**Figure 12.1** A middle-aged lady presented with sudden thunderclap headache. (**A**) Initial head CT demonstrates a small amount of right convexity subarachnoid blood. (**B**) Lateral and (**C**) magnified oblique images from DSA demonstrate classic, multifocal, segmental areas of vasoconstriction (arrows) in the anterior and middle cerebral artery branches that suggest the diagnosis of RVCS. These changes resolved completely on a follow-up DSA after 1 month.

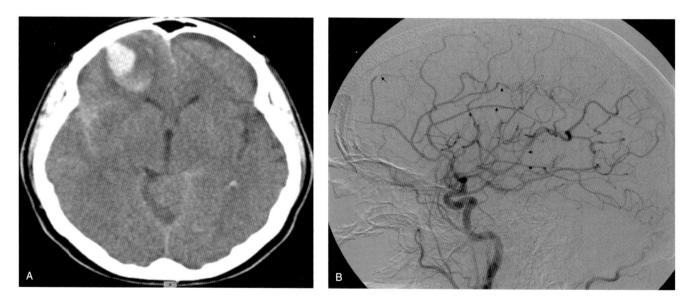

**Figure 12.2** (**A**) Axial CT image shows a right frontal intraparenchymal hematoma with a small amount of subarachnoid bleed in the Sylvian fissure. (**B**) Lateral projection of cerebral DSA performed on the same day shows multifocal short-segment stenoses (arrows). Follow-up angiography showed resolution of stenoses.

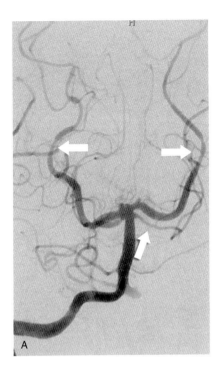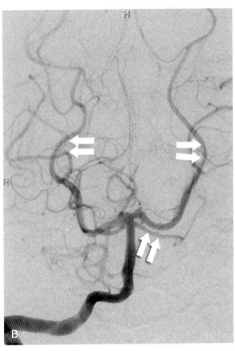

**Figure 12.3** (**A**) Right vertebral angiogram in another patient with RCVS demonstrates multifocal vasoconstriction involving the posterior cerebral and left superior cerebellar arteries (single arrows). (**B**) A follow-up study after 6 weeks demonstrates complete resolution of multifocal spasm (double arrows). The patient made an excellent recovery.

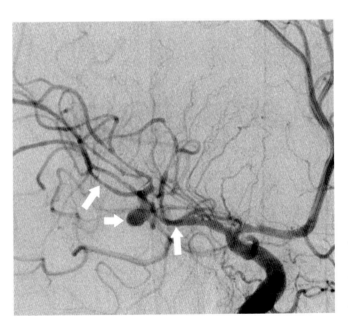

**Figure 12.4** In contrast to RCVS, the SAH-associated vasospasm tends to involve the proximal cisternal vessels and there is imaging evidence of a ruptured aneurysm. In this case, there is moderate diffuse spasm of distal M1 and proximal M2 branches of right MCA (arrows). Note also a right MCA bifurcation aneurysm (short arrow), the source of SAH in this patient.

# Moyamoya disease/syndrome

## Imaging description

Moyamoya disease is an idiopathic, progressive, occlusive disorder affecting the vessels of the circle of Willis. Although first described in Japan, it is now reported from all over the world [1].

Moyamoya disease features smooth narrowing of the distal internal carotid artery (ICA), often extending to the carotid terminus and proximal portions of the anterior and middle cerebral arteries (ACA and MCA). In contrast, moyamoya syndrome refers to a phenomenon similar in clinical presentation and anatomic findings but caused by various systemic disease entities. These include a long list of potential causes including hematological disorders (sickle cell disease, SLE, aplastic anemia), congenital syndromes (neurofibromatosis, Down's syndrome, tuberous sclerosis), and other vascular diseases (coarctation of aorta, radiation injury).

The imaging features on cross-sectional studies are dependent on the presenting features. Ischemic presentations are common in children, while adults more commonly present with hemorrhagic manifestations. CT and MRI help demonstrate the ischemic infarcts, which are commonly located in the watershed distribution between the ACA and MCA or MCA and posterior cerebral artery (PCA) territories. Infarcts of varying ages may be identified and generally related to progressive, ongoing ischemia. Generalized brain atrophy is not uncommon and occurs due to a chronic state of ischemia. On occasion, this atrophy is unilateral, if the disease is asymmetrically more advanced on one side compared to the other (Fig. 13.1).

Dilated cortical (pial) collaterals in this disease can be seen as areas of linear hyperintensity on FLAIR images in the cerebral sulci, the so-called "ivy sign" (Fig. 13.2). There may be an absence of flow void of the ICA or M1 segment of MCA, especially well visualized on T2-weighted sequences. Instead, one may note several, small and tortuous flow voids in the basal cisterns that correspond to the "puff-of-smoke" collateral vessels (Fig. 13.3). MRA and CTA have the potential to demonstrate the vascular alterations in this disease, but digital subtraction angiography (DSA) best characterizes the vascular abnormalities and provides information for treatment planning (Fig. 13.4).

The disease may be more advanced on one side than the other, and occasionally it can be unilateral. There may be additional involvement of the posterior circulation with narrowing of the P1 segments. Presence of collateral vessels at the basal aspect of the brain is virtually pathognomonic of this condition. These collaterals most commonly arise from the terminal ICA, ophthalmic artery, M1 segments, and occasionally P1 segments.

Hemorrhagic presentations are more common in adults, and hemorrhages can be either intraparenchymal or subarachnoid [2]. The hemorrhage is usually due to rupture of the fragile moyamoya collaterals or small pseudoaneurysms of the hypertrophied collateral vessels.

## Importance

Moyamoya is an important cause of stroke in young patients, but the diagnosis is often delayed because of a lack of awareness of this condition and/or its imaging signs.

## Typical clinical scenario

Highest incidence of moyamoya disease and syndrome is in the first decade of life. Children present most frequently with transient ischemic attacks (TIAs) or ischemic strokes. Intracranial hemorrhage is a more common mode of presentation in adults but can manifest in children. Symptomatic patients with moyamoya disease or phenomenon can be treated with a surgical procedure called encephalodural synangiosis (EDSA), a type of indirect bypass.

## Differential diagnosis

Differential diagnoses of moyamoya syndrome include other causes of pediatric stroke. Other causes of narrowing of ICA include vasculitides, post-radiation vasculopathy, and embolic disease.

### Teaching points

Bilateral steno-occlusive disease of ICA is characteristic, with frequent accompaniment of exuberant basal collateral vessels.

REFERENCES

1. Hoffman HJ. Moyamoya disease and syndrome. *Clin Neurol Neurosurg* 1997; **99** (Suppl 2): S39–44.

2. Gosalakkal JA. Moyamoya disease : a review. *Neurol India* 2002; **50**: 6–10.

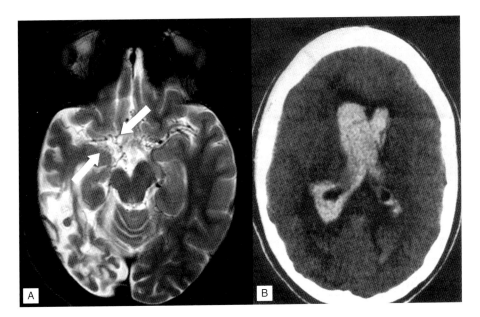

**Figure 13.1** (**A**) Chronic ischemia of right cerebral hemisphere has resulted in temporo-occipital infarcts and selective right cerebral atrophy. Note the absence of right ICA flow void and numerous tiny collateral vessels in the basal cisterns (arrows). (**B**) Hemorrhagic presentation in an adult with moyamoya disease. Note the intraventricular hemorrhage, which was a result of ruptured, fragile collateral vessels.

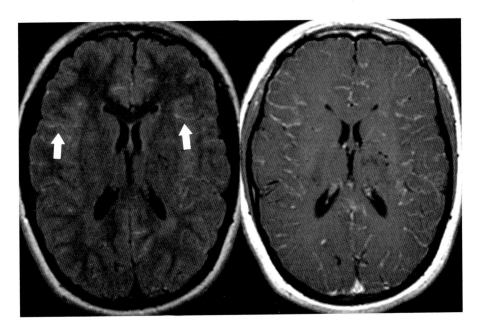

**Figure 13.2** FLAIR image reveals linear high signal in subarachnoid spaces (arrows), presumed to be from slow flow in dilated pial collaterals ("ivy sign"). These vessels enhance after contrast administration: note several flow voids in the basal ganglia, corresponding to basal collaterals arising from ICA.

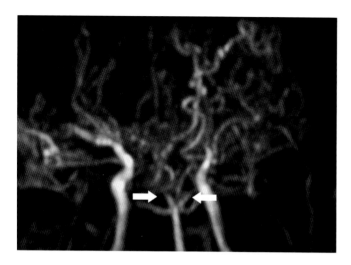

**Figure 13.3** Time-of-flight (TOF) MRA of the same patient as in Fig. 13.2 reveals complete tapered occlusion of ICAs and several hypertrophied collaterals. In this patient, bilateral PCAs are also occluded (arrows).

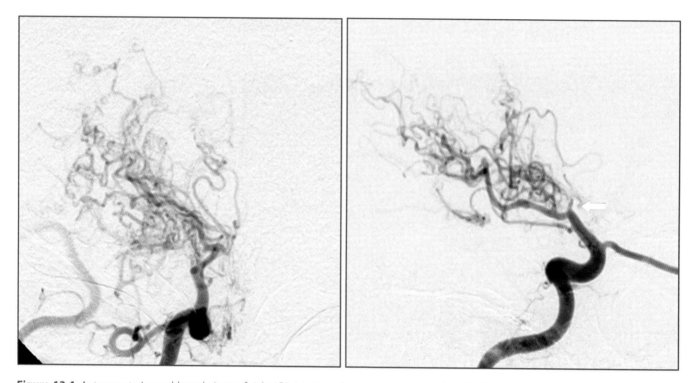

**Figure 13.4** Anteroposterior and lateral views of right ICA injection demonstrates the classic puff-of-smoke collaterals arising from the carotid terminus. Note the occlusion of ICA (arrow) beyond the take-off of the anterior choroidal artery.

# Cortical venous thrombosis

## Imaging description

Isolated cortical venous thrombosis (ICVT) is a rare but underdiagnosed occurrence. The difficulty in diagnosis arises because of variability in the cortical venous system, and the small size and peripheral location of the cortical veins. The "definitive imaging proof" of ICVT is the demonstration of thrombus in the cortical vein and lack of visualization of this vessel on CT or MR venography (CTV or MRV) [1].

Thrombus in the cortical vein may be visualized on CT as the "cord sign," with high density of the thrombus appearing similar to the hyperdense middle cerebral artery (MCA) sign in acute ischemic stroke. Signal-intensity changes on MRI depend on the age of the thrombus at the time of imaging. Acute thrombus has a predominantly isointense signal on T1-weighted and hypointense signal on T2-weighted sequences, reflecting the presence of deoxyhemoglobin. Accumulation of methemoglobin may result in hyperintense signal on T1- and T2-weighted sequences [1,2]. In general, the sequences that display sensitivity to the paramagnetic products of hemoglobin (T2*, susceptibility-weighted imaging) can play an important role in diagnosis by demonstrating a tubular area of hypointense signal in the thrombosed vessel (Figs. 14.1, 14.2) [3]. The vascular studies (MRV, CTV, or DSA) complement MRI in establishing the diagnosis by demonstrating lack of filling or partial opacification (Fig. 14.1) of the corresponding vein(s). Digital subtraction angiography (DSA) may be helpful in demonstrating the collateral pathways and their adequacy.

Parenchymal changes are frequently encountered in the territory of drainage of the thrombosed vein. These changes may consist of vasogenic edema, swelling, and/or hemorrhage (Figs. 14.1, 14.2) [1]. The hemorrhage, if encountered, can take the form of small petechial hemorrhages or frank lobar hematoma.

## Importance

ICVT should be considered in the differential diagnosis of other causes of focal edema or hemorrhage. Awareness of this condition and correct diagnosis will help with the institution of early therapy.

## Typical clinical scenario

Similar to dural sinus thrombosis, the predisposing conditions for ICVT can include dehydration, pregnancy, medications, and hypercoagulable states. The clinical features include sudden onset of headache followed by focal or generalized seizures and focal neurologic deficits including hemiparesis, aphasia, sensory deficits, or hemianopia. In a smaller number of patients, ICVT may also present with isolated subarachnoid hemorrhage. Clinical signs of increased intracranial pressure and mental obtundation may be present.

## Differential diagnosis

ICVT should be distinguished from other causes of lobar cerebral hemorrhage, such as hypertension and amyloid angiopathy amongst others. Cortical venous involvement may also occur as a part of more extensive dural venous thrombosis. Gradient echo (GRE) or susceptibility-weighted imaging (SWI) demonstrating a cord- or band-like hypo-intense structure can help in recognition of this condition.

Confusion may also arise in differentiating ICVT from cases of thrombosis of developmental venous anomaly (DVA). In cases of DVA thrombosis (see Case 15), thrombosed radicles or collector veins have an abnormal intramedullary course, compared to the subarachnoid location of the thrombosed vein in the setting of ICVT (Fig. 14.3).

> ### Teaching points
>
> ICVT is considered rare but the diagnosis may be missed because of a lack of awareness of this entity amongst clinicians as well as radiologists. GRE or SWI sequences must always be included in the protocol for imaging intracranial hemorrhage cases. Routine use of these sequences may help recognize ICVT, leading to early institution of therapy.

REFERENCES

1. Boukobza M, Crassard I, Bousser MG, Chabriat H. MR imaging features of isolated cortical vein thrombosis: diagnosis and follow-up. *AJNR Am J Neuroradiol* 2009; **30**: 344–8.
2. Chang R, Friedman DP. Isolated cortical venous thrombosis presenting as subarachnoid hemorrhage: a report of three cases. *AJNR Am J Neuroradiol* 2004; **25**: 1676–9.
3. Idbaih A, Boukobza M, Crassard I, *et al.* MRI of clot in cerebral venous thrombosis: high diagnostic value of susceptibility-weighted images. *Stroke* 2006; **37**: 991–5.

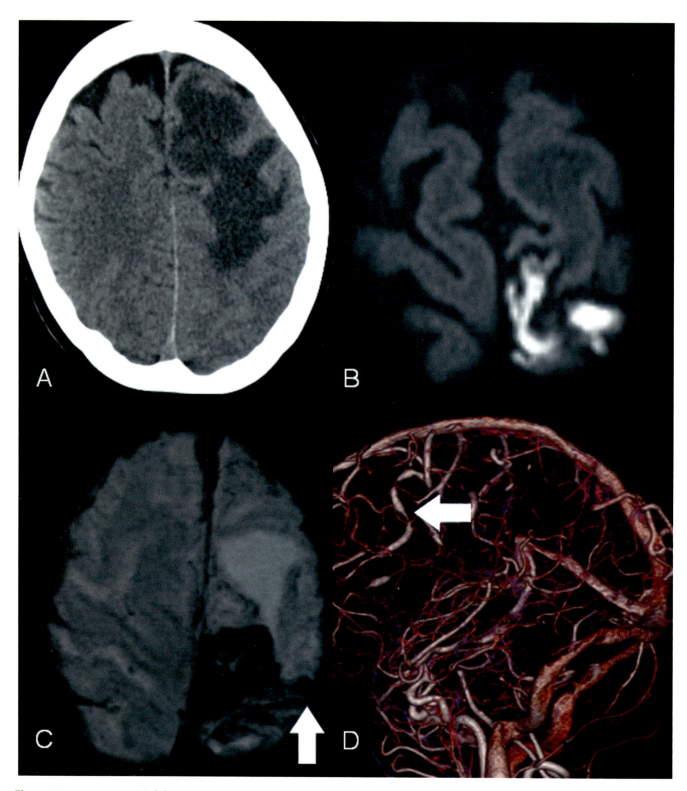

**Figure 14.1** A patient with left frontal AVM who previously underwent gamma knife therapy presented with right hemiparesis. (**A**) Non-contrast CT revealed edema and mass effect in the left frontal lobe. (**B**) A tubular structure is noted in the left parietal convexity on DWI sequence that restricts diffusion and is most consistent with an acute cortical vein thrombus. (**C**) The cortical venous thrombus is dark on GRE sequence (arrow). (**D**) CTV reveals a paucity of cortical veins in the left parietal region and also the presence of stenosis in some cortical veins (arrow), presumably changes of radiation vasculopathy.

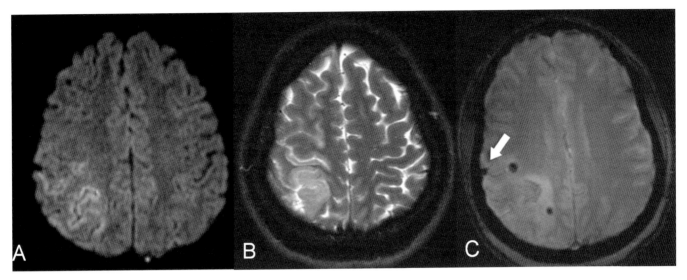

**Figure 14.2** (**A**) Axial DWI, (**B**) T2-weighted, and (**C**) GRE images of a patient who presented with acute-onset headache followed by neurologic deterioration show an area of parenchymal edema and ischemia. The GRE image shows the thrombosed cortical vein as a dark tubular structure outside the brain parenchyma (arrow). Also note small foci of parenchymal bleeds, which are commonly seen in this setting.

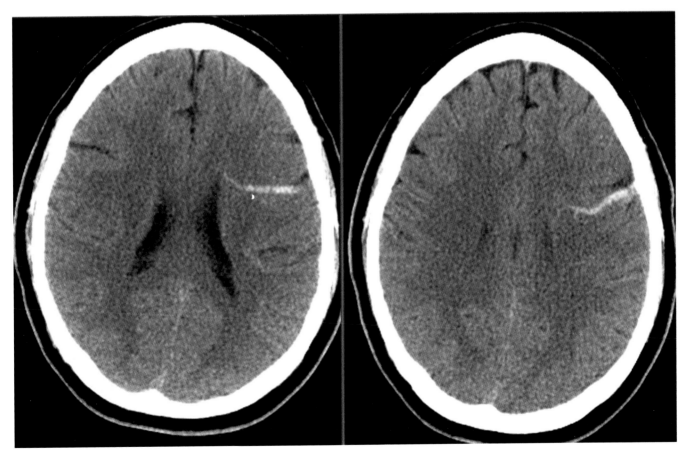

**Figure 14.3** Non-contrast CT demonstrates the "cord sign," but note that the vein courses via the brain parenchyma rather than into the subarachnoid space. This imaging appearance is very suggestive of spontaneous thrombosis of DVA rather than CVT. The diagnosis of thrombosed DVA was later confirmed on MRI and MRV (not shown).

# Developmental venous anomalies

## Imaging description

Developmental venous anomalies (DVAs) are the most common of the cerebral vascular malformations, with an incidence of up to 2.6% in the general population. They are believed to occur as a result of an embryological event that leads to interruption in the normal development of the venous system.

Normal cerebral veins may be anatomically divided into two distinct systems of drainage: superficial (pial, cortical) and deep (subependymal). The absence of development of normal pial or subependymal veins leads to an "anomalous venous disposition," in which the drainage patterns are reversed [1]. A DVA consists of a radial complex of venous radicles draining normal brain parenchyma that converge into a dilated collecting vein, resulting in its characteristic caput medusae (medusa head) appearance (Fig. 15.1). DVAs of the brain range from a small, single draining vein involving a small portion of the brain, to a large, essentially hemispheric venous anomaly. Contrast-enhanced CT or MRI can identify the collector vein of DVA as a linear or curvilinear focus of enhancement that courses from the deep white matter to a cortical vein or to a dural sinus (Fig. 15.2). Alternatively, the enhancement may course in the opposite direction in a deep draining DVA, in which the intracortical and superficial medullary veins drain toward the deep venous system.

MRI is particularly useful, and much superior to CT, for the evaluation of associated parenchymal abnormalities as well as for the detection of cavernous malformations (CMs) that are frequently associated with DVAs. A hemosiderin-sensitive sequence or susceptibility-weighted imaging (SWI) should be included in the imaging protocol to aid in the detection of the associated CM.

While the vast majority of DVAs are incidental and benign, there is growing realization that a small fraction of these lesions may be symptomatic [2]. DVAs can be associated with cortical dysplasias. In rare cases, the DVAs can undergo spontaneous thrombosis, resulting in brain edema, venous hypertension, and hemorrhagic infarction (Fig. 15.3). In general, conservative management is appropriate, but large hematomas may require surgical decompression.

## Importance

A typical DVA, if diagnosed correctly, does not need any further investigation or follow-up studies. However, it is also important to keep in mind that DVAs can occasionally be symptomatic due to associated abnormalities or locoregional venous hypertension.

## Typical clinical scenario

DVAs are typically benign and asymptomatic lesions. Symptomatic DVAs may however present with headaches, seizures, focal neurological deficits, or intracranial hemorrhage [2]. The sequelae of a DVA are likely related to regional venous hypertension that occurs in the vicinity of the DVA.

## Differential diagnosis

Familiarity with the imaging findings of DVA is all that is needed for correct diagnosis of this condition. The imaging findings are pathognomonic and there is no other vascular malformation that has similar characteristics. In clinical practice, perhaps the most common "mislabeled diagnosis" is a brain arteriovenous malformation (AVM). However, AVMs are associated with nidus within the brain parenchyma (Fig. 15.4), enlargement of the cortical arteries and draining veins, as well as structural changes in the brain such as edema or focal atrophy.

Additionally, it should be recognized that DVA is now the preferred terminology for these lesions. Other previously utilized terms such as venous angioma, cerebral venous malformation, and cerebral venous medullary malformation do not accurately describe this condition and should be abandoned.

---

### Teaching points

Enhancing, linear, venous radicles draining into a collector vein constitute the classic and pathognomonic "medusa head" appearance of DVAs. While the majority of these lesions are asymptomatic, a small fraction of DVAs indeed result in symptoms due to associated lesions (cavernous malformations, arteriovenous malformation, cortical dysplasia) or locoregional venous hypertension.

---

REFERENCES

1. Lasjaunias P, Burrows P, Planet C. Developmental venous anomalies (DVA): the so-called venous angioma. *Neurosurg Rev* 1986. **9**: 233–42.
2. Pearl M, Gregg L, Gandhi D. Cerebral venous development in relation to developmental venous anomalies and vein of Galen aneurysmal malformations. *Semin Ultrasound CT MR* 2011; **32**: 252–63.

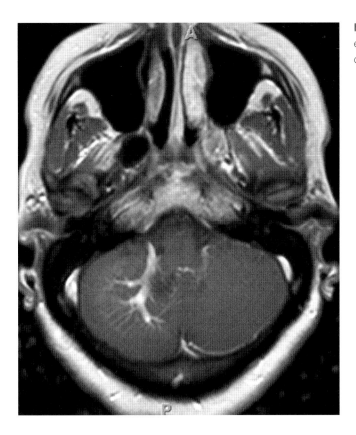

**Figure 15.1** A DVA of right cerebellum is seen on this T1-weighted enhanced image. Note the small venous radicles that converge onto the collector vein (caput medusae appearance).

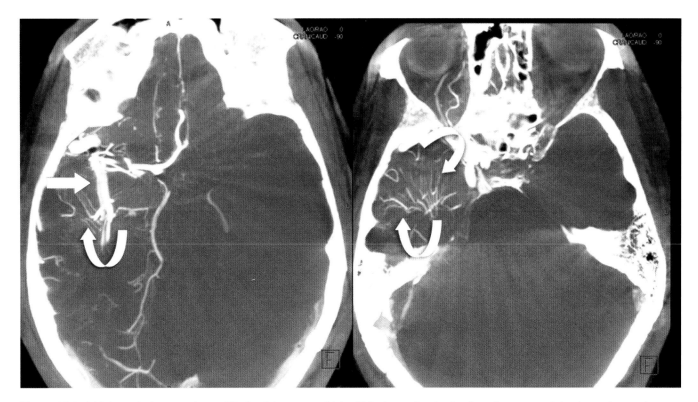

**Figure 15.2** A high-resolution cone-beam CT of a right temporal lobe DVA shows the details of small venous radicles (curved arrows) draining into a large venous collector (straight arrow).

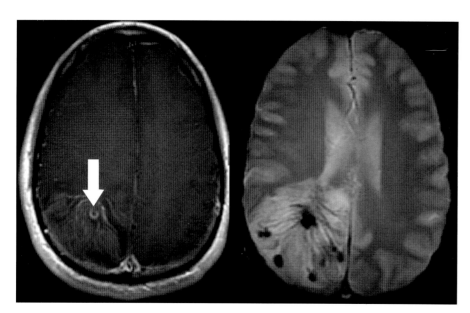

**Figure 15.3** Spontaneous thrombosis of DVA can rarely occur. A thrombus is seen as a filling defect in the collector vein (arrow), resulting in venous hypertension and focal enhancement of the parietal lobe. Gradient echo (GRE) sequence demonstrates a developing venous infarct with petechial hemorrhages.

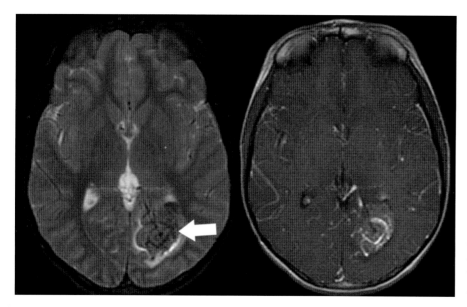

**Figure 15.4** DVAs are sometimes confused with arteriovenous malformations (AVMs), but the imaging characteristics of these two conditions are completely different. AVMs demonstrate a cluster of flow voids (nidus) within brain parenchyma (arrow). This is an acutely ruptured AVM.

# CASE 16 Dural arteriovenous fistula

## Imaging description

Adult dural arteriovenous fistulas (DAVFs), which represent the majority of lesions, are most common at the transverse, sigmoid, and cavernous sinuses [1,2]. The DAVF shunt is located in the dural leaflets, and these lesions receive their main arterial supply from meningeal arteries. For example, lesions in the transverse and sigmoid sinuses receive a supply predominantly from occipital, middle meningeal, and ascending pharyngeal arteries or the meningohypophyseal trunk (Fig. 16.1).

MRI (and CT/CTA) findings depend on the location, morphology, and severity of the fistula. MRI and CTA can demonstrate engorged vessels, dilated venous pouches, or abnormal vascular enhancement in the presence of a DAVF (Figs. 16.1, 16.2). Of note, these vessels are located in the osteodural complex and, in high-grade lesions, in the subarachnoid space. Several of these findings are the result of venous hypertension or retrograde cortical venous drainage (CVD), leading to medullary venous congestion. Venous hypertension in high-grade lesions is also thought to contribute to parenchymal abnormalities such as white matter T2 hyperintensity, intracranial hemorrhage (Fig. 16.3), or venous infarction. Parenchymal changes are better appreciated on MRI. Low-grade lesions may exhibit only flow-void clustering, engorged veins, or proptosis. Susceptibility-weighted imaging (SWI) can accurately depict retrograde CVD associated with DAVF.

MRA (especially with dynamic, time resolved techniques) and CTA are making rapid strides in the diagnosis of shunting lesions. Using these techniques, a high level of sensitivity can be achieved but reliable detection (and severity) of retrograde cortical reflux is still quite difficult. CTA may fail to detect very small lesions that are in close relation to the skull base.

Digital subtraction angiography (DSA) remains a gold standard for DAVF and allows detection of small lesions that may be missed by other modalities. The temporal resolution and ability to perform selective injections allow for precise identification of early dural venous sinus filling or cortical venous reflux (Fig. 16.3). Catheter angiography also provides the foundation for endovascular embolization, which has become a first-line therapy for DAVF treatment.

## Importance

Diagnosis of DAVFs is often delayed or missed due to the non-specific nature of associated clinical symptoms and imaging features. In high-grade subtypes of DAVFs (Borden types II and III), cortical venous reflux (CVR) may be present [2]. In these lesions, an annual mortality rate of 10.4%, an annual risk of intracranial hemorrhage of 8.1%, and an annual risk of non-hemorrhagic neurologic deficit of 6.9% are reported [1].

## Typical clinical scenario

The majority of patients with DAVF present in their fifth and sixth decades. These lesions are predominantly idiopathic, although a small percentage of patients have a previous history of craniotomy, trauma, or dural sinus thrombosis. Pulsatile tinnitus is common and results from increased blood flow through the dural venous sinuses. DAVFs involving the cavernous sinus may be associated with proptosis, chemosis, ophthalmoplegia, or decreased visual acuity. Hemorrhagic presentations are less common overall, but may be the first manifestation in high-grade lesions.

## Differential diagnosis

DAVFs are most commonly confused with parenchymal arteriovenous malformations (AVMs). The presence of dural arterial supply and absence of a nidus in the brain parenchyma are hallmarks of DAVFs and serve to distinguish these lesions from the parenchymal AVMs. Although DAVFs can occur anywhere within the dura mater, the majority are located in the transverse, sigmoid, cavernous and superior sagittal sinuses. In contrast, the parenchymal AVMs occur in the brain parenchyma and derive their blood supply from cortical (or pial) arteries.

> ### Teaching points
>
> DAVFs are commonly misdiagnosed and poorly understood lesions. The presence of excessive flow voids (or enhancing vessels) adjacent to the osteodural complex or subarachnoid space should raise a suspicion for DAVF.

REFERENCES

1. Gandhi D, Chen J, Pearl M, et al. Intracranial dural arteriovenous fistulas: classification, imaging findings, and treatment. AJNR Am J Neuroradiol 2012; 33: 1007–13.
2. Borden JA, Wu JK, Shucart WA. A proposed classification for spinal and cranial dural arteriovenous fistulous malformations and implications for treatment. J Neurosurg 1995; 82: 166–79.

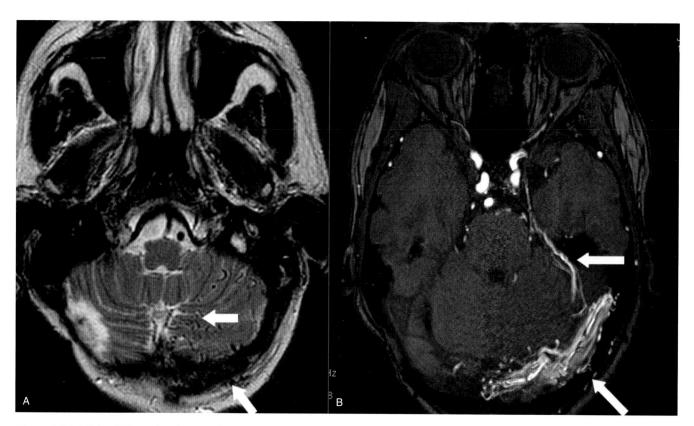

**Figure 16.1** (**A**) Axial T2-weighted image through the posterior fossa is suspicious for the presence of a DAVF. Several flow voids are depicted (arrows); some of the flow voids are in the subarachnoid space, while others are adjacent to the left occipital bone. (**B**) Source image from contrast-enhanced MRA revealing arterial vessels supplying the shunt in the left transverse sinus. Note hypertrophy of tentorial branch of meningohypophyseal artery and branches of occipital artery (arrows).

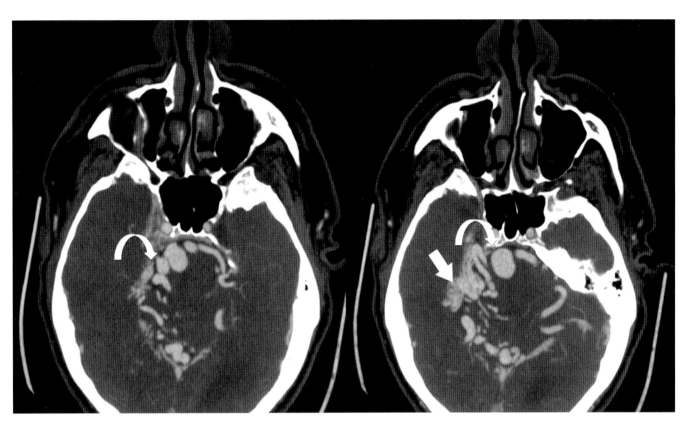

**Figure 16.2** A complex, high-grade DAVF with extensive retrograde cortical reflux. In this case, the primary shunt was in the superior petrosal sinus (straight arrow) and long-standing retrograde reflux has resulted in venous ectasia and several venous aneurysms (curved arrows).

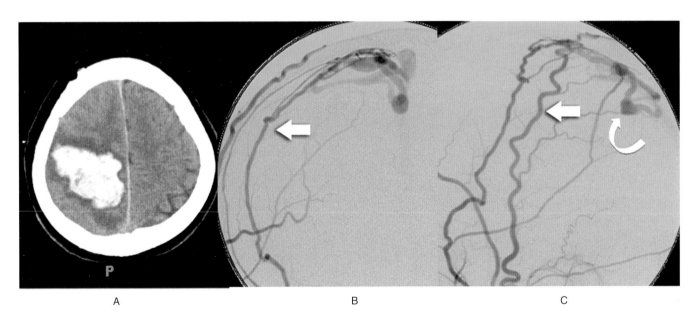

A                                          B                                          C

**Figure 16.3** Acute hemorrhagic presentation of DAVF. (**A**) CT shows a right frontoparietal hematoma, and MRI (not shown) displayed adjacent flow voids in the subarachnoid space. (**B**) Anteroposterior and (**C**) lateral views of right external carotid injection reveal a Borden type III (high-grade) DAVF of convexity cortical vein supplied by middle meningeal artery (arrow). The venous aneurysm (curved arrow) was the presumed site of rupture. The DAVF was successfully embolized.

# CASE 17 Cavernous malformation

## Imaging description

Cavernous malformations (CMs) are angiographically cryptic vascular malformations of the brain and spinal cord that consist of discrete, honeycomb-like masses of endothelial-lined sinusoidal spaces. These are circumscribed lesions and consist of thrombosed blood. While the majority of these lesions are solitary, multiplicity may occur in nearly 20% of patients. Multiple lesions are more common in genetic/familial forms of CMs.

Cross-sectional studies identify and characterize the majority of these lesions, and these are nearly always occult on angiography [1]. CT demonstrates well-defined, focal hyperdense masses that may have internal, speckled calcifications. There is a lack of mass effect or edema, differentiating these from brain neoplasms. MRI is far more sensitive, as well as more specific, in the diagnosis of CMs. The MR appearances parallel the pathoanatomic changes on histologic exam. There is internal heterogeneity, and "popcorn"-type areas of high T1 signal from subacute blood products (methemoglobin) are often noted [1]. There is a peripheral rim of hemosiderin around the lesion, generally indicative of seepage of blood breakdown products in the periphery of the mass. This rim is best noted on T2-weighted sequences, although even more marked blooming is observed on gradient echo (GRE) and susceptibility-weighted imaging (SWI) sequences (Fig. 17.1). There is no edema and generally no adjacent arterial vessels. CMs have a known association with developmental venous anomalies.

CMs are generally located in the cortex or subcortical white matter and frequently abut the subarachnoid or ventricular spaces (Fig. 17.2). Nearly 25% of lesions are infratentorial, split equally between brainstem and cerebellar locations. Within the brainstem, the pons is most commonly affected. CMs may result in intracranial hemorrhage (Fig. 17.3), although the hemorrhages are smaller and better tolerated than arteriovenous malformation (AVM)-related bleeds. Once the CM ruptures, it becomes more prone to rebleed and has a more aggressive course.

## Importance

Appropriate recognition of CMs will prevent additional work-up to exclude other lesions that are commonly confused with this lesion.

## Typical clinical scenario

Most CMs are detected incidentally on MRI, but these lesions can be symptomatic due to acute hemorrhage, seizures, or focal neurologic deficits [2]. The seizures are believed to be secondary to irritation of adjacent cortex, seepage of hemosiderin, or gliosis. CMs located in eloquent areas such as brainstem can result in focal neurologic deficits.

## Differential diagnosis

Lesions that contain blood products or create magnetic inhomogeneity and susceptibility effects can be mistaken for CMs. Hemorrhagic tumors may appear like CMs on account of internal hemorrhage, and occasionally a hemosiderin rim. However, a popcorn-like appearance on T1-weighted study and lack of "tumor-like" enhancement, mass effect, or edema help differentiate CMs from hemorrhagic neoplasms.

### Teaching points

Classic MRI features of CMs include a well-defined, discrete mass with internal subacute-chronic blood products, hemosiderin rim with lack of mass effect or edema. The imaging appearance is characteristic enough to make the firm diagnosis and avoid further work-up. The rate of spontaneous hemorrhage is relatively low, but once the hemorrhage has occurred there is a greater tendency for re-hemorrhage, and therefore treatment should be considered.

REFERENCES

1. Ide C, De Coene B, Baudrez V. MR features of cavernous angioma. *JBR-BTR* 2000; **83**: 320

2. Hauck EF, Barnett SL, White JA, Samson D. Symptomatic brainstem cavernomas. *Neurosurgery* 2009; **64**: 61–70.

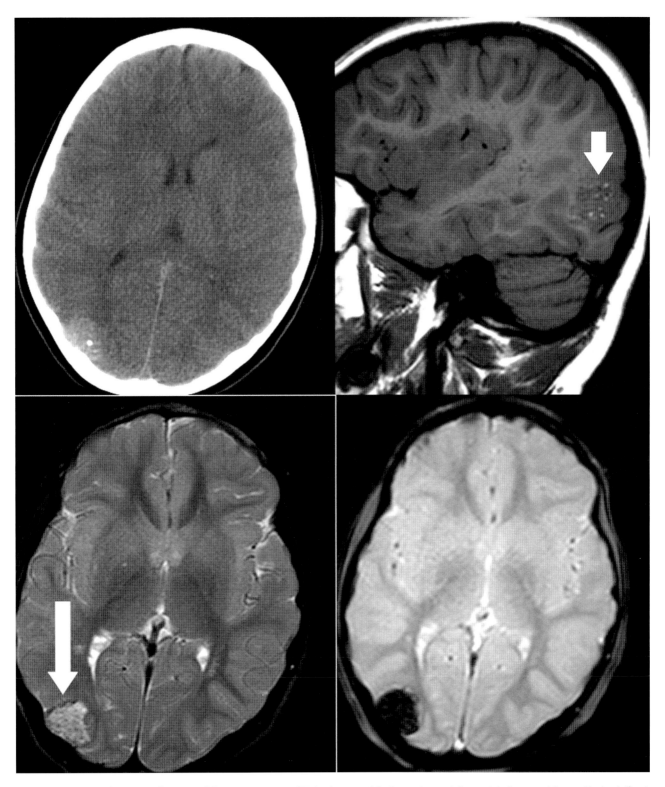

**Figure 17.1** Typical imaging features of CM. Non-contrast CT displays a mildly hyperdense right occipital mass with speckled calcification. The mass has a popcorn-like appearance on sagittal T1-weighted sequence (short arrow), high T2 signal with a faint hemosiderin rim (long arrow). Marked susceptibility effect is noted on GRE sequence.

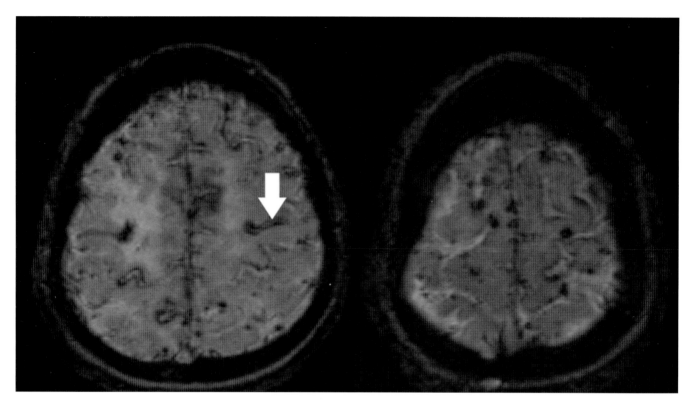

**Figure 17.2** Multiple CMs in a patient with familial CMs. Many of the lesions are located in the cortex and subcortical region. Chronic seepage of blood products in the subarachnoid space has resulted in chronic superficial siderosis (arrow).

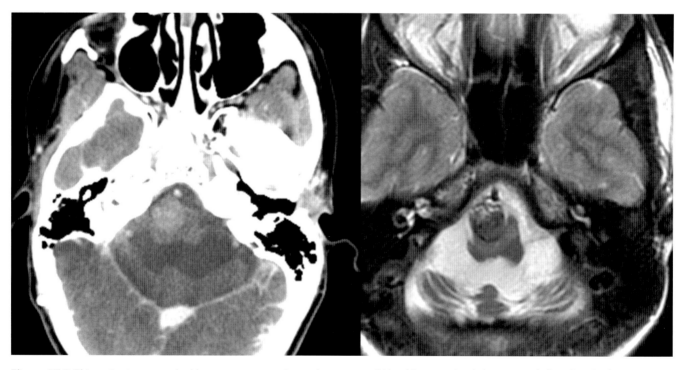

**Figure 17.3** This patient presented with acute motor weakness due to a small bleed in a previously known medullary CM. CT demonstrates a hyperdense mass in the right medulla. The presence of edema is noted around the CM on T2-weighted sequence, a feature that is generally absent in unruptured CMs.

# Tumefactive demyelinating lesion

## Imaging description

Demyelinating lesions are usually small and multiple. Occasionally demyelinating lesions can mimic neoplasms clinically, radiologically, and even histologically – hence the name tumefactive demyelinating lesion (TDL). TDLs usually present as large white matter lesions in the periventricular or subcortical regions [1]. In particular, solitary TDLs are often misdiagnosed as tumor, leading to unnecessary biopsy, surgery, and delay in treatment.

While TDLs show a spectrum of imaging abnormalities, certain features are commonly seen, and these help in differentiating TDLs from other lesions [2,3]. On CT, TDLs show hypoattenuation [4]. On post-contrast MRI, incomplete ring enhancement is a relatively characteristic feature, which may be present up to 70% of patients (Figs. 18.1, 18.2). The T2 signal is variable, but most lesions show a markedly increased T2 signal centrally and relatively decreased signal peripherally. Up to 50% of TDLs do not have mass effect or edema, which is a critical observation in differential diagnosis. When mass effect and/or edema present they are usually less pronounced than what would be expected from a high-grade glioma of similar size, although occasionally marked mass effect can be seen. Diffusion-weighted imaging (DWI) signal is also variable across the lesions, with central parts showing increased diffusivity and peripheral potions showing relative restricted diffusion (Fig. 18.1).

Perfusion studies may be helpful when they show diminished relative cerebral blood volume (rCBV), but significant overlap exists between rCBV values of high-grade tumors and TDLs [5]. MR spectroscopy is helpful in differential diagnosis and shows glutamate/glutamine peaks on short TE exams [1,2].

## Importance

Numerous reports describe TDLs undergoing biposy, surgical resection, and even radio- and chemotherapy because they were mistaken for brain tumors. Recognition of this entity can prevent unnecessary and potentially dangerous work-up and provide timely and proper treatment.

## Typical clinical scenario

Patients usually present with focal neurologic deficits and lack a history of prior similar episodes. TDL can occur in the very young and the elderly, but is most commonly seen in middle-aged women.

## Differential diagnosis

High-grade gliomas and lymphoma are considered in the differential diagnosis. Both of these entities can closely mimic TDL but usually show more mass effect and edema. Post-contrast enhancement is also more pronounced with gliomas and lymphoma. Incomplete ring enhancement of TDL is very characteristic. Both high-grade gliomas and TDL have similar DWI characteristics with enhancing parts of the lesions showing restricted diffusion. Perfusion-weighted imaging (PWI) features of these entities also show great overlap. On MR spectroscopy, presence of glutamate/glutamine favors TDL over glioma and lymphoma. Interestingly, unenhanced CT may be helpful in differential diagnosis: the enhancing parts of TDL are usually hypodense, in contrast to gliomas, which usually show relative hyperdensity in the enhancing parts.

> ## Teaching points
>
> TDL can present in any age group and mimic neoplasms. Incomplete ring of enhancement and relative lack of mass effect and edema around the lesion are characteristic features of TDL.

REFERENCES

1. Cianfoni A, Niku S, Imbesi SG. Metabolite findings in tumefactive demyelinating lesions utilizing short echo time proton magnetic resonance spectroscopy. *AJNR Am J Neuroradiol* 2007; **28**: 272–7.
2. Saini J, Chatterjee S, Thomas B, Kesavadas C. Conventional and advanced magnetic resonance imaging in tumefactive demyelination. *Acta Radiol.* 2011; **52**: 1159–68.
3. Kiriyama T, Kataoka H, Taoka T, *et al.* Characteristic neuroimaging in patients with tumefactive demyelinating lesions exceeding 30 mm. *J Neuroimaging* 2011; **21**: e69–77.
4. Kim DS, Na DG, Kim KH, *et al.* Distinguishing tumefactive demyelinating lesions from glioma or central nervous system lymphoma: added value of unenhanced CT compared with conventional contrast-enhanced MR imaging. *Radiology* 2009; **251**: 467–75.
5. Blasel S, Pfeilschifter W, Jansen V, *et al.* Metabolism and regional cerebral blood volume in autoimmune inflammatory demyelinating lesions mimicking malignant gliomas. *J Neurol.* 2011; **258**: 113–22.

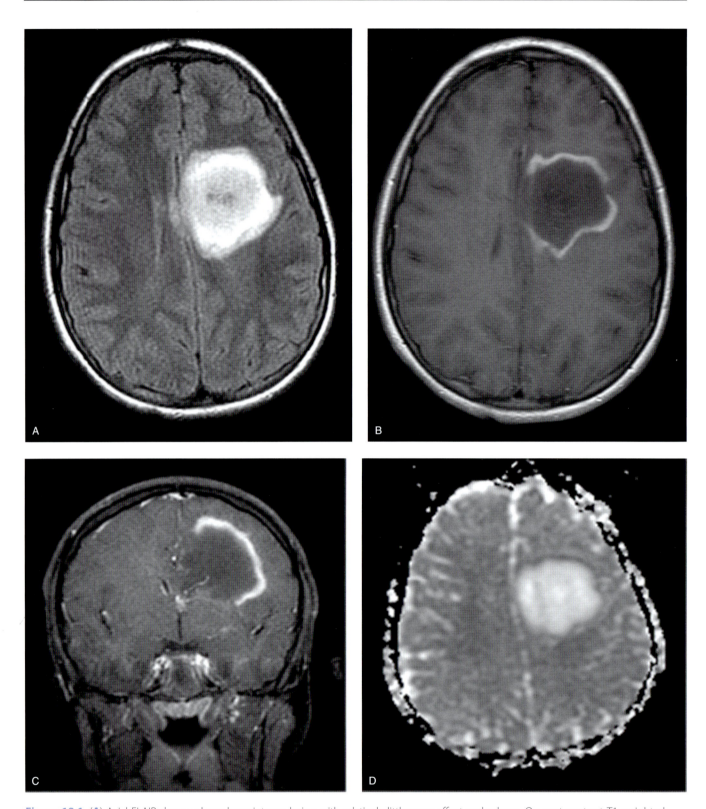

**Figure 18.1** (**A**) Axial FLAIR shows a large hyperintense lesion with relatively little mass effect and edema. On post-contrast T1-weighted (**B**) axial and (**C**) coronal images there is an "open ring" enhancement with the non-enhancing part facing the ventricle. (**D**) Apparent diffusion coefficient (ADC) map shows only minimal restriction of diffusion in the enhancing part of the lesion.

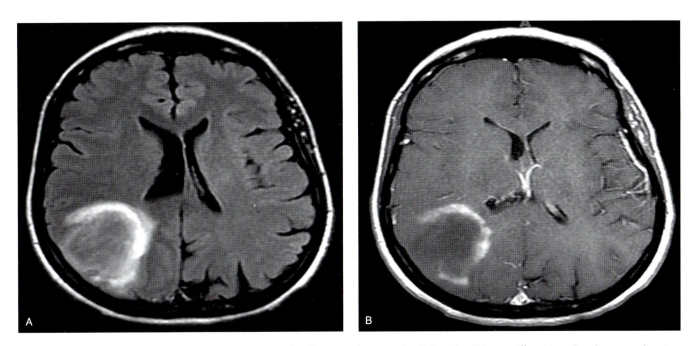

**Figure 18.2** (**A**) Axial FLAIR and (**B**) post-contrast T1-weighted images show another TDL with mild mass effect. Note that the non-enhancing part of the lesion faces the subcortical region in this patient.

# Acute disseminated encephalomyelitis

## Imaging description

Acute disseminated encephalomyelitis (ADEM) is an immune-mediated disorder of the CNS characterized by an inflammatory reaction and demyelination that predominantly involves the white matter of the brain and spinal cord [1]. ADEM is usually precipitated by a viral infection or vaccination. There is no specific biologic marker for ADEM; therefore the diagnosis is based on clinical and imaging features.

On MRI, ADEM lesions appear hyperintense on T2-weighted and FLAIR, and hypo- to isointense on T1-weighted imaging. Diffusion-weighted imaging (DWI) signal is variable, as is enhancement on post-contrast images, depending on the stage and degree of inflammation. The most common MRI pattern consists of multiple, 1–2 cm, bilateral and asymmetric lesions scattered throughout the cerebral hemispheres, cerebellum, brainstem, and occasionally the spinal cord (Fig. 19.1) [2]. The cortex is spared in the majority of cases but the deep gray matter nuclei are frequently involved (Fig. 19.2).

Sometimes ADEM presents with "tumefactive" lesion(s) that show(s) perilesional edema. Solitary lesions are uncommon but they require differentiation from primary tumors and infarcts (Fig. 19.3). Acute hemorrhagic ADEM is uncommon and presents with multiple hemorrhagic lesions. Sequential MRIs are important in establishing the diagnosis of ADEM; in most cases lesions show partial and complete resolution within a few months. ADEM is not expected to develop new lesions within the short-term follow-up period, although recurrent forms of ADEM have been described.

## Importance

The diagnosis of ADEM is never certain initially, and imaging plays a significant role in excluding mimickers. ADEM is monophasic in most cases and has a good outcome, although significant neurologic sequelae may remain in a minority of patients. Lethal forms of ADEM exist.

## Typical clinical scenario

The typical presenting features include an acute encephalopathy with multifocal neurologic signs and deficits with a history of a viral infection or vaccination in the previous 1–2 weeks. the majority of the patients are children.

## Differential diagnosis

In its most common form (i.e., multiple lesions scattered throughout) ADEM resembles multiple sclerosis. Neither clinically nor radiologically is there a definitive way of differentiating the two, although the following imaging features favor ADEM when present: (a) relative lack of corpus callosum involvement (MS frequently involves CC); (b) cortical involvement (MS spares the cortex); (c) many enhancing lesions (only a small portion of all lesions enhance in MS). Tumefactive ADEM lesions may mimic primary low-grade brain tumors. The presence of additional lesions strongly favors ADEM, as low-grade brain tumors are often unifocal. Lesional MR spectroscopy is not very helpful in differentiating tumor from ADEM, although MR spectroscopy may show extralesional metabolic derangement in visually normal-appearing white matter, which favors ADEM. Because ADEM lesions can have significantly restricted diffusion on DWI, acute infarct may be considered in the differential diagnosis (Fig. 19.4). If the lesion or lesions conform to a vascular territory MRI distinction may not be possible, although ischemic stroke is rare in pediatric populations.

> ## Teaching points
>
> ADEM usually afflicts children, and presents with variable imaging patterns that may mimic brain tumors and infarct.

REFERENCES

1. Tenembaum S, Chitnis T, Ness J, *et al.* Acute disseminated encephalomyelitis. *Neurology* 2007; **68** (16 Suppl 2): S23–36.
2. Rossi A. Imaging of acute disseminated encephalomyelitis. *Neuroimaging Clin N Am* 2008; **18**: 149–61; ix.

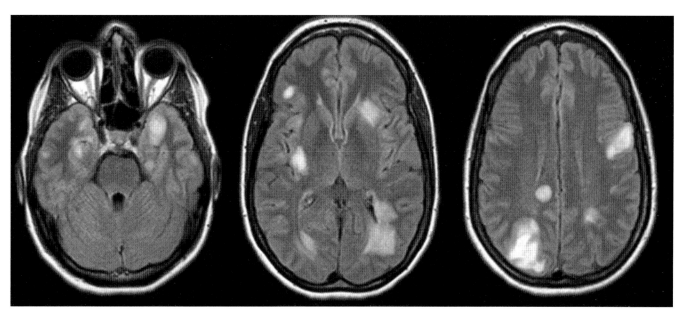

**Figure 19.1** Multiple FLAIR hyperintense lesions scattered throughout the subcortical white matter with some lesions involving the cortex as well. Infratentorial lesions were also present. Some of the lesions showed mild patch enhancement on post-contrast images (not shown).

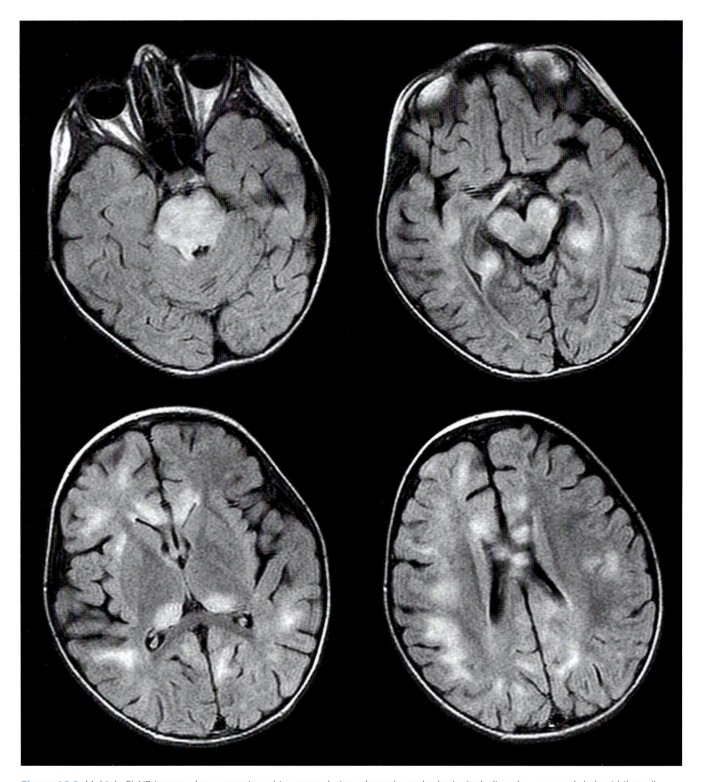

**Figure 19.2** Multiple FLAIR images show extensive white matter lesions throughout the brain, including the pons and thalami bilaterally.

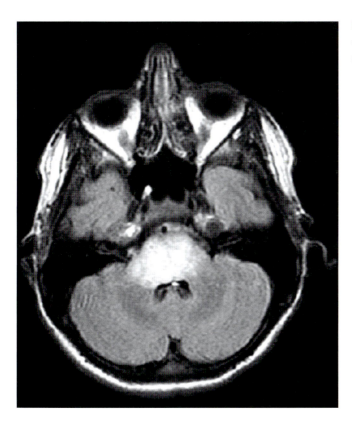

**Figure 19.3** Solitary pontine lesion on FLAIR image. No significant enhancement was present on post-contrast images. Follow-up showed complete resolution of this lesion with complete clinical recovery.

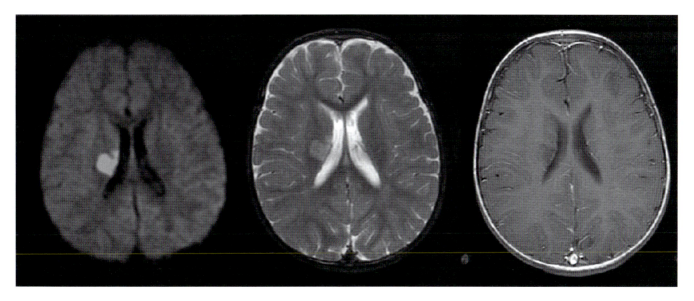

**Figure 19.4** A 2-year-old presented with acute onset of arm weakness and was thought to have acute infarct, given the location of the lesion and markedly restricted diffusion. No vascular lesion was found; clinical work-up including CSF analysis favored an inflammatory process. The patient completely recovered clinically and radiologically and received a diagnosis of ADEM.

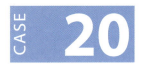

# Progressive multifocal leukoencephalopathy

## Imaging description

Progressive multifocal leukoencephalopathy (PML) is a demyelinating disorder of the brain caused by the JC virus (JCV). PML is most frequently seen in HIV/AIDS patients and patients with hematological malignancies [1]. On MRI, characteristic features of PML include unifocal or multifocal areas of hyperintensity on T2-weighted/FLAIR images, and corresponding areas of hypointensity on T1-weighted images with no associated mass effect or enhancement on post-contrast T1-weighted images [2]. Lesions can be patchy or confluent and involve the subcortical white matter including the U-fibers and the cerebellum (Fig. 20.1). The middle cerebellar peduncle is a common site of involvement (Fig. 20.2).

Diffusion-weighted imaging (DWI) may show variable signal; increased DWI signal corresponds to the sites of active infection [3]. Rarely, multiple sclerosis patients receiving natalizumab (a monoclonal antibody) may develop PML, which may show post-contrast enhancement. The diagnosis of PML is established by demonstrating the JCV DNA in CSF or brain biopsy.

## Importance

Many white matter lesions can be seen in immunocompromised patients, which require different diagnostic work-up and treatment. PML should be in the differential diagnosis of immunocompromised patients presenting with neurologic deficits. PML is lethal in about half of the cases, but recently the mortality rate has decreased due to the successful immune reconstitution treatments available (Fig. 20.3).

## Typical clinical scenario

PML develops in immunocompromised individuals, such as patients with HIV/AIDS or hematological malignancies, or patients receiving organ transplants. Recently, the monoclonal antibodies natalizumab, efalizumab, and rituximab, which are used for the treatment of multiple sclerosis, psoriasis, haematological malignancies, Crohn's disease, and rheumatic diseases, have been associated with PML. Patients present with various neurologic deficits depending on the site of demyelination.

## Differential diagnosis

Although various white matter lesions can occur in immunocompromised patients, including opportunistic infections and lymphoma, PML can be differentiated from these by its characteristic lack of mass effect, perilesional edema and post-contrast enhancement. HIV leukoencephalopathy can also present with similar white matter signal abnormalities but these tend to spare the subcortical U-fibers and have less pronounced signal change on T1-weighted images.

## Teaching points

In an immunocompromised patient with recent development of neurologic deficits and single or multiple subcortical white matter lesions without mass effect or enhancement, PML should be suspected.

REFERENCES

1. Brew BJ, Davies NW, Cinque P, Clifford DB, Nath A. Progressive multifocal leukoencephalopathy and other forms of JC virus disease. *Nat Rev Neurol* 2010; **6**: 667–79.

2. Tan CS, Koralnik IJ. Progressive multifocal leukoencephalopathy and other disorders caused by JC virus: clinical features and pathogenesis. *Lancet Neurol* 2010; **9**: 425–37.

3. Clifford DB, De Luca A, Simpson DM, *et al.* Natalizumab-associated progressive multifocal leukoencephalopathy in patients with multiple sclerosis: lessons from 28 cases. *Lancet Neurol* 2010; **9**: 438–46.

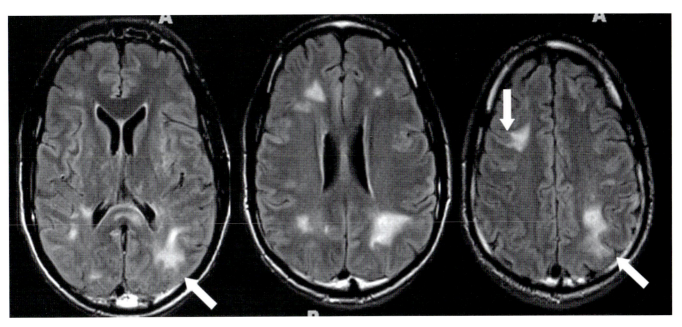

**Figure 20.1** Multiple patchy and confluent regions of FLAIR hyperintensity in the subcortical regions with involvement of the U-fibers (arrows). Note the absence of mass effect. No contrast enhancement was present. The patient had HIV/AIDS.

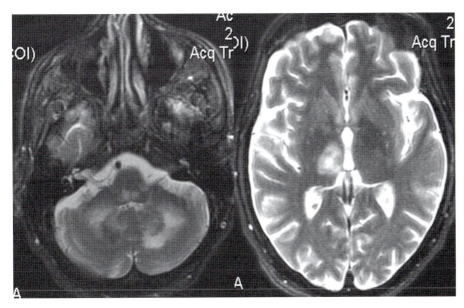

**Figure 20.2** In a patient with HIV/AIDS, axial T2-weighted images show bilateral confluent signal abnormalities in the middle cerebellar peduncles and posterior pons, as well as the right thalamus, compatible with PML. While the middle cerebellar peduncle is a common site of involvement with PML, the brainstem and deep gray matter involvement is unusual.

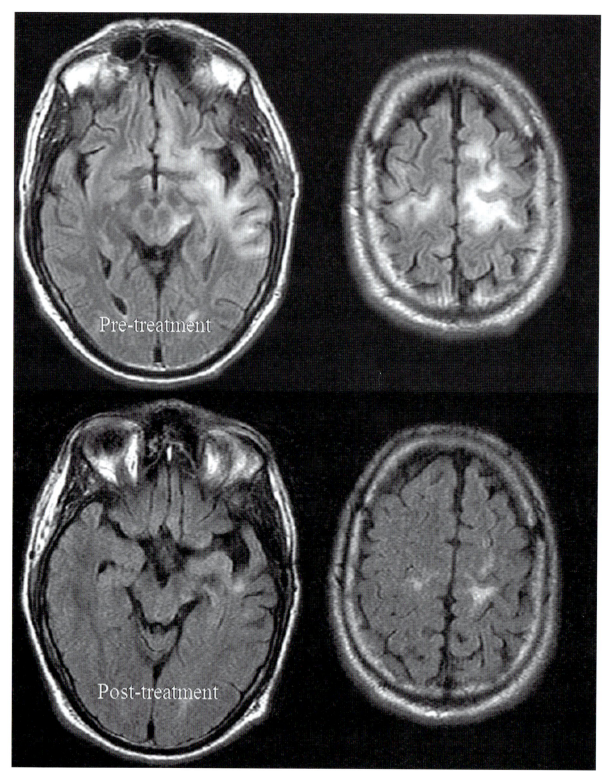

**Figure 20.3** FLAIR images of a patient with HIV/AIDS show typical findings of PML (upper row) which was confirmed with CSF polymerase chain reaction (PCR) analysis. Following highly active antiretroviral treatment (HAART) (lower row), lesions regressed.

# CASE 21

# Osmotic myelinolysis

## Imaging description

Osmotic myelinolysis (OM) is a distinctive clinical syndrome with classic symptoms of acute mental status change, pseudo-bulbar palsy, and spastic quadriparesis that can progress to coma and death if uncorrected. Previously known as central pontine myelinolysis (CPM) when described for the first time in 1959, it was thought to be a sequela of alcoholism or malnutrition. In the early 1980s, rapid correction of hyponatremia was established as the cause. The presumptive underlying pathophysiology is damage to the blood–brain barrier and changes in cellular volume as a response to rapid alteration in extracellular fluid osmolality, leading to loss of myelin sheath with relative sparing of axons and neurons and without inflammatory infiltrates [1]. It can also occur in the basal ganglia, thalami and supratentorial gray–white matter junction, whence the name extrapontine myelinolysis (EPM) [2,3].

CT scan may be nearly normal in the acute phase, with possible low attenuation seen in the subacute and chronic phases. On MRI, confluent hyperintense T2 and FLAIR signal can be seen (Fig. 21.1) spreading centrifugally from the median raphe, located in the dorsal basis pontis with relative sparing of tegmentum, corticospinal, and corticobulbar tracts, except in the most severe cases [2,4]. Contrast enhancement is occasionally seen in the subacute to late stages.

The most common extrapontine location is the basal ganglia, which are involved symmetrically (Fig. 21.2). Hyperintensity on diffusion-weighted images associated with a decrease in apparent diffusion coefficient (ADC) value in the acute phase has been reported [4]. However on recovery, ADC values normalize while diffusion-weighted images continue to show hyperintensity.

## Importance

The cause and pathogenesis of OM are not completely known. Some reports also indicate that many of the lesions are not demyelinating in the strictest sense. Frank necrosis with axonal lysis, especially in the central part of the lesions, is discovered by many investigators [2]. It is also reported in patients with chronic cirrhotic liver disease, those with orthotopic liver transplant, and those with surgical removal of pituitary gland [1,2]. With such a diverse clinical background, it is important to rule out other differential diagnostic conditions before committing to the diagnosis of OM.

## Typical clinical scenario

During initial hyponatremia, altered mental status and seizures are common. Hyponatremia may be associated with an alcoholic binge, excessive vomiting, burns, or hepatic and renal insufficiency, diabetes mellitus, and syndrome of inappropriate antidiuretic hormone secretion (SIADH). The symptoms may resolve initially with correction of sodium levels in serum. The syndrome of osmotic demyelination emerges a few days to weeks after the initial episode and presents with disorientation, altered consciousness, movement disorder of extra pyramidal type, dysarthria, pseudobulbar palsy, or dysphagia. The disorder may also be identified in children with mild malnutrition.

## Differential diagnosis

Ischemic infarction of the pons involves both the central and peripheral pontine fibers (Fig. 21.3). Perforating territory pontine infarcts tend to be unilateral, but when they are bilateral they may be difficult to distinguish from CPM, based only on imaging findings.

Areas of demyelination, as seen in multiple sclerosis or acute disseminated encephalomyelitis (ADEM), often involve pons and exhibit high T2 and FLAIR signal (Figs. 21.4, 21.5). However, it is rare to have diffusion restriction. Also look for areas of demyelination elsewhere in the brain.

Posterior reversible encephalopathy syndrome (PRES) may predominantly involve the pons, but often additional lesions are present in the cerebellar hemispheres and occipital subcortical regions.

## Teaching points

In the proper clinical setting, characteristic MRI findings of increased T2 signal in the central pons with sparing of the tegmentum posteriorly and corticospinal tracts anteriorly are diagnostic of OM. Extrapontine OM may be present with or without central pontine myelinolysis.

REFERENCES

1. King JD, Rosner MH. Osmotic demyelination syndrome. *Am J Med Sci* 2010; **339**: 561–7.
2. Chua GC, Sitoh YY, Lim CC, *et al.* MRI findings in osmotic myelinolysis. *Clin Radiol* 2002; **57**: 800–6.
3. Tatewaki Y, Kato K, Tanabe Y, Takahashi S. MRI findings of corticosubcortical lesions in osmotic myelinolysis: report of two cases. *Br J Radiol* 2012; **85**: e87–90.
4. Cramer SC, Stegbauer KC, Schneider A, *et al.* Decreased diffusion in central pontine myelinolysis. *AJNR Am J Neuroradiol* 2001; **22**: 1476–9.

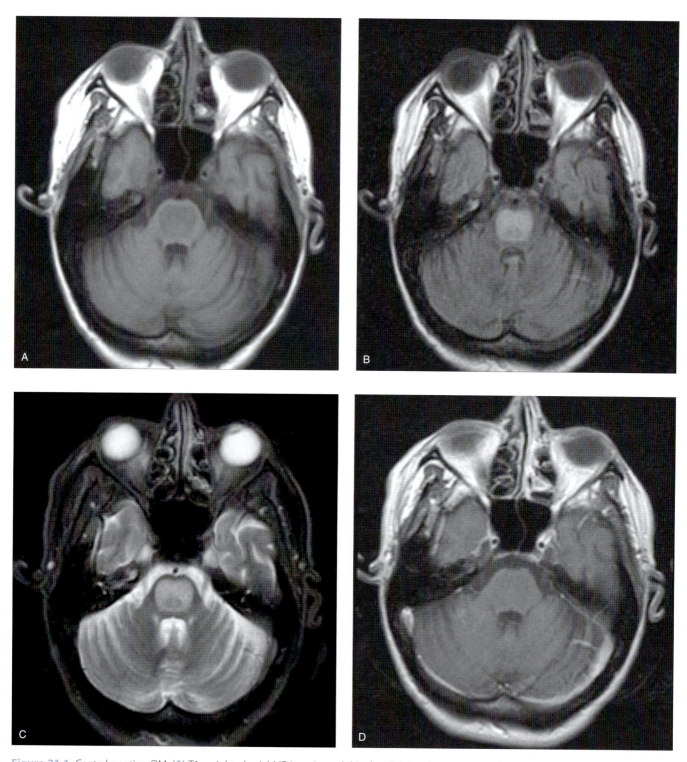

**Figure 21.1** Central pontine OM. (**A**) T1-weighted axial MR imaging exhibits low T1 signal area in central pons with mild loss of volume. Note mild prominence of cerebellar folia, which may be a sign of chronic alcoholism. (**B, C**) FLAIR and T2-weighted axial MR imaging exhibits high FLAIR and T2 signal in central pons, sparing the periphery. (**D**) Post-contrast T1-weighted axial MR imaging exhibits no significant post-contrast enhancement. (**E, F**) Areas of restricted diffusion are seen within the pons on DWI with increased ADC values.

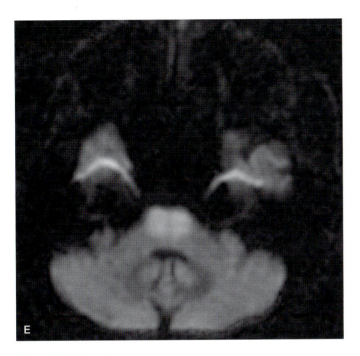

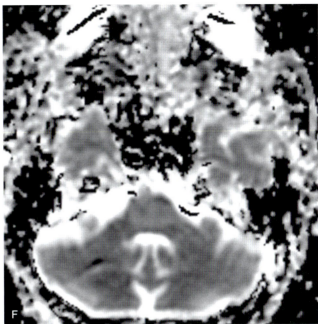

**Figure 21.1** (cont.)

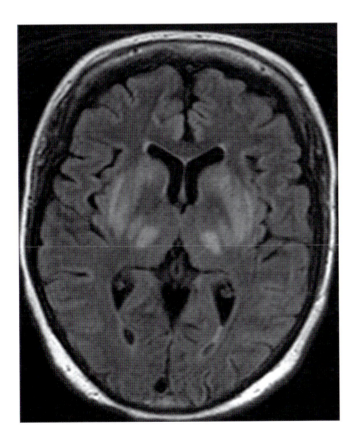

**Figure 21.2** Extrapontine OM. Axial FLAIR image shows bilateral and symmetric areas of increased signal in the corpus striatum, thalamus, and internal capsule secondary to OM.

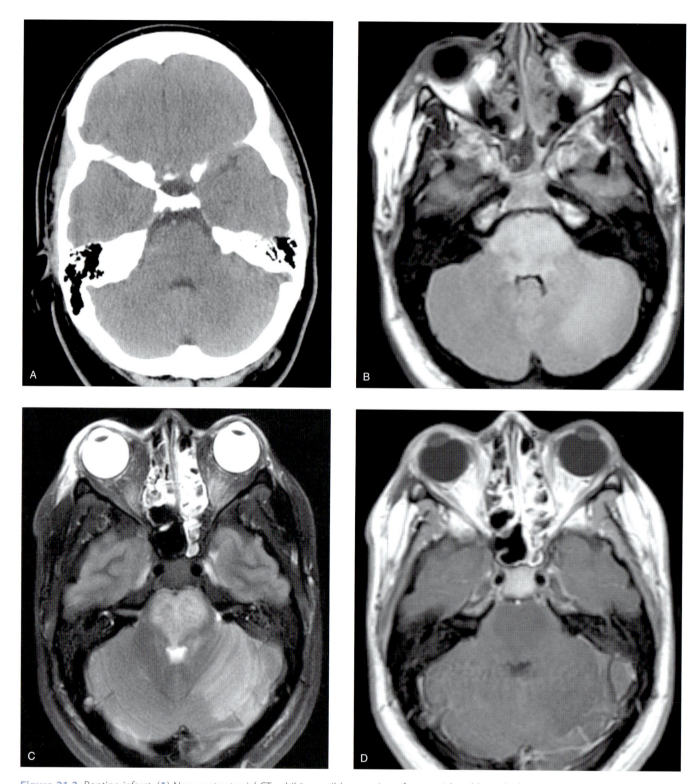

**Figure 21.3** Pontine infarct. (**A**) Non-contrast axial CT exhibits a mild expansion of pons with mild patchy low attenuation. (**B**, **C**) FLAIR and T2-weighted axial MR imaging exhibits diffuse high T2 and FLAIR signal in pons with mild expansion. Note patchy T2 signal hyperintensity involving left cerebellar hemisphere. Note involvement of the pons in a diffuse fashion. (**D**) Post-contrast T1-weighted axial MR imaging exhibits non-enhancing mildly decreased T1 signal lesion without significant abnormal post-contrast enhancement. (**E**, **F**) Areas of diffusion restriction are seen involving the pons as well as bilateral cerebellar hemispheres with corresponding diminished diffusion coefficient. (**G**) MRA of brain exhibits lack of signal at left vertebral artery with incomplete irregular filling of the basilar artery.

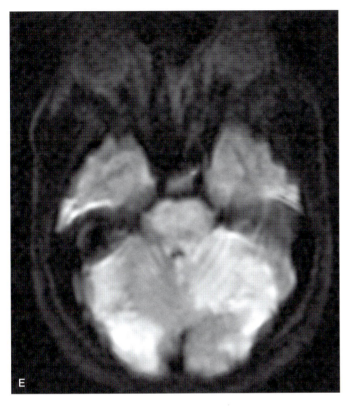

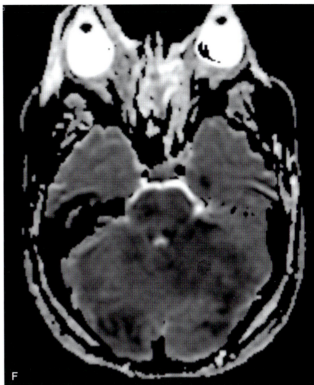

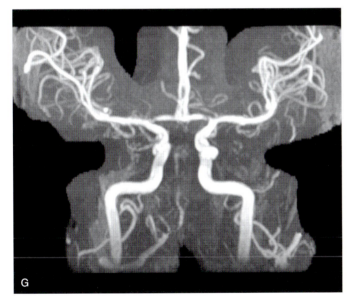

Figure 21.3 (cont.)

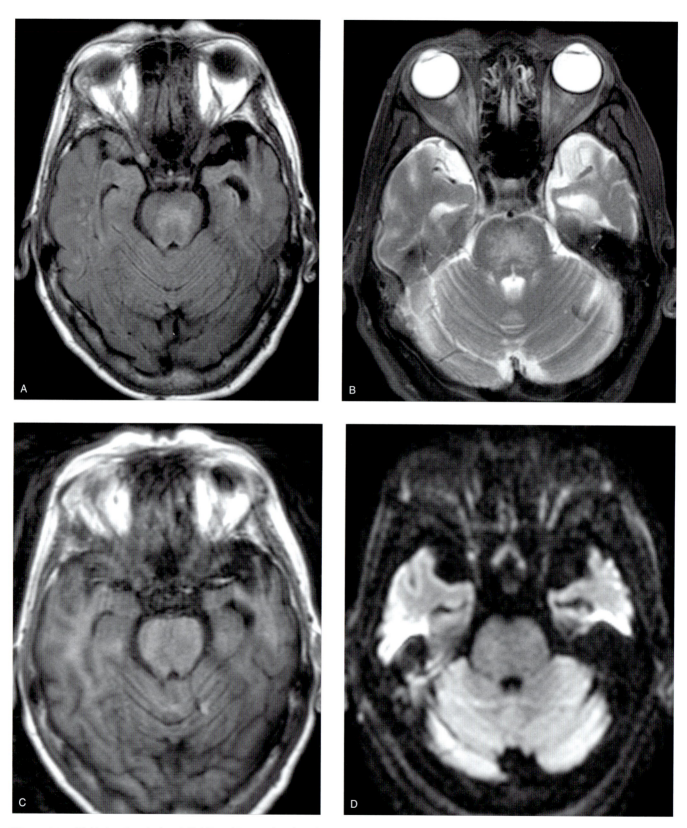

**Figure 21.4** Multiple sclerosis. (**A**, **B**) FLAIR and T2-weighted axial MR imaging exhibits patchy areas of high T2 and FLAIR signal involving the central pons. There were also demyelinating plaques in supratentorial white matter. (**C**) T1-weighted axial MR imaging exhibits isointense T1 signal of the pons. (**D**) No evidence for diffusion restriction is seen on DWI.

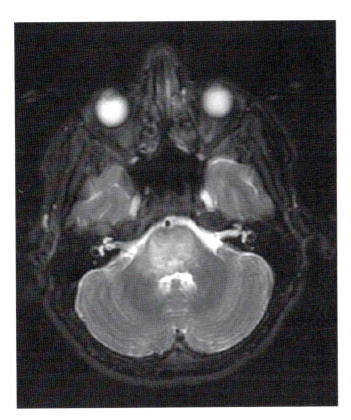

**Figure 21.5** ADEM. Axial T2-weighted image shows a diffusely hyperintense lesion in the pons which does not spare the periphery. The patient's symptoms and MRI findings resolved on follow-up.

## Imaging description

Evaluating a patient with multifocal neurologic symptoms is a diagnostic challenge for a neurologist [1]. Clinical symptomatology and imaging presentation of neurosarcoidosis is so diverse and varied, that it is one of the commonest differential diagnoses for a suitable case in board exams!

There is a wide spectrum of MR imaging findings in neurosarcoidosis. The spectrum of intracranial findings includes cranial nerve enhancement (Fig. 22.1), leptomeningeal enhancement (Fig. 22.2), and enhancing (Fig. 22.3) and non-enhancing parenchymal lesions [2]. Involvement of pituitary hypothalamic neuraxis (Fig. 22.4) is common, as is involvement of optic nerves (Fig. 22.4) [3]. Involvement of the brainstem (Fig. 22.5), the choroid plexus, and the ependymal lining of ventricular system (Fig. 22.5) can also be seen [4]. Involvement of the dura can lead to pachymeningeal thickening (Fig. 22.6) [5,6] and sometimes presence of dural-based extra-axial granulomatous mass that can mimic meningioma (Fig. 22.7). There can be intramedullary or extramedullary involvement of the spinal cord (Fig. 22.8) [7].

Gadolinium-enhanced MRI is the modality of choice for imaging diagnosis. FDG-PET can help the diagnoses of systemic sarcoidosis by showing increased metabolic activity in mediastinal adenopathy [8]. It is also proposed as a more sensitive early test for neurosarcoidosis [9].

## Importance

Sarcoidosis is a chronic inflammatory multisystem disorder of unknown etiology. No organ is immune to sarcoidosis, but in up to 90% of patients the lungs are involved [10]. Neurosarcoidosis is a serious and devastating complication of systemic sarcoidosis, occurring in 5–15% of the patients [4]. Isolated neurosarcoidosis without systemic involvement is thought to represent 15–17% of total cases of neurosarcoidosis [10]. The incidence of sarcoidosis in North America is estimated at 3–10 per 100 000 in the Caucasian population and 35–80 per 100 000 amongst African-Americans.

A typical presentation of pulmonary sarcoidosis is bilateral hilar lymphadenopathy and erythema nodosum. The disease typically affects adults between the age of 20 and 40 years [4]. Neurosarcoidosis can manifest as an acute-onset monophasic illness or as a slow, chronic illness. The pathological hallmark of sarcoidosis is non-caseating granuloma [1], which is a collection of activated macrophages and their derivative epithelioid and giant cells surrounded by mononuclear infiltrates [4]. The cranial nerves, hypothalamus, and pituitary gland are more commonly involved, but sarcoid granulomas can affect the meninges, the brain parenchyma, the brainstem, the choroid plexus, and the subependymal layer of the ventricular system or the peripheral nerves [4]. It can also mimic idiopathic hypertrophic pachymeningitis [5,6].

Patients with known systemic sarcoidosis who are neurologically symptomatic and have a documented imaging diagnosis receive treatment for a trial period with close monitoring, if infectious and neoplastic disorders have been excluded [1]. Corticosteroids offer first-line treatment for sarcoidosis; however, for long-term treatment, steroid-sparing immunosuppressive agents are utilized.

## Typical clinical scenario

The presenting neurologic symptoms depend upon the location of the granuloma in neuraxis. Cranial nerve palsies are the most frequent presentation, found in 50–75% of symptomatic patients [1]. Cranial nerve VII and the optic nerve are the cranial nerves most affected in neurosarcoidosis. Headaches, visual impairment, and seizures are present in about 25–30% of patients [2]. Inflammation and granuloma formation in the leptomeninges is seen in about 10–20% of patients with neurosarcoidosis [1]. Diplopia, paresthesias, memory impairment, and hypopituitarism are seen in 10–15% of patients. Other presenting symptoms include hearing impairment, dysphagia, muscle weakness, psychosis, and movement disorders. A third of patients with neurosarcoidosis have multiple neurological lesions [4].

## Differential diagnosis

The commonest manifestations of neurosarcoidosis, cranial nerve enhancement (Fig. 22.1) or leptomeningeal enhancement (Fig. 22.2), can also be seen in cases of infectious meningitis or meningeal carcinomatosis. However, CSF analysis can show the presence of infection or infective agent in the case of meningitis, and malignant cells in the case of meningeal carcinomatosis. Enhancement of the pituitary stalk (Fig. 22.4) can mimic infundibular histiocytosis; however, the age of onset in this condition is younger, 6–14 years. Parenchymal neurosarcoidosis (Fig. 22.3) can mimic intracranial metastatic secondary deposits. However, in that case, there may not be presence of mediastinal lymphadenopathy and the laboratory findings would be different. FLAIR changes in cases of parenchymal neurosarcoidosis (Fig. 22.6) can mimic periventricular white matter disease; however, the symptomatology and laboratory results would be different. Pachymeningeal thickening in neurosarcoidosis (Fig. 22.6) can mimic idiopathic hypertrophic pachymeningitis; however, dural biopsy would have different findings. A dural-based extra-axial granuloma (Fig. 22.7) can mimic a dural-based benign mass such as meningioma; however, in that case there would not be any parenchymal or leptomeningeal imaging findings. Finally, lymphoma involvement of the CNS can have very similar appearance to essentially all forms of sarcoidosis involvement.

## Teaching points

Neurologic manifestations are frequently the presenting symptoms of systemic sarcoidosis. MR imaging is used for both diagnosis and follow-up to assess the response to immunosuppressive therapy or in surveillance for new lesions. Correlating MRI findings with a chest x-ray can be beneficial. Non-enhancing white matter lesions, cranial nerve enhancement, and pachymeningeal involvement can be clinically silent in neurosarcoidosis and vice versa. However, follow-up imaging studies with improvement or worsening of imaging abnormalities show excellent correlation with clinical improvement or worsening on immunosuppressive therapy.

REFERENCES

1. Vargas DL, Stern BJ. Neurosarcoidosis: diagnosis and management. *Semin Respir Crit Care Med* 2010; **31**: 419–27.

2. Shah R, Roberson GH, Curé JK. Correlation of MR Imaging Findings and Clinical Manifestations in Neurosarcoidosis. *AJNR Am J Neuroradiol* 2009; **30**: 953–61.

3. Langrand C, Bihan H, Raverot G, *et al.* Hypothalamo-pituitary sarcoidosis: a multicenter study of 24 patients. *QJM* 2012; **105**: 981–95.

4. Hoitsma E, Faber CG, Drent M, Sharma OP. Neurosarcoidosis: a clinical dilemma. *Lancet Neurology* 2004; **3**: 397–407.

5. Kupersmith MJ, Martin V, Heller G, Shah A, *et al.* Idiopathic hypertrophic pachymeningitis. *Neurology* 2004; **62**: 686–94.

6. Rossi S, Giannini F, Cerase A, *et al.* Uncommon findings in idiopathic hypertrophic cranial pachymeningitis. *J Neurol* 2004; **251**: 548–55.

7. Alraies MC, Desai R, Alraiyes AH. Unusual presentation of sarcoidosis: involving testis, spinal cord and the brain. *QJM* 2013; **106**: 781–2.

8. Mañá J, Gámez C. Molecular imaging in sarcoidosis. *Curr Opin Pulm Med* 2011; **17**: 325–31.

9. Huang JF, Aksamit AJ, Staff NP. MRI and PET imaging discordance in neurosarcoidosis. *Neurology* 2012; **79**: 1070.

10. Pawate S, Moses H, Sriram S. Presentations and outcomes of neurosarcoidosis: a study of 54 cases. *QJM* 2009; **102**: 449–60.

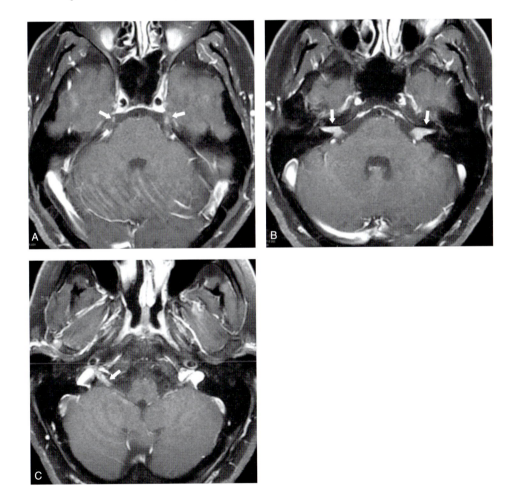

**Figure 22.1** Multiple enhancing cranial nerves in a 42-year-old male with recent-onset trigeminal neuralgia, ataxia, hearing loss, and dysphagia. (**A**) Post-contrast T1-weighted axial MR imaging exhibits patchy post-contrast enhancement of the cisternal portion of bilateral cranial nerve V (arrows). (**B**) Post-contrast T1-weighted axial MR image also exhibits mass-like thickening and enhancement of intracanalicular portion of bilateral cranial nerves VII and VIII (arrows). (**C**) At a lower level, enhancement of right-sided cranial nerves IX–XI is also seen (arrow).

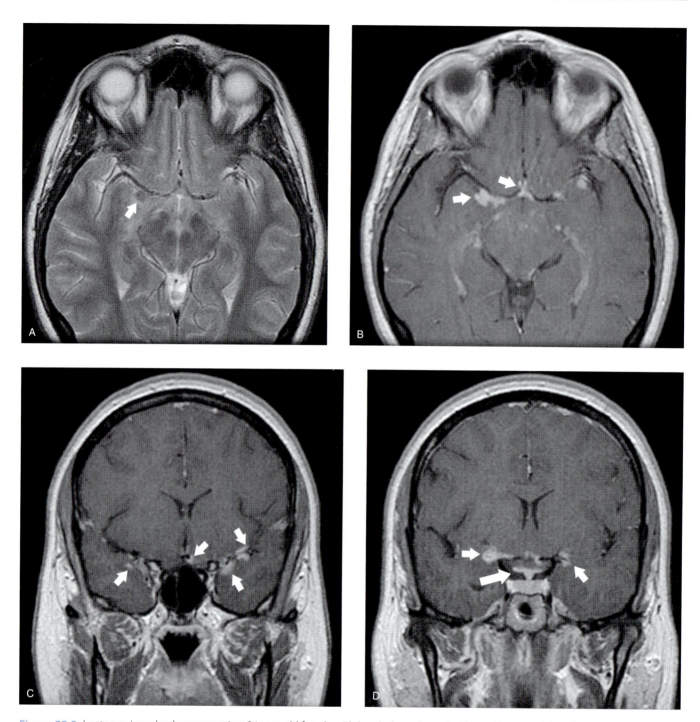

**Figure 22.2** Leptomeningeal enhancement in a 34-year-old female with headaches, photophobia, and hormonal disturbance. (**A**) T2-weighted axial MR image exhibits a low T2 signal nodularity along the posterior margin of M1 segment of right MCA (short arrow). (**B**) Post-contrast T1-weighted axial MR image exhibits patchy and nodular enhancement along the bilateral ACA and right MCA (short arrows). Similar nodular enhancement is also seen at the anterior margin of the superior portion of bilateral cerebral peduncles. (**C**) Post-contrast T1-weighted coronal MR image exhibits patchy leptomeningeal enhancement along the basal cistern and also along the Sylvian cistern (short arrows). (**D**) Post-contrast T1-weighted coronal MR image exhibits patchy and nodular enhancement along the basal cisterns (short arrows), along the inferior surface of the optic chiasm (long arrow), and also extending onto the pituitary stalk.

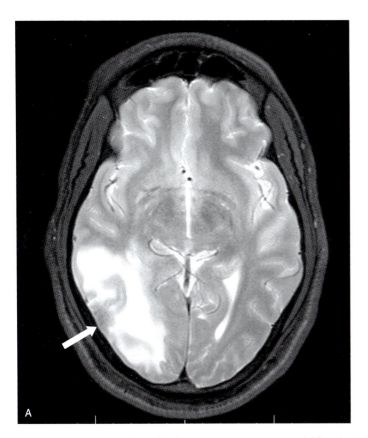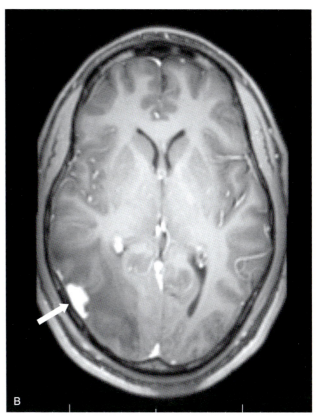

**Figure 22.3** Intraparenchymal enhancing mass in a 22-year-old female with headaches, vomiting, and visual disturbances. (**A**) T2-weighted axial MR image exhibits a low T2 signal nodular mass (arrow) along the superficial surface of the right occipital lobe with a large amount of surrounding irregular high T2 signal vasogenic edema. (**B**) Post-contrast T1-weighted axial MR image exhibits intense enhancement of the nodular mass (arrow) with surrounding low T1 signal edema.

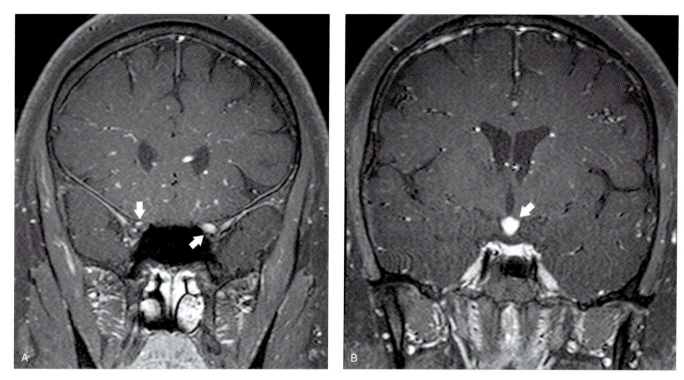

**Figure 22.4** Enhancement of bilateral optic nerves and pituitary stalk in a 38-year-old female with visual disturbance and hormonal disturbance. (**A**) Post-contrast fat-saturated T1-weighted coronal MR image shows patchy and nodular enhancement of bilateral optic nerves (short arrows) at the level of the orbital apex. Note the mild nodularity of leptomeningeal enhancement. (**B**) More posterior coronal section exhibits intense mass-like midline enhancement along the inferior hypothalamus and pituitary stalk (short arrow).

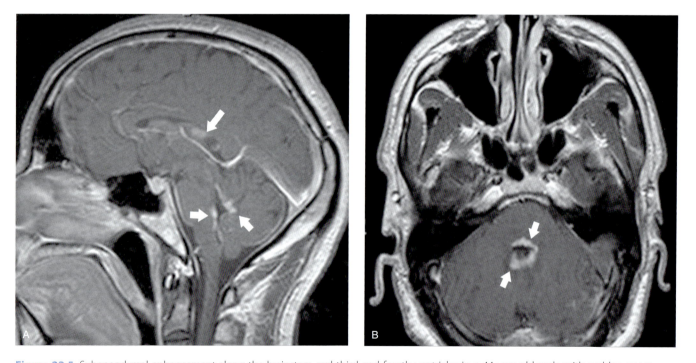

**Figure 22.5** Subependymal enhancement along the brainstem and third and fourth ventricles in a 44-year-old male with sudden-onset headaches, nausea, and ataxia. (**A**) Post-contrast T1-weighted sagittal MR image exhibits patchy and nodular post-contrast enhancement along the floor and roof of the fourth ventricle (short arrows) as well as within the third ventricle (long arrow). (**B**) Post-contrast T1-weighted axial MR imaging exhibits thick rind of enhancement along the subependymal region at the anterior and posterior margin of the fourth ventricle (short arrows).

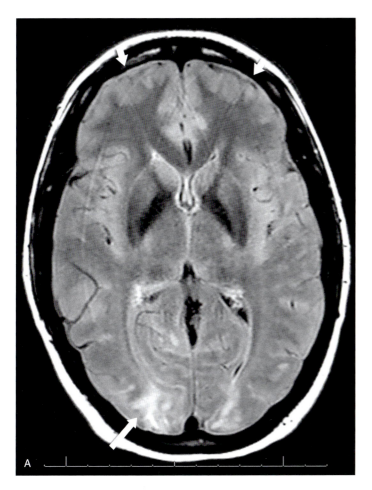

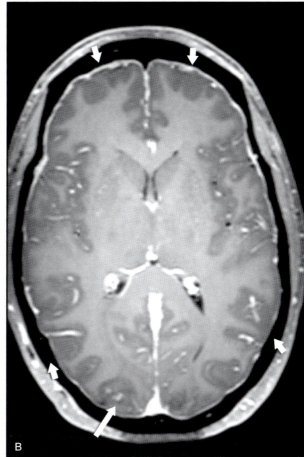

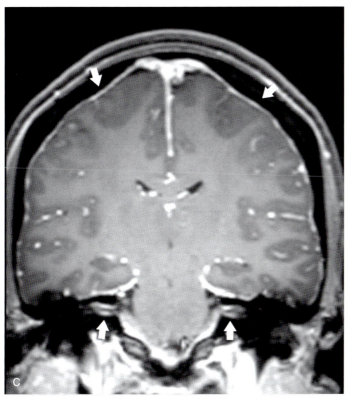

**Figure 22.6** Pachymeningeal thickening, parenchymal enhancement, and bilateral cranial nerve VII/VIII enhancement in a 32-year-old male with chronic headaches, visual disturbances, and hearing loss. (**A**) FLAIR-weighted axial MR image exhibits patchy intraparenchymal high FLAIR signal at the subcortical region of bilateral occipital lobes (long arrow) with mild thickening and high FLAIR signal of the dura (short arrows) that can mimic a tiny subdural collection. (**B**) Post-contrast T1-weighted axial MR image shows patchy post-contrast enhancement at the subcortical region of the right occipital lobe (long arrow) without any significant enhancement on the left side. There is pachymeningeal thickening and enhancement of the dural reflections (short arrows). (**C**) Post-contrast T1-weighted coronal MR image exhibits pachymeningeal thickening and enhancement at bilateral high convexity (arrows) and basilar part of the middle cranial fossa, which extends along the intracanalicular portion of bilateral cranial nerves VII and VIII (arrows).

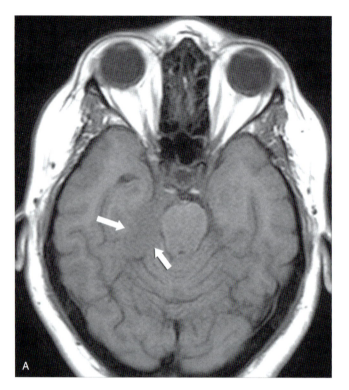

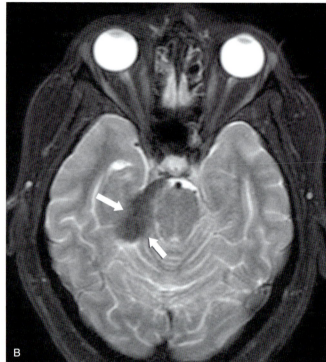

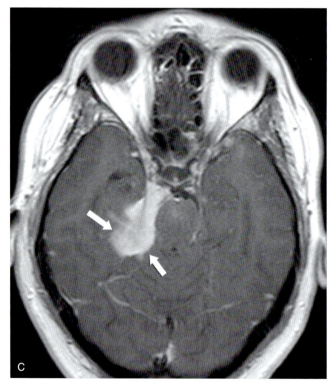

**Figure 22.7** Extra-axial dural-based enhancing mass in a 46-year-old male with headaches and right-sided hearing loss. (**A**) T1-weighted axial MR image exhibits a mass-like lesion that is isointense to brain parenchyma (arrows) at the right prepontine cistern and perimesencephalic cistern. (**B**) T2-weighted axial MR image shows the extra-axial mass having low T2 signal (arrows). (**C**) Post-contrast T1-weighted axial MR image shows intense enhancement of the extra-axial mass (arrows).

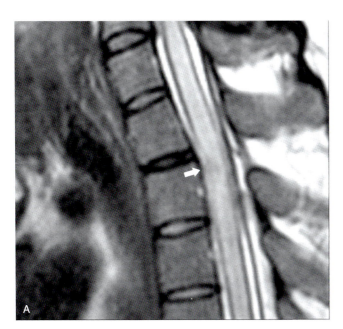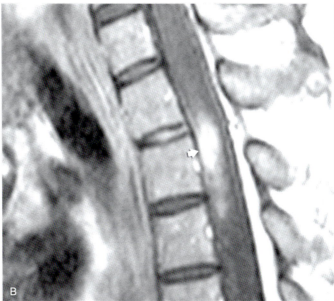

**Figure 22.8** Intramedullary enhancing lesion with edema of the thoracic cord in a 24-year-old female with bilateral lower-extremity weakness and paresthesias. (**A**) T2-weighted sagittal MR image of upper thoracic spine exhibits intramedullary high T2 signal and expansion of the spinal cord (arrow). (**B**) Post-contrast T1-weighted sagittal MR image shows patchy intramedullary enhancing lesion (arrow).

# Posterior fossa masses in children

## Imaging description

Posterior fossa tumors account for approximately 50% of pediatric brain tumors [1]. While supratentorial location predominates in infants, infratentorial tumors are more frequent in children older than 4 years of age [2]. Common pediatric posterior fossa tumors include juvenile pilocytic astrocytoma (JPA), ependymoma, medulloblastoma (MB), and brainstem gliomas; uncommon tumors include atypical teratoid rhabdoid tumor (ATRT), glioblastoma, hemangioblastoma, and gangliocytoma. Essentially all of these tumors with the exception of brainstem gliomas either arise from or secondarily involve the cerebellum.

MB is the most common childhood CNS tumor, accounting for 12–25% of all childhood CNS tumors (Fig. 23.1) [3]. MBs are associated with a rapid growth and early subarachnoid spread that may extend into the spinal canal. Different histologic subtypes exist; the great majority of MBs arise from midline inferior vermis and exhibit a classic histologic type, whereas desmoplastic MBs tend to occur off-midline and in older children. Children less than 3 years of age have an inferior survival rate [4]. Typical imaging features of MBs include hyperdensity on CT, decreased T2 signal and elevated DWI signal with accompanying decreased apparent diffusion coefficient (ADC) values. About half of MBs include cysts and non-enhancing regions.

Ependymomas arise from the roof or floor of the fourth ventricle (Fig. 23.2). They tend to grow in the ventricle and extend through the foramina of Luschka and Magendie, resulting in the classic "toothpaste" sign [2]. Ependymomas appear more heterogeneous and are more likely to exhibit areas of calcification and hemorrhage.

Pilocytic astrocytomas are benign tumors that typically consist of a large cyst and a small enhancing nodule, although variable imaging features include solid and heterogeneous tumors with necrosis and hemorrhage (Fig. 23.3).

## Importance

Regardless of the histologic type, hydrocephalus is frequently present and the reason for clinical presentation. Hydrocephalus may have to be addressed before definitive treatment of the posterior fossa tumor. Cerebellar masses are treated with surgical resection with adjuvant chemotherapy and radiation therapy depending on histology and completeness of resection [4,7]. Presence of CSF dissemination affects treatment decisions and should be routinely evaluated with whole spine imaging in MB before surgery. Ependymomas can also show CSF dissemination.

## Typical clinical scenario

Signs and symptoms of increased intracranial pressure, such as headaches and vomiting, are the most common presentation of these tumors as they cause obstructive hydrocephalus due to obstruction of the CSF pathway at the level of the fourth ventricle. In case of MB, destruction of cerebellar vermis may lead to truncal ataxia and nystagmus as presenting signs. It is more commonly seen in children <5 years of age with 2.5:1 male to female predominance. Ependymoma manifests in the age group of 1–5 years, presenting with headaches, vomiting, ataxia, visual disturbance, and torticollis. Pilocytic astrocytoma affects children from 5 to 15 years of age and is the most common primary brain tumor (supratentorial and infratentorial combined) in children. It presents with headache, nausea, vomiting, ataxia, and cerebellar signs.

## Differential diagnosis

Atypical teratoid rhabdoid tumor (ATRT) is rare and often indistinguishable from MB. When a pediatric posterior fossa mass looks like MB, and the age is less than 1–2 years, ATRT should be considered in the differential (Fig. 23.4). High-grade tumors (anaplastic astrocytoma and glioblastoma) are rare, and more commonly seen in older children (Fig. 23.5). They exhibit more heterogeneous signal intensity, prominent heterogeneous and ring-like enhancement with poorly defined margins, and multicentricity or extra-axial metastasis [2]. Choroid plexus papilloma of the fourth ventricle can mimic an intra-fourth-ventricular mass, like ependymoma; however, they exhibit a much more avid enhancement and often frond-like margins (Fig. 23.6). Hemangioblastoma is seen mostly in young adults and may be associated with von Hippel–Lindau syndrome (Fig. 23.7).

## Teaching points

The great majority of cerebellar masses in children represent MB, ependymoma, or JPA. MBs are hyperdense on CT and show decreased ADC values in their solid component on MRI. Ependymomas are soft tumors that spread through the outlets of the fourth ventricle and do not show decreased ADC. Most JPAs have a large cyst and a small nodule. Presurgical assessment of CSF dissemination is imperative in MBs and ependymomas.

REFERENCES

1. Rasalkar DD, Chu WC, Paunipagar BK, *et al*. Paediatric intra-axial posterior fossa tumours: pictorial review. *Postgrad Med J* 2013; **89**: 39–46.
2. Poretti A, Meoded A, Huisman TA. Neuroimaging of pediatric posterior fossa tumors including review of the literature. *J Magn Reson Imaging* 2012; **35**: 32–47.
3. Bartlett F, Kortmann R, Saran F. Medulloblastoma. *Clin Oncol (R Coll Radiol)* 2013; **25**: 36–45.

4. Sridhar K, Sridhar R, Venkatprasanna G. Management of posterior fossa gliomas in children. *J Pediatr Neurosci* 2011; **6** (Suppl 1): S72–7.

5. Steffen-Smith EA, Venzon DJ, Bent RS, *et al.* Single- and multivoxel proton spectroscopy in pediatric patients with diffuse intrinsic pontine glioma. *Int J Radiat Oncol Biol Phys* 2012: **84**: 774–9.

6. Hankinson TC, Campagna EJ, Foreman NK, *et al.* Interpretation of magnetic resonance images in diffuse intrinsic pontine glioma: a survey of pediatric neurosurgeons. *J Neurosurg Pediatr* 2011; **8**: 97–102.

7. Forbes JA, Reig AS, Smith JG, *et al.* Findings on preoperative brain MRI predict histopathology in children with cerebellar neoplasms. *Pediatr Neurosurg* 2011; **47**: 51–9.

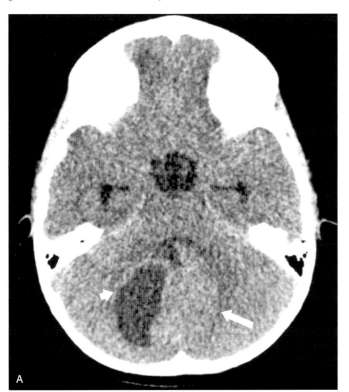

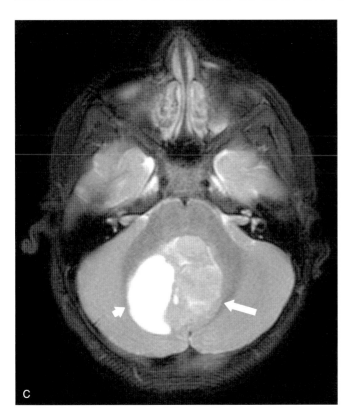

**Figure 23.1** Medulloblastoma. (**A**) Non-contrast axial CT scan exhibits a mildly hyperdense solid mass (arrow) within the fourth ventricle with an intramural cyst (short arrow) and resultant compression of fourth ventricle. (**B**) T1-weighted axial MR image exhibits a heterogeneously hypointense T1 signal mass (arrow) with adjacent intramural cyst (short arrow). (**C**) T2-weighted axial MR image shows a mass marginally hyperintense to gray matter (arrow) and a hyperintense T2 signal cyst (short arrow).

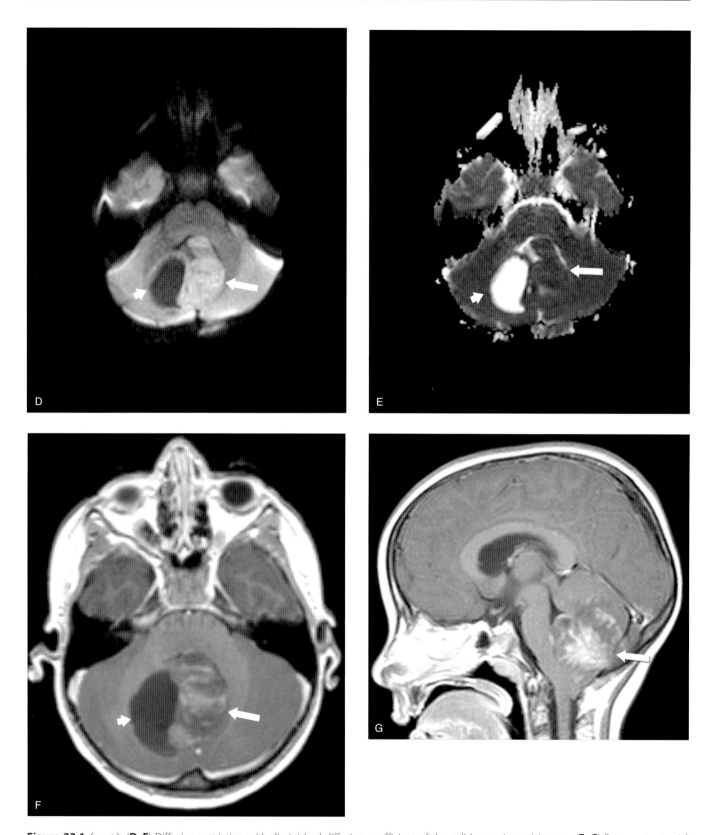

**Figure 23.1** (cont.) (**D**, **E**) Diffusion restriction with diminished diffusion coefficient of the solid mass (arrow) is seen. (**F**, **G**) Post-contrast axial and sagittal T1-weighted MR images exhibit a heterogeneous contrast enhancement of the solid midline cerebellar vermian mass (arrow) with a non-enhancing cyst (short arrow).

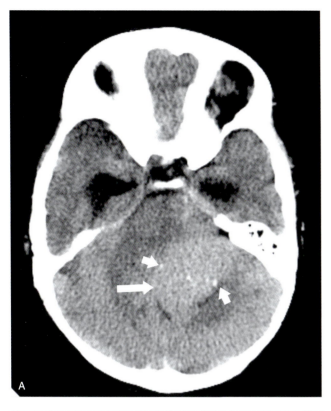

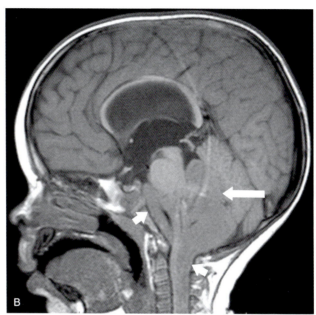

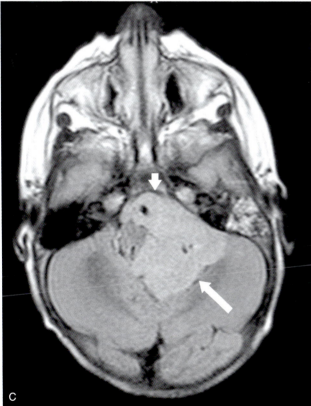

**Figure 23.2** Ependymoma. (**A**) Non-contrast axial CT exhibits hyperdense intra-fourth-ventricular mass (arrow) extending into left cerebellopontine angle (CPA) through left foramen of Luschka. Areas of punctate calcification (short arrows) are seen. There is dilatation of bilateral temporal horns due to obstructive hydrocephalus. (**B**) T1-weighted sagittal MR image exhibits large heterogeneous, iso- to hypointense T1 signal mass (arrow) within the fourth ventricle, extending into prepontine cistern and cisterna magna (short arrow). There is resultant marked hydrocephalus with dilatation of the aqueduct of Sylvius. (**C**) FLAIR-weighted axial MR image exhibits large high FLAIR signal mass (arrow) extending from the fourth ventricle into the left foramen of Luschka with a large exophytic component in left CPA and pontomedullary cistern (short arrow), enveloping the basilar artery. The sharp interface between CSF and the mass is seen on FLAIR-weighted imaging.

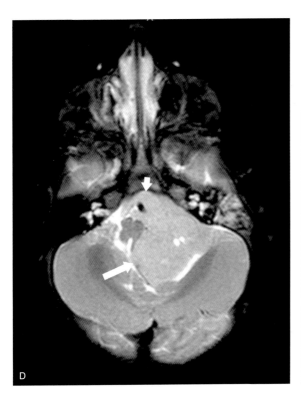

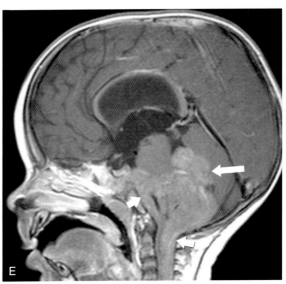

**Figure 23.2** (cont.) (**D**) T2-weighted axial MR image exhibits a heterogeneous, iso- to marginally hyperintense T2 signal mass (arrow) extending extra-axially (short arrow), with presence of small cystic foci. (**E**) Post-contrast T1-weighted sagittal MR image exhibits heterogeneous moderate enhancement of the large posterior fossa mass (arrow).

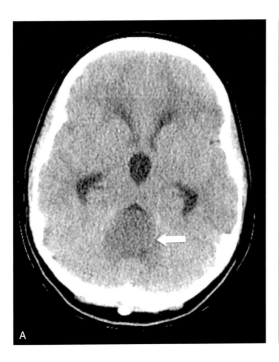

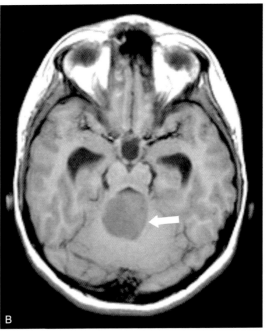

**Figure 23.3** Juvenile pilocytic astrocytoma. (**A**) Non-contrast axial CT exhibits a discrete hypodense mass (arrow) extending into the fourth ventricle with obstructive hydrocephalus. (**B**) T1-weighted axial MR image exhibits hypointense T1 signal mass (arrow) extending into the fourth ventricle with obstructive hydrocephalus. (**C**) FLAIR-weighted axial MR image exhibits hyperintense signal of the mass (arrow). (**D**) T2-weighted axial MR image exhibits hyperintense T2 signal of a relatively well-defined mass (arrow). (**E**) Post-contrast T1-weighted sagittal MR image exhibits an anteroinferior intensely enhancing solid portion (short arrow) of the mass (arrow).

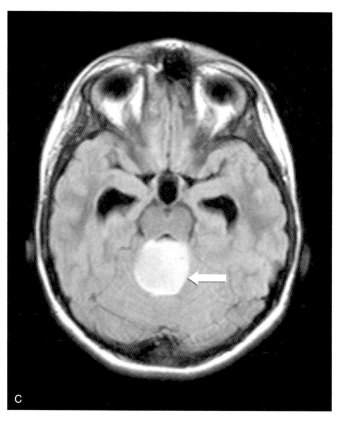

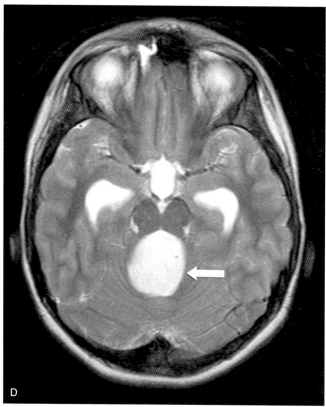

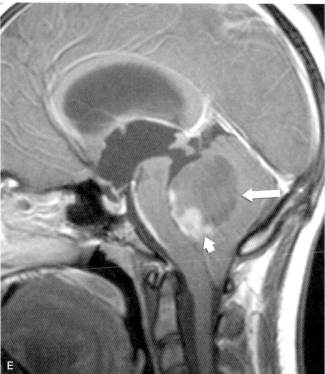

**Figure 23.3** (cont.)

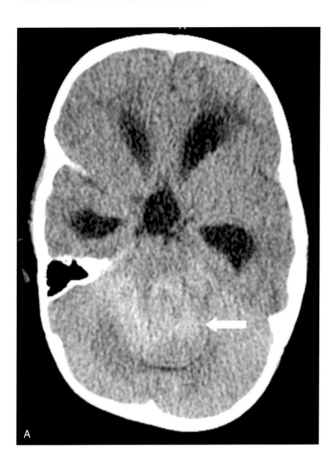 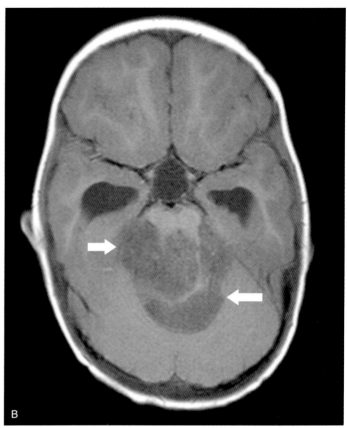

**Figure 23.4** ATRT. (**A**) Non-contrast axial CT exhibits irregular heterogeneous ring hyperdense vermian mass (arrow), extending into fourth ventricle with resultant obstructive hydrocephalus. (**B**) T1-weighted axial MR image exhibits large heterogeneously hypointense T1 signal mass (arrows). (**C**) T2-weighted axial MR image exhibits a heterogeneously hyperintense T2 signal mass (arrows) with resultant hydrocephalus. (**D**, **E**) Post-contrast T1-weighted axial and sagittal MR images exhibit large heterogeneously enhancing cerebellar vermian mass (arrow) compressing the fourth ventricle with resultant hydrocephalus.

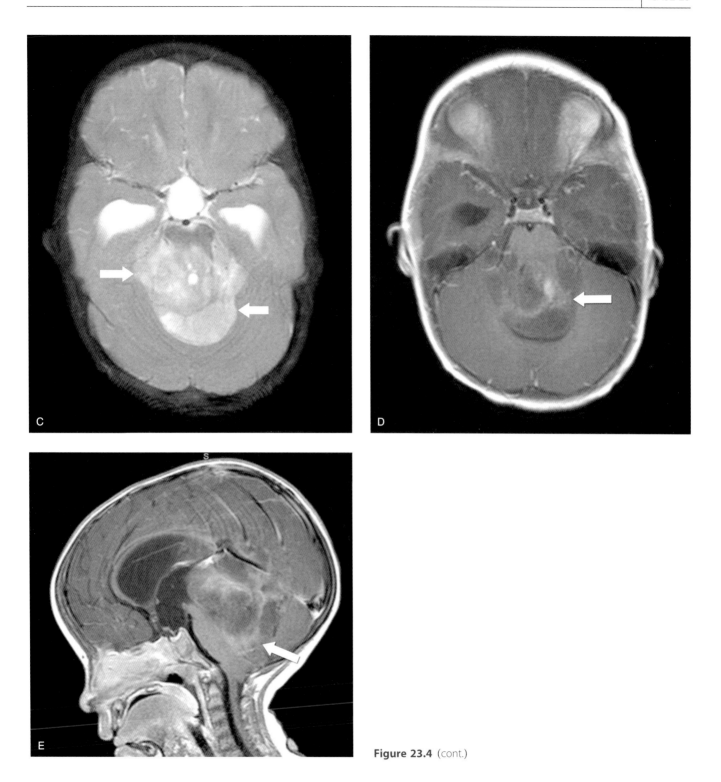

**Figure 23.4** (cont.)

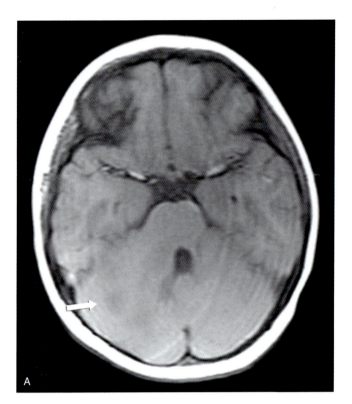

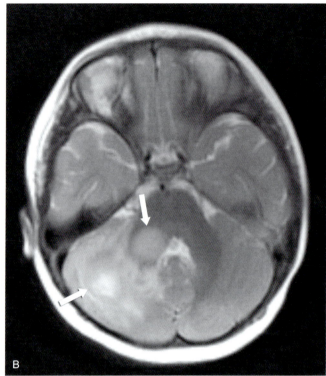

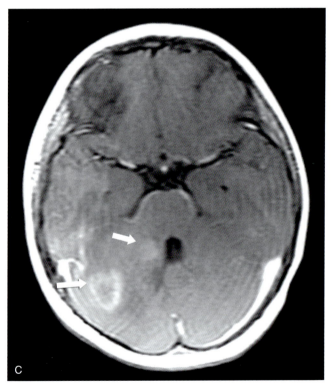

**Figure 23.5** Anaplastic astrocytoma of cerebellum and pons. (**A**) T1-weighted axial MR image exhibits an ill-defined heterogeneously hypointense T1 signal mass (arrow) at the right side of cerebellum and right brachium pontis. (**B**) T2-weighted axial MR image exhibits multicentricity of ill-defined heterogeneously high T2 signal mass (arrows). (**C**) Post-contrast T1-weighted axial MR image exhibits patchy and heterogeneous post-contrast enhancement (arrows).

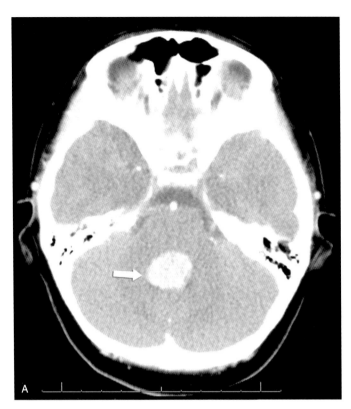
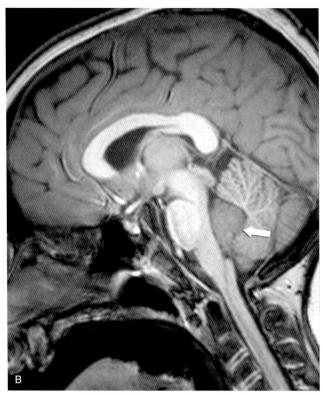

**Figure 23.6** Choroid plexus papilloma. (**A**) Post-contrast axial CT exhibits densely enhancing intra-fourth-ventricle mass (arrow). (**B**) T1-weighted sagittal MR image exhibits a well-defined lobulated hypointense T1 signal mass within the fourth ventricle (arrow). (**C**) FLAIR-weighted axial MR image exhibits rounded high FLAIR signal mass within the fourth ventricle with crenated margins (arrow) and presence of flow voids. (**D**) T2-weighted axial MR image exhibits mildly hyperintense T2 signal mass (arrow) within the fourth ventricle with central flow voids. (**E**) Post-contrast T1-weighted axial MR image exhibits intense post-contrast enhancement of the mass (arrow).

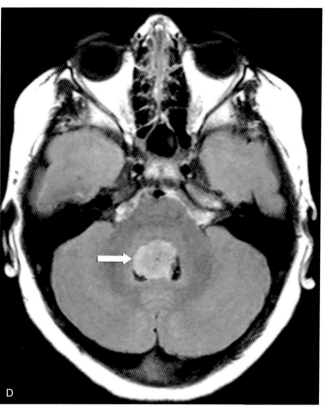

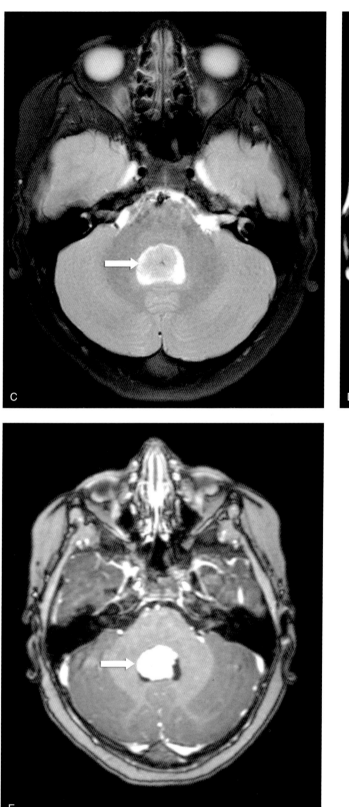

Figure 23.6 (cont.)

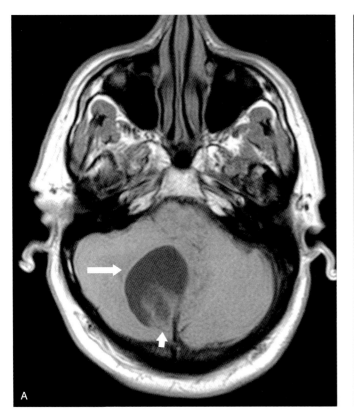

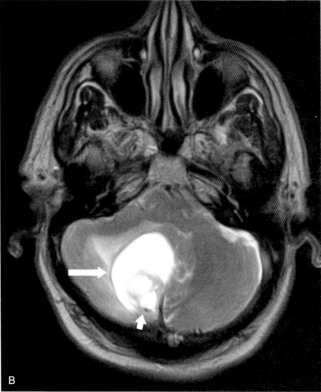

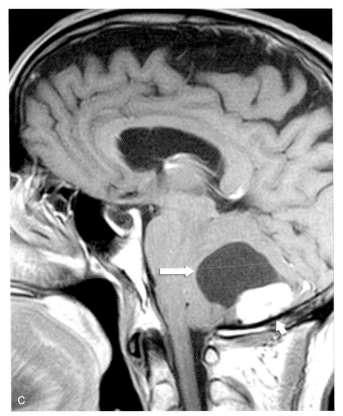

**Figure 23.7** Hemangioblastoma. (**A**) T1-weighted axial MR image exhibits a large cyst (arrow) within the right cerebellar hemisphere with a mural nodule (short arrow). (**B**) T2-weighted axial MR image exhibits hyperintense T2 signal right cerebellar cyst (arrow) with surrounding edema and a mural nodule (short arrow). (**C**) Post-contrast T1-weighted sagittal MR image exhibits a large cerebellar cyst (arrow) with intensely enhancing mural nodule (short arrow).

# 24 Low-grade glioma

## Imaging description

An expansile hyperintense T2 signal mass with symptoms of increased intracranial pressure and sometimes seizures is an imaging conundrum. It may represent a relatively low-grade glioma, or it may represent higher-grade neoplasms. Gliomas are classified into WHO grades I–IV according to histologic criteria. Low-grade gliomas (LGGs) affect both children and adults. The predominant histologic type of glioma found in children is a grade I tumor, juvenile pilocytic astrocytoma (JPA) (Fig. 24.1), which is often curable if completely resectable. However, LGGs in adults, known as WHO grade II gliomas, are infiltrative and may not be completely resected surgically [1].

The LGG accounts for about 20–30% of all gliomas in adults [2]. An LGG is a slow-growing, diffusely infiltrating astrocytic or oligodendrocytic neoplasm with a high degree of cellular differentiation. The recent discovery of isocitrate dehydrogenase 1 and 2 (IDH1 and IDH2) mutations in glioma has provided reproducible prognostic biomarkers and novel therapeutic targets [3]. More than 60% are associated with p53 mutation; they are also associated with a few chromosomal abnormalities. About two-thirds are supratentorial, predominantly involving the frontal and temporal lobes. About half of the infratentorial brainstem gliomas are low-grade astrocytomas. On non-contrast CT, they appear as ill-defined isodense to hypodense masses without significant enhancement (Fig. 24.2). About 20% exhibit areas of calcification, with rare cyst formation. On MRI, they appear as homogeneous hypointense T1 signal, predominantly white matter mass, which can be expansile and may appear well circumscribed (Fig. 24.3) but infiltrates the surrounding brain parenchyma. Hemorrhage and surrounding edema are rarely seen [4]. On FLAIR-weighted imaging, a homogeneous hyperintense mass is seen and no significant post-contrast enhancement is seen.

However, it is sometimes difficult to differentiate LGG from anaplastic astrocytoma or oligodendroglioma, based only on MR findings. Lack of enhancement, diffusion restriction and relatively lower rCBV and low permeability values help differentiate LGGs from high-grade tumors [5]. High choline and low NAA resonance on MR spectroscopy are typical but not specific [4]. The most common histologic variant is fibrillary (Fig. 24.2), while the gemistocytic type (Fig. 24.4) is more aggressive and likely to progress to anaplastic astrocytoma or glioblastoma multiforme (GBM).

## Importance

During their natural course, LGGs tend to progress to a higher grade of malignancy, leading to neurological disability and ultimately to death [6]. During the low-grade phase, these tumors exhibit a continuous and spontaneous radiological growth which can be measured by quantitative MRI. The velocity of expansion is supposed to have a strong diagnostic significance regarding progression-free and overall survival. The median survival is 6–10 years; death is due to progression in the grade of tumor, and rarely due to spread of low-grade mass. Surgical resection is the primary treatment, but recurrent disease is associated with malignant transformation in a majority of cases. According to a recent study, treatment at a center that favored early surgical resection was associated with better overall survival than treatment at a center that favored biopsy and watchful waiting [7]. Adjuvant chemotherapy and radiotherapy can be performed at the time of recurrence or progression.

## Typical clinical scenario

LGG can occur at all ages and has slight male predominance. However, a majority occur between the ages of 20 and 50 years. The most common symptoms of LGG are those of increased intracranial pressure, namely nausea, vomiting, and headaches. When it involves the cortical structures, seizures are common. Other focal neurological signs vary with tumor location and include behavioral changes and focal neurological deficits.

## Differential diagnosis

Anaplastic astrocytoma (Fig. 24.5) can sometimes appear as a focal or diffuse mass, predominantly white matter in origin but also involving overlying cortex or the gray matter. It can lack post-contrast enhancement and may be difficult to distinguish without biopsy. However, advanced imaging sequences including diffusion and perfusion and spectroscopy can be helpful. Oligodendroglioma (Fig. 24.6) is a cortically based mass with variable post-contrast enhancement. It is divided into WHO grade II and anaplastic grade III tumors. Presence of calcification is very common. Brain inflammation such as cerebritis and herpes encephalitis can present with acute onset. Herpes encephalitis (Fig. 24.7) commonly involves the limbic system and medial temporal lobes with possible areas of hemorrhage and post-contrast enhancement. Vascular territory ischemic infarction would exhibit diffusion restriction, vascular territory distribution, and acute onset, and would involve both gray and white matter.

## Teaching points

LGGs can be indistinguishable from high-grade tumors (WHO grade III) on conventional imaging. Advanced imaging techniques such as MR spectroscopy, diffusion-weighted images, and perfusion-weighted images are helpful for better differentiation. Interval change in imaging features of a low-grade tumor is usually indicative of dedifferentiation to a higher grade.

REFERENCES
1. Markert JM. The role of early resection vs biopsy in the management of low-grade gliomas. *JAMA* 2012; **308**: 1918–19.
2. Udaka YT, Yeh-Nayre LA, Amene CS, *et al.* Recurrent pediatric central nervous system low-grade gliomas: the role of surveillance neuroimaging in asymptomatic children. *J Neurosurg Pediatr* 2013; **11**: 119–26.
3. Theeler BJ, Yung WK, Fuller GN, De Groot JF. Moving toward molecular classification of diffuse gliomas in adults. *Neurology* 2012; **79**: 1917–26.
4. Lemort M, Canizares-Perez AC, Van der Stappen A, *et al.* Progress in magnetic resonance imaging of brain tumours. *Curr Opin Oncol* 2007; **19**: 616–22.
5. Bisdas S, Kirkpatrick M, Giglio P, *et al.* Cerebral blood volume measurements by perfusion-weighted MR imaging in gliomas: ready for prime time in predicting short-term outcome and recurrent disease? *AJNR Am J Neuroradiol* 2009; **30**: 681–8.
6. Pallud J, Taillandier L, Capelle L, *et al.* Quantitative morphological magnetic resonance imaging follow-up of low-grade glioma: a plea for systematic measurement of growth rates. *Neurosurgery* 2012; **71**: 729–39.
7. Jakola AS, Myrmel KS, Kloster R, *et al.* Comparison of a strategy favoring early surgical resection vs a strategy favoring watchful waiting in low-grade gliomas *JAMA.* 2012; **308**: 1881–8.

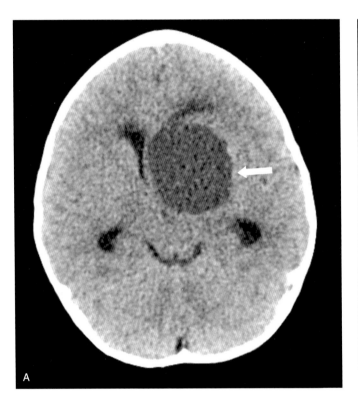 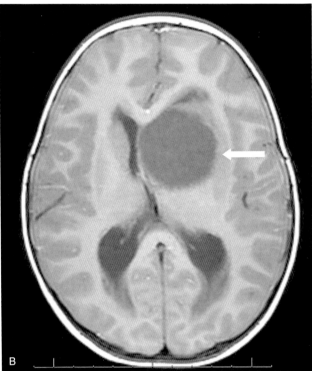

**Figure 24.1** Pilocytic astrocytoma, WHO grade I tumor. (**A**) Non contrast axial CT exhibits a relatively well-defined expansile mass (arrow) at deep left frontal lobe with mass effect on the ventricular system. (**B**) T1-weighted axial MR image exhibits hyperintense T1 signal rounded mass (arrow) with irregular margins at left deep frontal lobe with ventricular compression. (**C**) T2-weighted axial MR image exhibits hyperintense T2 signal mass (arrow) with irregular margins, ventricular compression, and patchy periventricular high T2 signal due to hydrocephalus. (**D**) There is no evidence for diffusion restriction of the large left deep frontal lobe mass (arrow). (**E**) Post-contrast T1-weighted axial MR image exhibits mild peripheral enhancement of the hypointense T1 signal deep left frontal lobe mass (arrow).

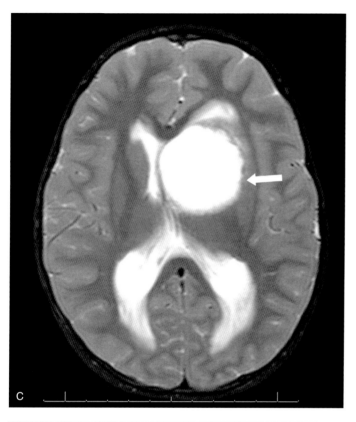

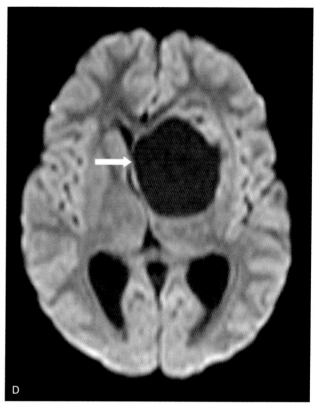

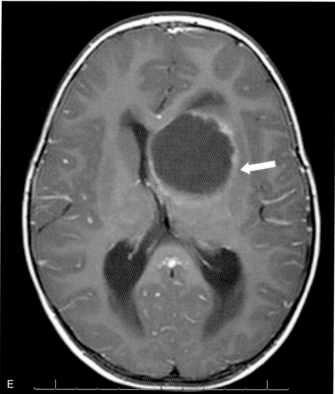

Figure 24.1 (cont.)

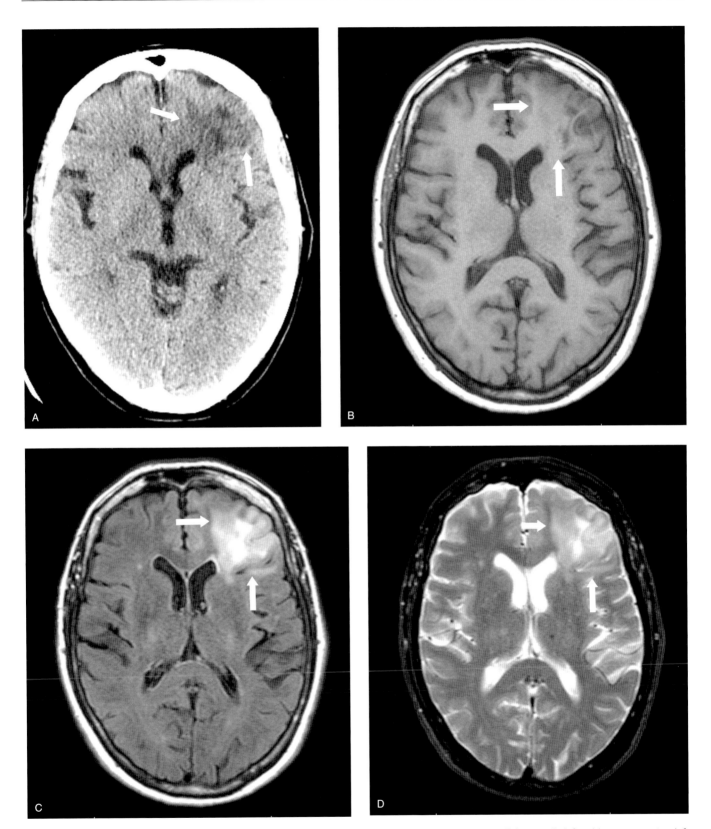

**Figure 24.2** Fibrillary low-grade astrocytoma, WHO grade II tumor. (**A**) Non-contrast T1 axial image exhibits an ill-defined low-attenuating left deep frontal lobe lesion (arrows). (**B**) T1-weighted axial MR image exhibits an iso- to marginally hypointense T1 signal area (arrows) at left frontal lobe. (**C**) FLAIR-weighted axial MR image exhibits patchy high FLAIR signal, predominantly involving the left frontal white matter, but also infiltrating the overlying gray matter (arrows). (**D**) T2-weighted axial MR image exhibits the mass having heterogeneously hyperintense T2 signal (arrows). (**E**) Post-contrast T1 axial imaging exhibits lack of significant post-contrast enhancement (arrow). (**F**) Lack of diffusion restriction is seen on diffusion-weighted imaging (arrow). (**G**) rCBV map exhibits lack of increased perfusion (arrow).

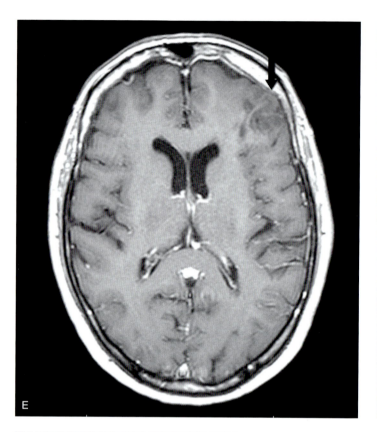

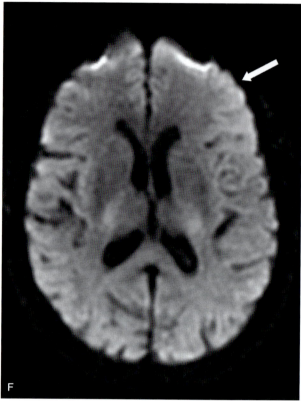

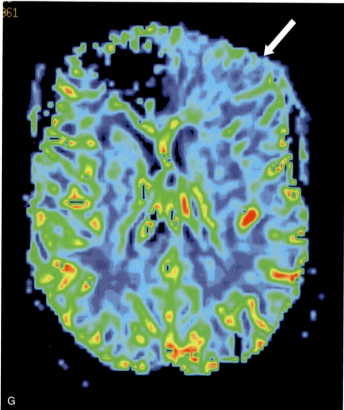

**Figure 24.2** (cont.)

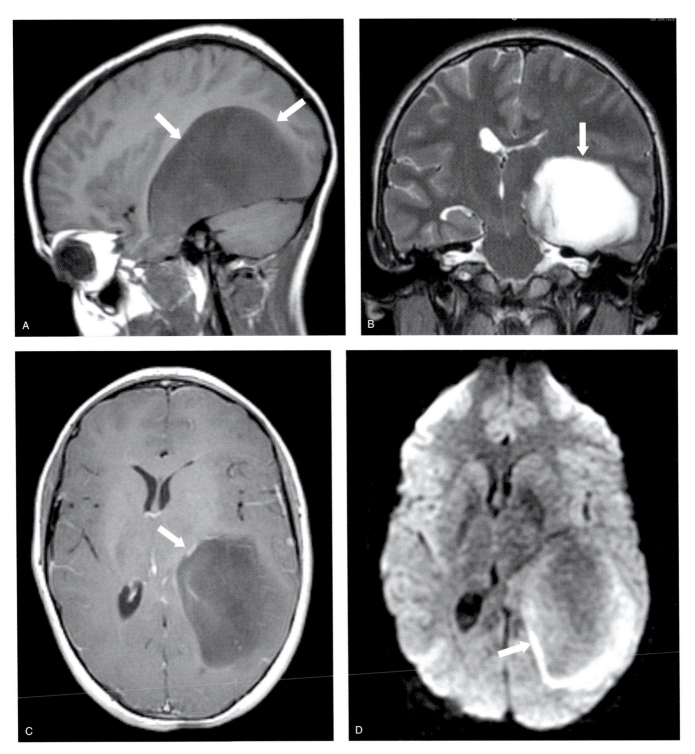

**Figure 24.3** Low-grade glioma (LGG). WHO grade II tumor. (**A**) T1-weighted parasagittal MR image exhibits a well marginated hypointense T1 signal mass (arrows) at left temporal lobe. (**B**) T2-weighted coronal image exhibits hyperintense T2 signal mass involving the left temporal lobe (arrow). (**C**) Post-contrast T1-weighted axial imaging exhibits lack of significant post-contrast enhancement (arrow). (**D**, **E**) Diffusion-weighted axial image and ADC map exhibit lack of diffusion restriction (arrow).

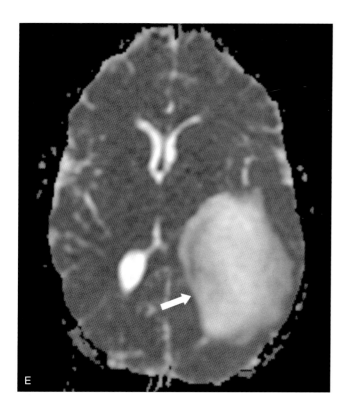

E

**Figure 24.3** (cont.)

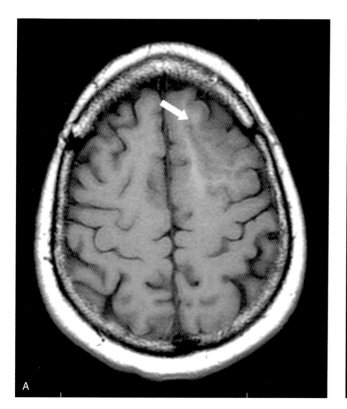

A

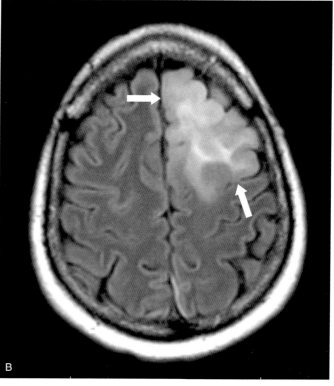

B

**Figure 24.4** Gemistocytic low-grade astrocytoma. WHO grade II tumor. (**A**) T1-weighted axial MR image exhibits an irregular hypointense T1 signal area at high-convexity left frontal lobe (arrow). (**B**) FLAIR-weighted axial MR image exhibits irregular, infiltrating high T2 signal mass involving no white matter and expanding overlying cerebral sulci (arrows). (**C**) T2-weighted axial MR image exhibits heterogeneously high T2 signal of the mass (arrows). (**D**) Post-contrast T1-weighted axial image exhibits lack of significant post-contrast enhancement (arrows). (**E**) rCBV map exhibits areas of decreased MR perfusion (arrow).

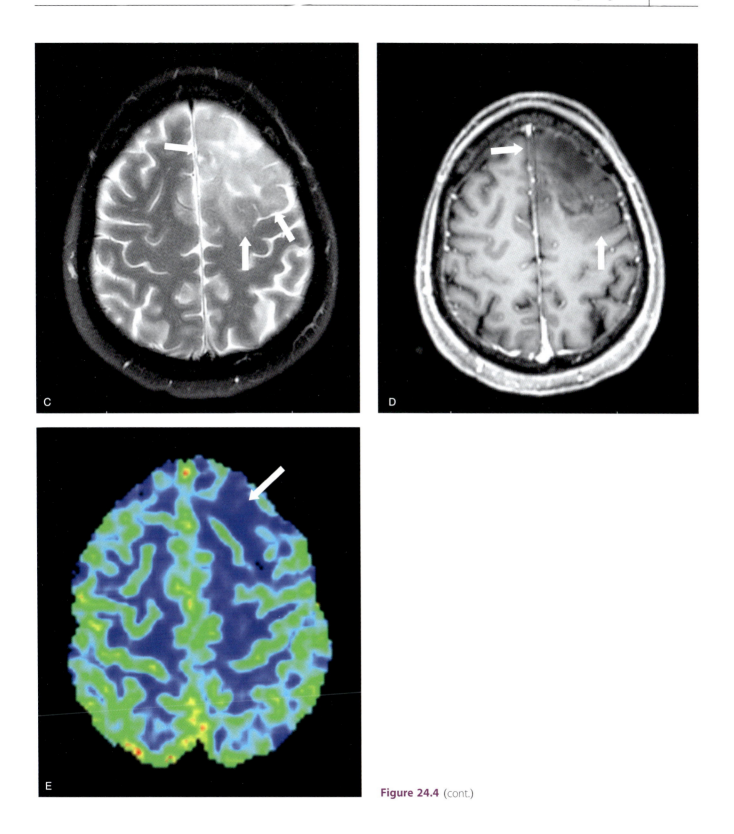

**Figure 24.4** (cont.)

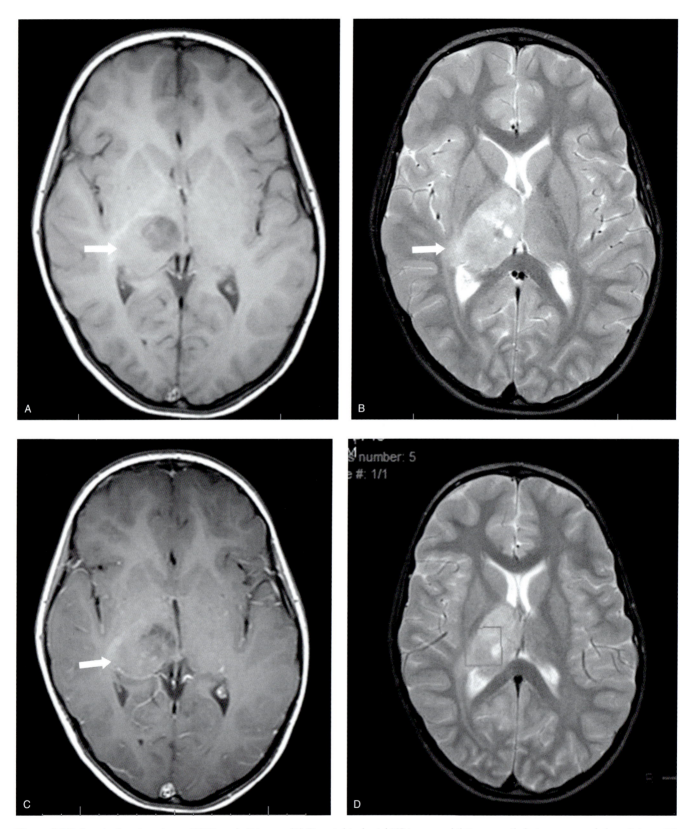

**Figure 24.5** Anaplastic astrocytoma. WHO grade III tumor. (**A**) T1-weighted axial MR image exhibits expansile heterogeneously hypointense T1 signal mass involving the right thalamus and surrounding white matter (arrow). (**B**) T2-weighted axial MR image exhibits heterogeneously hyperintense T2 signal mass (arrow). (**C**) On post-contrast T1-weighted axial MR image, mild patchy post-contrast enhancement is seen within the lateral component of the lesion (arrow). (**D**, **E**) MR spectroscopy exhibits increased choline resonance with diminished NAA peak. (**F**, **G**) True diffusion restriction of the more lateral component is seen on diffusion-weighted images and ADC map (arrow).

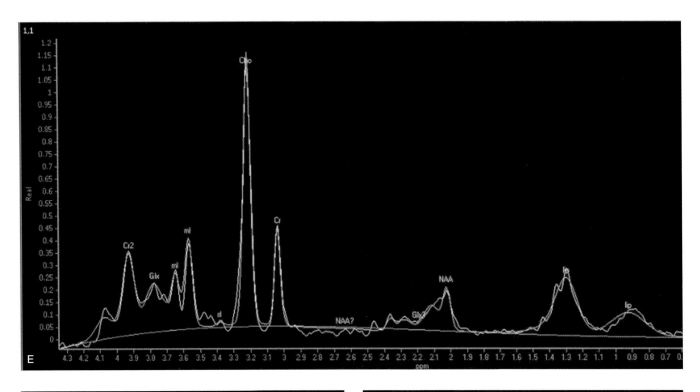

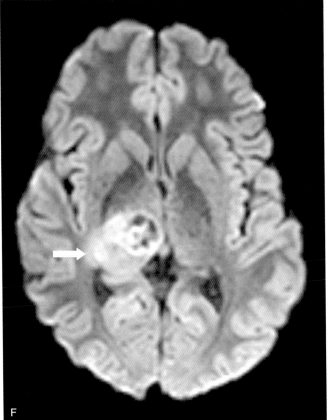

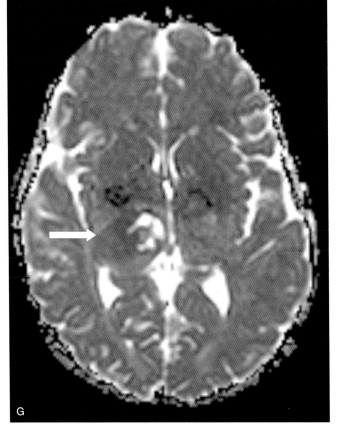

**Figure 24.5** (cont.)

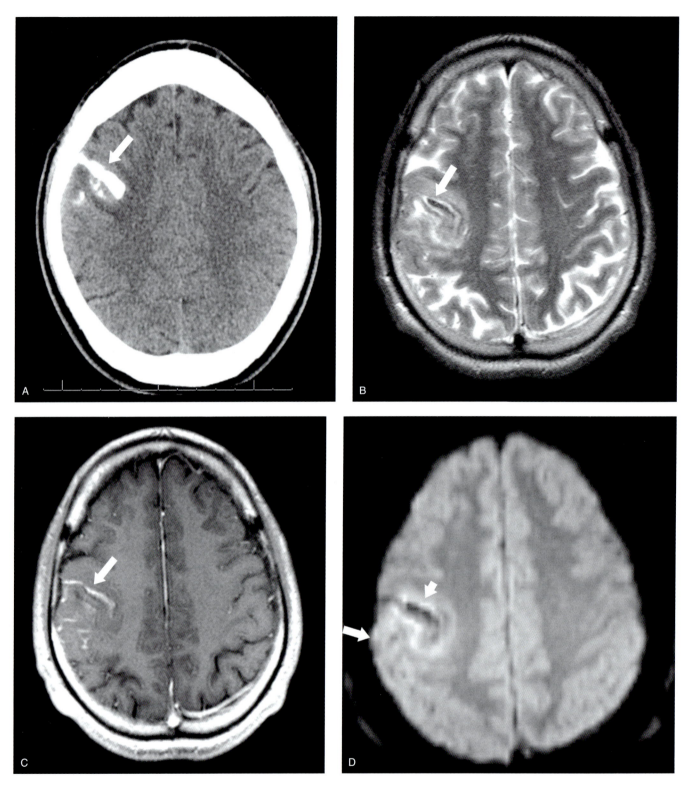

**Figure 24.6** Oligodendroglioma. WHO grade II tumor. (**A**) Non-contrast axial CT exhibits cortical calcification along high-convexity right frontal sulci (arrow) with surrounding irregular hypodense lesion. (**B**) T2-weighted axial MR image exhibits low T2 signal linear calcification (arrow) surrounded by irregular hyperintense T2 signal lesion. (**C**) Post-contrast T1-weighted axial MR image exhibits irregular enhancement along the high convexity sulci (arrow). (**D**, **E**) There is no evidence for true diffusion restriction of the surrounding area (arrow), while the linear cortical calcification displays low signal (short arrow). (**F**) rCBV map exhibits normal cortical perfusion along the area of calcification (short arrow) with decreased perfusion of the surrounding lesion (arrow).

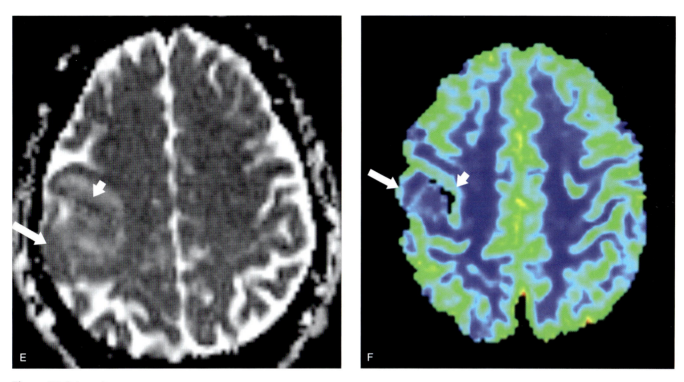

**Figure 24.6** (cont.)

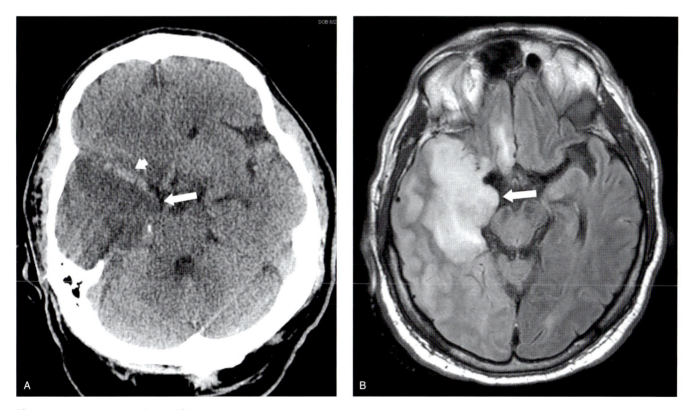

**Figure 24.7** Herpes encephalitis. (**A**) Non-contrast axial CT exhibits expansile low-attenuating lesion at right temporal lobe (arrow) with effacement of right temporal horn. There is a peripheral area of hemorrhage (short arrow). (**B**) FLAIR-weighted axial MR image exhibits expansile high FLAIR signal area at right temporal and basifrontal lobes (arrow). (**C**) T2-weighted axial MR imaging exhibits hyperintense T2 signal lesion (arrow). (**D**) Diffusion-weighted images exhibit diffusion restriction, predominantly at the involved cerebral sulci (arrows). (**E**) Post-contrast T1-weighted axial MR imaging exhibits patchy post-contrast enhancement (short arrows) of the right temporal lobe lesion (arrow).

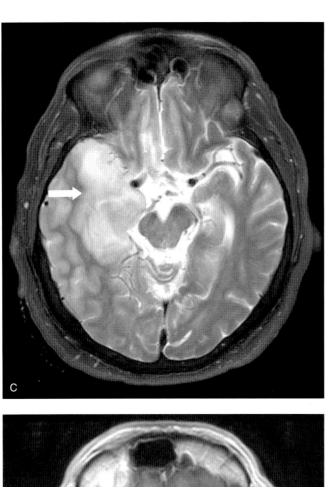

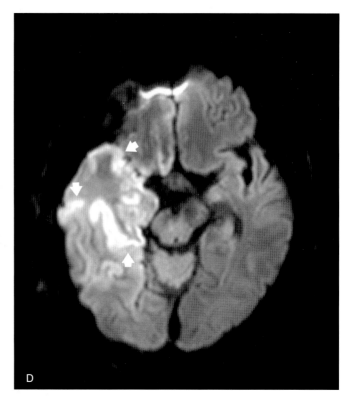

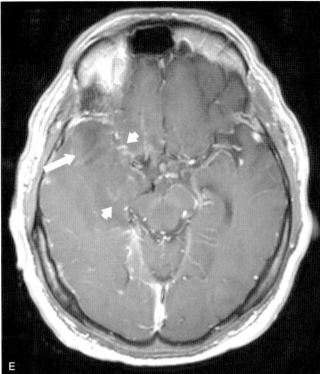

Figure 24.7 (cont.)

# Diffuse intrinsic pontine glioma

## Imaging description

Brainstem gliomas are 10–20% of all CNS tumors in the pediatric population, with 80% being diffuse intrinsic pontine gliomas (DIPGs). Because of the risks associated with biopsying DIPGs, currently the diagnosis is based on MRI features alone, with biopsy reserved for atypical cases [1]. Median survival is approximately 9–12 months, and 90% of the patients die before 2 years. Radiotherapy is considered to be the standard treatment modality, with many chemotherapy protocols being tried although there is no treatment currently available that has a significant impact on outcome. Proponents of biopsy diagnosis argue that modern steriotactic methods have decreased risk and obtaining tissue and studying molecular features of these tumors may help facilitate novel treatments. Regardless, MRI remains the main tool in diagnosis and management of these children.

The classic MRI features of DIPG include T1 hypointense and T2 heterogeneously hyperintense, ill-defined lesions occupying more than 50% of the cross-sectional surface area of the pons but not extending outside the brainstem (Fig. 25.1). They tend to grow and extend superiorly and inferiorly with progressive expansion of the brainstem. Exophytic growth is common, particularly anteriorly, engulfing the basilar artery. They might compress the fourth ventricle, but hydrocephalus is rare at presentation. Contrast enhancement is usually absent; when present it's usually minimal and patchy. While conventional MRI features are helpful in establishing the diagnosis, they cannot predict outcome, with the possible exception of enhancement. Lately, functional MRI methods are used to predict outcome; increased rCBV on susceptibility-weighted perfusion MRI, increased choline/NAA ratio on MR spectroscopy, and enhancement on post-contrast T1-weighted images are associated with shorter mean survival time [2,3].

## Importance

DIPG has a worse prognosis than many other brainstem lesions, and MRI plays a significant role in diagnosis and management of these children because most cases are managed without tissue diagnosis.

## Typical clinical scenario

Peak age is between 5 and 10 years, and the classic clinical triad at presentation consists of ataxia, pyramidal signs, and cranial nerve deficits. Cranial nerves VI and VII are most frequently involved.

## Differential diagnosis

Juvenile pilocytic astrocytoma (JPA) is another brainstem mass in children that has a better prognosis. JPAs usually contain areas of cysts and intense enhancement (Fig. 25.2). Acute disseminated encephalomyelitis (ADEM) is common in the pediatric age group and typically presents with multifocal non-enhancing signal abnormalities. When a solitary ADEM lesion is limited to the pons it may be very difficult to differentiate it from DIPG (Fig. 25.3). ADEM, however, shows a relatively quick evolution of MRI findings and often results in complete resolution. Central pontine myelinolysis may have a similar imaging appearance to DIPG but the clinical context is different. Posterior reversible encephalopathy syndrome (PRES) may involve the brainstem but usually presents with multifocal lesion (Fig. 25.4). Clinical context is also helpful in differentiating PRES from other brainstem lesions. Spongiform changes of neurofibromatosis type 1 may present within the pons, but rarely large enough to mimic DIPG.

## Teaching points

In a child with a short duration of neurologic symptoms and a diffusely infiltrating pontine T2 hyperintensity, expansion of the pons and engulfing of the basilar artery should allow a diagnosis of DIPG and preclude biopsy. In addition to conventional MRI, spectroscopy and perfusion imaging should be performed to help predict outcome.

REFERENCES

1) Hankinson TC, Campagna EJ, Foreman NK, Handler MH. Interpretation of magnetic resonance images in diffuse intrinsic pontine glioma: a survey of pediatric neurosurgeons. *J Neurosurg Pediatr* 2011; **8**: 97–102.

2) Hipp SJ, Steffen-Smith E, Hammoud D, *et al.* Predicting outcome of children with diffuse intrinsic pontine gliomas using multiparametric imaging. *Neuro Oncol* 2011; **13**: 904–9.

3) Dellaretti M, Reyns N, Touzet G, *et al.* Diffuse brainstem glioma: prognostic factors. *J Neurosurg* 2012; **117**: 810–14.

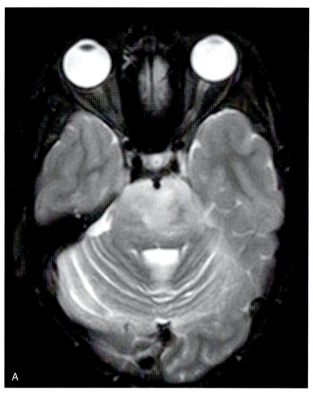

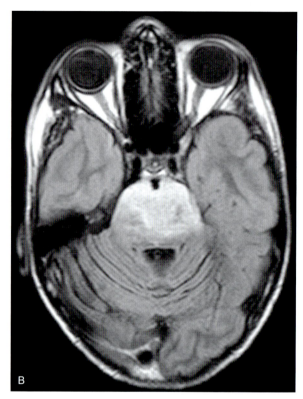

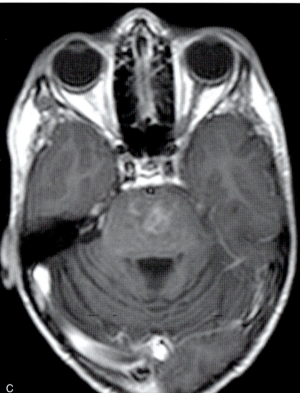

**Figure 25.1** Diffuse intrinsic pontine glioma (DIPG). Axial (**A**) T2-weighted, (**B**) FLAIR, and (**C**) post-contrast T1-weighted images show an expansile infiltrating mass in the pons with characteristic engulfing of the basilar artery. Patchy enhancement is an uncommon feature, as most DIPGs do not show any enhancement.

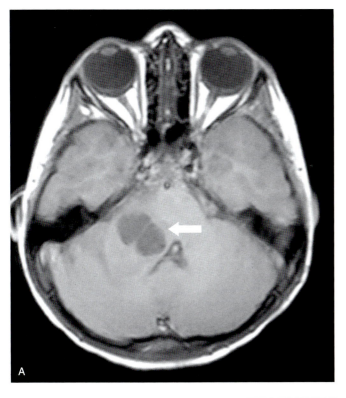

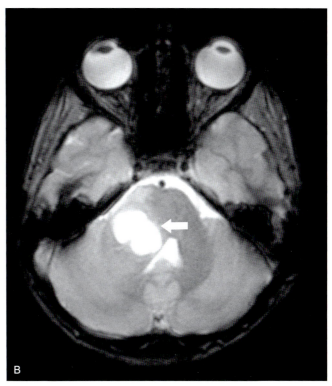

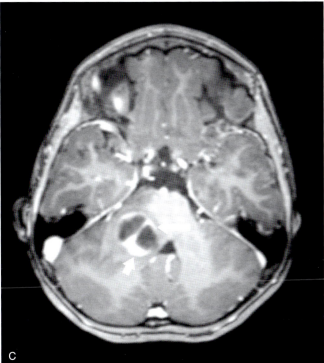

**Figure 25.2** Pilocytic astrocytoma. Axial (**A**) T1-weighted, (**B**) T2-weighted, and (**C**) post-contrast T1-weighted images show a cystic and solid mass with avid enhancement.

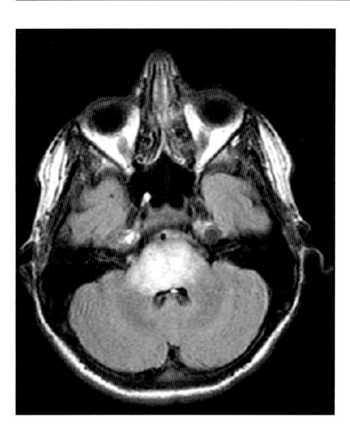

**Figure 25.3** Acute disseminated encephalomyelitis (ADEM). Axial FLAIR image shows an infiltrating hyperintense lesion in the pons in a child who presented with relatively acute-onset neurologic findings. DIPG and ADEM are considered in differential diagnosis. Follow-up imaging showed resolution of the finding.

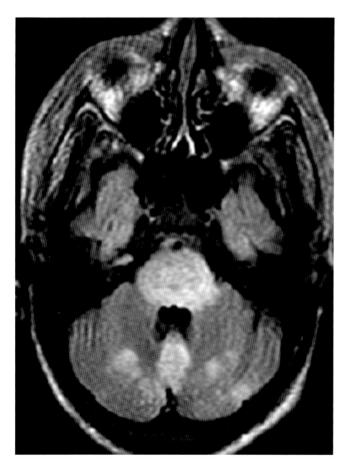

**Figure 25.4** Posterior reversible encephalopathy syndrome (PRES). Axial FLAIR image shows multifocal signal abnormalities in the cerebellum along with diffuse pontine abnormality in this patient with a history of hypertension who presented with seizure and encephalopathy.

## Imaging description

Radiologists rely on enhancement in evaluating treatment response in glioblastoma multiforme (GBM). According to the widely used Macdonald criteria, >25% increase in enhancing tissue indicates tumor progression. Surgery when feasible followed by concurrent temozolomide (TMZ) and radiotherapy (RT) became the standard of care for GBMs. Recently, there has been an increasing awareness of progressive and enhancing lesions on MR images shortly after TMZ+RT treatment that improve or stabilize on follow-up imaging in the absence of further treatment [1]. This is termed "pseudoprogression" as it mimics true tumor progression. Up to 30% of GBM patients exhibit this phenomenon, and present with increased enhancement, edema, and mass effect within 3–4 months of treatment.

Conventional MRI sequences are not helpful in making a distinction between pseudo and true progression (Fig. 26.1) [2]. The definitive diagnosis is based on demonstration of the lesion getting better on follow-up MRI or biopsy, although perfusion images may show decreased rCBV and increased apparent diffusion coefficient (ADC) values, in contrast to true tumor progression (Fig. 26.2) [3].

## Importance

Whether to continue with standard adjuvant chemotherapy or to switch to an alternative therapy is decided based on response determined by MRI. Mistaking pseudoprogression for true progression may result in cessation of effective treatment. MGMT is a DNA repair gene found in GBMs which is silenced when it is methylated. Methylated MGMT has been associated with better response to therapy in GBMs [4]. Also, methylation of MGMT promoter is associated with a much higher incidence of pseudoprogression. Therefore, pseudoprogression may potentially become an indirect indicator of longer survival.

## Typical clinical scenario

Pseudoprogression usually occurs within the first 3 months after completing treatment, but it may occur from the first few weeks to 6 months after treatment. Most patients are asymptomatic (i.e., no new symptoms), but some will present with worsening symptoms, probably as a result of mass effect [5].

## Differential diagnosis

Pathologically, pseudoprogression shows gliosis and reactive radiation-induced changes without evidence of viable tumor, and it presumably represents an inflammatory response against the tumor. While pseudoprogression is considered to be a type of radiation-related injury, it is different than the typical radiation necrosis, which occurs 18–24 months post-treatment.

Increased enhancement can be induced by microischemic changes that occur during surgery and result in blood–brain barrier disruption. Although these cannot be differentiated from tumor, they usually lack the exuberant enhancement and edema present in tumor progression or pseudoprogression.

## Teaching points

Approximately 30% of GBM patients who are treated with TMZ+RT will present with increasing enhancement and edema in the tumor bed which resolves on the follow-up MRIs, hence the name pseudoprogression. Pseudoprogression occurs in patients with methylated MGMT promoter. Conventional MRI cannot differentiate this from true tumor progression. While ADC maps and susceptibility-weighted perfusion studies provide the correct diagnosis with 70–80% accuracy, definitive diagnosis is based on clinical follow-up or biopsy.

REFERENCES

1. Gerstner ER, McNamara MB, Norden AD, et al. Effect of adding temozolomide to radiation therapy on the incidence of pseudo-progression. J Neurooncol 2009; 94: 97–101.
2. Young RJ, Gupta A, Shah AD, et al. Potential utility of conventional MRI signs in diagnosing pseudoprogression in glioblastoma. Neurology 2011; 76: 1918–24.
3. Kong DS, Kim ST, Kim EH, et al. Diagnostic dilemma of pseudoprogression in the treatment of newly diagnosed glioblastomas: the role of assessing relative cerebral blood flow volume and oxygen-6-methylguanine-DNA methyltransferase promoter methylation status. AJNR Am J Neuroradiol 2011; 32: 382–7.
4. Brandes AA, Tosoni A, Franceschi E, et al. Recurrence pattern after temozolomide concomitant with and adjuvant to radiotherapy in newly diagnosed patients with glioblastoma: correlation with MGMT promoter methylation status. J Clin Oncol 2009; 27: 1275–9
5. Hygino da Cruz LC, Rodriguez I, Domingues RC, et al. Pseudoprogression and pseudoresponse: imaging challenges in the assessment of posttreatment glioma. AJNR Am J Neuroradiol 2011; 32: 1978–85.

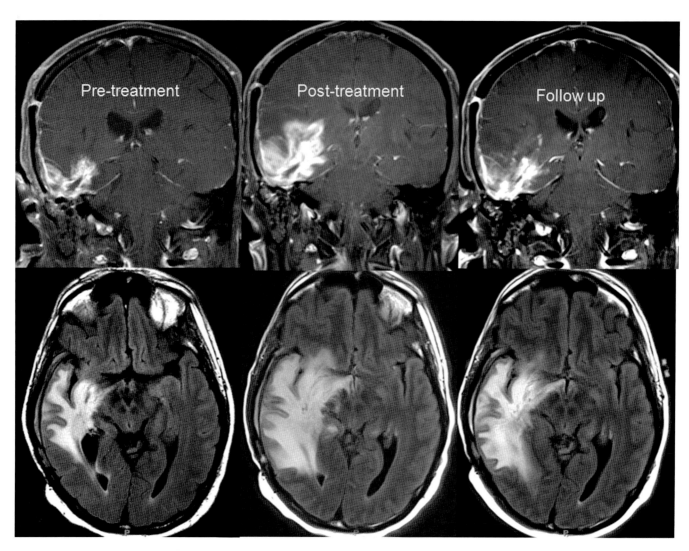

**Figure 26.1** Pseudoprogression of GBM. Post-contrast T1-weighted and corresponding FLAIR images of a patient with GBM, before TMZ+RT (left), 6 weeks after treatment start (middle), and at 12-week follow-up (right). Note the marked increase in enhancement, edema, and mass effect associated with the right temporal lesion on the early follow-up MRI (middle), which decreased subsequently without any change in treatment. This lesion was later removed, and pathology showed treatment effect with minimal viable tumor.

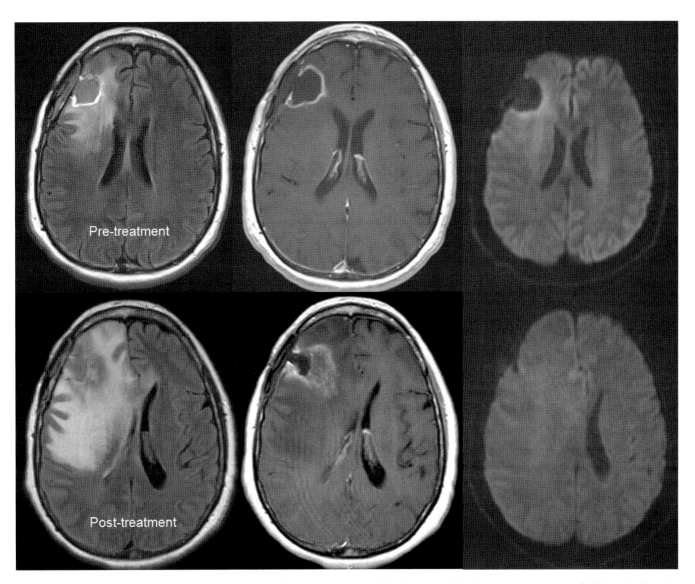

**Figure 26.2** FLAIR (left), post-contrast T1-weighted (middle), and DWI (right) MRI of a patient following surgical resection of GBM and before the initiation of TMZ+RT (upper row) and 4 weeks after treatment started (lower row). Marked increase in edema, mass effect, and enhancement suggested tumor recurrence, although DWI showed no diffusion restriction as would be expected from a cellular tumor. Biopsy showed pure treatment effect with no viable tumor identified.

# Pseudoresponse in treatment of GBM

## Imaging description

Radiologists rely on enhancement in evaluating treatment response in glioblastoma multiforme (GBM). According to the widely used Macdonald criteria, >50% decrease in enhancing tissue indicates treatment response. Currently, anti-VGEF agents such as bevacizumab are commonly used for recurrent GBM treatment [1]. Antiangiogenic properties of this agent result in a rapid and dramatic decrease in the degree and amount of enhancement in the tumor bed with decreasing edema and mass effect and some improvement in clinical performance scores [1,2]. This translates to marked improvement in radiographic response rates and some improvement in disease-free survival rates, but no significant improvement is seen in overall survival rate in these patients (Figs. 27.1, 27.2, 27.3) [1]. While contrast-enhancing lesions decrease in size, FLAIR and DWI images may show enlargement of the tumor and are more reliable than contrast-enhanced images in evaluating treatment response [3,4].

## Importance

The rapid decrease in contrast enhancement is secondary to stabilization of the blood–brain barrier rather than true tumor reduction [5]. Caution should be exercised in interpreting this as true response.

## Typical clinical scenario

Bevacizumab is usually used as an alternative to the standard temozolomide and radiotherapy (TMZ+RT) or in cases of recurrent tumor, and it may generate a rapid "response," sometimes within a few days. Enhancement and edema usually rebound with cessation of treatment enhancement and decrease with restarting of treatment.

## Differential diagnosis

Response in the setting of bevacizumab treatment should be confirmed with FLAIR and DWI findings. Enlargement of infiltrative signal abnormalities on FLAIR and DWI should be interpreted as progression even when the enhancing tumor is decreasing.

> ## Teaching points
>
> Response to treatment with anti-VEGF agents is best evaluated with FLAIR and DWI/ADC images, as contrast enhancement decreases as a result of blood–brain barrier normalization rather than actual tumor reduction.

REFERENCES

1. Butowski N. Anti-angiogenic therapy in glioma. *Clin Transl Oncol* 2011; **13**: 294–300.
2. Norden AD, Young GS, Setayesh K, *et al.* Bevacizumab for recurrent malignant gliomas: efficacy, toxicity, and patterns of recurrence. *Neurology* 2008; **70**: 779–87
3. Pope WB, Kim HJ, Huo J, *et al.* Recurrent glioblastoma multiforme: ADC histogram analysis predicts response to bevacizumab treatment. *Radiology* 2009; **252**: 182–9
4. Gerstner ER, Chen PJ, Wen PY, *et al.* Infiltrative patterns of glioblastoma spread detected via diffusion MRI after treatment with cediranib. *Neuro Oncol* 2010; **12**: 466–72
5. Batchelor TT, Sorensen AG, di Tomaso E, *et al.* AZD2171, a pan-VEGF receptor tyrosine kinase inhibitor, normalizes tumor vasculature and alleviates edema in glioblastoma patients. *Cancer Cell* 2007; **11**: 83–95.

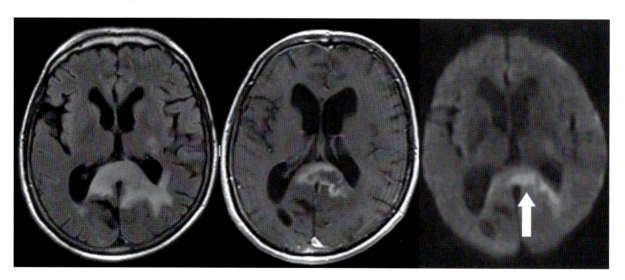

**Figure 27.1** FLAIR (left), post-contrast T1-weighted (middle), and DWI (right) MRI of a patient with recurrent GBM shows an enhancing necrotic mass centered in the splenium of the corpus callosum with small areas of restricted diffusion present (arrow).

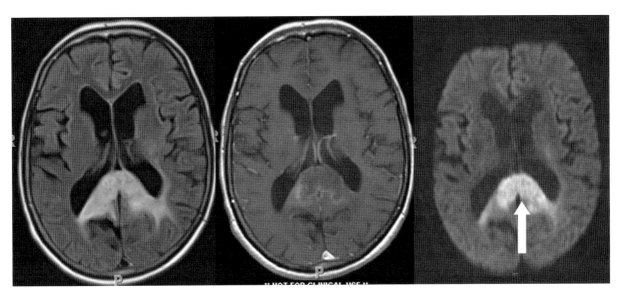

**Figure 27.2** Follow-up MRI of the same patient as in Fig. 27.1 shortly after treatment with bevacizumab shows interval growth of the DWI abnormality (arrow) and no significant change in FLAIR signal compatible with tumor progression. Marked reduction in contrast enhancement is secondary to antiangiogenic treatment.

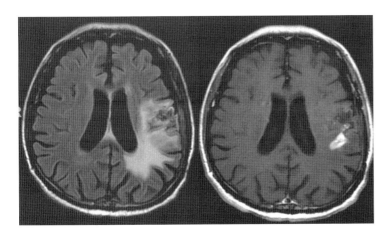

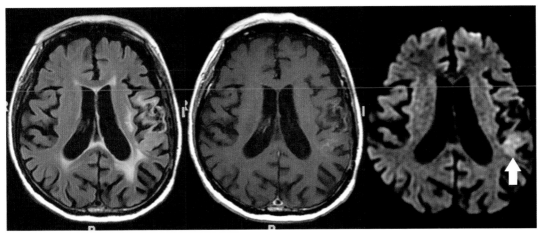

**Figure 27.3** Axial FLAIR and post-contrast T1-weighted images of a patient with recurrent GBM before the start of bevacizumab (top row), and follow-up MRI study with additional DWI (bottom row) demonstrating marked reduction in FLAIR signal abnormality and nearly resolved contrast enhancement, with persistent DWI abnormality in the previously enhancing lesion suggesting pseudoresponse. Pseudoresponse was confirmed on later follow-up, which showed tumor growth in the same area.

# Low-grade oligodendroglioma

## Imaging description

Relative cerebral blood volume (rCBV) measurement derived from perfusion-weighted imaging (PWI) is shown to predict the grade of gliomas [1,2]. WHO grade II gliomas show lower rCBV than WHO grade III and IV gliomas. This is based on rCBV's ability to accurately predict microvascular density (MVD) within a tumor. MVD is a measure of angiogenesis and is associated with various cytogenetic and molecular features including vascular endothelial growth factor (VEGF) and epidermal growth factor receptor (EGFR) expression/overexpression. Although demonstration of high rCBV within a brain tumor appears to be a good predictor of aggressive behavior and higher grade, limitations do exist, presumably because of the heterogeneity present between various types of tumors and their cytogenetic features.

One such limitation is apparent in the evaluation of oligodendrogliomas (ODGs) [3]. Certain low-grade ODGs show increased rCBV (Figs. 28.1, 28.2). The most common cytogenetic aberrations in ODGs are losses on chromosomes 1p (60%), 19q (60–70%), and 10q (25%). In particular, combined allelic loss (loss of heterozygosity, LOH) on chromosomes 1p and 19q is associated with both chemosensitivity and longer survival after chemotherapy. Recently, it has been shown that WHO grade II ODGs that have 1p and 19q LOH (which is associated with better outcome) demonstrate higher rCBV values on PWI MRI as compared to ODGs that have intact 1p and 19q (which is associated with worse outcome), in stark contrast to astrocytomas, in which increased rCBV predicts higher grade [4].

## Importance

Treatment of patients with brain tumors relies on histopathological type and grade. ODGs account for 5% of intracranial primary tumors and 25–30% of gliomas. In general, ODGs have a better outcome than astrocytic tumors. In particular, ODGs with co-deleted 1p and 19q have a more favorable outcome than ODGs of the same grade with intact 1p and 19q chromosomes and astrocytomas, due to their greater response to chemotherapy. Increased rCBV in astrocytomas is associated with higher WHO grade and worse outcome, whereas increased rCBV in grade II ODGs is associated with 1p 19q LOH status and better outcome. Because grade III ODGs also have increased rCBV, PWI is not as powerful in predicting ODG grade as it is in predicting astrocytoma grade, but when combined with histopathological features PWI can provide important prognostic information.

## Typical clinical scenario

Clinical presentation of brain tumors is variable, depending on many features including the location and biological behavior of the tumor. Once a brain tumor is identified on MRI, radiologists should try to determine the histological type and grade to help with management decisions.

## Differential diagnosis

Low-grade ODGs are generally well-defined, cortically based T2 hyperintense and non-enhancing lesions that are easily recognized as being a primary brain tumor, although initially they may be mistaken for infarct and encephalitis. Short-term follow-up MRIs usually show a stable lesion with ODGs and rapidly changing lesions with infarct and encephalitis. It is often difficult to differentiate a low-grade astrocytoma from a low-grade ODG, although ODGs usually involve the peripheral brain (cortical-based) and show more heterogeneity on conventional MRI than astrocytomas, which are usually deeper and more homogeneous. The heterogeneity of ODGs may in part be secondary to a high incidence of calcifications. Rarer low-grade brain tumors such as gangliogliomas and dysembryoplastic neuroepithelial tumors (DNET) are also in the differential diagnosis.

## Teaching points

PWI MRI can predict the grade of an astrocytic tumor, but its use in ODG is limited by the fact that ODGs with 1p 19q LOH often show increased rCBV despite their more favorable nature compared to other ODGs and astrocytomas.

REFERENCES

1. Law M, Yang S, Wang H, et al. Glioma grading: sensitivity, specificity, and predictive values of perfusion MR imaging and proton MR spectroscopic imaging compared with conventional MR imaging. *AJNR Am J Neuroradiol* 2003; **24**: 1989–98.

2. Preul C, Kuhn B, Lang EW, et al. Differentiation of cerebral tumors using multi-section echo planar MR perfusion imaging. *Eur J Radiol* 2003; **48**: 244–51.

3. Whitmore RG, Krejza J, Kapoor GS, et al. Prediction of oligodendroglial tumor subtype and grade using perfusion weighted magnetic resonance imaging. 2007 *J Neurosurg* **107**: 600–9.

4. Kapoor GS, Gocke TA, Chawla S, et al. Magnetic resonance perfusion-weighted imaging defines angiogenic subtypes of oligodendroglioma according to 1p19q and EGFR status. *J Neurooncol* 2009; **92**: 373–86.

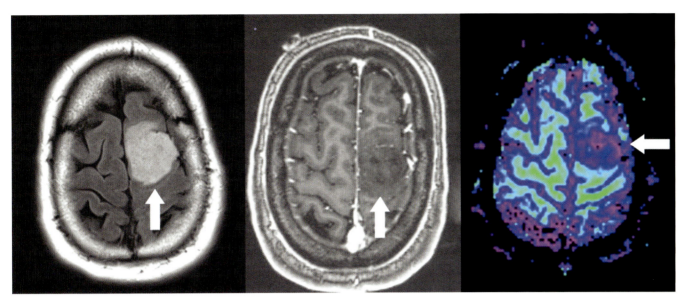

**Figure 28.1** Axial FLAIR (left) and post-contrast T1-weighted (middle) images show a well-defined cortical-based mass with uniform signal intensity and no enhancement suggesting a low-grade glioma, probably an oligodendrioglioma (ODG), given its location. Accompanying PWI (right) shows increased rCBV to the tumor (arrow), which turned out to be a grade II ODG with 1p and 19q LOH. Increased rCBV would be worrisome for a higher-grade tumor if this were an astrocytoma.

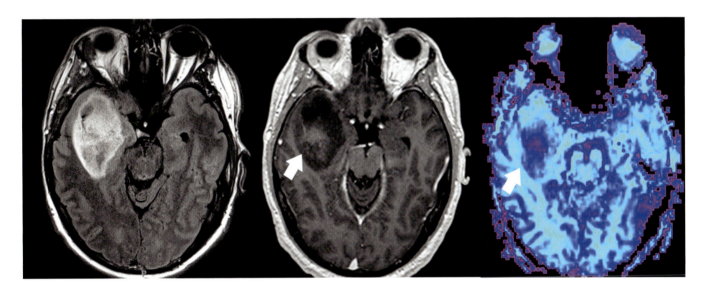

**Figure 28.2** Axial FLAIR (left), post-contrast T1-weighted (middle), and PWI (right) images show a large intra-axial tumor with well-defined borders and some signal heterogeneity. A central area of minimal enhancement is noted compared to pre-contrast images (arrow), which shows markedly increased rCBV, features suggesting a tumor grade potentially greater than WHO grade II. Pathologic assessment was consistent with WHO grade II ODG.

# Primary CNS lymphoma

## Imaging description

Primary CNS lymphoma (PCNSL), a malignant brain neoplasm composed of B lymphocytes, occurs only in the CNS in most cases, in contrast to secondary involvement of CNS by systemic lymphoma, in immunocompromised patients with a history of prior infection with Epstein–Barr virus, and occasionally in immunocompetent patients [1]. As brain does not have lymphoid tissue or lymphatic circulation, the site of origin is something of a mystery [1].

Typical PCNSL presents as a solitary or multiple solid mass (es) in the periventricular regions and corpus callosum with avid and homogeneous enhancement, decreased T2 signal, and decreased water diffusivity secondary to increased cellularity with a variable degree of surrounding vasogenic edema [2]. On CT, PCNSL, unlike many other masses, shows hyperattenuation (Fig. 29.1). Deviation from this classic imaging appearance is common, however, particularly in severely immunocompromised patients, and non-enhancing, heterogeneously enhancing, or ring-enhancing lesions present a diagnostic challenge (Fig. 29.2).

Interestingly, PCNSL, unlike most malignant masses, shows decreased rCBV in perfusion imaging, which may be very helpful in differential diagnosis (Fig. 29.3) [3]. They are also seen in subependymal locations with diffuse post-contrast enhancement. When the CNS is secondarily affected due to systemic lymphoma, the imaging findings include dural-based enhancing masses (Fig. 29.4), leptomeningeal and cranial nerve enhancement, pituitary infudibular involvement, and subependymal/intraventricular enhancing lesions (Fig. 29.5) [3].

## Importance

CNS lymphoma has poor long-term prognosis, with median survival of about 3 years in AIDS patients. There is high association with AIDS and post-transplant status. There is a dramatic response to steroids, with shrinkage of volume and improvement in intensity of post-contrast enhancement. However, relapse is very common. It is important to have CSF analysis as part of the diagnostic work-up [4].

## Typical clinical scenario

The clinical manifestations are related to increased intracranial pressure with nausea, vomiting, and headaches. Altered mental status and focal neurological deficits are almost always seen. Cognitive changes and psychiatric disturbances may be present before and after treatment [5]. PCNSL is seen in an elderly population, commonly in the sixth or seventh decade of life. In immunocompromised patients, however, including recent transplant recipients and patients with AIDS, it may be seen in young adults or the middle-aged.

## Differential diagnosis

Glioblastoma is a malignant glial tumor of the brain that commonly involves the corpus callosum and crosses the midline (Fig. 29.6). It generally displays hypointense T2 signal with heterogeneous post-contrast enhancement. Areas of tumor necrosis and ring enhancement are seen in the majority of cases. Increased rCBV on PWI is helpful in differentiating PCNSL. An abscess (Fig. 29.7) can present as a focal parenchymal mass with hypointense T2 signal rim and peripheral ring enhancement with central necrosis. However, it almost always displays restricted diffusion and diminished diffusion coefficient in the central part of the lesion rather than at the wall. Neurosarcoidosis typically exhibits leptomeningeal enhancement and sometimes parenchymal lesions, and mimics secondary CNS involvement by systemic lymphoma (Fig. 29.8). Active demyelination as seen in multiple sclerosis can exhibit an incomplete ring enhancement which may involve the corpus callosum. However, it displays hyperintense T2 signal and has comparatively little mass effect.

## Teaching points

Imaging features of PCNSL differ from that of secondary CNS involvement by systemic lymphoma. PCNSL is generally hyperdense on non-contrast CT, frequently associated with diffusion restriction, and exhibits hypointense T2 signal with intense post-contrast enhancement and decreased rCBV. Typical imaging features of PCNSL may not be seen in patients with immunocmpromised status. Treatment with steroids causes a rapid and dramatic decrease in the size of the mass as well as the intensity of contrast enhancement.

REFERENCES

1. Ricard D, Idbaih A, Ducray F, et al. Primary brain tumours in adults. Lancet 2012; 379: 1984–96.
2. Yap KK, Sutherland T, Liew E, et al. Magnetic resonance features of primary central nervous system lymphoma in the immunocompetent patient: a pictorial essay. J Med Imaging Radiat Oncol 2012; 56: 179–86.
3. Brar R, Prasad A, Sharma T, Vermani N. Multifocal lateral and fourth ventricular B-cell primary CNS lymphoma. Clin Neurol Neurosurg 2012; 114: 281–3.
4. Baraniskin A, Deckert M, Schulte-Altedorneburg G, Schlegel U, Schroers R. Current strategies in the diagnosis of diffuse large B-cell lymphoma of the central nervous system. Br J Haematol 2012; 156: 421–32.
5. Correa DD, Shi W, Abrey LE, et al. Cognitive functions in primary CNS lymphoma after single or combined modality regimens. Neuro Oncol 2012; 14: 101–8.

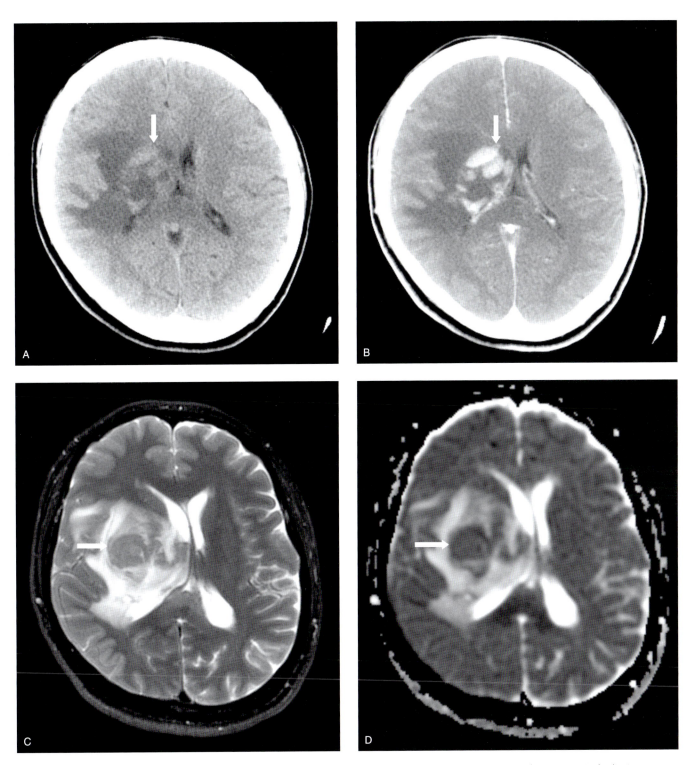

**Figure 29.1** Primary CNS lymphoma. (**A**) Non-contrast axial CT exhibits patchy mildly hyperdense areas in right periventricular brain parenchyma (arrow), surrounded by low-attenuating white matter edema. (**B**) Post-contrast axial CT exhibits dense enhancement of solid periventricular masses (arrow). (**C**) T2-weighted axial MR image exhibits low T2 signal of the periventricular masses (arrow). (**D**) On ADC map, diminished diffusion coefficient of the solid mass is seen (arrow). (**E**) On post-contrast axial MR image, there is intense enhancement of the solid masses (arrow). (**F**) Post-contrast T1-weighted coronal image shows the extent and periventricular location of the densely enhancing right cerebral solid lesions (arrow).

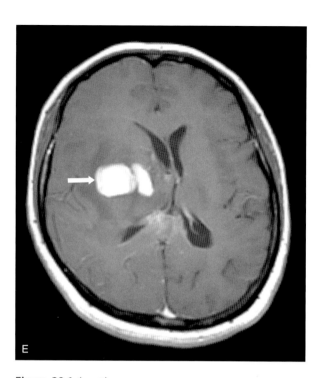
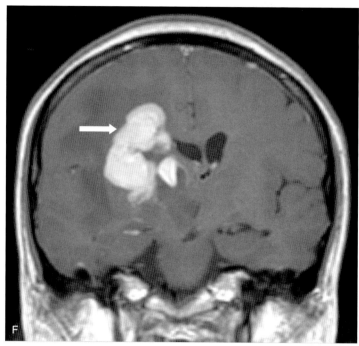

**Figure 29.1** (cont.)

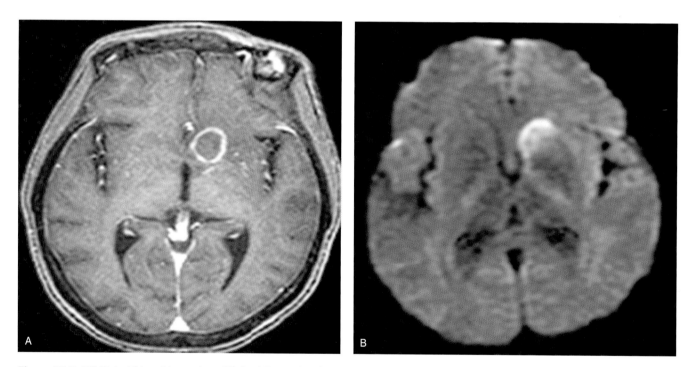

**Figure 29.2** PCNSL in HIV-positive patient. (**A**) Axial T1-weighted post-contrast image shows a single ring-enhancing mass in the left caudate nucleus region which was proven by biopsy to be PCNSL. (**B**) Axial DWI image shows increased signal in the wall of the necrotic lesion, a finding which is not expected in toxoplasmosis.

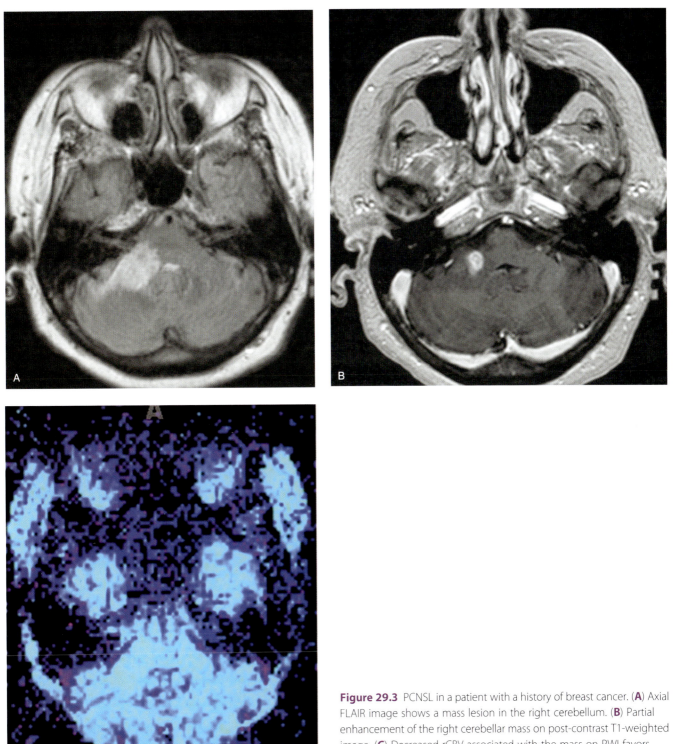

**Figure 29.3** PCNSL in a patient with a history of breast cancer. (**A**) Axial FLAIR image shows a mass lesion in the right cerebellum. (**B**) Partial enhancement of the right cerebellar mass on post-contrast T1-weighted image. (**C**) Decreased rCBV associated with the mass on PWI favors PCNSL over breast carcinoma metastasis, which is typically associated with increased rCBV.

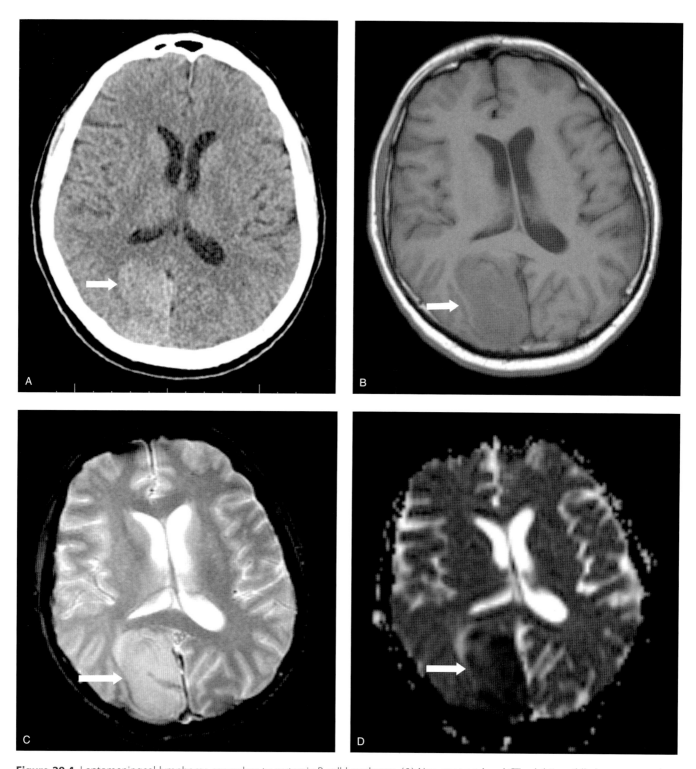

**Figure 29.4** Leptomeningeal lymphoma secondary to systemic B-cell lymphoma. (**A**) Non-contrast head CT exhibits mildly hyperattenuating right occipital mass (arrow). (**B**) T1-weighted axial MR image exhibits hypointense T1 signal mass (arrow). (**C**) T2-weighted axial MR image shows mildly hyperintense T2 signal right occipital mass (arrow). (**D**) ADC map exhibits diminished diffusion coefficient of the mass (arrow). (**E**) Post-contrast T1-weighted axial MR image exhibits patchy heterogeneous enhancement of the mass with gyriform pattern (arrow). (**F**) Post-contrast T1-weighted axial MR image at a high level exhibits enhancement within the leptomeninges (short arrows).

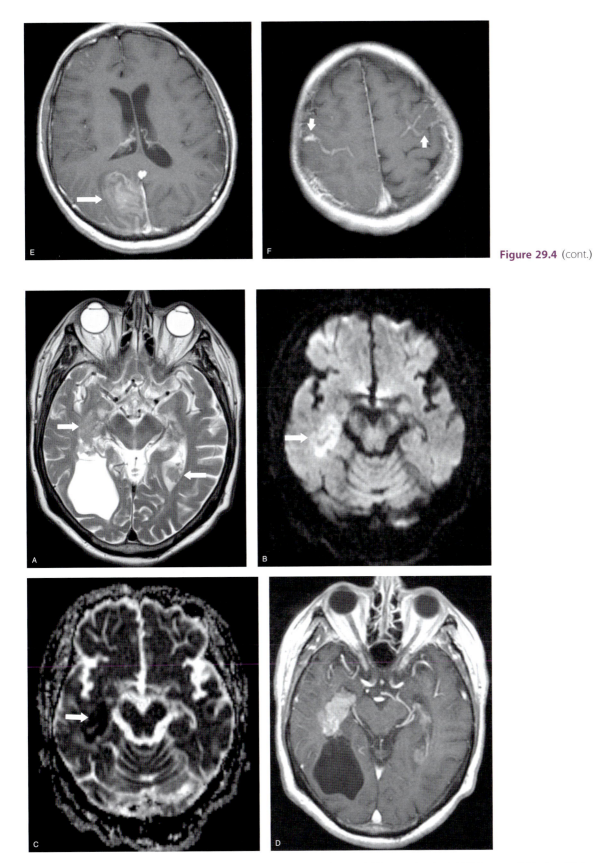

**Figure 29.4** (cont.)

**Figure 29.5** Intraventricular metastases from systemic B-cell lymphoma. (**A**) T2-weighted axial MR image exhibits low T2 signal nodular masses at bilateral lateral ventricles (arrow). (**B**, **C**) There is evidence for diffusion restriction and diminished diffusion coefficient of the visualized right temporal horn mass (arrow). (**D**) Post-contrast T1-weighted axial MR image exhibits intense post-contrast enhancement of the intraventricular masses.

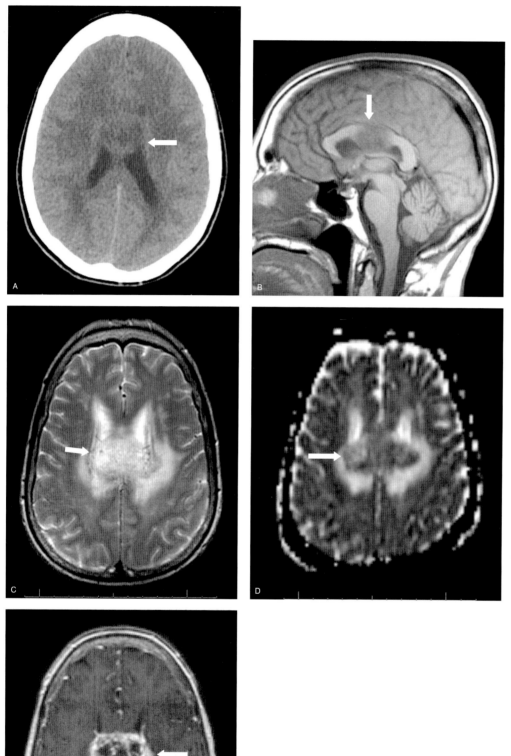

**Figure 29.6** Glioblastoma multiforme (GBM). (**A**) Non-contrast axial CT exhibits a heterogeneous expansile mass (arrow) at corpus callosum. (**B**) T1-weighted sagittal MR image exhibits expansile hypointense T1 signal mass at corpus callosum (arrow). (**C**) T2-weighted axial MR image exhibits heterogeneously high T2 signal mass involving the corpus callosum (arrow) with hyperintense T2 signal edema in the periventricular white matter. (**D**) ADC map exhibits diminished diffusion coefficient (arrow). (**E**) Post-contrast T1-weighted axial image exhibits irregular ring enhancement of the mass (arrow) with central non-enhancing necrotic component.

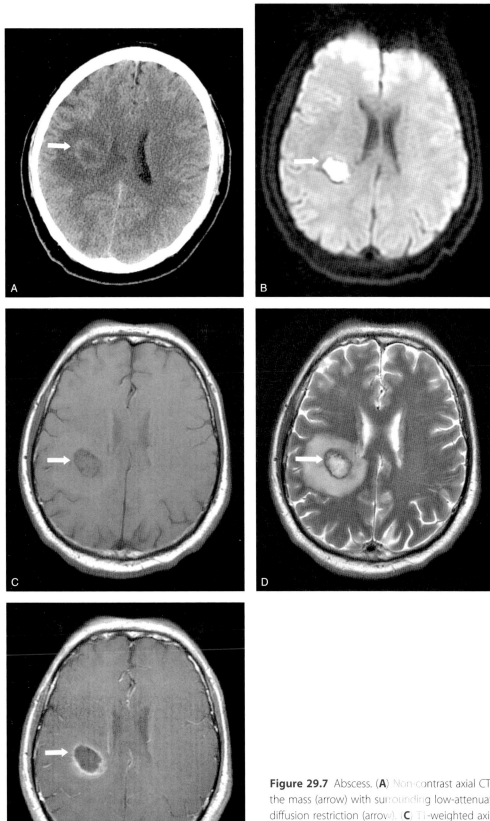

**Figure 29.7** Abscess. (**A**) Non-contrast axial CT exhibits mildly hyperdense capsule of the mass (arrow) with surrounding low-attenuating edema. (**B**) There is evidence for diffusion restriction (arrow). (**C**) T1-weighted axial MR image exhibits iso- to hypointense T1 signal central core of the mass (arrow). (**D**) T2-weighted axial MR image exhibits high T2 signal mass surrounded by irregular low T2 signal capsule (arrow). (**E**) Post-contrast T1-weighted axial MR image exhibits irregular rim enhancement of the right periventricular mass (arrow).

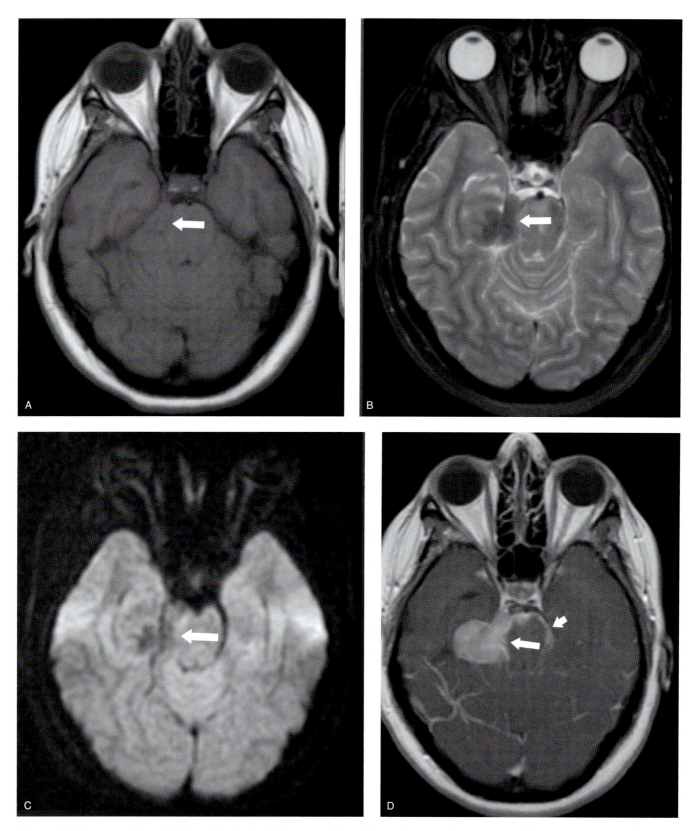

**Figure 29.8** Neurosarcoidosis. (**A**) T1-weighted axial MR image exhibits a lobulated extra-axial mass in the right prepontine cistern that is isointense to brain parenchyma (arrow). (**B**) T2-weighted axial MR image exhibits hypointense T2 signal of the mass (arrow). (**C**) There is no evidence for diffusion restriction within the mass (arrow). (**D**) Post-contrast T1-weighted axial MR image exhibits intense post-contrast enhancement of the extra-axial mass (arrow) as well as of the leptomeninges on the dorsal and left lateral surface of the pons (short arrow).

## Imaging description

The pineal gland develops as a diverticulum in the roof of the third ventricle between 4 and 8 weeks of gestational age. However, it is not redundant, like an appendix, and secretes melatonin, which controls diurnal rhythm [1]. Normally, it has a pinecone-like shape, measures about 8–10 mm, and does not have a blood–brain barrier, enhancing normally on post-contrast imaging. Histologically, lobules of pineocytes, which are specialized neurons, and a small amount of astrocytes, along with fibrovascular stroma, make up the normal gland.

Mass lesions of the pineal region make up less than 1% of intracranial masses in adults. However, in the pediatric age group they account for about 3–8% of intracranial neoplasms [2]. Tumors of pineal parenchymal origin account for about 14–27% of pineal masses [3] and include low-grade pineocytoma (Fig. 30.1), intermediate-grade pineal parenchymal tumor of intermediate differentiation (PPTID) (Fig. 30.2), and highly malignant pineoblastoma (Fig. 30.3).

Pineocytomas are more commonly found in adults, with an excellent (85–100%) 5-year survival rate following gross total resection. PPTID is a WHO grade II/III neoplasm that exhibits slight female preponderance, makes up at least 20% of all the pineal parenchymal tumors, peaks in early adulthood, and has a 5-year survival of 40–74% [4].

Pineoblastomas, embryonal primitive neuroectodermal tumors of the pineal gland, are highly malignant WHO grade IV lesions, accounting for 40% of pineal parenchymal tumors and most commonly occurring in the first two decades of life. Cerebrospinal fluid (CSF) dissemination is commonly seen and is the most common cause of death. Five-year survival is only 60%. Papillary tumor of the pineal region (PTPR) is a rare neuroepithelial neoplasm, arising from specialized ependymocytes in the pineal region, that occurs in both children and adults (Fig. 30.4).

## Importance

Mass lesions of the pineal region include a diverse group of entities, presenting with not hugely dissimilar clinical findings. The imaging appearance of pineal masses, in correlation with laboratory evaluation, helps to narrow down the differential diagnosis. Imaging is also useful to evaluate the extent of tumor infiltration into the surrounding brain parenchyma and to assess possible complications, including hydrocephalus and CSF dissemination.

## Typical clinical scenario

The most classic presentation of pineal region mass is Parinaud's syndrome, a complex mix of ophthalmological signs consisting of up-gaze palsy, pseudo-Argyll Robertson pupil, convergence retraction nystagmus, eyelid retraction, and conjugate down-gaze in primary position. It is also associated with blepharospasm, internuclear ophthalmoplegia, cranial nerve IV palsy, and bilateral papilledema. In case of a large mass obstructing the aqueduct of Sylvius, hydrocephalus with resulting headache, nausea, and vomiting due to increased intracranial pressure is common. Germ cell tumors (GCTs), which are more common in males, are also associated with precocious puberty.

## Differential diagnosis

GCTs (Fig. 30.5) are neoplastic derivatives of multipotent embryonic germ cells, and the commonest neoplasm of the pineal region, accounting for about 40–50% of all the pineal region tumors [4]. They are further classified into germinomatous and non-germinomatous GCTs, the latter including teratomas, yolk sac tumor, choriocarcinoma, and embryonal carcinoma.

Germinomas represent more than half of GCTs, and teratomas are the second most common. Ninety percent of patients present in the first two decades of life, with 3 times greater male preponderance in the pineal region [5]. Serum or CSF oncoproteins are high in GCTs. Synchronous pineal and suprasellar germinomas (Fig. 30.6) are found only in 5–10% of all the GCTs [6].

Pineal cysts (Fig. 30.7) are typically asymptomatic and generally 2–15 mm in size. They are mostly seen in adults, with incidence peaking in the fifth decade and a female predominance, and they remain stable in size over time [7]. The fluid in the cyst is proteinaceous and may contain hemorrhagic components (Fig. 30.8). Typically cysts >10 mm are followed up with imaging studies to document stability; however, it is very rare for a tumor to mimic a pineal cyst [8].

Many other neoplasms in the pineal region derive from the cell types in the vicinity. These include meningioma (Fig. 30.9), ependymoma, primitive neuroectodermal tumor (Fig. 30.10), choroid plexus tumors, metastatic lesions (Fig. 30.11), ganglioglioma, lipoma (Fig. 30.12), and epidermoid and dermoid cysts [3]. Astrocytomas in the pineal region commonly arise from tectal plate, corpus callosum, or thalamus, but rarely may arise from the neuronal elements within the pineal gland. Tectal gliomas (Fig. 30.13) are usually low-grade (pilocytic, WHO grade I or II), occur more frequently in childhood, and usually require only shunting for long-term survival [9]. However, close imaging follow-up is performed to ensure stability. Diffusely infiltrating WHO grade II–IV astrocytomas are also seen arising from neural elements of the pineal gland (Fig. 30.14).

## Teaching points

The pineal parenchymal neoplasms account for about 30% of all pineal tumors. GCTs account for 40% of all pineal neoplasms. Pineocytoma is more common in adults and has excellent prognosis. Pineoblastoma (with bad prognosis) and GCT (with relatively better prognosis) are more common in the first two decades of life and are associated with CSF dissemination. Pineocytoma and pineoblastoma exhibit exploding calcification at the periphery of the mass, while hyperattenuating germinoma engulfs a central area of calcification. Pineoblastoma, germinomas, and epidermoid may exhibit diffusion restriction. Pineal germinomas are three times more common in males than in females. Pineal cysts rarely mimic a tumor and do not require a follow-up if <10 mm in size or non-obstructive. Presence of lipid within a tiny mass is indicative of a teratoma, dermoid cyst, or lipoma. Tectal gliomas are generally low-grade astrocytomas and are not treated surgically. Fat saturation and gradient echo (GRE) sequences can help differentiate between lipid and hemorrhage.

REFERENCES

1. Preslock JP. The pineal gland: basic implications and clinical correlations. *Endocr Rev* 1984; **5**: 282–308.
2. Drummond KJ, Rosenfeld JV. Pineal region tumours in childhood: a 30-year experience. *Childs Nerv Syst* 1999; **15**: 119–26.
3. Smith AB, Rushing EJ, Smirniotopoulos JG. From the archives of the AFIP: lesions of the pineal region: radiologic–pathologic correlation. *Radiographics* 2010; **30**: 2001–20.
4. Srinivasan N, Pakala A, Mukkamalla C, Oswal A. Pineal germinoma. *South Med J* 2010; **103**: 1031–7.
5. Korogi Y, Takahashi M, Ushio Y. MRI of pineal region tumors. *J Neurooncol* 2001; **54**: 251–61.
6. Jennings M, Gelman R., Hochberg F. Intracranial germ-cell tumors: natural history and pathogenesis. *J Neurosurg* 1985; **63**: 155–67.
7. Cauley KA, Linnell GJ, Braff SP, Filippi CG. Serial follow-up MRI of indeterminate cystic lesions of the pineal region: experience at a rural tertiary care referral center. *AJR Am J Roentgenol* 2009; **193**: 533–7.
8. Pastel DA, Mamourian AC, Duhaime AC. Internal structure in pineal cysts on high-resolution magnetic resonance imaging: not a sign of malignancy. *J Neurosurg Pediatr* 2009; **4**: 81–4.
9. Dağlıoğlu E, Cataltepe O, Akalan N. Tectal gliomas in children: the implications for natural history and management strategy. *Pediatr Neurosurg* 2003; **38**: 223–31.

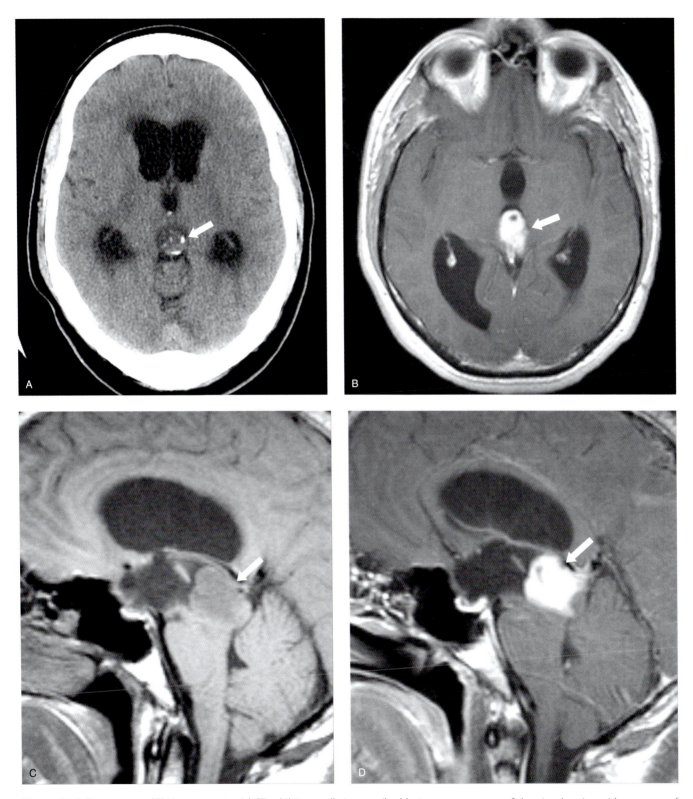

**Figure 30.1** Pineocytoma. (**A**) Non-contrast axial CT exhibits a well-circumscribed heterogeneous mass of the pineal region with presence of fragmented calcium along the periphery (arrow). Lateral ventricles are dilated due to obstructive hydrocephalus. (**B**) Post-contrast T1-weighted axial MR image exhibits intense enhancement of the pineal mass (arrow). (**C**) T1-weighted sagittal MR image exhibits a well-circumscribed mildly hypointense T1 signal pineal region mass (arrow) with marked enlargement of both the lateral and third ventricles. (**D**) Post-contrast T1-weighted sagittal MR image exhibits intense enhancement of the pineal mass (arrow) with hydrocephalus.

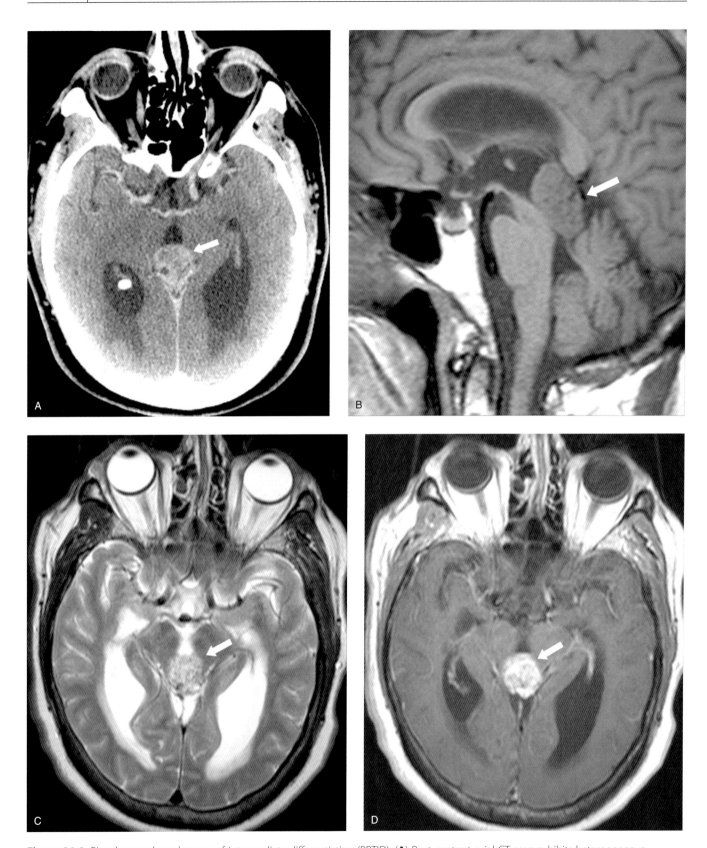

**Figure 30.2** Pineal parenchymal tumor of intermediate differentiation (PPTID). (**A**) Post-contrast axial CT scan exhibits heterogeneous contrast enhancement of the enlarged pineal gland (arrow) with obstructive hydrocephalus. (**B**) T1-weighted sagittal MR image exhibits a heterogeneously iso- to mildly hypointense T1 signal pineal mass (arrow). (**C**) T2-weighted axial MR image exhibits a hyperintense mass (arrow) involving the pineal region with hydrocephalus. (**D**) Post-contrast T1-weighted axial image exhibits intense enhancement of the mass (arrow).

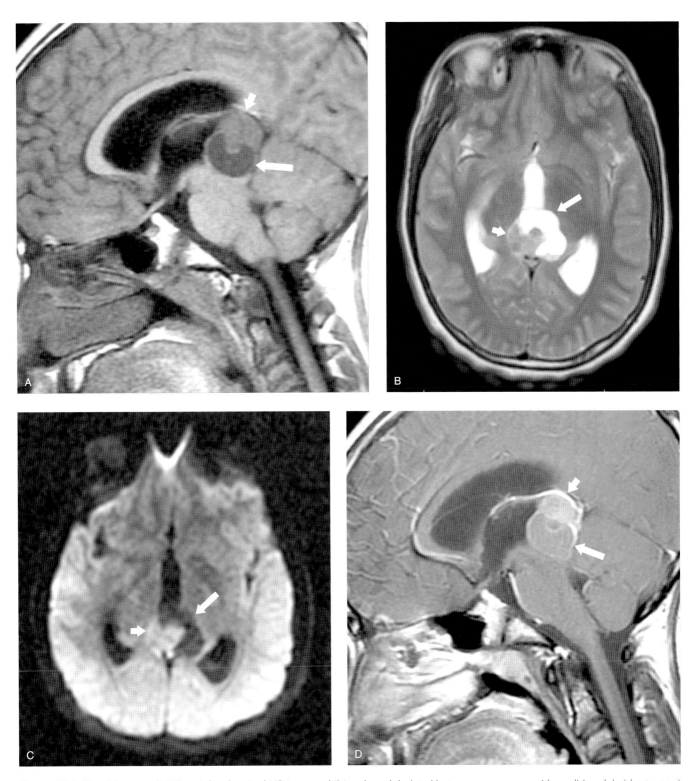

**Figure 30.3** Pineoblastoma. (**A**) T1-weighted sagittal MR image exhibits a large lobulated heterogeneous mass with a solid nodule (short arrow) and a cystic necrotic component (arrow). There is effacement of the aqueduct of Sylvius. Lack of hydrocephalus is due to previous placement of a ventriculostomy shunt. (**B**) T2-weighted axial MR image exhibits mildly hypointense heterogeneous solid nodule (short arrow) with a peripheral cystic component (arrow). (**C**) Diffusion-weighted MR image shows hyperintensity within the solid nodule (short arrow) with low signal of the cystic component (arrow). The nodule had low signal intensity on ADC map. (**D**) Post-contrast T1-weighted sagittal image exhibits intense enhancement of the solid nodule (short arrow) with peripheral enhancement of the cystic component (arrow).

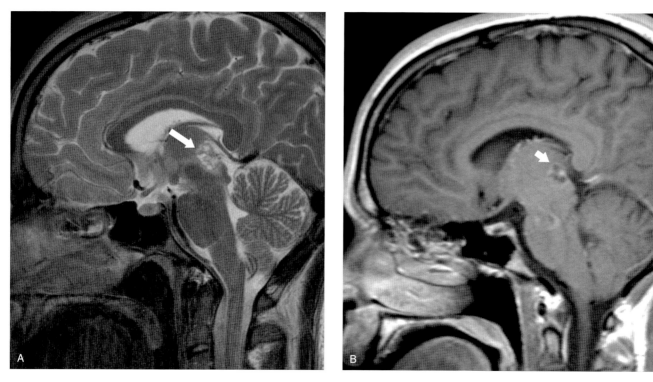

**Figure 30.4** Papillary tumor of the pineal region (PTPR). (**A**) T2-weighted sagittal MR image exhibits a heterogeneous, multicystic pineal mass (arrow). (**B**) Post-contrast T1-weighted sagittal MR image shows a small enhancing nodule with peripheral enhancement of the cystic mass (short arrow).

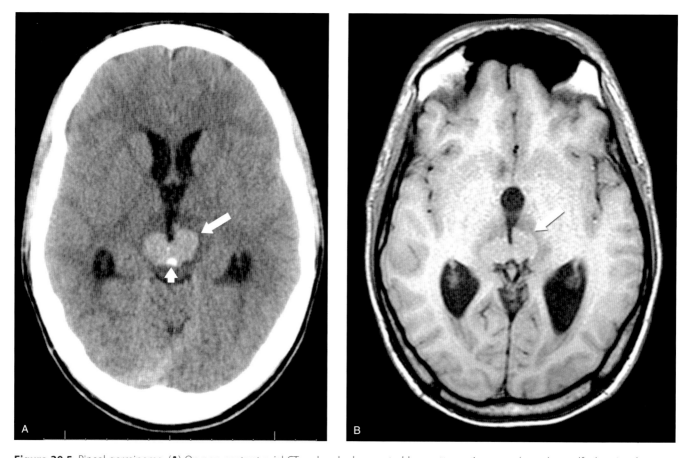

**Figure 30.5** Pineal germinoma. (**A**) On non-contrast axial CT, a sharply demarcated hyperattenuating mass (arrow) engulfs the pineal calcification (short arrow). (**B**) T1-weighted axial MR image exhibits infiltrating mildly high T1 signal mass (arrow) with surrounding edema.

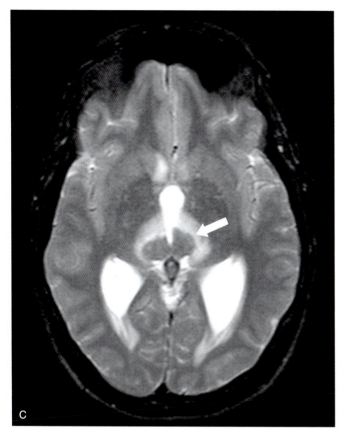

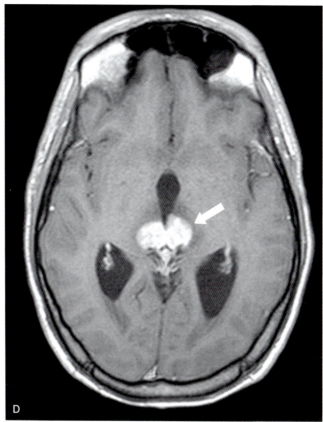

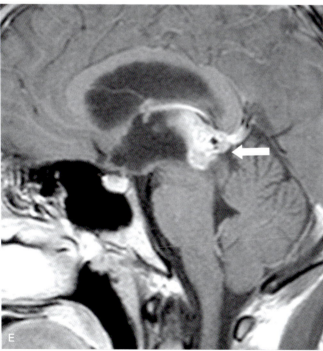

**Figure 30.5** (cont.) (**C**) T2-weighted axial MR image exhibits the low T2 signal infiltrating mass (arrow) with surrounding high T2 signal edema. (**D**, **E**) Post-contrast T1-weighted axial and sagittal imaging exhibits intense post-contrast enhancement of the pineal mass (arrow).

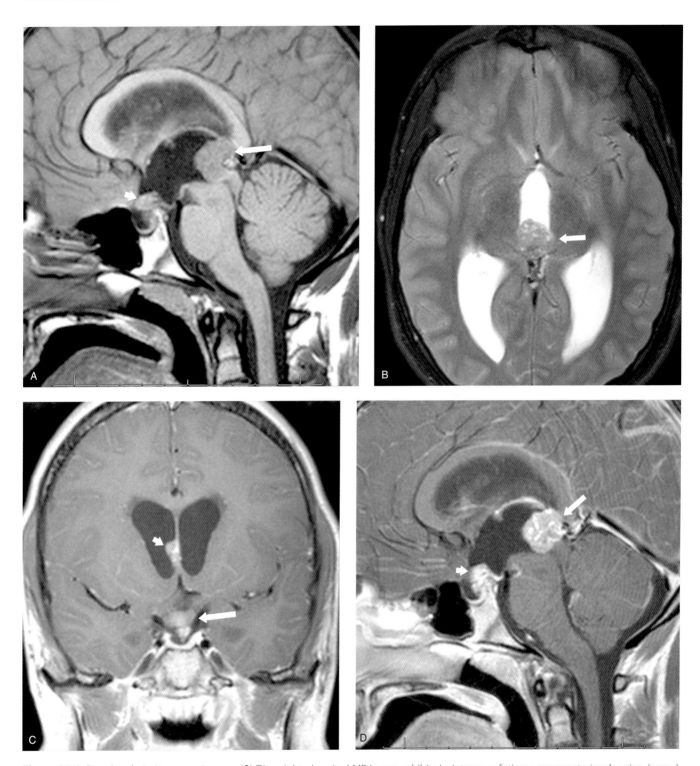

**Figure 30.6** Pineal and pituitary germinomas. (**A**) T1-weighted sagittal MR image exhibits isointense soft tissue masses at pineal region (arrow) and suprasellar region (short arrow) with marked hydrocephalus. (**B**) T2-weighted axial MR image exhibits iso- to mildly hypointense T2 signal of the pineal mass (arrow). (**C**) Post-contrast T1-weighted coronal MR image exhibits enhancing nodules at suprasellar region along the optic chiasm (arrow) and along the septum pellucidum (short arrow), likely due to CSF dissemination. (**D**) Post-contrast T1-weighted sagittal image exhibits intense patchy enhancement of the pineal (arrow) and suprasellar mass (short arrow).

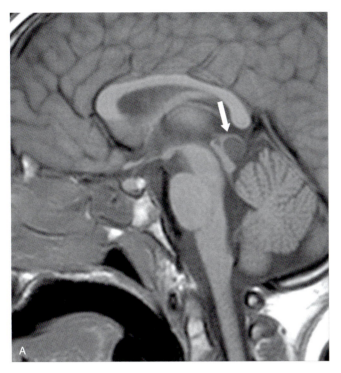

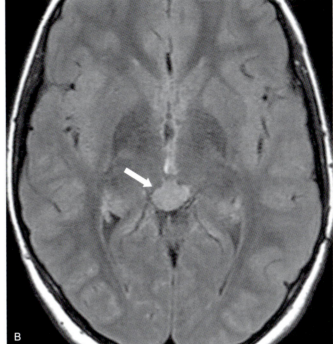

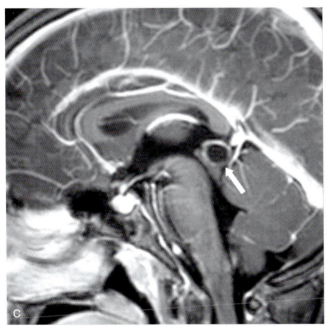

**Figure 30.7** Pineal cyst. (**A**) T1-weighted sagittal MR image exhibits small rounded low T1 signal pineal mass (arrow). (**B**) FLAIR-weighted axial MR image exhibits hyperintensity of the rounded lesion (arrow), likely due to proteinaceous content. (**C**) Post-contrast T1-weighted MR image exhibits peripheral capsular enhancement of the pineal cyst (arrow).

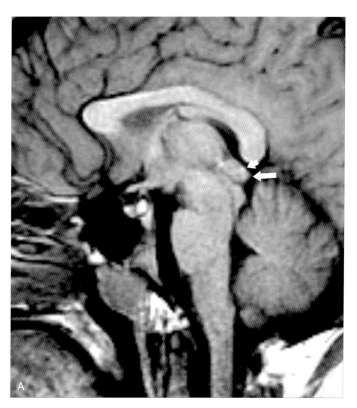

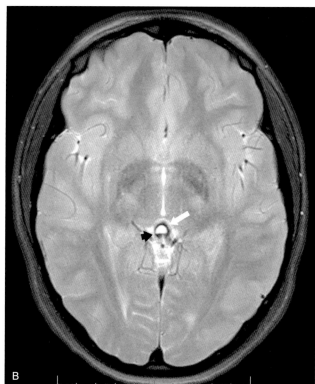

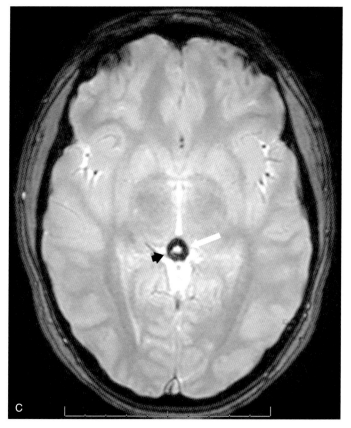

**Figure 30.8** Hemorrhage within pineal cyst. (**A**) T1-weighted sagittal MR image exhibits small iso to hypointense pineal mass (arrow) with a punctate area of high T1 signal (short arrow). (**B**) T2-weighted axial image exhibits a fluid level within the pineal cyst (white arrow) with low T2 signal at the dependent portion (short black arrow), likely hemorrhagic blood products. (**C**) Gradient echo T2*-weighted axial MR image exhibits blooming susceptibility of the capsule of the pineal cyst (white arrow), more posteriorly (short black arrow).

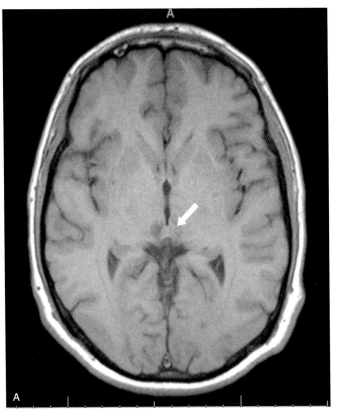

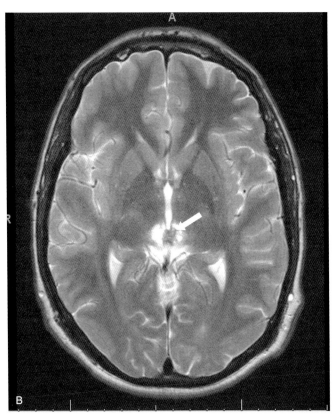

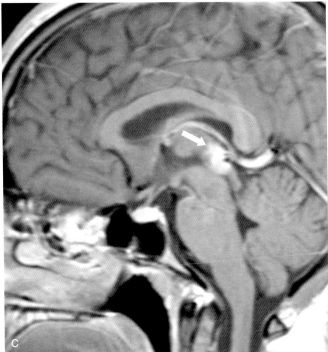

**Figure 30.9** Pineal meningioma. (**A**) T1-weighted axial MR image exhibits a small iso-T1 signal mass of the pineal gland (arrow). (**B**) T2-weighted axial MR image shows that the mass is isointense to brain parenchyma (arrow). (**C**) Post-contrast T1-weighted sagittal MR image exhibits intense enhancement of the small pineal mass (arrow).

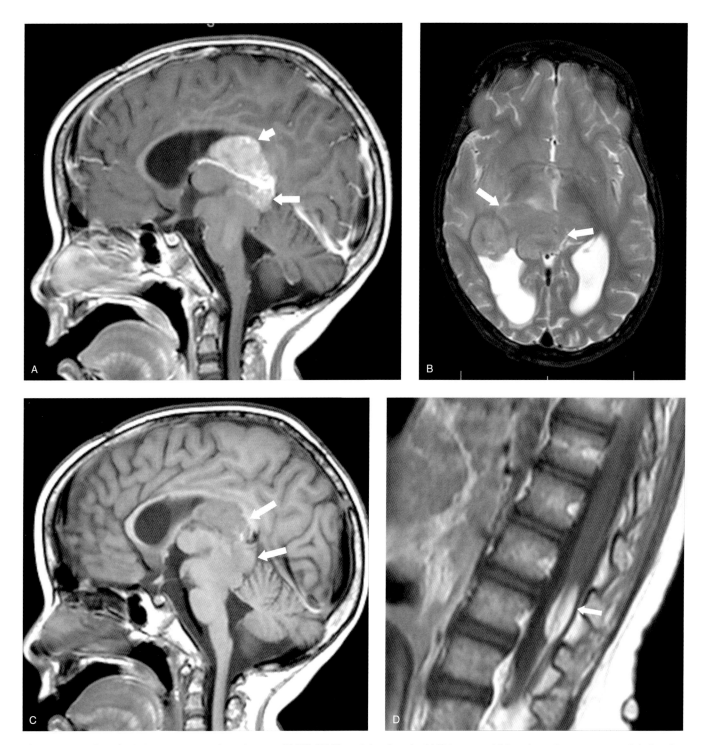

**Figure 30.10** Pineal primitive neuroectodermal tumor (PNET). (**A**) T1-weighted sagittal MR image exhibits a large heterogeneous lobulated mass iso- to hypointense to brain parenchyma at the pineal region (arrow), posterior third ventricle, and within the posterior part of the lateral ventricles (short arrow). (**B**) T2-weighted axial MR image exhibits large irregular low T2 signal mass at pineal region, infiltrating thalamus and seen within the right lateral ventricle (arrows). (**C**) Post-contrast T1-weighted sagittal image exhibits intense enhancement of the lobulated mass (arrows). (**D**) Post-contrast T1-weighted sagittal image exhibits an enhancing drop metastasis at the level of conus medullaris (arrow).

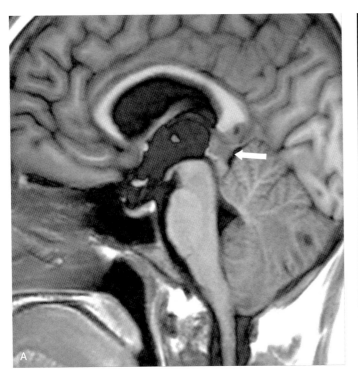

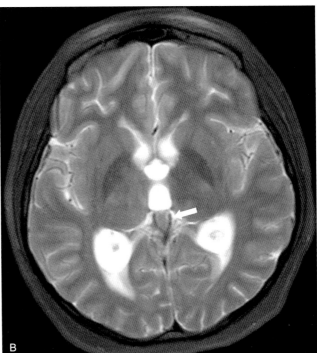

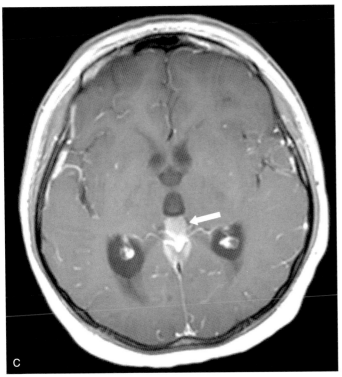

**Figure 30.11** Metastatic chloroma of pineal region in a patient with acute lymphoblastic leukemia (ALL). (**A**) T1-weighted sagittal MR image exhibits iso- to hypointense T1 signal mass at the pineal region (arrow). (**B**) T2-weighted axial MR image shows that the mass is iso- to hypointense to brain parenchyma (arrow). (**C**) Post-contrast T1-weighted axial image shows intense enhancement of the pineal mass (arrow).

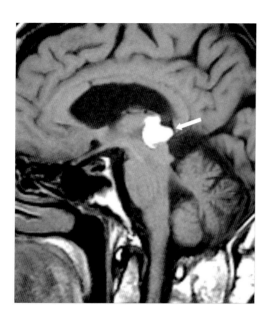

**Figure 30.12** Pineal lipoma. T1-weighted sagittal MR image exhibits irregular lobulated high T1 signal mass at the pineal region (arrow).

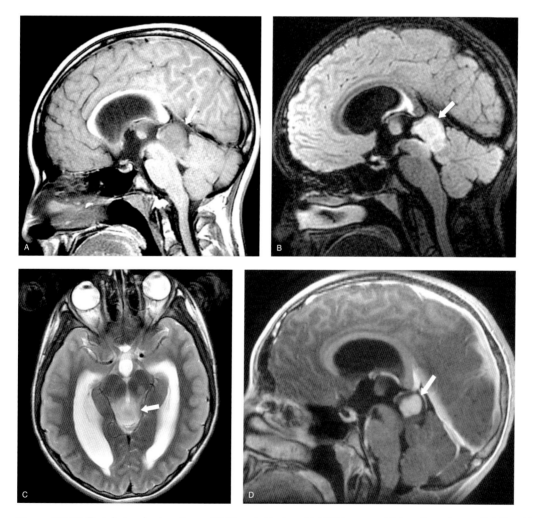

**Figure 30.13** Tectal pineal astrocytoma. (**A**) T1-weighted sagittal MR image exhibits a large but well-defined hypointense mass (arrow) at the pineal region and tectal plate with resultant aqueduct stenosis and hydrocephalus. (**B**) FLAIR-weighted sagittal MR image exhibits hyperintense signal of the large lobulated mass (arrow) causing aqueduct stenosis. (**C**) T2-weighted axial MR image exhibits hyperintense T2 signal mass (arrow) at the region of tectum with aqueduct stenosis and hydrocephalus. (**D**) Post-contrast T1-weighted sagittal MR image exhibits intense post-contrast enhancement of the mass (arrow).

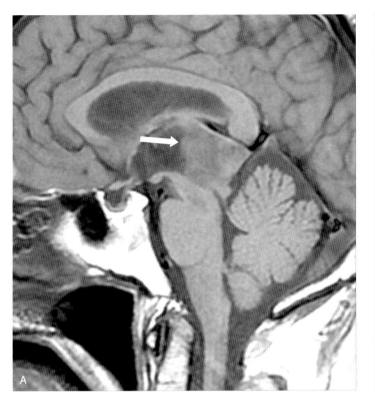

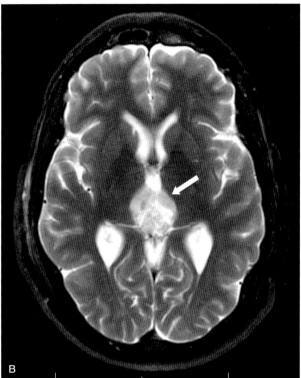

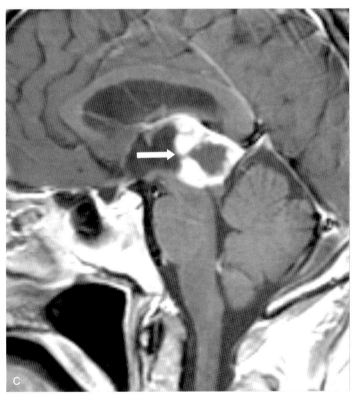

**Figure 30.14** Pineal GBM. (**A**) T1-weighted sagittal MR image exhibits an irregular expansile hypointense mass (arrow) at pineal region. (**B**) T2-weighted axial MR image exhibits a heterogeneous infiltrating mass (arrow) at the pineal region. (**C**) Post-contrast T1-weighted sagittal MR image exhibits shaggy peripheral rim enhancement of the mass (arrow).

## Imaging description

Intraventricular tumors (IVTs) have diverse demographics and histogenesis. Ependymomas (Fig. 31.1) and choroid plexus tumors (Figs. 31.2, 31.3) are relatively common entities, particularly in the pediatric group, and should be considered first in the differential diagnosis. Although considered to be prototypical IVTs, subependymomas and neurocytomas (Fig. 31.4) are actually much less common than meningiomas (Fig. 31.5) and metastases (Fig. 31.6). Chordoid glioma of the third ventricle and rosette-forming glioneural tumor of the fourth ventricle are unique IVTs, although they are much less common than astrocytomas, oligigodendrogliomas, and glioblastomas (Figs. 31.7, 31.8). Lateral ventricular neoplasms account for 50% of all intraventricular tumors in adults and 25% in children.

Although these neoplasms are easily detected with CT and MRI, both techniques are relatively non-specific in identifying the type of tumor [1]. Per anatomic location, supratentorial intraventricular masses can be classified into ependymal, subependymal, choroid plexus, parenchymal, septum pellucidum, foramen of Monro, third ventricular, or aqueductal in origin. Infratentorial intraventricular masses can be ependymal, subependymal, vermian, cerebellar, or choroid plexus in origin. Correlation of demographic, clinical, and imaging features of IVTs allows creating a comprehensive differential diagnosis [2].

Most ependymomas will occur in the fourth ventricle. When supratentorial in location, intraventricular ependymomas are less common than parenchymal ependymomas. They are associated with calcifications or cyst formation in 50% of the cases and hemorrhage in about 10% [2]. They are associated with high incidence of incomplete tumor resection and permanent neurological complications associated with their removal [3].

Choroid plexus papillomas occur most frequently in the lateral and fourth ventricles. They avidly enhance and demonstrate frond-like borders. Choroid plexus carcinomas may be very similar in appearance to papillomas; peritumoral edema favors carcinoma over papilloma, however.

Intraventricular meningiomas can be clinically classified as spontaneously arising meningiomas (SAM), neurofibromatosis-2-associated meningiomas (NF2-M), and radiation-induced meningiomas (RIM) [4]. A majority of intraventricular meningiomas are located in trigone, arising from the stroma of the choroid plexus or from the tela choroidea with 2:1 female preponderance [5]. Central neurocytoma is a rare intraventricular benign neoplasm with prominent neuronal differentiation affecting young adults within the lateral ventricles near the foramen of Monro [6]. Typically, it has a favorable prognosis after adequate surgical intervention [7], but calcifications or

adhesions can affect gross total resection, in which case radiotherapy or radiosurgery can be chosen as a salvage treatment in case of recurrence [8].

## Importance

Radiological diagnosis has a great bearing on further treatment planning. Endoscopic intraventricular surgery is increasingly employed as a minimally invasive alternative to open transcranial surgery for specific ventricular tumors [9]. A solid tumor <2cm in size and a cystic lesion with even larger size can be surgically removed endoscopically [10]. Detailed radiological evaluation of possible calcification, adhesions, cyst formation, and vascularity help in planning the type of surgery. Dynamic susceptibility contrast-enhanced MRI (DSC-MRI) of intraventricular tumors can provide additional information on the vascularization of intraventricular masses and help in differential diagnosis [11]. Poorly vascularized tumors include ependymoma and subependymoma, intermediately vascularized tumors include central neurocytoma and lung metastasis, while highly vascularized tumors include choroid plexus papilloma, carcinoma, meningioma, and renal carcinoma metastasis [11].

## Typical clinical scenario

The spectrum of clinical presentation varies widely according to the underlying etiology. However, the commonest complication of an intraventricular mass is focal dilatation of ventricles around the mass with possible intraventricular obstructive hydrocephalus. In that case, signs of increased intracranial pressure such as nausea, vomiting, headaches, visual disturbances, and papilledema are common. It can occur at any age, from neonatal to elderly populations.

## Differential diagnosis

A choroid plexus cyst (Fig. 31.9) with or without prior hemorrhage or xanthogranulomatous change is the most common intraventricular mass, without any clinical significance. It is a common incidental finding in older patients with about 40% prevalence. Between 3% and 11% of cases of intracranial cavernous hemangioma (Fig. 31.10) are intraventricular, and they generally arise from the subependymal region or septum pellucidum [12]. Presence of calcification and a hemosiderin rim are common findings. Both primary CNS lymphoma (PCNSL) and intracranial metastasis of systemic lymphoma can involve the corpus callosum and extend into the ventricles along the ependymal surfaces (Fig. 31.11). Infectious conditions such as neurocysticercosis can also present as intraventricular cystic mass. Anterior third ventricular masses include pituitary macroadenomas with suprasellar extension and craniopharyngiomas (Fig. 31.12).

## Teaching points

Meningiomas, metastases, and even astrocytomas and oligodendrogliomas should be considered in the differential diagnosis of intraventricular masses, in addition to more prototypical tumors such as ependymomas, subependymomas, choroid plexus tumors, and neurocytomas.

REFERENCES

1. Delmaire C, Boulanger T, Leroy HA, *et al.* Imaging of lateral ventricle tumors. *Neurochirurgie* 2011; **57**: 180–92.

2. Fenchel M, Beschorner R, Naegele T, *et al.* Primarily solid intraventricular brain tumors. *Eur J Radiol* 2012; **81**: e688–96.

3. Nowak A, Marchel A. Surgical treatment of intraventricular ependymomas and subependymomas. *Neurol Neurochir Pol* 2012; **46**: 333–43.

4. Pinto PS, Huisman TA, Ahn E, *et al.* Magnetic resonance imaging features of meningiomas in children and young adults: a retrospective analysis. *J Neuroradiol* 2012; **39**: 218–26.

5. Bertalanffy A, Roessler K, Koperek O, *et al.* Intraventricular meningiomas: a report of 16 cases. *Neurosurg Rev* 2006; **29**: 30–5.

6. Chen H, Zhou R, Liu J, Tang J. Central neurocytoma. *J Clin Neurosci* 2012; **19**: 849–53.

7. Chen CL, Shen CC, Wang J, *et al.* Central neurocytoma: a clinical, radiological and pathological study of nine cases. *Clin Neurol Neurosurg* 2008; **110**: 129–36.

8. Qian H, Lin S, Zhang M, Cao Y. Surgical management of intraventricular central neurocytoma: 92 cases. *Acta Neurochir (Wien)* 2012; **154**: 1951–60.

9. Qiao L, Souweidane MM. Purely endoscopic removal of intraventricular brain tumors: a consensus opinion and update. *Minim Invasive Neurosurg* 2011; **54**: 149–54.

10. Schroeder HW. Intraventricular tumors. *World Neurosurg* 2013; **79**(2 Suppl): S17.e15–19.

11. Holveck A, Grand S, Boini S, *et al.* Dynamic susceptibility contrast-enhanced MRI evaluation of cerebral intraventricular tumors: preliminary results. *J Neuroradiol* 2010; **37**: 269–75.

12. Kasliwal MK, Sharma BS. Giant intraventricular mass arising from the septum pellucidum. Cavernoma. *J Clin Neurosci* 2011; **18**: 1108, 1145.

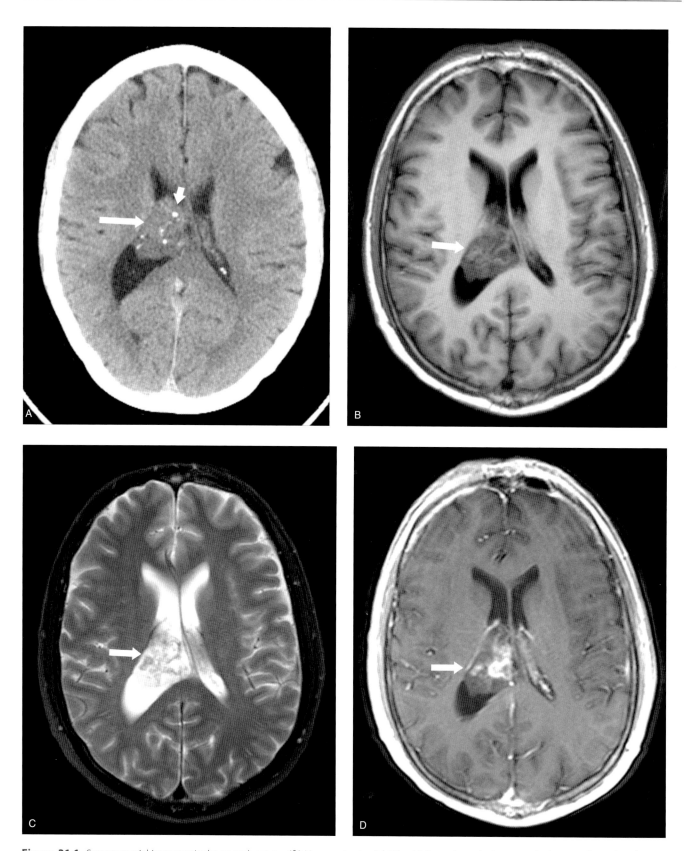

**Figure 31.1** Supratentorial intraventricular ependymoma. (**A**) Non-contrast axial CT exhibits an irregular intraventricular mass (arrow) with areas of calcification (short arrow) and expansion of right lateral ventricle. (**B**) T1-weighted axial MR image exhibits a heterogeneous hypo- to isointense T1 signal mass within the lateral ventricle (arrow). (**C**) T2-weighted axial MR image exhibits heterogeneous hypo- to hyperintense T2 signal intraventricular mass (arrow). (**D**) Post-contrast T1-weighted axial MR image exhibits heterogeneous patchy enhancement of the mass (arrow).

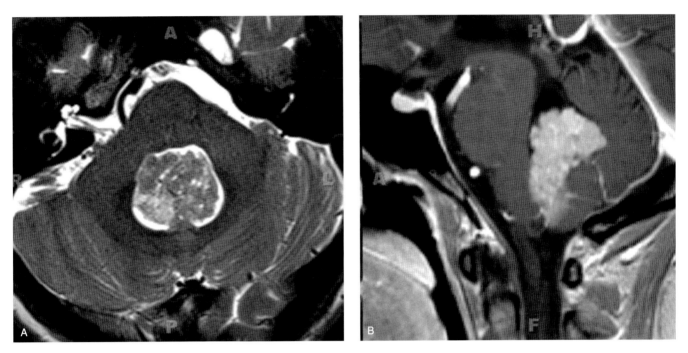

**Figure 31.2** Choroid plexus papilloma. (**A**) Axial T2-weighted image shows a well-defined intraventricular mass with mixed signal intensity. (**B**) Sagittal post-contrast T1-weighted image shows avid enhancement of the mass, which has a frond-like contour.

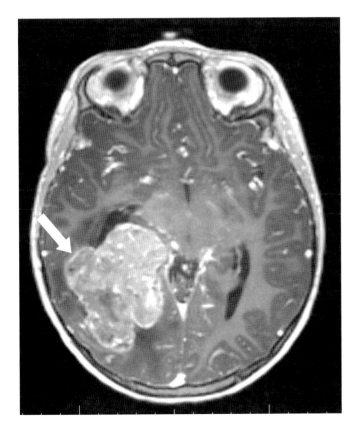

**Figure 31.3** Choroid plexus carcinoma. A large lobulated intensely and heterogeneously enhancing choroid plexus mass within the right atrium (arrow) also infiltrates the surrounding brain parenchyma.

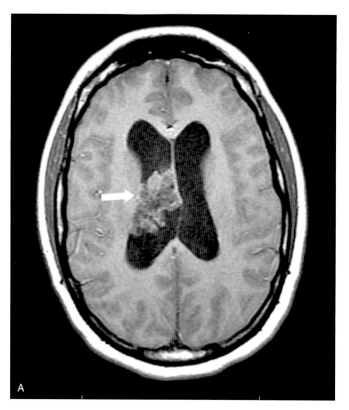

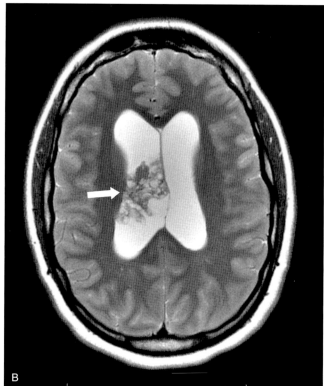

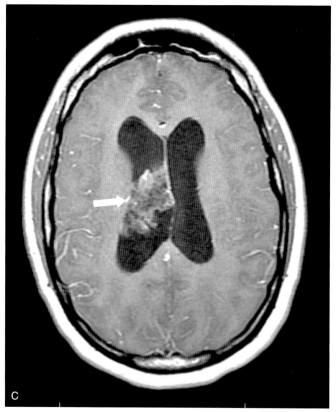

**Figure 31.4** Central neurocytoma. (**A**) T1-weighted axial MR image exhibits a heterogeneous hypointense to marginally hyperintense T1 signal mass within the right lateral ventricle (arrow) extending from septum pellucidum to subependymal region. (**B**) T2-weighted axial MR image exhibits multiple rounded cystic areas within the heterogeneous mass (arrow). (**C**) Post-contrast T1-weighted axial MR image exhibits patchy post-contrast enhancement of the heterogeneous mass (arrow).

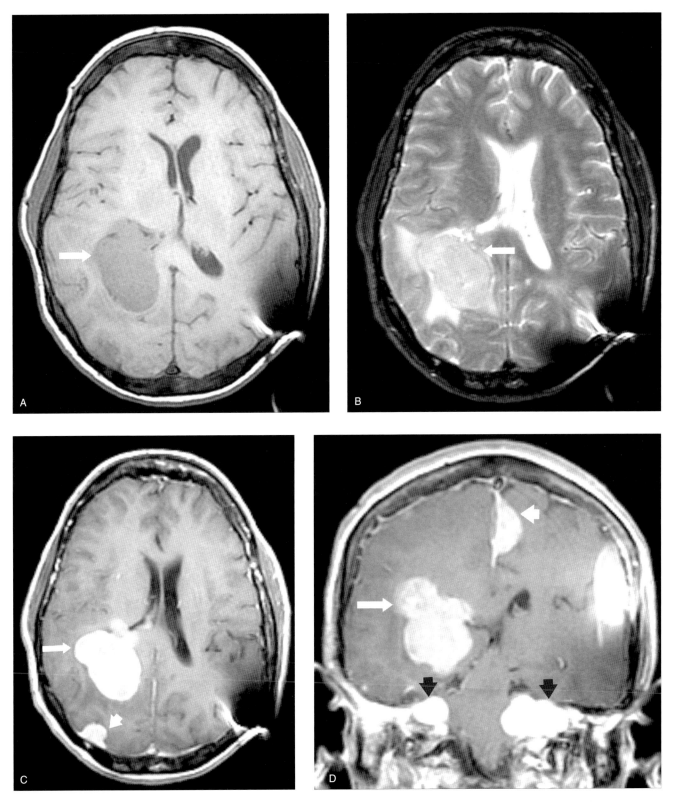

**Figure 31.5** NF2-associated intraventricular meningioma. (**A**) T1-weighted axial MR image exhibits a lobulated mass (arrow) isointense to gray matter expanding the right atrium. (**B**) T2-weighted axial MR image exhibits the mass (arrow) to be isointense to gray matter, with presence of periventricular high T2 signal due to transependymal CSF migration caused by focal obstruction at right atrium. (**C**) Post-contrast T1-weighted axial MR image exhibits intense enhancement of the mass (arrow) with presence of an enhancing dural-based meningioma (short arrow). (**D**) Post-contrast T1-weighted coronal MR image exhibits large lobulated intraventricular mass (white arrow) with a lobulated parafalcine meningioma (short white arrow) and bilateral vestibular schwannomas (short black arrows).

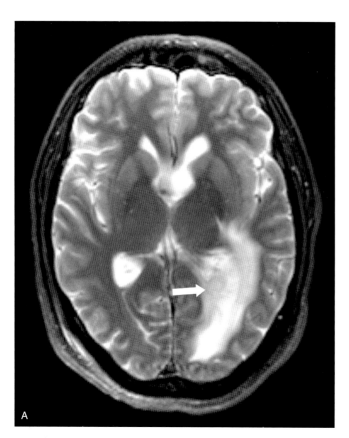
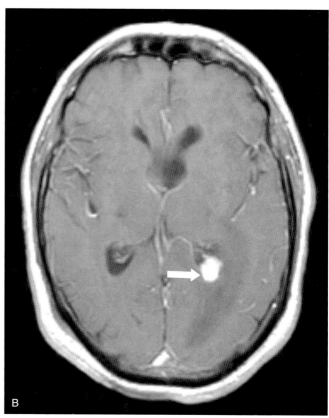

**Figure 31.6** Metastatic renal cell carcinoma to choroid plexus. (**A**) T2-weighted axial MR image exhibits an irregular hyperintense T2 signal mass (arrow) at left atrium with a large amount of surrounding parenchymal edema in a patient with known metastatic renal cell carcinoma. (**B**) Post-contrast T1-weighted axial MR image exhibits intense enhancement of left choroid plexus nodular mass (arrow).

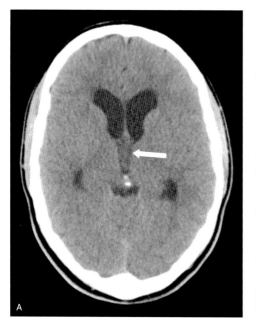
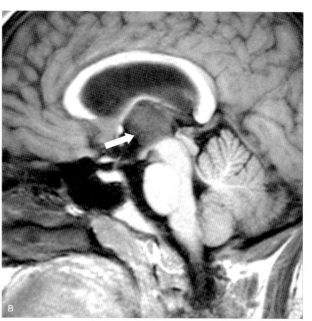

**Figure 31.7** Third ventricular oligoastrocytoma. (**A**) Non-contrast axial CT exhibits low-attenuating soft tissue mass (arrow) within the anterior third ventricle. (**B**) T1-weighted sagittal MR image exhibits an expansile hypointense T1 signal mass (arrow) within the third ventricle. (**C**) FLAIR-weighted axial MR image exhibits hyperintense FLAIR signal of the lobulated mass (arrow). (**D**) T2-weighted axial MR image exhibits hyperintense T2 signal expansile mass (arrow) within the anterior third ventricle. (**E**) Post-contrast T1-weighted axial MR image exhibits mild patchy enhancement of the mass (arrow).

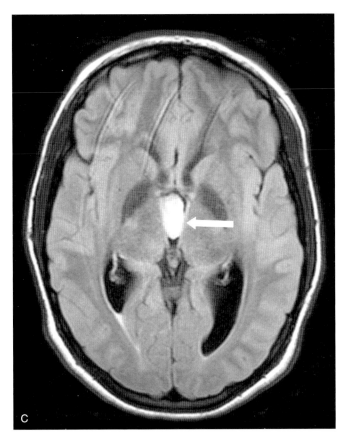

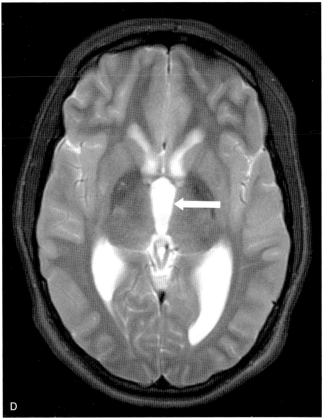

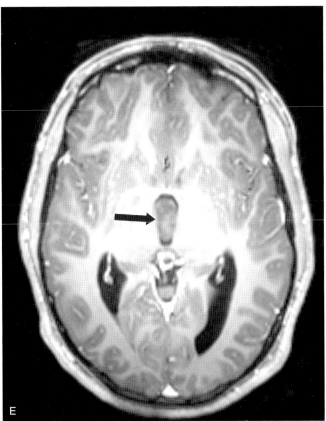

**Figure 31.7** (cont.)

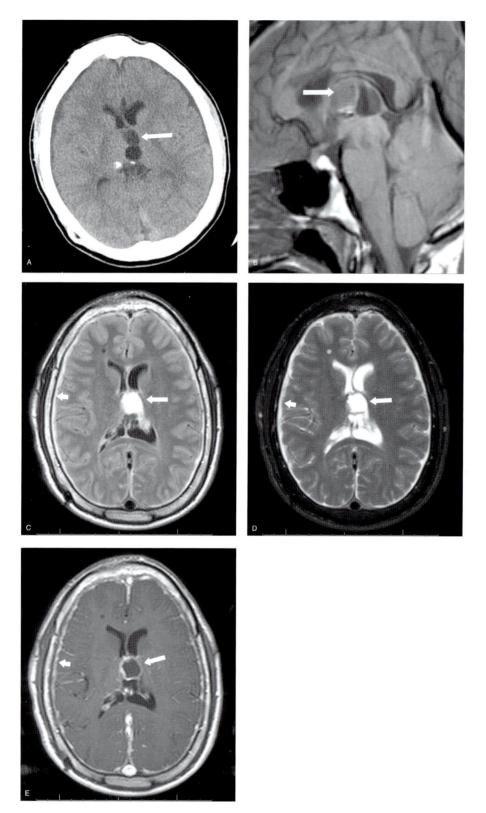

**Figure 31.8** Third ventricular ganglioglioma. (**A**) Non-contrast axial CT exhibits a cystic mass within the anterior third ventricle (arrow). (**B**) T1-weighted sagittal MR image exhibits intermediate T1 signal rounded mass within anterior third ventricle (arrow). (**C**) FLAIR-weighted axial imaging exhibits high signal within the rounded mass due to proteinaceous content (arrow). Note high FLAIR signal pachymeningeal thickening (short arrow), likely due to long-standing ventriculostomy shunt. (**D**) T2-weighted axial MR image exhibits rounded cystic mass within anterior third ventricle (arrow) with pachymeningeal thickening (short arrow). (**E**) Post-contrast T1-weighted axial MR image exhibits peripheral ring-enhancing anterior third ventricular cystic mass (arrow) with enhancing pachymeningitis (short arrow).

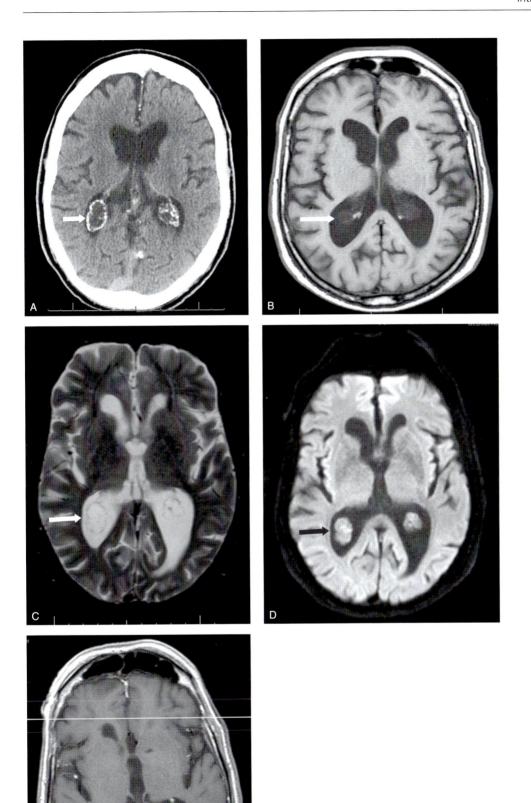

**Figure 31.9** Choroid plexus cyst. (**A**) Non-contrast axial CT exhibits rounded enlargement of bilateral choroid plexus with calcific rim (arrow). (**B**) T1-weighted axial MR image exhibits rounded hypointense T1 signal choroid plexus cysts (arrow). (**C**) T2-weighted axial MR image exhibits thin hypointense rim of the choroid plexus cyst (arrow). (**D**) High signal within the mass (arrow) on diffusion-weighted images is likely due to xanthogranulomatous changes. (**E**) Post-contrast T1-weighted axial MR imaging exhibits faint enhancement of the capsule of the choroid plexus cyst (arrow).

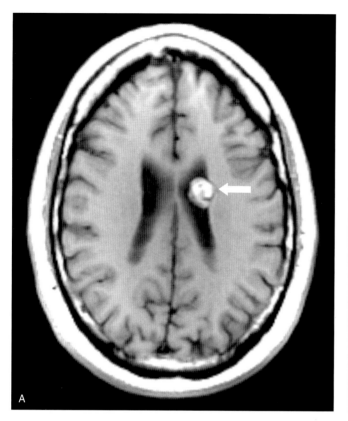

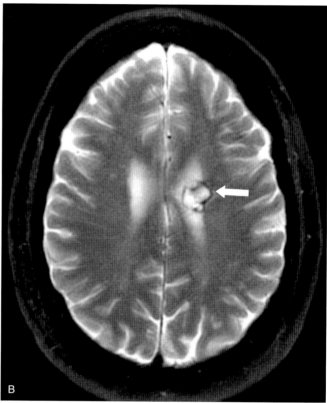

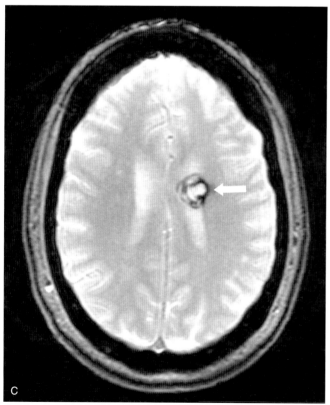

**Figure 31.10** Intraventricular cavernous hemangioma. (**A**) T1-weighted axial MR image exhibits a lobulated hyperintense T1 signal subependymal mass with low T1 signal hemosiderin rim (arrow). (**B**) T2-weighted axial MR image exhibits irregular hyperintense T2 signal mass with low T2 signal hemosiderin rim (arrow). (**C**) Gradient echo T2*-weighted axial MR image exhibits enhanced susceptibility of the hemosiderin rim (arrow).

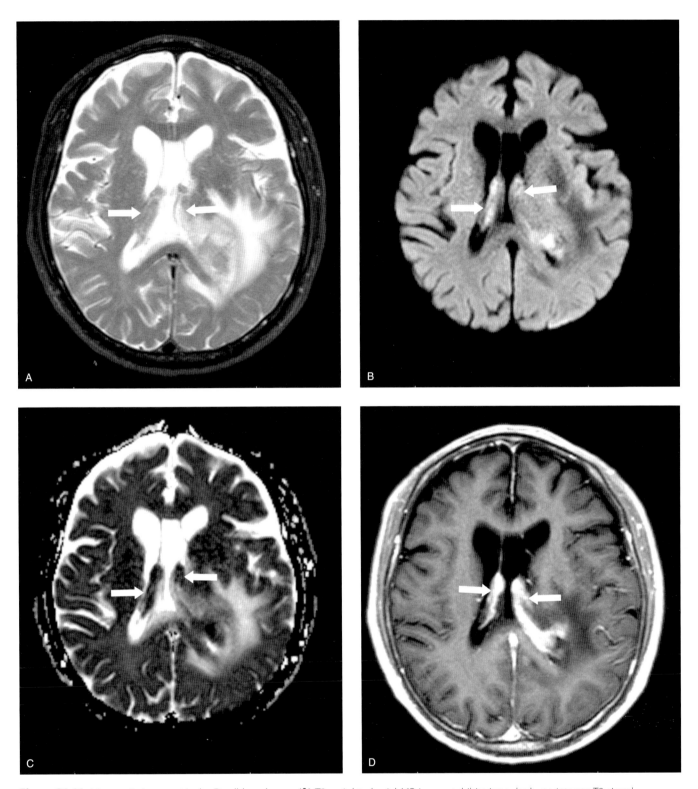

**Figure 31.11** Metastatic intraventricular B-cell lymphoma. (**A**) T2-weighted axial MR image exhibits irregular hyperintense T2 signal intraventricular masses (arrows) along the choroid plexus bilaterally with white matter edema at left cerebral hemisphere likely due to ependymal and parenchymal infiltration in a patient with known B-cell lymphoma. (**B**) Restricted diffusion of the masses (arrows) is seen on diffusion-weighted images. (**C**) Diminished diffusion coefficient of the masses (arrows) is seen on ADC map. (**D**) Post-contrast T1-weighted axial MR image exhibits intense patchy post-contrast enhancement (arrows).

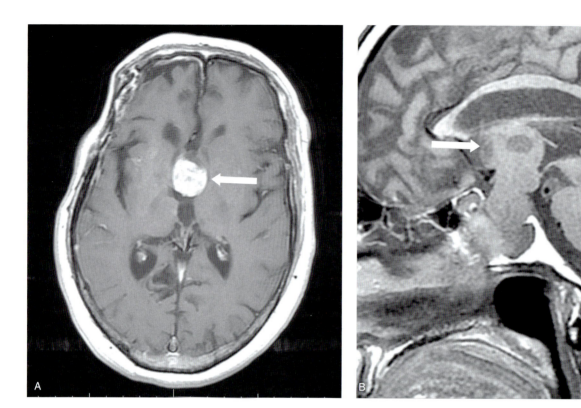

**Figure 31.12** Pituitary macroadenoma. (**A**) Post-contrast T1-weighted axial MR image exhibits an intensely enhancing lobulated mass (arrow) at the region of foramen of Monro. (**B**) T1-weighted sagittal MR image exhibits a large lobulated sellar mass with suprasellar extension (arrow) extending into third ventricle and reaching up to the foramina of Monro.

## Imaging description

Colloid cysts are congenital intracranial masses, derived from embryonic foregut, with an outer fibrous capsule and inner single-layer mucin-producing epithelium, containing mucoid and gelatinous material [1]. They are classically located in the anterior third ventricle, posterior and inferior to the crus of the fornix, which wraps around the cyst. Because of their unique location, they have the potential to impede the flow of CSF at the foramen of Monro, causing obstructive hydrocephalus [1,2].

On CT scan, colloid cysts are seen as oval or rounded anterior third ventricular masses measuring 1 mm to 3 cm. They may be hyperdense (Figs. 32.1A, 32.2A, 32.5A), isodense (Fig. 32.3A), or hypodense (Fig. 32.4A), depending on hydration state and proteinaceous content [3,4]. However, up to two-thirds display mild to moderate hyperdensity. On T1-weighted MR imaging, the colloid cyst may be isointense (Fig. 32.2B) or hypointense (Fig. 32.3B), but up to two-thirds appear to be hyperintense (Figs. 32.1B, 32.5B). On T2-weighted MR imaging, there may be hypointense (Figs. 32.1C, 32.2C) or hyperintense (Fig. 32.3C) [3,4]. On post-contrast imaging, there may be mild patchy enhancement of the capsule of the colloid cyst, but the content of the cyst does not exhibit any significant enhancement (Fig. 32.3B). When it is associated with cyst apoplexy, a part of the cyst may appear hyperdense on CT scan and hyperintense on T1-weighted MR imaging (Fig. 32.4A), and may be associated with rapid clinical deterioration [5]. A double density appearance of colloid cyst on CT and MRI due to different consistency of proteinaceous content is also described (Fig. 32.4) [6].

## Importance

Apart from the classic location in the anterior third ventricle, colloid cysts can be seen elsewhere in the brain. They are variously reported in the posterior third ventricle (Fig. 32.5), fourth ventricle [7], cavum interpositum [8], sella turcica, and within the lateral ventricle. It is not a neoplastic process, and considered a benign entity. However, because of its strategic location, it can result in sudden hydrocephalus and brain herniation with adverse clinical outcome. Even in the absence of hydrocephalus, it can be associated with diffuse myocardial injury leading to sudden death [1]. This may be secondary to direct stimulation by the cyst of hypothalamic structures, which play a key role in neuroendocrine and autonomic cardiovascular control. The preferred treatment is surgical resection with a transcallosal transforaminal approach [9]. However, the newer neuroendoscopic technique is associated with decreased morbidity and complications [10].

## Typical clinical scenario

Colloid cysts are more commonly detected in adults, peaking in the third and fourth decades of life. Up to 50% of patients with colloid cysts are asymptomatic, with incidental discovery on imaging of brain performed due to other indications. In the rest, headache is the most common manifestation. Nausea, vomiting, visual disturbance, ataxia, and syncope are also reported. In rare cases, rapid clinical deterioration due to onset of hydrocephalus with acute obstruction at foramina of Monro can lead to transtentorial herniation and death [2]. Sudden death even without hydrocephalus, likely due to direct stimulation of hypothalamus, is reported [1].

## Differential diagnosis

Presence of hemorrhage within the cyst can lead to variable appearance on CT and MR imaging with mixed density and heterogeneous T1 and T2 intensities (Fig. 32.4). Apart from the anterior third ventricle, atypical locations of colloid cyst such as posterior third ventricle (Fig. 32.5), cavum interpositum, sella turcica, and fourth ventricle should also be considered. Subependymal giant cell astrocytoma (SEGA) occurs in up to 15% of individuals with tuberous sclerosis complex, but is more likely to occur during childhood or adolescence (Fig. 32.6). They are slow-growing intraventricular neoplasms generally discovered near the foramen of Monro with heterogeneously low T1 and high T2 signal, and they exhibit patchy and variable post-contrast enhancement. However, they are more likely to be within the lateral ventricle. Central neurocytoma can present as non-enhancing heterogeneously iso- to hyperintense T1 signal midline mass with iso- to hyperintense T2 signal (Fig. 32.7). However, it is more likely seen with relation to the septum pellucidum and more often seen within the fourth ventricle than the third.

## Teaching points

Colloid cysts, localized characteristically in the anterior third ventricle, are easier to visualize on CT than MRI, when they are hyperattenuating, although they demonstrate variable CT attenuation and MRI signal. It may be useful to perform CT when findings on MRI are equivocal, and vice versa. One must keep in mind the possible unusual locations and complications such as hemorrhage, calcification, rupture, and meningitis. Progressive enlargement or spontaneous regression of a colloid cyst is possible [12]. Given the possibility of sudden deterioration and unpredictable outcomes, it is important to promptly communicate the finding of colloid cyst, even when incidental, to the referring physician.

REFERENCES

1. Turillazzi E, Bello S, Neri M, Riezzo I, Fineschi V. Colloid cyst of the third ventricle, hypothalamus, and heart: a dangerous link for sudden death. *Diagn Pathol* 2012; **7**: 144.

2. Silva D, Matis G, Chrysou O, *et al.* Sudden death in a patient with a third ventricle colloid cyst. *Arq Neuropsiquiatr* 2012; **70**: 311.

3. Armao D, Castillo M, Chen H, Kwock L. Colloid cyst of the third ventricle: imaging-pathologic correlation. *AJNR Am J Neuroradiol.* 2000; **21**: 1470–7.

4. Algin O, Ozmen E, Arslan H. Radiologic manifestations of colloid cysts: a pictorial essay. *Can Assoc Radiol J* 2013; **64**: 56–60.

5. Carrasco R, Pascual JM, Medina-López D, Burdaspal-Moratilla A. Acute hemorrhage in a colloid cyst of the third ventricle: a rare cause of sudden deterioration. *Surg Neurol Int* 2012; **3**: 24.

6. Dahdaleh NS, Dlouhy BJ, Kirby PA, Greenlee JD. Unusual "double density" colloid cysts. *J Clin Neurosci* 2012; **19**: 612–14.

7. Wang Z, Yan H, Wang D, *et al.* A colloid cyst in the fourth ventricle complicated with aseptic meningitis: a case report. *Clin Neurol Neurosurg* 2012; **114**: 1095–8.

8. Morris TC, Santoreneos S. Colloid cyst of velum interpositum: a rare finding. *J Neurosurg Pediatr* 2012; **9**: 206–8.

9. Symss NP, Ramamurthi R, Rao SM, *et al.* Management outcome of the transcallosal, transforaminal approach to colloid cysts of the anterior third ventricle: an analysis of 78 cases. *Neurol India* 2011; **59**: 542–7.

10. Boogaarts HD, Decq P, Grotenhuis JA, *et al.* Long-term results of the neuroendoscopic management of colloid cysts of the third ventricle: a series of 90 cases. *Neurosurgery* 2011; **68**: 179–87.

11. Goldberg EM, Schwartz ES, Younkin D, *et al.* Atypical syncope in a child due to a colloid cyst of the third ventricle. *Pediatr Neurol* 2011; **45**: 331–4.

12. Gbejuade H, Plaha P, Porter D. Spontaneous regression of a third ventricle colloid cyst. *Br J Neurosurg* 2011; **25**: 655–7.

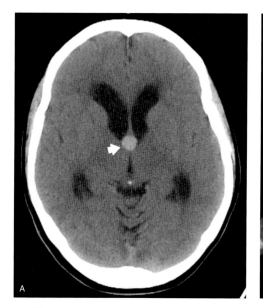
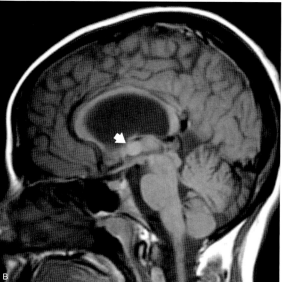
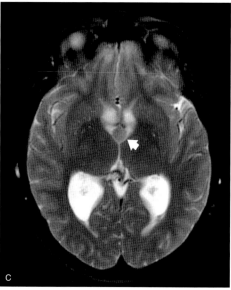

**Figure 32.1** 35-year-old male with intense headaches, nausea, and vomiting. (**A**) Non-contrast axial CT exhibits a rounded hyperdense anterior third ventricular mass (short arrow) with obstruction of foramen of Monro. There is dilatation of both the lateral ventricles, with periventricular lucencies suggesting transependymal CSF migration. (**B**) T1-weighted sagittal image exhibits a rounded hyperintense signal mass at the anterior and superior part of the third ventricle (short arrow) abutting the region of hypothalamus. (**C**) T2-weighted axial image exhibits hyperintense signal of the rounded mass (short arrow) at the level of foramen of Monro.

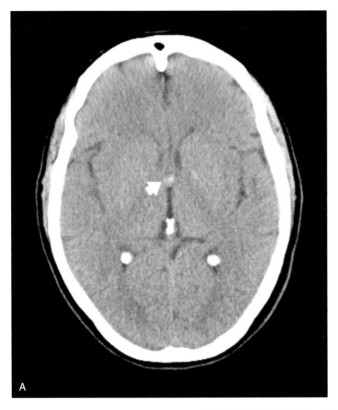

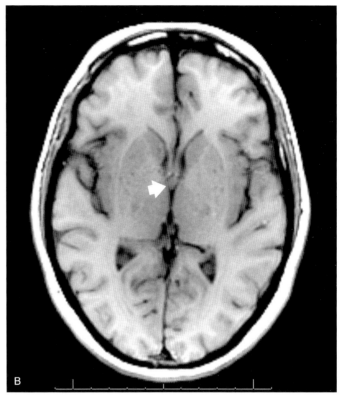

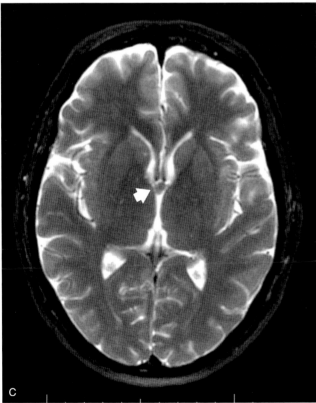

**Figure 32.2** 65-year-old male with mild trauma. (**A**) Non-contrast axial CT exhibits incidental finding of a small rounded hyperdense lesion at anterior third ventricle at the level of foramen of Monro without obstructive changes (short arrow). (**B**) T1-weighted axial image exhibits isodense nodularity (short arrow). (**C**) T2-weighted axial image exhibits the lesion to be hypointense (short arrow).

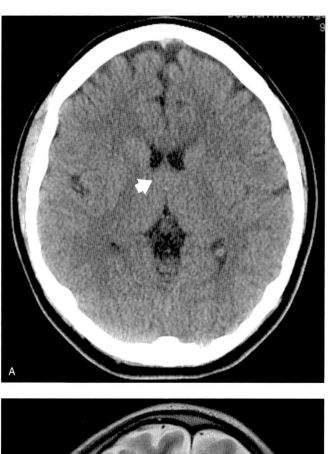

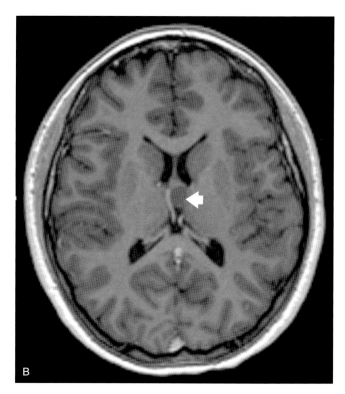

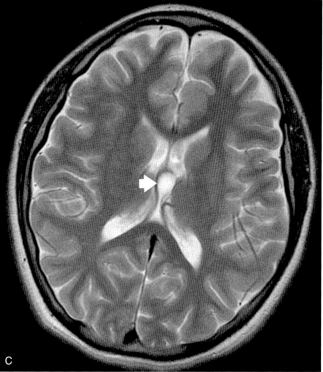

**Figure 32.3** 14-year-old male with intermittent headaches.
(**A**) Non-contrast axial CT exhibits a rounded lesion isodense to brain parenchyma (short arrow) at the level of foramen of Monro with normal size of ventricles. (**B**) Post-contrast T1-weighted axial image exhibits hypointense T1 signal cyst (short arrow), draped by internal cerebral veins with minimal enhancement of the capsule.
(**C**) T2-weighted axial image exhibits hyperintense signal cyst (short arrow).

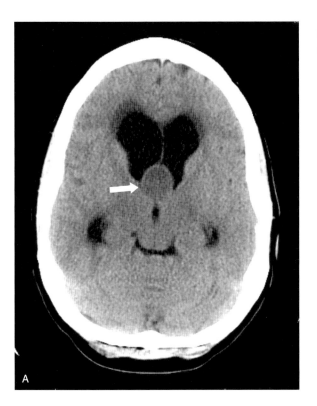

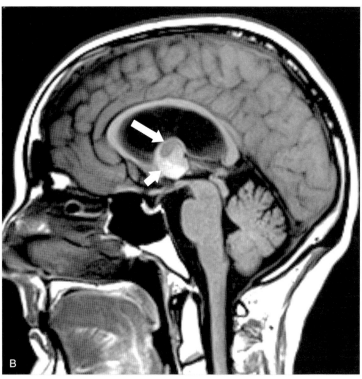

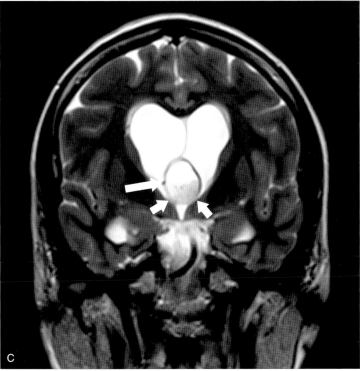

**Figure 32.4** 42-year-old female with sudden-onset vomiting and refractory headaches. (**A**) Non-contrast axial CT exhibits a large oval lesion at the level of foramen of Monro that is predominantly hypoattenuating (arrow) with resultant obstructive hydrocephalus. (**B**) T1-weighted sagittal image exhibits a mixed-intensity oval lesion at anterior third ventricle wedged into foramen of Monro with a superior hypointense T1 signal component (arrow) and a more inferior hyperintense T1 signal component (short arrow). (**C**) T2-weighted coronal image exhibits a fluid level with a superior cystic high T2 signal component (arrow) and an inferior hypointense T2 signal region (short arrows).

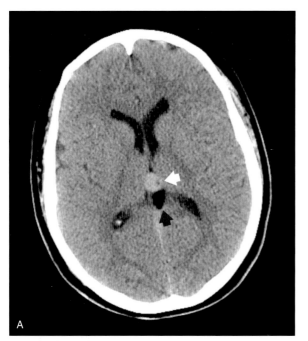

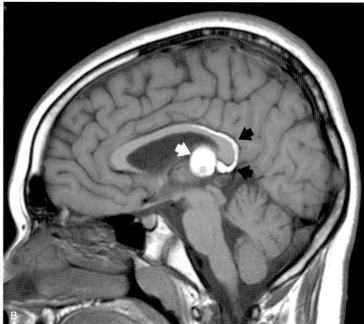

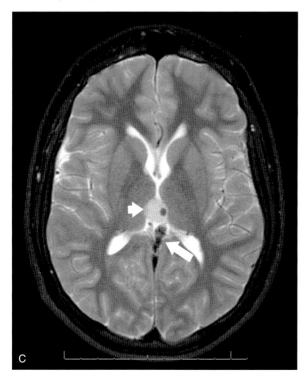

**Figure 32.5** 18-year-old female with history of concussion following motor vehicle accident. (**A**) Non-contrast axial CT exhibits an incidental rounded hyperdense mass in posterior third ventricle (short white arrow) with an oblong low-attenuating lesion posterior to it (short black arrow).
(**B**) T1-weighted sagittal image exhibits an oblong high T1 signal mass at posterior third ventricle (short white arrow). Note the incidental lipoma of corpus callosum (short black arrows) that ends just posterior to it.
(**C**) T2-weighted fat-saturated axial image exhibits intermediate T2 signal of the posterior third ventricular mass (short arrow) with low T2 signal of the lipoma of corpus callosum (long arrow).

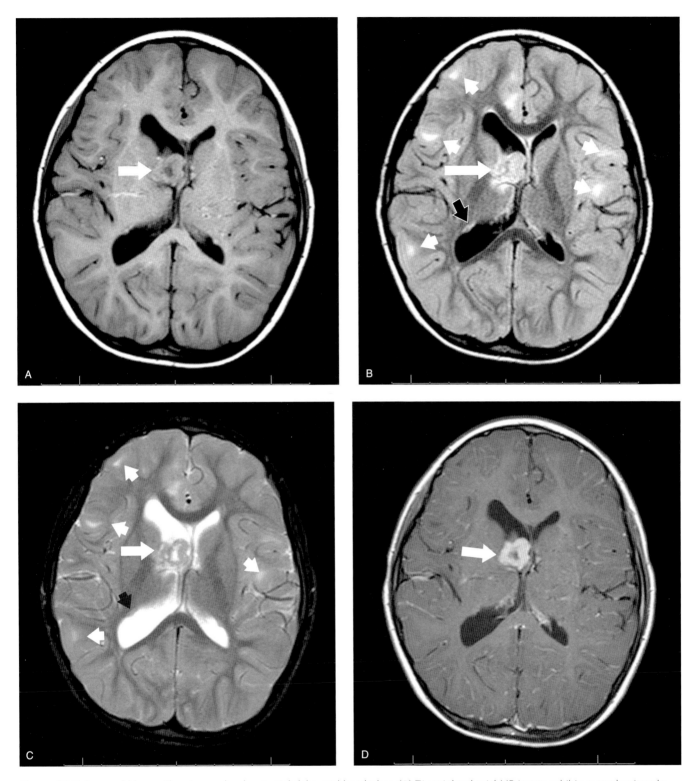

**Figure 32.6** 6-year-old boy with seizures, developmental delay and headaches. (**A**) T1-weighted axial MR image exhibits a predominantly isointense T1 signal mass within the right frontal horn, at the level of foramen of Monro (arrow). (**B**) Axial FLAIR image exhibits numerous peripheral patchy high-signal areas, likely cortical tubers (short white arrows). There is a subependymal nodule at posterior right lateral ventricle (short black arrow). The mass exhibits high FLAIR signal (arrow) and likely represents a subependymal giant cell astrocytoma (SEGA) in a patient with tuberous sclerosis. (**C**) T2-weighted axial MR image exhibits a heterogeneously hypointense mass at the foramen of Monro on the right (arrow). The cortical tubers (short white arrows) and subependymal nodule (short black arrow) are seen. (**D**) Post-contrast T1-weighted axial MR image exhibits intense heterogeneous enhancement of the mass (arrow).

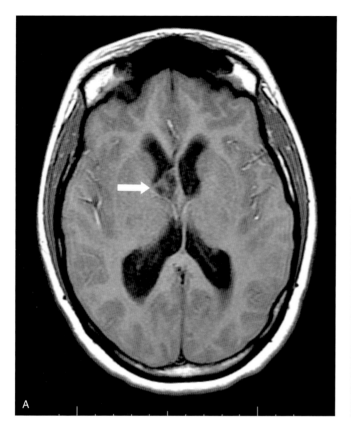

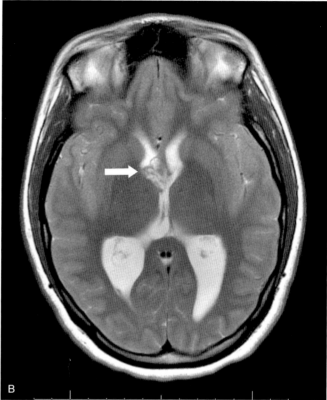

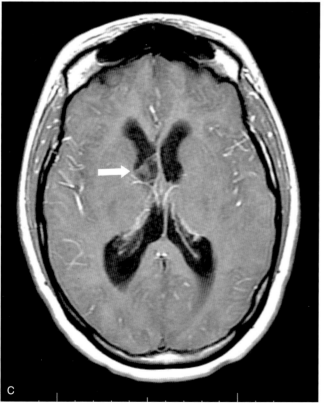

**Figure 32.7** 26-year-old female with intermittent headaches and central neurocytoma. (**A**) T1-weighted axial MR image exhibits irregular heterogeneous predominantly isointense mass at the right frontal horn with relation to septum pellucidum and foramina of Monro (arrow). There is mild prominence of lateral ventricles. (**B**) T2-weighted axial MR image shows a cystic mass with multiple septa (arrow). (**C**) Post-contrast T1-weighted axial MR image does not exhibit any significant post-contrast enhancement of the mass (arrow).

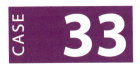

# CASE 33  Primary intraosseous meningioma

## Imaging description

Meningiomas are common benign masses that are easily recognized on the basis of their typical dural-based location. About 1–2% of menigiomas arise from extradural locations and pose a diagnostic challenge [1]. The most common extradural location is the calvarium (Fig. 33.1) [3–5]. Primary intraosseous meningiomas (PIMs) require differentiation from other bone lesions, ranging from benign process such as fibrous dysplasia to highly malignant masses such as osteosarcoma [2]. Although initially presumed to arise from meningothelial cells trapped in sutures or fracture lines, only 8% of the calvarial meningiomas are found along the cranial sutures [4] and only 15% of the PIMs have a history of trauma to the head [3]. They probably arise from multipotent mesenchymal cell precursors, likely as a reaction to an unidentified stimulus [4].

Most of the PIMs tend to present with hyperostosis, but they may present with osteolytic or mixed appearance on CT scans, generating a differential diagnosis depending on distinguishing subtype [6]. On MRI there is always soft tissue enhancement adjacent to the bone lesion. Soft tissue enhancement may be intra- and/or extracranial, and it may range from mild dural thickening to sizable masses. It may be difficult to distinguish an intradural plaque such as meningioma with associated reactive hyperostosis from a true PIM with imaging (Fig. 33.2). Most PIMs are benign, although osteolytic skull lesions and extracranial soft tissue masses are associated with more aggressive histologic subtypes [4,6].

## Importance

Even though biologically benign and slow-growing, the incidence of aggressive features is higher in intraosseous meningiomas (11%) than in intradural meningiomas (2%) [4,5]. PIMs should be treated with wide surgical excision and reconstruction of the bone [3] whereas meningiomas with reactive hyperostosis can be managed without bone removal. Adjuvant radiotherapy may be performed in patients who show progression of residual mass or progression in symptoms [4].

## Typical clinical scenario

Sphenoid wings and frontoparietal convexity are the two most common locations for intraosseous meningiomas. They are usually slow-growing, firm, and painless. Sphenoid wing PIMs are associated with proptosis and optic nerve compression. Convexity masses may present as palpable scalp masses. They predominantly occur later in life, from the fifth to the seventh decade.

## Differential diagnosis

Fibrous dysplasia may be indistinguishable from PIM on CT (Fig. 33.3), but it lacks the enhancing soft tissue component on MRI. When present, spiculated bone margins suggest PIM, because the cortex is smooth in fibrous dysplasia. On angiography, fibrous dysplasias do not have a tumor blush, which is seen in PIM. En plaque and globular meningiomas are frequently associated with hyperostosis of the overlying calvarium (Fig. 33.4). However, the hyperostotic component does not enhance in en plaque meningioma, while in intraosseous meningioma there is often intense gadolinium enhancement of the intradiploic mass [1,4,6].

Primary intraosseous cavernous hemangiomas are slow-growing benign tumors arising from intrinsic vasculature of the bone (Fig. 33.5); they account for 10% of benign skull tumors and 0.2% of all bone tumors [7,8], and they present with a characteristic "honeycomb" pattern of ossification on CT.

Other osteolytic skull lesions include eosinophilic granuloma (Fig. 33.6), plasmacytoma, or metastatic deposits from lymphoma (Fig. 33.7) or other cancer (Fig. 33.8). Metastatic deposits from prostate cancer can be osteoblastic and may be associated with reactive enhancement and thickening of underlying dura (Fig. 33.9). Eosinophilic granuloma is more commonly seen in children. Metastatic deposits from lymphoma or other cancer may be multifocal, while blastic deposits from prostate can be focal or diffuse. Osteosarcoma of calvarium is a rare primary malignant bone tumor and is sometimes seen following long-term radiation therapy.

## Teaching points

PIMs are rare but require differentiation from other sclerotic bone lesions such as fibrous dysplasia, as their treatment is different. The osteolytic subtype of PIM is more likely to have aggressive features than the sclerotic variety. PIMs with associated intracranial and extracranial soft tissue masses should be differentiated from metastases.

REFERENCES

1. Agrawal V, Ludwig N, Agrawal A, Bulsara KR. Intraosseous intracranial meningioma. *AJNR Am J Neuroradiol* 2007; **28**: 314–15.
2. El Mahou S, Popa L, Constantin A, *et al.* Multiple intraosseous meningiomas. *Clin Rheumatol* 2006; **25**: 553–4.
3. Devi B, Bhat D, Madhusudhan H, *et al.* Primary intraosseous meningioma of orbit and anterior cranial fossa: a case report and literature review. *Australas Radiol* 2001; **45**: 211–14.

4. Tokgoz N, Oner YA, Kaymaz M, *et al.* Primary intraosseous meningioma: CT and MRI appearance. *AJNR Am J Neuroradiol* 2005; **26**: 2053–6.

5. Lang FF, Macdonald OK, Fuller GN, DeMonte F. Primary extradural meningiomas: a report on nine cases and review of the literature from the era of computerized tomography scanning. *J Neurosurg* 2000; **93**: 940–50.

6. Elder JB, Atkinson R, Zee CS, Chen TC. Primary intraosseous meningioma. *Neurosurg Focus* 2007; **23**: E13.

7. Liu JK, Burger PC, Harnsberger HR, Couldwell WT. Primary Intraosseous Skull Base Cavernous Hemangioma: Case Report. *Skull Base* 2003; **13**: 219–28.

8. Naama O, Gazzaz M, Akhaddar A, *et al.* Cavernous hemangioma of the skull: 3 case reports. *Surg Neurol* 2008; **70**: 654–9.

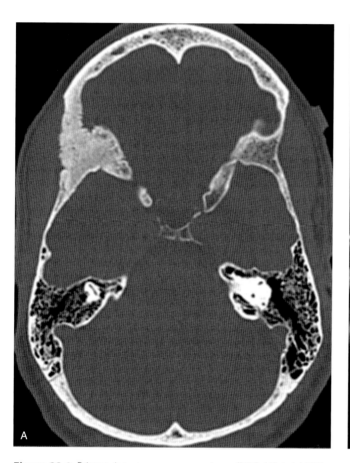
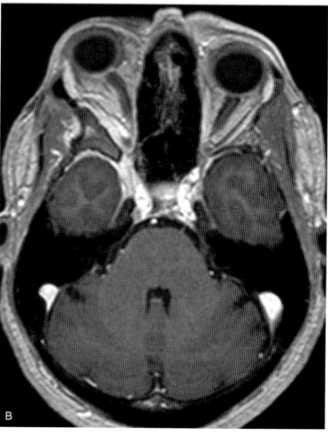

**Figure 33.1** Primary intraosseous meningioma (PIM). (**A**) Axial CT image shows a markedly sclerotic lesion expanding the right sphenoid wing. Note mildly spiculated margins. (**B**) Post-contrast T1-weighted MR image reveals some enhancement within the sclerotic lesion and prominent soft tissue enhancement along the dura, extraconal orbit, and temporalis muscle without an obvious mass.

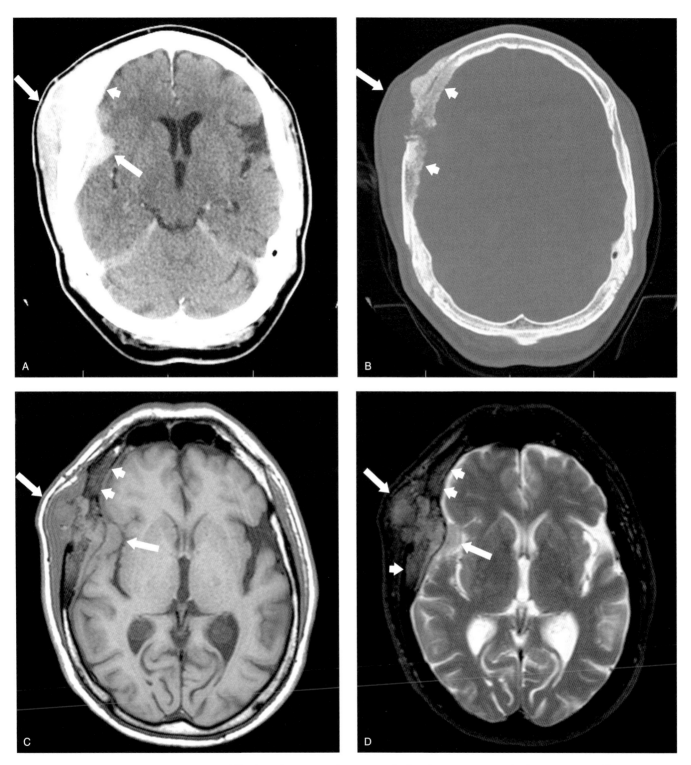

**Figure 33.2** Intraosseous meningioma: it is difficult in this case to determine whether this is a PIM or a dural meningioma infiltrating the bone. (**A**, **B**) Contrast-enhanced axial CT exhibits densely enhancing lobulated intracranial extra-axial and extracranial masses (arrows) on both sides of expanded right frontoparietal calvarium (short arrows) with relation to right coronal suture. (**C**) T1-weighted axial MR image exhibits intracranial and extracranial soft tissue masses (arrows), isointense to brain parenchyma with a heterogeneous iso to hypointense T1 signal calvarial mass (short arrows) resulting in expansion of the diploic spaces. (**D**) T2-weighted axial MR image exhibits iso- to marginally hypointense T2 signal of the soft tissue masses (arrows) with hypo- to isointense T2 signal of the intradiploic component (short arrows). (**E**, **F**) Post-contrast T1-weighted axial and coronal MR imaging exhibits intense enhancement of intracranial dural-based mass (arrow) with reactive thickening of dura underlying homogeneously enhancing calvarial mass (short arrows) with extracranial soft tissue extension (arrow).

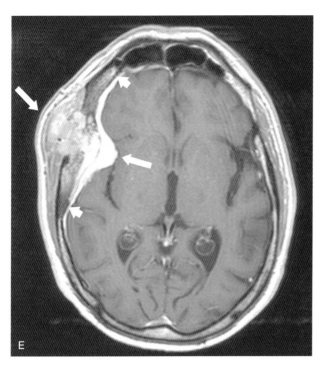
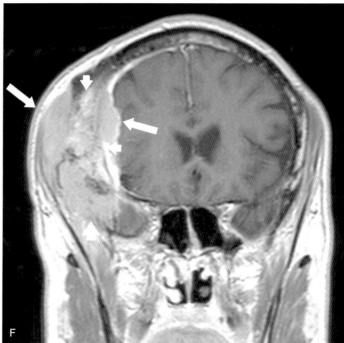

**Figure 33.2** (cont.)

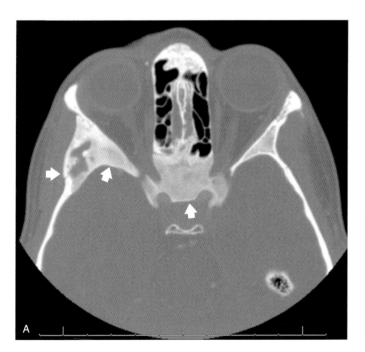
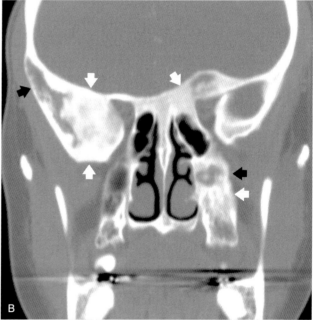

**Figure 33.3** Fibrous dysplasia. (**A**, **B**) There is thickening and expansion with ground-glass appearance of the skull base involving basisphenoid and right greater wing of the sphenoid bone with ground-glass matrix (short white arrows). Note the intact cortical margins and abrupt transition between the normal and abnormal bone. Areas of increased fibrous content appear to be lytic and hypodense (short black arrows).

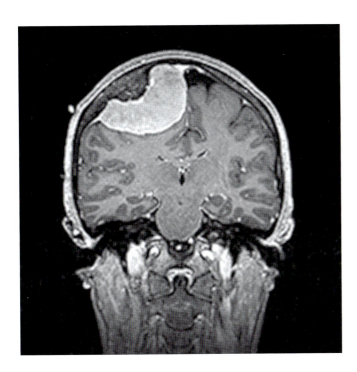

**Figure 33.4** Meningioma with hyperostosis. Large meningioma with a focal hyperostosis of the overlying bone. Notice the lack of enhancement in the bone. No evidence of meningioma was present in bone on pathologic evaluation.

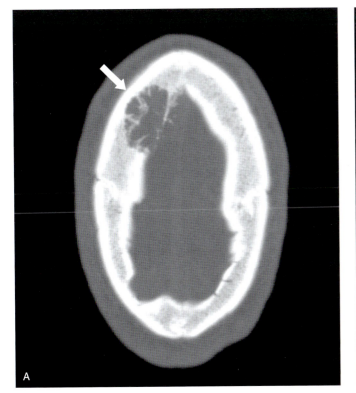

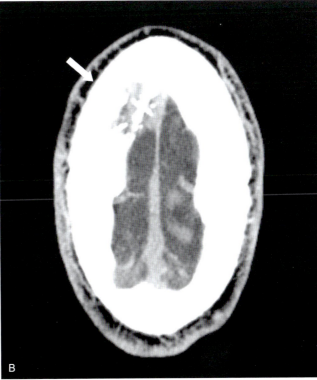

**Figure 33.5** Cavernous hemangioma. (**A**, **B**) Post-contrast axial CT exhibits enhancing lytic lesion of high-convexity right frontal calvarium with intradiploic honeycomb pattern (arrow).

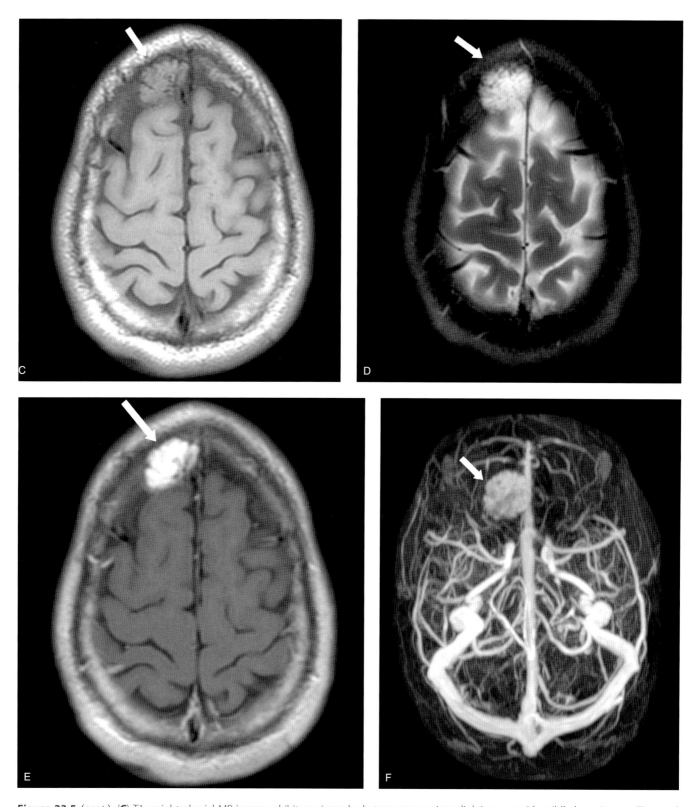

**Figure 33.5** (cont.) (**C**) T1-weighted axial MR image exhibits an irregular heterogeneous intradiploic mass with mildly hyperintense T1 signal (arrow). (**D**) Fat-saturated T2-weighted axial MR image exhibits hyperintense T2 signal with mottled appearance (arrow). (**E**) Post-contrast T1-weighted axial MR image exhibits intense post-contrast enhancement (arrow). (**F**) Gadolinium-enhanced MR venography exhibits a mottled mass in the vicinity of the superior sagittal sinus (arrow).

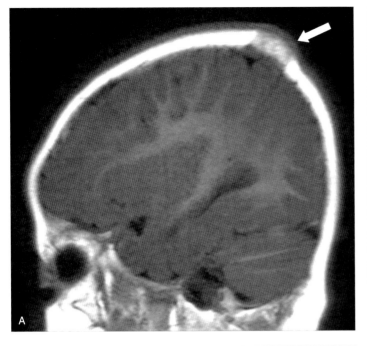

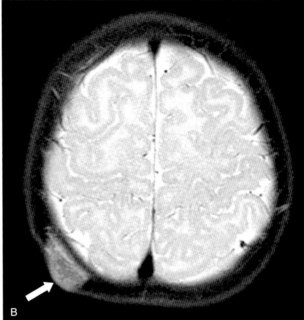

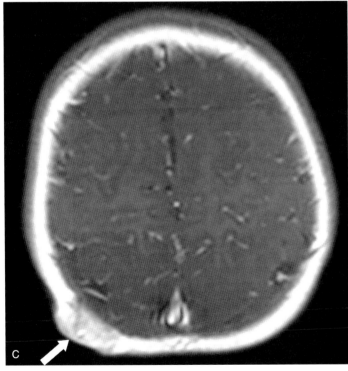

**Figure 33.6** Eosinophilic granuloma. (**A**) T1-weighted sagittal MR image exhibits a right high-convexity calvarial mass extending into overlying scalp (arrow). (**B**) T2-weighted axial MR image exhibits low T2 signal calvarial mass extending into overlying scalp (arrow). (**C**) Post-contrast T1-weighted axial MR image exhibits mild patchy enhancement of the mass (arrow).

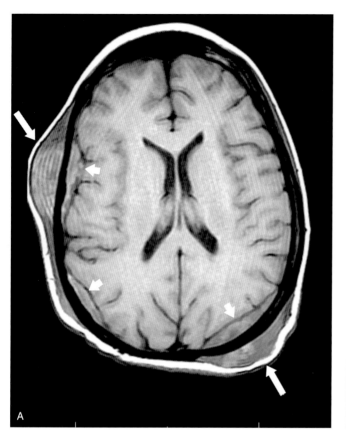

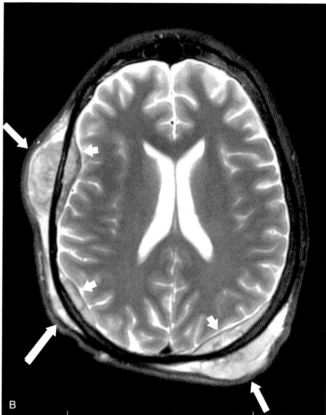

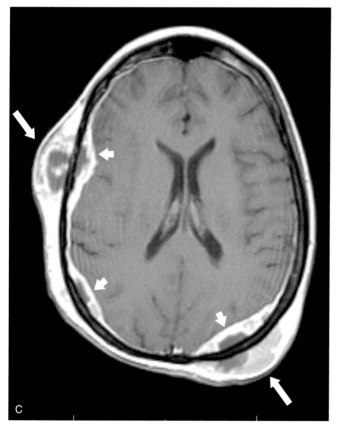

**Figure 33.7** Deposits from B-cell lymphoma. (**A**) T1-weighted axial MR image exhibits lobulated mildly hyperintense T1 signal intracranial extra-axial (short arrows) and extracranial (arrows) multifocal masses on both sides of the calvarium. There is no evidence for calvarial expansion. (**B**) T2-weighted axial MR image exhibits heterogeneously hypo- to mildly hyperintense T2 signal of the intracranial (short arrows) and extracranial (arrows) masses. (**C**) Post-contrast T1-weighted axial image exhibits patchy variable post-contrast enhancement of these intracranial masses with reactive thickening and enhancement of underlying dura (short arrows) and intense variable enhancement of extracranial masses (arrows). There is no evidence for significant enhancement or expansion of the calvarium.

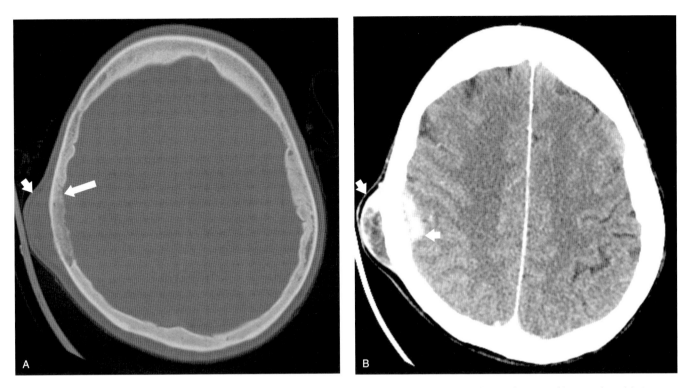

**Figure 33.8** Metastatic deposit from rectal carcinoma. (**A**, **B**) Post-contrast axial CT scan exhibits a lytic right parietal bone calvarial lesion (arrow) with a densely enhancing irregular intracranial mass (short arrow) as well as a heterogeneously enhancing extracranial mass (short arrow).

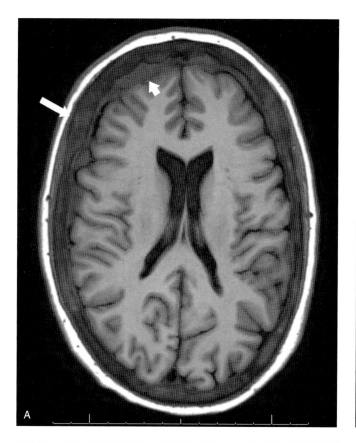

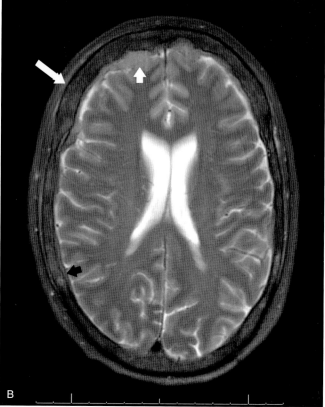

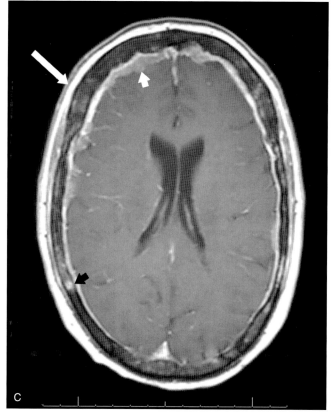

**Figure 33.9** Metastatic deposit from prostate carcinoma. (**A**) T1-weighted axial MR image exhibits generalized expansion of calvarium with hypointense T1 signal (arrow). Note the iso- to hypointense T1 signal extra-axial mass (short arrow). (**B**) Fat-saturated T2-weighted axial MR image exhibits expansion of the calvarium (arrow) and presence of dural-based extra-axial mass (short white arrow). Rounded high T2 signal within the calvarium likely represents intradiploic vessel (short black arrow). (**C**) Post-contrast T1-weighted axial MR image exhibits low T1 signal expanded calvarium (arrow) with thickening and enhancement of underlying dura (short white arrow). Enhancing intradiploic vessel is seen (short black arrow).

# 34 Suprasellar meningioma

## Imaging description

Tumors involving the sella and suprasellar cistern have diverse origin although their clinical presentation is very similar. Most common sellar and suprasellar tumor is pituitary macroadenoma. Suprasellar meningiomas commonly arise from diaphragma sellae or tuberculum sellae (Fig. 34.1); however, large meningiomas originating along the planum sphenoidale (Fig. 34.2) or greater wing of the sphenoidal bone (Fig. 34.3) may also extend into the suprasellar cistern or parasellar region [1].

The suprasellar meningiomas account for 10% of all the chiasmal tumors [2], and the position of the chiasm related to the tumor determines the pattern of visual loss [3]. Histologically, they consist of elongated bipolar cells with eosinophilic cytoplasm, arranged in syncytial configuration with whirls. When present, psammoma bodies (concentrically laminated calcifications) are a distinguishing feature. On CT, a suprasellar meningioma appears as iso- to mildly hyperdense, intensely enhancing, lobulated mass with or without areas of calcification. They are generally isointense to cortical gray matter on both T1-weighted and T2-weighted images, but atypical features such as cystic areas or hemorrhage are frequently seen. On post-contrast study, homogeneous and intense enhancement is seen, with frequent presence of a dural tail.

## Importance

Suprasellar masses without involvement of sella turcica have traditionally been surgically excised by a transcranial approach, whereas pituitary adenomas that extend to the suprasellar region are treated with endoscopic trans-sphenoidal approaches. For the non-pituitary suprasellar masses, recently, supraorbital craniotomy [4], a supraorbital endoscopic approach, and endoscopic endonasal extended transsphenoidal approaches that protect the normal pituitary gland [5] have been suggested. A large suprasellar meningioma can also be embolized before the surgery to minimize blood loss [6]. With the popularity of minimally invasive surgery that can shorten hospital stay, radiologists will be increasingly responsible for identifying the relationship of adjacent critical vascular structures and optic apparatus.

## Typical clinical scenario

Suprasellar meningiomas commonly present with visual disturbance in the form of reduced visual acuity, loss of color vision, and visual field defects, most commonly bitemporal hemianopsia due to compression of the inferior chiasmatic fibers [2]. Tumors involving the floor of the anterior cranial fossa and involving the olfactory tracts can result in anosmia.

## Differential diagnosis

A large intrasellar pituitary macroadenoma can extend into the suprasellar cistern (Fig. 34.4). It can cause significant mass effect on the optic chiasm and third ventricle. A craniopharyngioma (Fig. 34.5) can be predominantly suprasellar, or suprasellar and intrasellar, but rarely only intrasellar. Ninety percent of craniopharyngiomas exhibit cystic component, areas of calcification, and variable post-contrast enhancement. Pilocytic astrocytoma (Fig. 34.6) is more commonly seen in infants and the pediatric age group, but can also be seen in young adults. It expands the hypothalamus and optic chiasm and may extend into the optic nerves and tracts. Calcification is uncommon in hypothalamic pilocytic astrocytoma. Germinoma is morphologically homologous to neoplasm arising in gonads and extragonadal sites. CNS germinomas (Fig. 34.7) are seen along the midline near the third ventricle, with about 25–35% also seen in the suprasellar region. Proliferating Langerhans cell histiocytes form granulomas within the skull or infundibulum/hypothalamus region. A thick enhancing pituitary stalk is the most common CNS manifestation of Langerhans cell histiocytosis (LCH) (Fig. 34.8).

## Teaching points

While imaging features of pituitary macroadenomas that extend to the suprasellar region and suprasellar non-pituitary tumors that extend into the sella may overlap, there is a significant difference in surgical approaches to these tumors. Macroadenomas are treated via an endoscopic transsphenoidal approach, and non-pituitary sellar/suprasellar tumors are treated with transcranial or modified endoscopic approaches that protect the pituitary gland. When dealing with a sellar and suprasellar mass, if even a small part of the normal pituitary gland is visualized it indicates a non-pituitary tumor, as large macroadenomas almost invariably replace the entire gland, rendering it invisible on imaging.

REFERENCES

1. Johnsen DE, Woodruff WW, Allen IS, *et al*. MR imaging of the sellar and juxtasellar regions. *Radiographics* 1991; **11**: 727–58.

2. Kadis GN, Mount LA, Ganti SR. The importance of early diagnosis and treatment of the meningiomas of the planum sphenoidale and tuberculum sellae: a retrospective study of 105 cases. *Surg Neurol* 1979; **12**: 367–71.

3. Shapey J, Danesh-Meyer HV, Kaye AH. Suprasellar meningioma presenting with an altitudinal field defect. *J Clin Neurosci* 2012; **19**: 155–8.

4. McLaughlin N, Ditzel Filho LF, *et al*. The supraorbital approach for recurrent or residual suprasellar tumors. *Minim Invasive Neurosurg* 2011; **54**: 155–61.

5. Chowdhury FH, Haque MR, Goel AH, Kawsar KA. Endoscopic endonasal extended transsphenoidal removal of tuberculum sellae meningioma (TSM): an experience of six cases. *Br J Neurosurg* 2012; **26**: 692–9.

6. Lefkowitz M, Giannotta SL, Hieshima G, *et al*. Embolization of neurosurgical lesions involving the ophthalmic artery. *Neurosurgery* 1998; **43**: 1298–303.

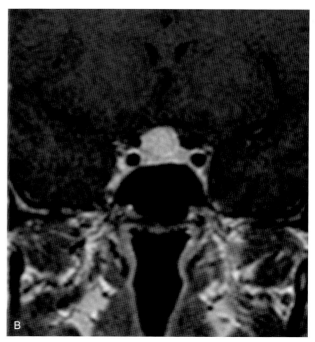

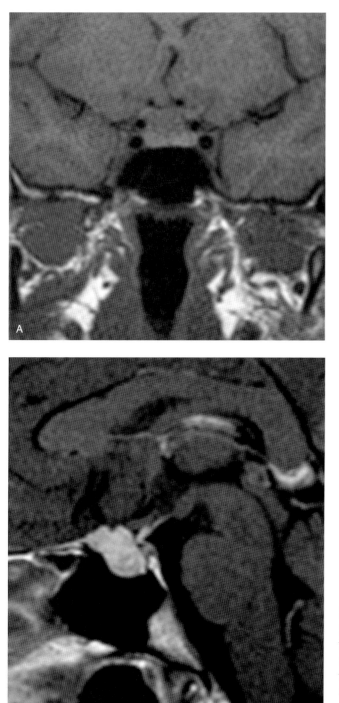

**Figure 34.1** Diaphragma sellae meningioma. (**A**, **B**) Coronal pre- and post-contrast T1-weighted MR images show a well-defined mass in the sella and suprasellar region which could be mistaken for a pituitary macroadenoma. Note that there is a subtle difference between the pituitary gland and the mass, virtually excluding the possibility of macroadenoma. (**C**) Sagittal post-contrast T1-weighted image shows the suprasellar mass and pituitary separately. Also note that a pituitary adenoma of this size would usually expand the sella more.

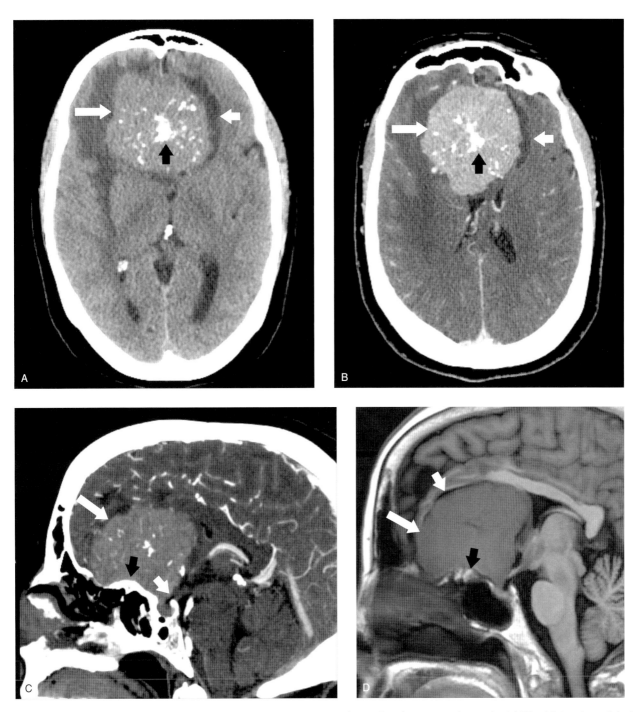

**Figure 34.2** Planum sphenoidale meningioma. (**A**, **B**) Non-contrast-enhanced and contrast-enhanced axial CT exhibits a large lobulated suprasellar mass (arrow) isodense to brain parenchyma with areas of speckled calcification (short black arrow) and surrounding cystic space (short white arrow). Low-attenuating white matter edema is seen at right frontal lobe. (**C**) Sagittal reconstruction non-contrast-enhanced CT exhibits a large lobulated suprasellar planum sphenoidale meningioma (arrow), predominantly anterior to the optic chiasm (short white arrow). There is mild hyperostosis of the floor of the anterior cranial fossa (short black arrow). The pituitary gland is separately visualized within the sella turcica. (**D**) T1-weighted sagittal MRA exhibits a large planum sphenoidale meningioma (arrow) with iso- to marginally hypointense T1 signal elevating the optic nerve and the corpus callosum (short white arrow). Hyperintense T1 signal of bone marrow is seen from hyperostotic floor of anterior cranial fossa (short black arrow). The pituitary gland is separately visualized within the sella turcica. (**E**) Fat-saturated T2-weighted coronal MR image exhibits a large lobulated suprasellar mass (arrow) iso- to mildly hyperintense to brain parenchyma with surrounding cystic space (short arrows). Hyperintense T2 signal white matter edema is seen at right frontal lobe. (**F**) Fat-saturated post-contrast T1-weighted sagittal MR image exhibits a large suprasellar mass (arrow) elevating the corpus callosum with superior small cystic space (short arrow). The mass appears to be anterior to optic chiasm and separate from pituitary gland.

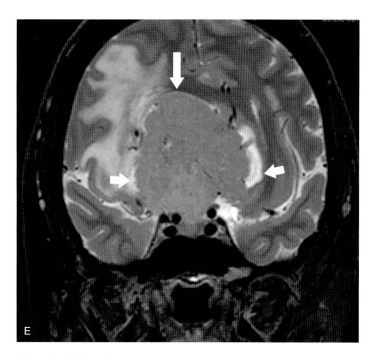
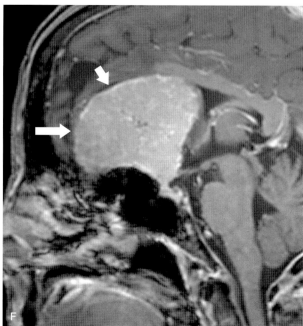

**Figure 34.2** (cont.)

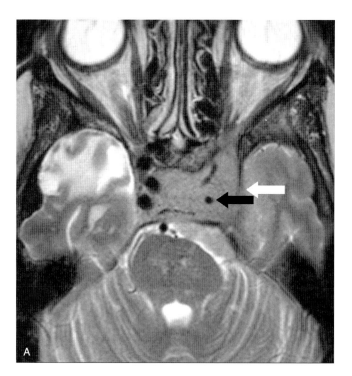
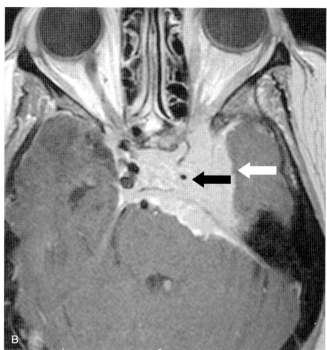

**Figure 34.3** Cavernous sinus meningioma. (**A**) T2-weighted axial MR image exhibits a low T2 signal left cavernous sinus mass (white arrow), isointense to brain parenchyma with exophytic extension in prepontine cistern. There is narrowing of the lumen of the intracavernous left internal carotid artery (black arrow). (**B**, **C**) Post-contrast T1-weighted axial and coronal images show left cavernous sinus meningioma (white arrow) extending into left middle cranial fossa and prepontine cistern with narrowing of the lumen of intracavernous left internal carotid artery (black arrow).

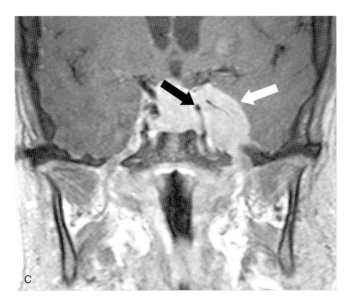

**Figure 34.3** (cont.)

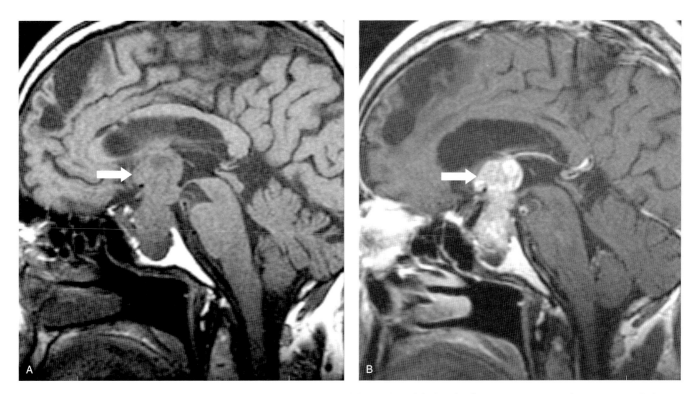

**Figure 34.4** Pituitary adenoma. (**A**) T1-weighted sagittal MR image exhibits a large lobulated soft tissue mass arising from an expanded sella turcica and extending into the suprasellar region (arrow), reaching up to the floor of the lateral ventricles. (**B**) Post-contrast T1-weighted sagittal MR image exhibits an intensely enhancing large lobulated sellar and suprasellar mass (arrow).

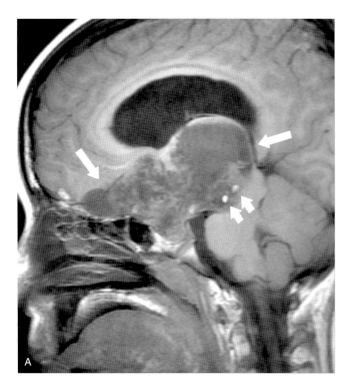

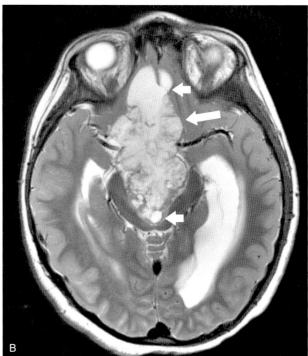

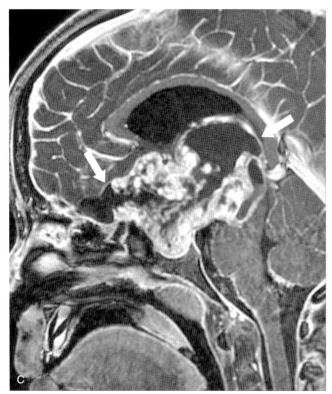

**Figure 34.5** Craniopharyngioma. (**A**) T1-weighted sagittal MR image exhibits a large heterogeneous sellar/suprasellar mass with an anterior cystic component along the planum sphenoidale (arrow) and a posterior cystic component in the mass extending within the third ventricle (arrow). Rounded hyperintense T1 signal areas (short arrows) may represent presence of cholesterol versus dystrophic calcification. (**B**) T2-weighted axial MR image exhibits a large, heterogeneously hyperintense T2 signal, suprasellar mass (arrow) extending into interpeduncular cistern splaying the cerebral peduncles with presence of anterior and posterior cystic components (short arrows). (**C**) Post-contrast fat-saturated T1-weighted sagittal image exhibits heterogeneous intense enhancement of the solid portion of the mass with areas of non-enhancing cystic components (arrow).

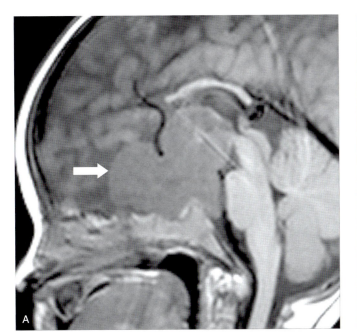

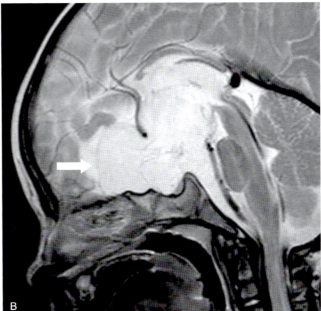

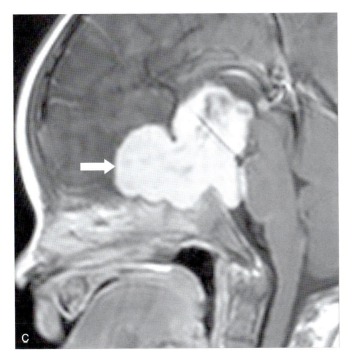

**Figure 34.6** Pilocytic astrocytoma. (**A**) T1-weighted sagittal MR image exhibits a large lobulated suprasellar mass (arrow) with iso- to hypointense T1 signal. (**B**) T2-weighted sagittal MR image exhibits marked hyperintense T2 signal of the mass (arrow). (**C**) Post-contrast T1-weighted sagittal image exhibits intense post-contrast enhancement (arrow).

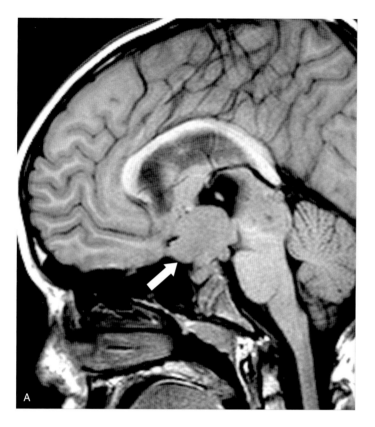

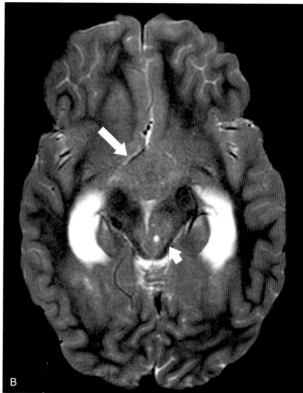

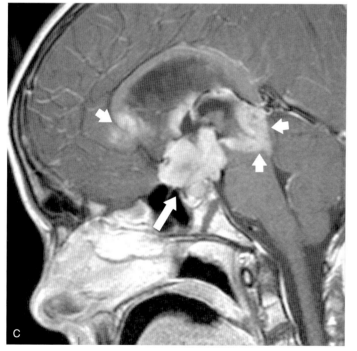

**Figure 34.7** Germinoma. (**A**) T1-weighted sagittal MR image exhibits a large lobulated isointense T1 signal suprasellar mass (arrow). Soft tissue expansion of the pineal region and along the floor of the lateral ventricle is also seen. (**B**) Fat-saturated T2-weighted axial MR image exhibits iso- to mildly hyperintense T2 signal suprasellar mass (arrow) with another focus in periaqueductal region and cerebral peduncles (short arrow), likely from pineal lesion. There is marked enlargement of both the temporal horns due to obstructive hydrocephalus. (**C**) Post-contrast T1-weighted sagittal MR image exhibits strong and homogeneous enhancement of the suprasellar mass (arrow), the pineal lesion (short arrows), the lesion along the floor of the lateral ventricle, and along the genu of corpus callosum (short arrow).

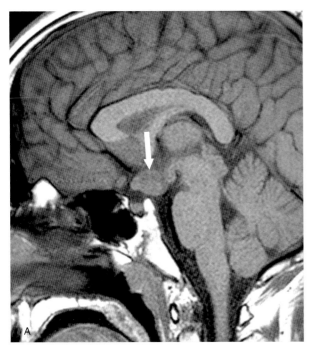

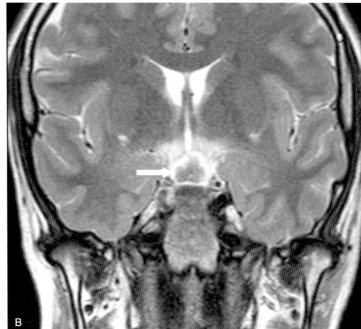

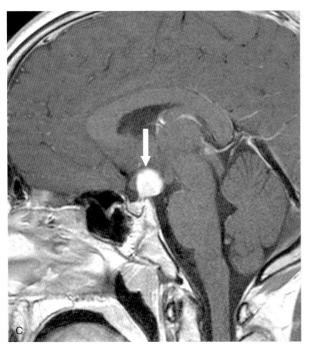

**Figure 34.8** Langerhans cell histiocytosis. (**A**) T1-weighted sagittal MR image exhibits isointense soft tissue mass (arrow) at hypothalamus. (**B**) T2-weighted coronal MR image exhibits hypointense T2 signal suprasellar mass (arrow). (**C**) Post-contrast T1-weighted sagittal MR image shows intense enhancement of the hypothalamic nodule (arrow) extending into pituitary stalk.

## Imaging description

The adenoma arises from the hypophyseal cells in the anterior pituitary, and when more than 1 cm in diameter it is considered a macroadenoma. More than 30% of patients with macroadenoma have one or more hormone deficiencies at the time of presentation, most commonly growth hormone (GH) deficiency. The following laboratory studies are routinely performed: ACTH, free cortisol, thyrotroponin, thyroxine, prolactin, GH, IGF-1, testosterone, LH, FSH, and estradiol [1].

Histologically, pituitary adenomas are benign in nature, but they may enlarge and invade surrounding structures. They may be diagnosed early when they are endocrinologically active [1], but neurologically silent pituitary macroadenomas can extend into the suprasellar region (Fig. 35.1), invade surrounding structures, encase the internal carotid artery (ICA) (Fig. 35.2), invade the cavernous sinus, and extend into the sphenoidal sinuses (Fig. 35.3). Recently, two potential molecular markers, EMMPRIN and galectin-3, were found to be associated with aggressiveness and invasion by pituitary adenoma [2].

The presence of symptomatic pituitary adenoma is estimated to be close to 94 cases per 100 000 population. The pituitary adenomas represent about 10% of all intracranial neoplasms [3]. MRI is currently the diagnostic imaging modality of choice for pituitary macroadenomas, allowing for superior soft tissue differentiation and the ability to evaluate possible invasion of surrounding structures. The pituitary macroadenomas appear to be hypo- to isointense to gray matter, while on T2-weighted images they most commonly appear isointense to gray matter (Fig. 35.1). Some of the GH-producing adenomas display hypointense T2 signal. Post-contrast enhancement is generally strong but heterogeneous. Depending on the possibility of cystic degeneration and intratumoral hemorrhage, there may be small areas of fluid-fluid levels (Fig. 35.1E) or pituitary apoplexy within the macroadenoma (Fig. 35.4) [3,4].

## Importance

MRI is extremely important in evaluating the presence of cavernous sinus invasion in pituitary macroadenoma [5,6], as endocrinologic remission is rarely obtained after microsurgery alone in patients with invasive tumors [6]. Various precise criteria for cavernous sinus invasion have been suggested, including absence of periarterial enhancement and encasement of the angle of the intracavernous ICA by the tumor [5], the status of cavernous sinus venous compartments, the size of cavernous sinus, bulging of the lateral wall of the cavernous sinus, displacement of intracavernous ICA by adenoma, grade of parasellar extension, and percentage of intracavernous ICA encasement by the tumor [6].

Macrocystic and macrohemorrhagic adenomas and solid tumors with enhanced diffusivity are more likely to be successfully managed with a trans-sphenoidal hypophysectomy [7]. MRI is also invaluable for volumetric classification of pituitary macroadenomas, as it predicts the outcome and morbidity following endoscopic endonasal trans-sphenoidal surgery. Pituitary macroadenomas with volume $> 10 \, cm^3$ and cavernous sinus invasion are associated with a higher likelihood of subtotal resection and postoperative morbidity [8]. In such cases, a combined endoscopic trans-sphenoidal transventricular approach helps to achieve a gross total removal of the mass [9]. MRI is also useful to evaluate the presence of postoperative pituitary apoplexy within the immediate postoperative period, which has been reported to occur in pituitary macroadenomas $> 4 \, cm$ in diameter after subtotal resection (Fig. 35.1G) [10].

## Typical clinical scenario

Close to 25% of the macroadenomas are not endocrinologically active, but close to 65% of functional adenomas are classified as macroadenomas. The endocrinological manifestations include acromegaly, Cushing's disease, hyperprolactinemia, and rarely hyperthyroidism. Frequently, endocrinological symptoms lead to early diagnosis of small lesions. However, when functionally silent, they present with symptoms related to local mass effect. They generally present with headaches and visual field defects, which vary according to the position of the tumor in relation to the optic chiasm and bilateral optic nerves. The commonest visual defect is bitemporal hemianopsia. Other manifestations include hydrocephalus from obstruction of the third ventricle resulting in headache, nausea, and vomiting, and, ironically, hypopituitarism due to compression of normal pituitary gland.

## Differential diagnosis

Up to 50% of females of age 18–35 years have a hyperplastic pituitary gland, which may measure $> 10 \, mm$ with a convex superior margin (Fig. 35.5). It is important to note that the post-contrast enhancement is homogeneous, without evidence for an area of low contrast uptake, and the pituitary gland is functionally normal.

Meningioma, which accounts for 18% of all intracranial tumors, is the second most common neoplasm of the sellar region after pituitary adenoma [11]. Frequent origins of parasellar meningiomas include the tuberculum sella, diaphragma sellae, dorsum sellae, and clinoid processes (Fig. 35.6).

Intrasellar craniopharyngioma (Fig. 35.7) generally displays a solid nodule, and a cyst with rim and nodular enhancement is more common than solid enhancement. Areas of calcification may also be seen. It is more commonly seen in children than adults.

Langerhans cell histiocytosis (LCH) (Fig. 35.8) is a rare disorder in which granulomatous deposits occur at multiple sites within the body, but which often involves the hypothalamo-pituitary axis [12]. Diabetes insipidus is a well-recognized complication. A chordoma (Fig. 35.9) can rarely present as a predominantly sellar and suprasellar lesion. An aneurysm in the sellar or parasellar region (Fig. 35.10) is always an important differential diagnosis of pituitary macroadenoma. Germinoma, metastatic disease, chondrosarcoma, and epidermoid cyst are some of the other differential diagnoses of a sellar mass.

## Teaching points

Pituitary macroadenoma may or may not be endocrinologically active. Bilateral temporal hemianopsia is most common presentation of suprasellar mass. The possibility of suprasellar extension, intraventricular extension, cavernous sinus invasion, ICA encasement and sphenoidal sinus invasion must be evaluated in all cases as these impact the surgical management.

REFERENCES

1. Hofstetter C, Ananad VK, Schwartz TH. Endoscopic transsphenoidal pituitary surgery. *Oper Tech Otolaryngol* 2011; **22**: 206–14.

2. Zhang Y, He N, Zhou J, Chen Y. The relationship between MRI invasive features and expression of EMMPRIN, galectin-3, and microvessel density in pituitary adenoma. *Clin Imaging* 2011; **35**: 165–73.

3. Johnsen DE, Woodruff WW, Allen IS, *et al.* MR imaging of the sellar and juxtasellar regions. *Radiographics* 1991; **11**(5): 727–58.

4. Bonneville F, Cattin F, Marsot-Dupuch K, *et al.* T1 signal hyperintensity in the sellar region: spectrum of findings. *Radiographics* 2006; **26**: 93–113.

5. Sol YL, Lee SK, Choi HS, *et al.* Evaluation of MRI criteria for cavernous sinus invasion in pituitary macroadenoma. *J Neuroimaging* 2012; doi: 10.1111/j.1552–6569.2012.00710.x.

6. Vieira JO, Cukiert A, Liberman B. Evaluation of magnetic resonance imaging criteria for cavernous sinus invasion in patients with pituitary adenomas: logistic regression analysis and correlation with surgical findings. *Surg Neurol* 2006; **65**: 130–5.

7. Boxerman JL, Rogg JM, Donahue JE, *et al.* Preoperative MRI evaluation of pituitary macroadenoma: imaging features predictive of successful transsphenoidal surgery. *AJR Am J Roentgenol* 2010; **195**: 720–8.

8. Hofstetter CP, Nanaszko MJ, Mubita LL, *et al.* Volumetric classification of pituitary macroadenomas predicts outcome and morbidity following endoscopic endonasal transsphenoidal surgery. *Pituitary* 2012; **15**: 450–63.

9. Romano A, Chibbaro S, Marsella M, *et al.* Combined endoscopic transsphenoidal-transventricular approach for resection of a giant pituitary macroadenoma. *World Neurosurg* 2010; **74**: 161–4

10. Patel SK, Christiano LD, Eloy JA, Liu JK. Delayed postoperative pituitary apoplexy after endoscopic transsphenoidal resection of a giant pituitary macroadenoma. *J Clin Neurosci* 2012; **19**: 1296–8.

11. Abele TA, Yetkin ZF, Raisanen JM, *et al.* Non-pituitary origin sellar tumours mimicking pituitary macroadenomas. *Clin Radiol* 2012; **67**: 821–7.

12. Kaltsas GA, Powles TB, Evanson J, *et al.* Hypothalamo-pituitary abnormalities in adult patients with langerhans cell histiocytosis: clinical, endocrinological, and radiological features and response to treatment. *J Clin Endocrinol Metab* 2000; **85**: 1370–6.

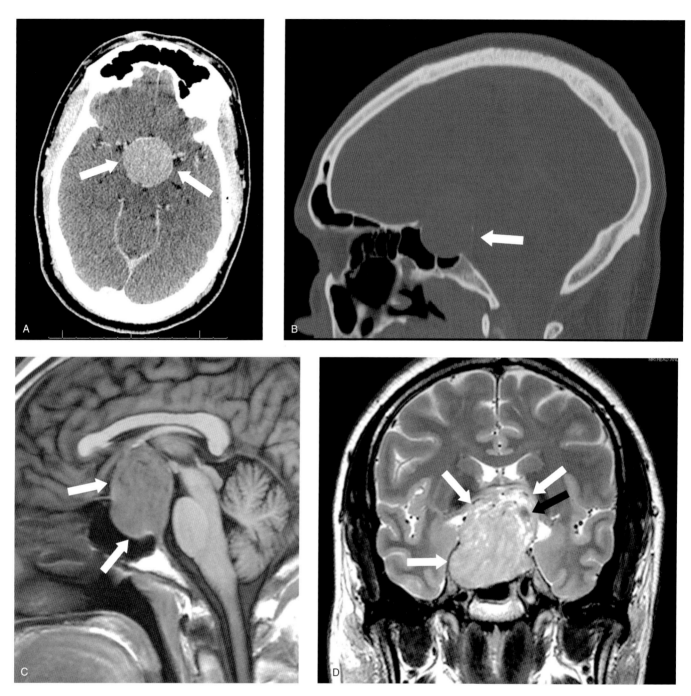

**Figure 35.1** Pituitary macroadenoma. (**A**) Post-contrast axial CT demonstrates a rounded densely enhancing mass (arrows) in the suprasellar region. (**B**) Sagittal reconstruction of bone window of head CT exhibits marked expansion of sella turcica with remodeling and erosion of the posterior clinoid process (arrow). (**C**) T1-weighted sagittal MR image exhibits a large lobulated mass isointense to brain parenchyma, arising from the sella turcica with suprasellar extension (arrows). There is elevation of mammillary bodies, optic chiasm, and floor of lateral ventricles. (**D**) T2-weighted coronal MR image exhibits a large sellar/suprasellar mass iso- to mildly hyperintense to brain parenchyma (white arrows). A focal low T2 signal area exhibits intratumoral hemorrhage (black arrow). (**E**) FLAIR-weighted axial MR image exhibits high FLAIR signal of the suprasellar mass (white arrows) with area of intratumoral hemorrhage seen as blood-fluid level (black arrow). (**F**) Post-contrast fat-saturated T1-weighted coronal image exhibits heterogeneously enhancing large suprasellar mass (white arrows). The intratumoral high T1 signal area (black arrow) corresponds to intratumoral hemorrhage. (**G**) T1-weighted sagittal MR image, following endoscopic trans-sphenoidal surgery, exhibits an area of postsurgical apoplexy within known pituitary macroadenoma (arrows).

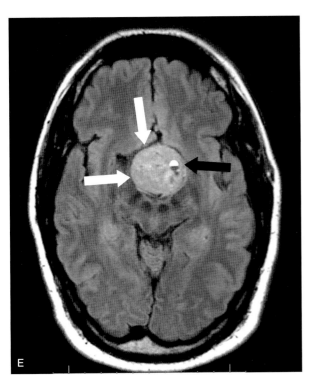

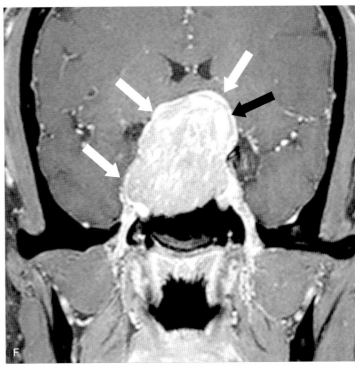

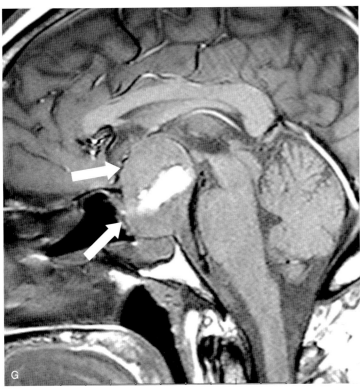

**Figure 35.1** (cont.)

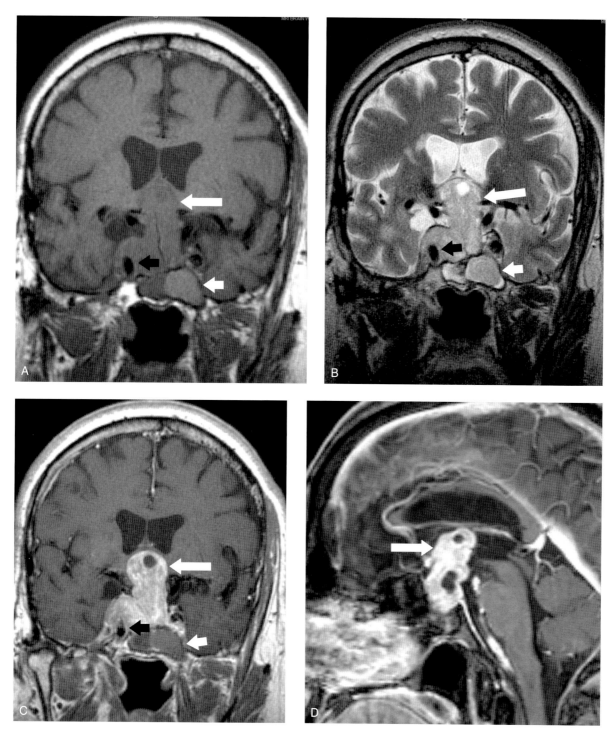

**Figure 35.2** Invasive pituitary macroadenoma. (**A**) T1-weighted coronal MR images exhibits a sellar mass that is isointense to brain parenchyma with suprasellar extension (white arrow) that invades the right cavernous sinus and envelops the intracavernous right ICA (short black arrow), which exhibits normal caliber. Note the mildly hyperintense T1 signal area of inspissated mucus within the sphenoidal sinus (short white arrow). (**B**) T2-weighted coronal MR image shows that the tumor has mildly hyperintense T2 signal (white arrow) and a cystic area within the suprasellar component. The lesion envelops the intracavernous right ICA (short black arrow). The area of inspissated mucus within the sphenoidal sinus exhibits low T2 signal (short white arrow). (**C**) Post-contrast T1-weighted coronal MR image exhibits heterogeneous enhancement of the large sellar/suprasellar mass (white arrow) invading the right cavernous sinus and enveloping the right ICA (short black arrow). The area of inspissated mucus does not show any enhancement (short white arrow). (**D**) Post-contrast T1-weighted sagittal MR image exhibits a large lobulated sellar mass with suprasellar extension reaching up to the floor of third ventricle (arrow) with two lobulated non-enhancing cystic areas within it.

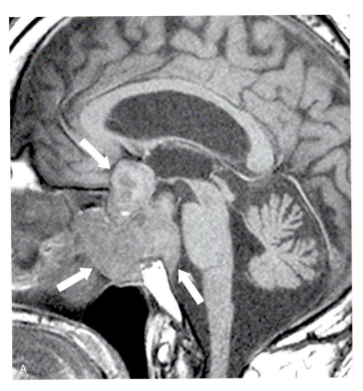

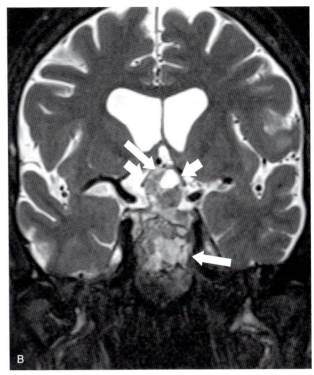

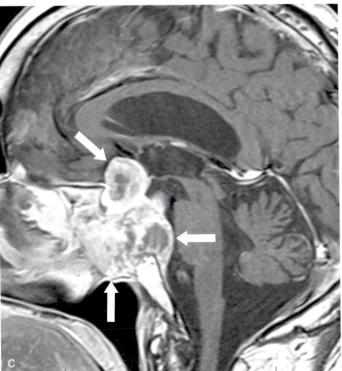

**Figure 35.3** Invasive pituitary macroadenoma. (**A**) T1-weighted sagittal MR imaging exhibits a large lobulated sellar mass (arrow) with suprasellar extension invading the sphenoidal sinus extending into prepontine cistern. The lesion exhibits isointense T1 signal. (**B**) T2-weighted coronal MR image exhibits large sellar/suprasellar mass that appears to be isointense to brain parenchyma (arrows) with intratumoral cystic areas (short arrows). (**C**) Post-contrast T1-weighted sagittal MR image exhibits heterogeneous enhancement of the mass (arrows).

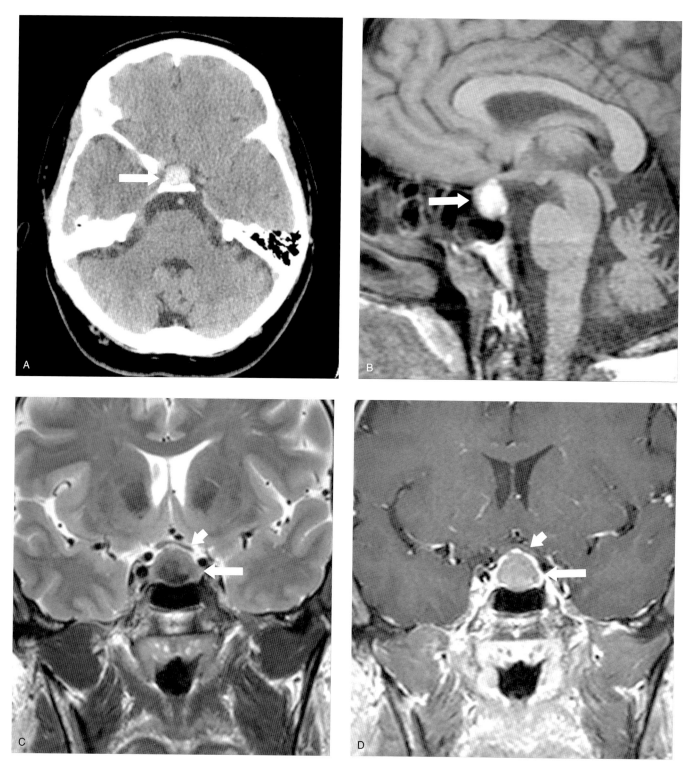

**Figure 35.4** Pituitary apoplexy. (**A**) Non-contrast axial CT exhibits hyperattenuating rounded sellar mass (arrow). (**B**) T1-weighted sagittal MR image exhibits hyperintense T1 signal sellar mass (arrow) with convex superior margin. (**C**) T2-weighted coronal MR image exhibits expanded pituitary gland appears to be isointense to brain parenchyma with area of low T2 signal at the dependent portion (arrow). There is bowing of optic chiasm (short arrow) due to suprasellar extension of the mass. (**D**) Post-contrast T1-weighted coronal MR image exhibits a central hypoenhancing pituitary macroadenoma with patchy high T1 signal hemorrhage at the dependent portion (arrow). Note the mass effect on the optic chiasm (short arrow).

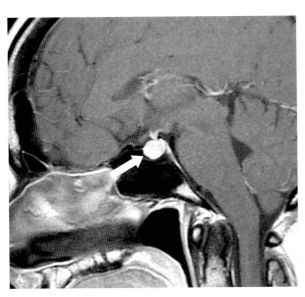
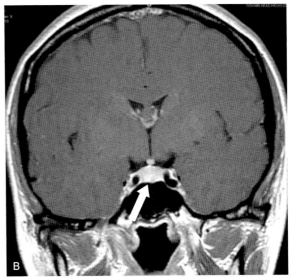

**Figure 35.5** Pituitary hyperplasia. (**A**) Post-contrast T1-weighted sagittal image exhibits homogeneously enhancing enlarged pituitary gland (arrow). (**B**) Post-contrast T1-weighted coronal image exhibits homogeneous enhancement of enlarged pituitary gland (arrow) with convex superior margin but without evidence for a focal area of hypoenhancement within the pituitary parenchyma to suggest pituitary adenoma.

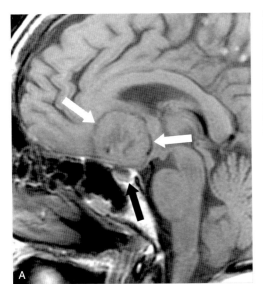
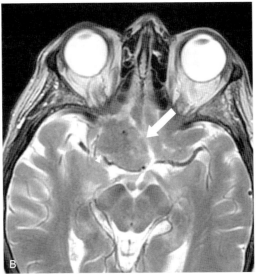

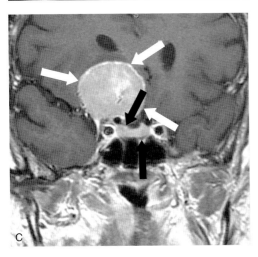

**Figure 35.6** Anterior clinoid meningioma. (**A**) T1-weighted sagittal MR image exhibits a rounded suprasellar mass (white arrows) isointense to brain parenchyma. The pituitary gland is seen separately within the sella turcica (black arrow). (**B**) T2-weighted axial MR image exhibits a right paracentral suprasellar mass (arrow), isointense to brain parenchyma with posterior displacement of right ACA. (**C**) Post-contrast T1-weighted coronal MR image exhibits a right paracentral homogeneously and intensely enhancing suprasellar mass (white arrows) arising from right anterior clinoid process, enveloping the supraclinoid right ICA. The pituitary gland can be seen within the sella turcica (black arrows).

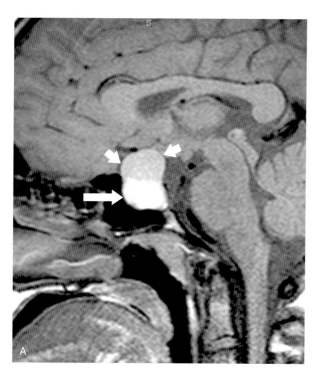

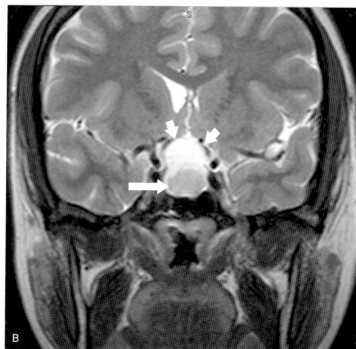

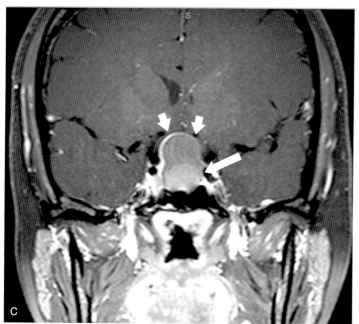

**Figure 35.7** Craniopharyngioma. (**A**) T1-weighted sagittal MR image exhibits a heterogeneous sellar/suprasellar mass with high T1 signal proteinaceous content at the dependent portion (arrow) and mildly high T1 signal cystic superior lobulation (short arrows). (**B**) T2-weighted coronal MR image exhibits T2 signal of the inferior content (arrow) with a high T2 signal superior cystic component (short arrows). (**C**) Post-contrast fat-saturated T1-weighted coronal image exhibits peripheral enhancement of the capsule of the mass (short arrows) with hypointense T1 signal of the inferior proteinaceous content (arrow).

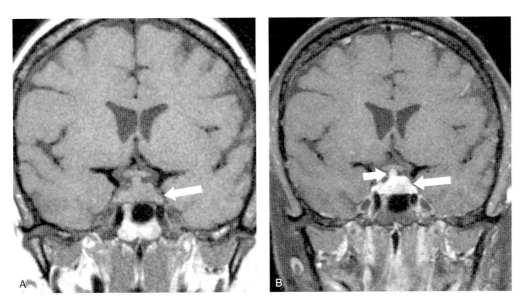

**Figure 35.8** Langerhans cell histiocytosis (LCH). (**A**) T1-weighted coronal MR image exhibits isointense mass on the left side of the pituitary gland (arrow). (**B**) Post-contrast T1-weighted coronal MR image exhibits mildly hypoenhancing intrasellar granuloma (arrow). There is thickening and enhancement of the pituitary stalk (short arrow).

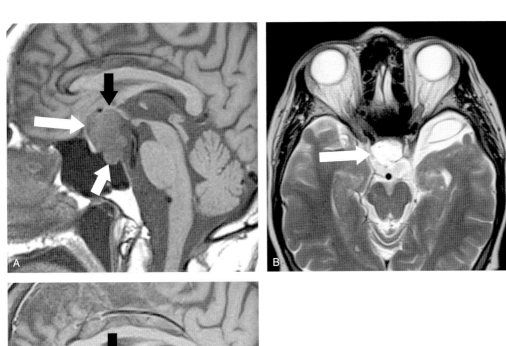

**Figure 35.9** Suprasellar chordoma. (**A**) T1-weighted sagittal MR image exhibits a lobulated sellar mass (short white arrow) with suprasellar extension (arrow) hypointense to brain parenchyma, with elevation of optic chiasm (short black arrow). (**B**) T2-weighted axial MR image exhibits hyperintense T2 signal of the sellar mass (arrow). (**C**) Post-contrast T1-weighted sagittal MR imaging exhibits patchy heterogeneous enhancement of the sellar (short white arrow) and suprasellar (arrow) mass with elevation of optic chiasm (short black arrow).

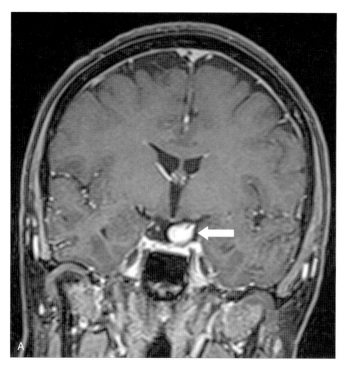

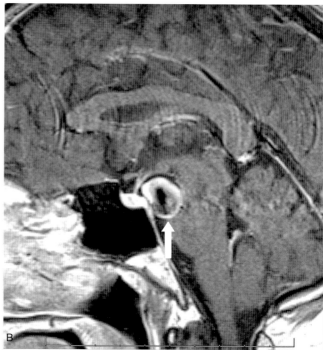

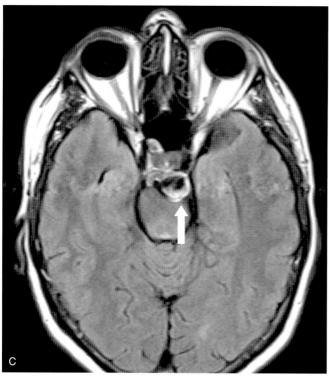

**Figure 35.10** Parasellar aneurysm. (**A**) Post-contrast fat-saturated T1-weighted coronal MR image exhibits rounded enhancing suprasellar and left parasellar mass (arrow). (**B**) Post-contrast T1-weighted sagittal MR image shows rounded heterogeneous enhancing mass superior and posterior to the sella turcica (arrow). (**C**) FLAIR-weighted axial MR image exhibits heterogeneous left parasellar mass extending into prepontine cistern central flow void (arrow), compatible with aneurysm of left posterior communicating artery.

# 36 Brain abscess

## Imaging description

Brain abscesses are uncommon compared to primary and secondary brain tumors in the developed countries. The imaging features of brain abscesses can be very similar to glioblastoma multiforme (GBM) and metastases, however. The typical brain abscess in an immunocompetent individual has a cystic/necrotic center, an enhancing wall, and surrounding edema with mass effect. Brain abscesses are usually of hematogenous origin and located in the deep white matter. They can be solitary or multiple. On MRI, abscesses show markedly restricted diffusion in their cystic regions and decreased perfusion in their walls (Fig. 36.1). These features allow differentiation of abscesses from GBM and metastases with greater than 95% accuracy (Fig. 36.2) [1–3]. Essentially all pyogenic abscesses show restricted diffusion on DWI, but non-pyogenic abscesses such as tuberculomas and toxoplasmomas have variable DWI signal [4]. However, GBMs rarely show restricted diffusion centrally, which may lead to erroneous diagnosis of abscess.

## Importance

Prompt diagnosis of brain abscess allows prompt treatment, which can be life-saving and negates expensive and time-consuming work-up for metastatic and primary tumors.

## Typical clinical scenario

Acute-onset seizure or focal neurologic deficits are the most common presenting symptoms. Systemic signs of infection are often absent. Recent history of dental procedures, endocarditis, sinonasal and otologic infections may be present.

## Differential diagnosis

In an immunocompetent adult presenting with a ring-enhancing centrally cystic or necrotic brain mass with associated surrounding edema and mass effect the differential diagnoses include abscess, GBM, and metastasis. Pyogenic abscesses show markedly and homogeneously increased DWI signal in their center. Rarely, GBMs may have central restricted diffusion in their cystic component, but this is usually less pronounced and more heterogeneous than that of abscesses. The wall of an abscess shows normal or diminished relative cerebral blood volume (rCBV), compared to the elevated rCBV seen in the walls of GBMs and metastases. Tuberculomas and cysticercosis lesions have variable DWI signal but they are often multiple. In immunocompromised patients, toxoplasmosis and lymphoma should be considered in the differential diagnosis; they demonstrate more variable imaging features (Fig. 36.3).

## Teaching points

A pyogenic abscess can reliably be differentiated from GBM and metastasis in most cases by identifying the markedly and homogeneously elevated central DWI signal and diminished rCBV in its wall.

REFERENCES

1. Reddy JS, Mishra AM, Behari S, et al. The role of diffusion-weighted imaging in the differential diagnosis of intracranial cystic mass lesions: a report of 147 lesions. Surg Neurol 2006; 66: 246–50.

2. Erdogan C, Hakyemez B, Yildirim N, Parlak M. Brain abscess and cystic brain tumor: discrimination with dynamic susceptibility contrast perfusion-weighted MRI. J Comput Assist Tomogr 2005; 29: 663–7.

3. Muccio CF, Esposito G, Bartolini A, Cerase A. Cerebral abscesses and necrotic cerebral tumours: differential diagnosis by perfusion-weighted magnetic resonance imaging. Radiol Med 2008; 113: 747–57.

4. Gupta RK, Prakash M, Mishra AM, et al. Role of diffusion weighted imaging in differentiation of intracranial tuberculoma and tuberculous abscess from cysticercus granulomas-a report of more than 100 lesions. Eur J Radiol 2005; 55: 384–92.

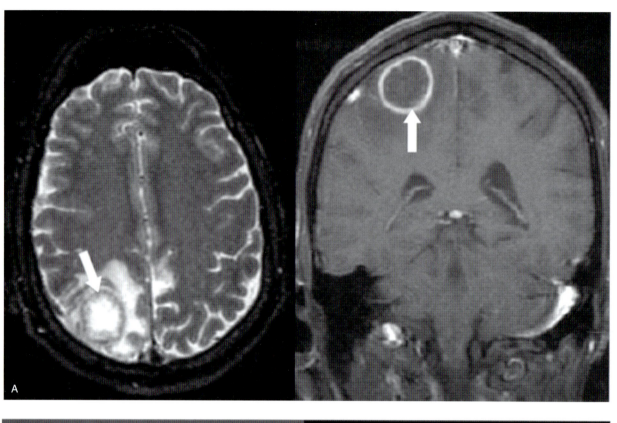

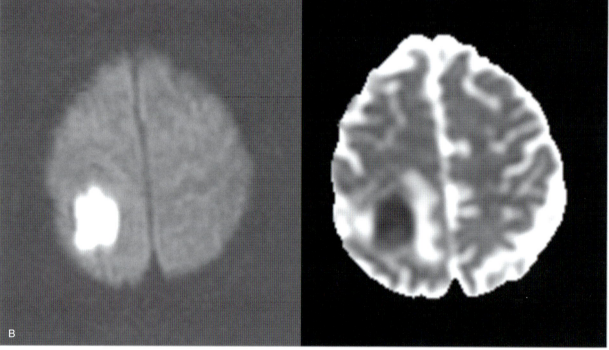

**Figure 36.1** (**A**) A solitary brain abscess shows centrally hyperintense signal with surrounding edema on T2-weighted imaging and a thin wall (arrow) that appears isointense to the brain. Post-contrast T1-weighted coronal image shows enhancement of the wall. (**B**) Axial DWI and ADC images show markedly restricted diffusion in the central non-enhancing component of the lesion.

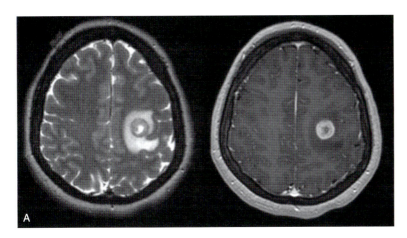

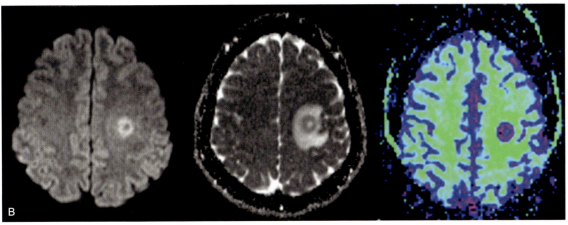

**Figure 36.2** (**A**) A solitary brain lesion with a central hyperintensity on T2-weighted imaging and a relatively thick wall shows enhancement on the post-contrast T1-weighted image. (**B**) DWI, ADC, and PWI images show mild restriction of diffusion within the wall of the lesion (compared to the central T2 hyperintense part in Fig. 36.1). There is increased diffusion in the central part of the lesion. Increased blood flow to the lesion wall is noted on PWI. These features would favor high-grade glioma or metastasis over pyogenic abscess. Biopsy revealed glioblastoma.

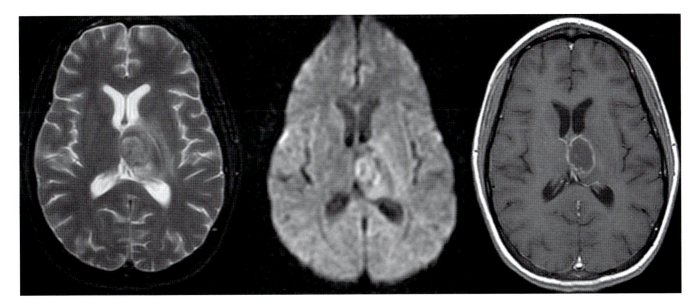

**Figure 36.3** A solitary left thalamic lesion with surrounding edema, hypointense wall, and central heterogeneous but mostly hyperintense T2 signal, some restriction of diffusion on DWI and wall enhancement on post-contrast T1-weighted image. The patient had HIV/AIDS. Biopsy revealed toxoplasmosis.

# **37** Neurocysticercosis

## Imaging description

The imaging spectrum of neurocysticercosis is broad, which may create challenges in differential diagnosis. Cysticercosis involvement of the central nervous system (CNS) may be divided into parenchymal and extraparenchymal categories [1]. Parenchymal lesions include four stages of evolution of infestation:

(1) Vesicular stage – parenchymal cysts and the scolex within them are identified on both CT and MRI. Cysts usually measure <1 cm, cyst signal follows that of CSF, and thus the scolex is usually best seen on FLAIR images. No significant enhancement is present at this stage, although minimal cyst wall enhancement and scolex enhancement may be seen on MRI (Fig. 37.1).
(2) Colloidal vesicular stage – early degeneration of cysts results in change in signal of cyst fluid. Rupture of cyst and release of antigens results in inflammatory reaction, edema, and ring enhancement seen both on MRI and CT. T2-weighted images may show decreased signal associated with the cyst wall (Fig. 37.2).
(3) Granular nodular stage – late degeneration of still active cyst results in decreasing edema. Enhancement becomes more nodular, and cysts get smaller or transform into small nodules, which may start showing calcification (Fig. 37.3).
(4) Nodular calcified stage – completion of degeneration results in an inactive lesion with resolution of edema and calcification of nodule, which shows decreased T1 and T2 signal and may be difficult to see on MRI. CT is more sensitive at this stage.

Extraparenchymal neurocysticercosis may present as (1) intraventricular cysts or (2) subarachnoid cysts. An intraventricular cyst results in hydrocephalus and may be impossible to identify on CT and difficult to see on MRI depending on the signal associated with the scolex (Fig. 37.4). Cysts are most commonly found in the fourth ventricle but they may move within the ventricles. Subarachnoid cysts usually present with a completely degenerated and therefore invisible scolex and form clusters of poorly visible cysts (racemose form), typically in the basilar cisterns. There may be enhancement of the adjacent meninges due to secondary inflammation.

Parenchymal and extraparenchymal forms may or may not be found together. Typically there are multiple parenchymal lesions found in cortical locations, but basal ganglia and cerebellar lesions may occur as well. Lesions may be in the same or different stages of evolution. Solitary lesions may also occur, and these require a broader differential diagnosis. Isolated intraventricular lesions may be difficult to diagnose.

## Importance

Cysticercosis is the most common parasitic disease worldwide, and it continues to be a significant problem in developed countries, partly because of immigration and travel, although approximately one-third of neurocysticercosis cases seen in developed countries occur in individuals with no history of travel.

## Typical clinical scenario

The most common clinical manifestation of neurocysticercosis is seizure. Obstructive hydrocephalus, intracranial hypertension, focal neurologic signs, and cerebral infarction may also occur. An acute encephalitis-like presentation has been described in the pediatric population.

## Differential diagnosis

When multiple lesions in different stages of evolution are found the diagnosis is straightforward. Multiple or single ring-enhancing lesions of the colloidal vesicular stage and nodular enhancing lesions of the granular nodular stage require differential diagnosis from abscesses and metastases. Neurocysticercosis lesions do not show restricted diffusion of DWI, which helps to differentiate them from pyogenic abscesses. Perfusion-weighted images show increased relative cerebral blood volume (rCBV) associated with metastases, which is not seen in neurocysticercosis.

> ### Teaching points
>
> Neurocysticercosis may be parenchymal and/or extraparenchymal, and multiple lesions may present at the same or different stages of disease. Ring-enhancing lesions can be differentiated from abscess and metastasis by DWI and PWI. Intraventricular and subarachnoid cysts can result in hydrocephalus and are difficult to diagnose, particularly with CT, because they resemble CSF.

REFERENCES
1. Lerner A, Shiroishi MS, Zee CS, Law M, Go JL. Imaging of neurocysticercosis. *Neuroimaging Clin N Am* 2012; **22**: 659–76.

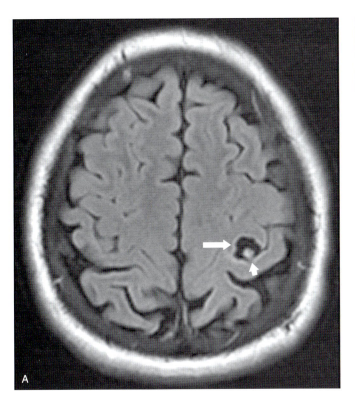

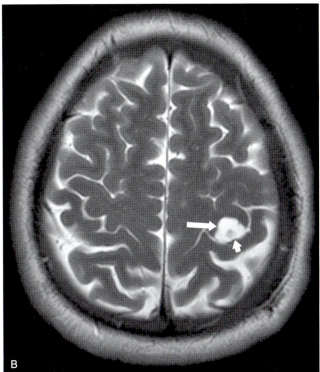

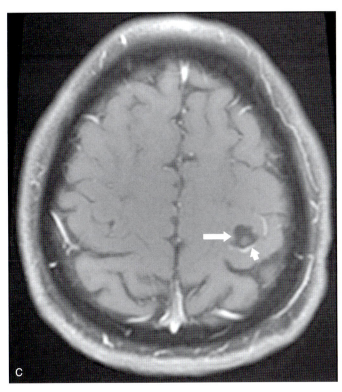

**Figure 37.1** Parenchymal vesicular neurocysticercosis. (**A**) Axial FLAIR, (**B**) T2-weighted, and (**C**) post-contrast T1-weighted images exhibit a CSF intensity left high-convexity posterior frontal lesion (arrow) with mildly high FLAIR signal of the scolex (short arrow) and no significant edema or enhancement. The linear enhancement along the posterior margin of the cyst likely represents a cortical vein.

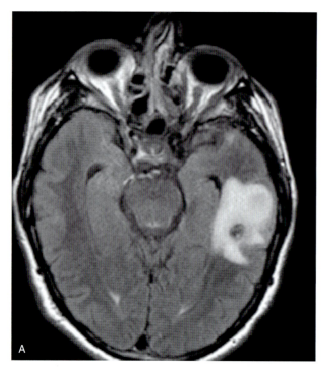

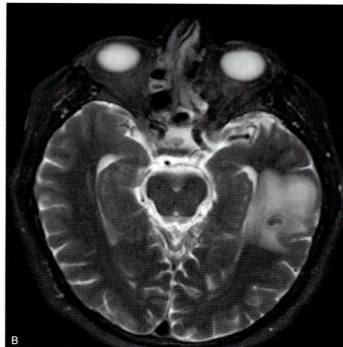

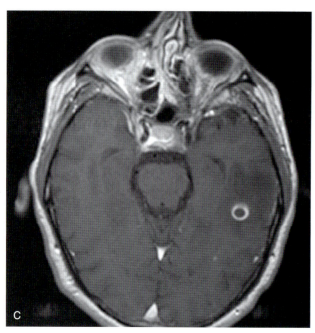

**Figure 37.2** Parenchymal colloidal vesicular neurocysticercosis. (**A**) Axial FLAIR, (**B**) T2-weighted, and (**C**) post-contrast T1-weighted images show a ring-enhancing lesion in the left temporal lobe with marked surrounding edema and T2 hypointense cyst in this patient, who presented with seizures.

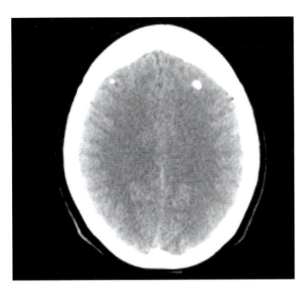
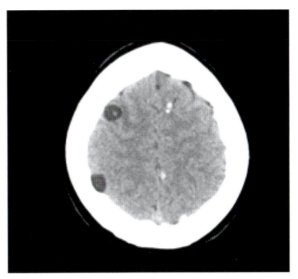

**Figure 37.3** Parenchymal neurocysticercosis, vesicular and nodular calcified stage. Axial CT images show multiple calcified nodules bilaterally in cortical locations with two vesicular-stage lesions seen in the right frontal lobe. Note the scolex within the more anterior vesicle.

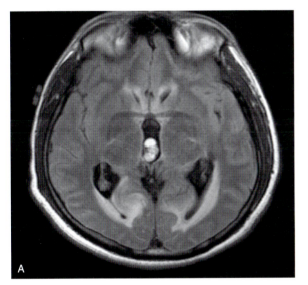
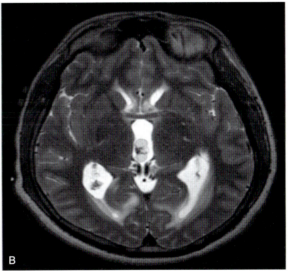
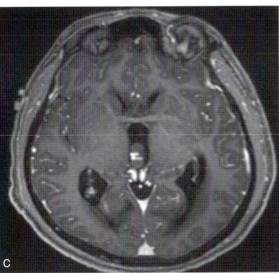

**Figure 37.4** Intraventricular neurocysticercosis. (**A**) Axial FLAIR, (**B**) T2-weighted, and (**C**) post-contrast T1-weighted images show an intraventricular cyst causing hydrocephalus and ependymitis resulting in periventricular signal changes. Note that the cyst has different signal than CSF and shows enhancement, making it easy to see.

## Imaging description

Tuberculosis of the central nervous system (CNS) accounts for 2% of HIV-negative and 19% of HIV-positive patients infected with pulmonary tuberculosis [1]. It is thought to be due to reactivation of a dormant "Rich focus" due to primary pulmonary tuberculosis [2,3]. Tuberculous meningitis (TBM) (Fig. 38.1), considered a medical emergency, is a common manifestation of CNS tuberculosis, presenting with meningeal inflammation, basal exudates, vasculitis, and hydrocephalus [4,5].

Basal exudates or meningeal inflammation may not be apparent on non-contrast CT or MRI; only possible hydrocephalus or patchy multifocal vasculitis may be seen; however, intense basilar leptomeningeal enhancement is seen on post-contrast studies [1,5,6]. Depending on the stage of response of the immune system, a parenchymal granuloma may or may not exhibit caseating necrosis [1]. A solid non-caseating granuloma (Fig. 38.2) appears as a solid isodense and isointense T1 signal mass-like lesion with a characteristic hypointense T2 signal and solid or complete ring enhancement [1,6,7]. Due to a cell-mediated delayed hypersensitivity reaction, the core undergoes a coagulative and liquefactive necrosis called caseation [1]. A caseating tuberculous granuloma (Fig. 38.3) with necrotic center exhibits a central hyperintense T2 signal within a hypointense T2 signal lesion and peripheral rim enhancement.

Complications of CNS tuberculosis include vasculitis, ischemia, ventriculitis, choroid plexitis, pachymeningitis, and arachnoiditis [3,6,7]. On MR angiography, vessel irregularity, narrowing, and occlusion may be seen. MR spectroscopy has a characteristic lipid peak with lack of other discernible resonances (Fig. 38.4) [2]. Heterogeneous-appearing tuberculoma may show choline resonance at 3.22 ppm along with lipid peak [6]. Tuberculous abscess is a rare condition that is seen more frequently in immunocompromised patients. On imaging, it is indistinguishable from a pyogenic abscess [1,3].

## Importance

TBM is considered a medical emergency. The diagnosis of TBM is best made with CSF analysis. Leucocytosis (predominantly lymphocytes), raised CSF proteins, and CSF plasma glucose <50% are considered diagnostic. However, mycobacterial culture or polymerase chain reaction (PCR) is necessary for bacteriological confirmation [4]. Treatment delay is strongly associated with death, and empirical anti-tuberculosis therapy should be started promptly in all patients in whom the diagnosis of TBM is suspected without waiting for microbiological or molecular diagnostic confirmation [7,8]. However, imaging is essential for the diagnosis of cerebral tuberculoma [8].

According to British Infection Society guidelines, the treatment consists of four drugs (isoniazid, rifampicin, pyrazinamide, ethambutol) for 2–4 months followed by two drugs (isoniazid, rifampicin) for 8–10 months. Adjunctive corticosteroids (either dexamethasone or prednisolone) should be given to all patients with TBM, regardless of disease severity. All patients with suspected or proven tuberculosis should be tested for HIV infection [8]. MRI is the modality of choice to monitor treatment response. Paradoxical expansion of intracranial tuberculoma or appearance of new lesions following treatment is considered a rare multifactorial response [6] but can also be seen due to multi-drug-resistant tuberculosis (MDR-TB). Addition of second-line of drugs and prolonged medical therapy up to 30 months are advocated [1].

## Typical clinical scenario

Tuberculous infection of brain is an uncommon disease with rising incidence and varied clinical manifestations [1,2]. It is more commonly seen in patients under the age of 15 years [1]. The spectrum extends from mild meningitis with no neurological deficits to coma. When presenting as meningitis, the signs and symptoms include headache, neck rigidity, and photophobia. Lethargy, anorexia, weight loss, confusion, myalgia, and fever are also typically present [4]. Cranial nerve palsies may also be encountered due to basal meningitis. Parenchymal tuberculoma presents with mass-like symptoms. Seizures, papilledema, nausea, and vomiting are commonly seen. Depending on the location within the brain, motor weakness and visual disturbances may also be seen. Paraparesis or paraplegia may be present due to parenchymal tuberculoma or possible radiculomyelitis.

## Differential diagnosis

Acute pyogenic meningitis (Fig. 38.5) is more common in children and is associated with neutropenic leukocytosis, increased protein, and lower glucose levels on CSF analysis [9]. It is usually associated with generalized swelling of the brain and diffuse leptomeningeal enhancement, which is more common at high convexity than at the basal cistern. In neonates, group B streptococci are more common and devastating infective agents. There is also presence of focal hyperintense T2 signal parenchymal abnormalities secondary to brain ischemia [9]. CNS involvement occurs in 5–10% of systemic sarcoidosis cases (Fig. 38.6). MRI demonstrates nodular and enhancing leptomeningeal lesions, particularly involving the basal cistern and the leptomeninges. Pyogenic abscess (Fig. 38.7) tends to be more common amongst males than females, for unknown reasons, and more commonly occurs during the first four decades of life [10].

Metastatic deposits from lung (Fig. 38.8) can present as multiple small nodular and ring-enhancing lesions, which may be parenchymal and periventricular. In the initial stages, there may be lack of significant perilesional edema. However, they tend to be T2 hyperintense. CNS lymphoma (see Case 29) and highly malignant metastatic deposits, such as from adenocarcinoma of breast (Fig. 38.9), can exhibit hypointense T2 signal due to high nuclear to cytoplasm ratio.

## Teaching points

Tuberculosis of the brain is a great mimic for various neoplasms and infections and a popular differential diagnosis in certification exams! Imaging findings of a combination of meningitis and intraparenchymal lesions suggest the diagnosis of tuberculosis. Intraparencyhmal tuberculosis lesions show characteristic hypointense T2 signal with or without a central hyperintense T2 signal, isointense T1 signal, and solid or ring enhancement on post-contrast T1-weighted images. Sequential imaging is recommended to monitor therapy response and to identify unexpected or asymptomatic complications during treatment.

REFERENCES

1. Shah GV. Central nervous system tuberculosis: imaging manifestations. *Neuroimaging Clin N Am* 2000; **10**: 355–74.

2. Patkar D, Narang J, Yanamandala R, *et al.* Central nervous system tuberculosis: pathophysiology and imaging findings. *Neuroimaging Clin N Am* 2012; **22**: 677–705.

3. Rodrigues MG, da Rocha AJ, Masruha MR, Minett TS. Neurotuberculosis: an overview. *Cent Nerv Syst Agents Med Chem* 2011; **11**: 246–60.

4. Garg RK. Tuberculous meningitis. *Acta Neurol Scand* 2010; **122**: 75–90.

5. Galimi R. Extrapulmonary tuberculosis: tuberculous meningitis new developments. *Eur Rev Med Pharmacol Sci* 2011; **15**: 365–86.

6. Trivedi R, Saksena S, Gupta RK. Magnetic resonance imaging in central nervous system tuberculosis. *Indian J Radiol Imaging* 2009; **19**: 256–65.

7. Bernaerts A, Vanhoenacker FM, Parizel PM, *et al.* Tuberculosis of the central nervous system: overview of neuroradiological findings. *Eur Radiol* 2003; **13**: 1876–90.

8. Thwaites G, Fisher M, Hemingway C, *et al.* British Infection Society guidelines for the diagnosis and treatment of tuberculosis of the central nervous system in adults and children. *J Infect* 2009; **59**: 167–87.

9. Mohan S, Jain KK, Arabi M, Shah GV. Imaging of meningitis and ventriculitis. *Neuroimaging Clin N Am* 2012; **22**: 557–83.

10. Rath TJ, Hughes M, Arabi M, Shah GV. Imaging of cerebritis, encephalitis, and brain abscess. *Neuroimaging Clin N Am* 2012; **22**: 585–607.

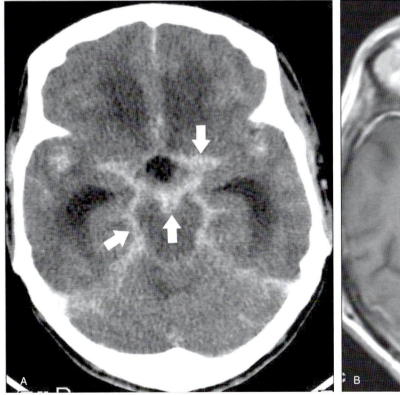
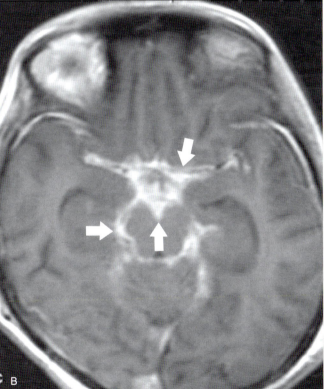

**Figure 38.1** Tuberculous meningitis. (**A**) Post-contrast axial CT exhibits irregular and heterogeneous leptomeningeal enhancement at the basilar cistern and perimesencephalic cistern (short arrows). There is resultant hydrocephalus with dilatation of both the temporal horns and third ventricle with periventricular low-attenuating areas, suggesting transependymal CSF migration. (**B**) Post-contrast T1-weighted axial MR image following ventricular shunting exhibits intense and nodular enhancement of the basal cistern.

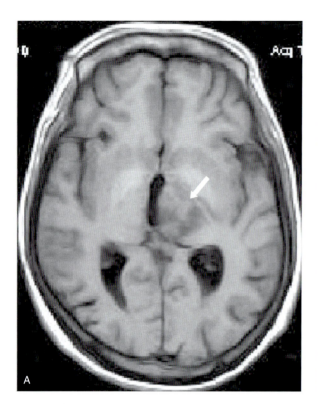

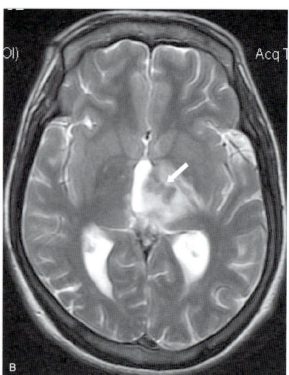

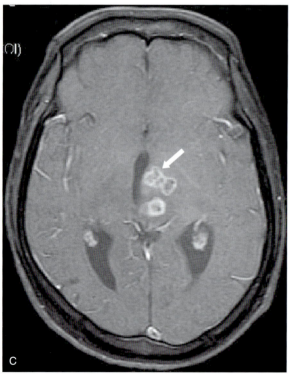

**Figure 38.2** Non-caseating tuberculous granuloma. (**A**) T1-weighted axial MR image exhibits a nodular left thalamic lesion, isointense to brain parenchyma (arrow), surrounded by hypointense T1 signal perilesional edema. (**B**) T2-weighted axial MR image exhibits hypointense T2 signal left thalamic lesion (arrow) with hyperintense T2 signal surrounding edema. (**C**) Fat-saturated post-contrast T1-weighted axial MR image exhibits peripheral ring enhancement (arrow).

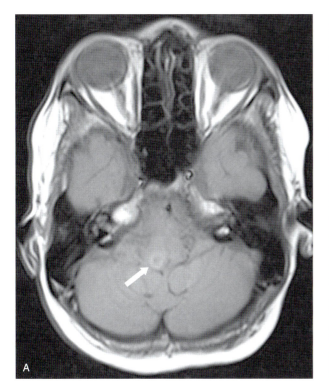

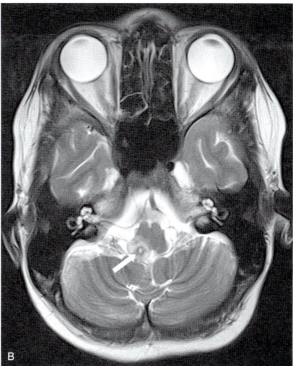

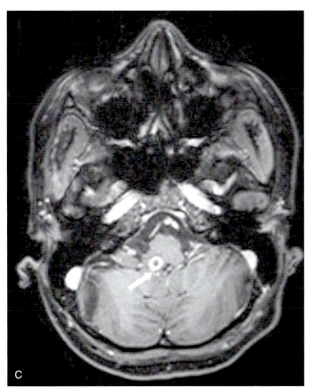

**Figure 38.3** Caseating tuberculous granuloma. (**A**) T1-weighted axial MR image exhibits mildly hyperintense T1 signal mass (arrow) with central mildly hypointense T1 signal core at right medulla oblongata. (**B**) T2-weighted axial MR image exhibits a hyperintense T2 signal mass with a central focal hyperintensity (arrow) and surrounding hyperintense T2 signal edema at the right medulla. (**C**) Post-contrast T1-weighted axial MR image exhibits a complete paracentral rim enhancement of the small right medullary lesion (arrow).

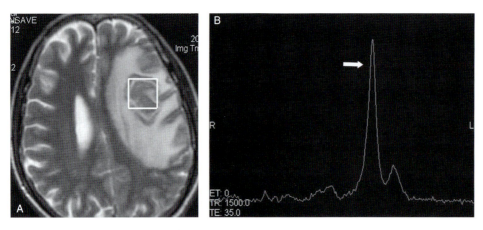

**Figure 38.4** Non-caseating tuberculous granuloma. (**A**) T2-weighted axial MR image exhibits an irregular lesion with a T2 hypointense rim and a large amount of surrounding hyperintense T2 signal edema in the left periventricular region. (**B**) Short TE MR spectroscopy of the lesion exhibits a large lipid peak (arrow) with lack of other resonances.

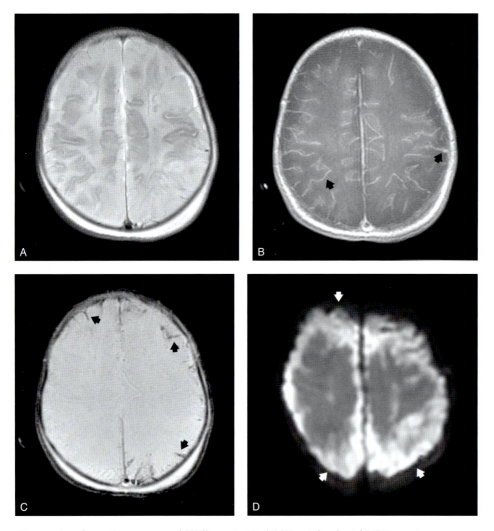

**Figure 38.5** Group B streptococcal (GBS) meningitis. (**A**) T2-weighted axial MR image in a neonate presenting with fever and meningeal signs exhibits extensive diffuse bilateral hyperintense T2 signal edema. (**B**) Post-contrast T1-weighted axial MR image exhibits extensive leptomeningeal enhancement at bilateral high convexity (short arrows). (**C**) Gradient echo T2*-weighted axial MR image exhibits enhanced susceptibility at a few cortical venous structures (short arrows), compatible with thrombotic changes. (**D**) Extensive areas of predominantly cortical diffusion restriction are seen bilaterally (short arrows).

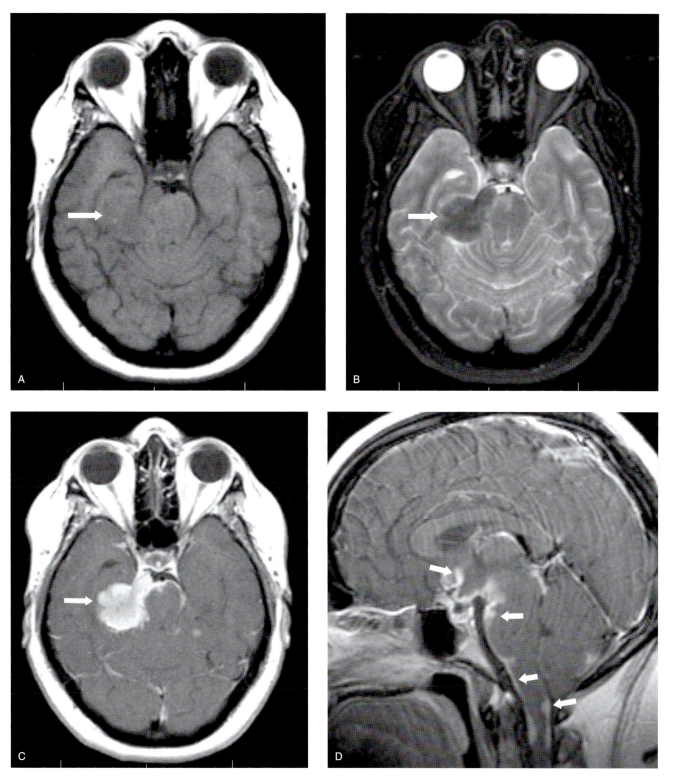

**Figure 38.6** Neurosarcoidosis. (**A**) T1-weighted axial MR image exhibits extra-axial nodular mass (arrow), marginally hypointense to isointense to brain parenchyma at left peripontine cistern. (**B**) T2-weighted axial MR image exhibits a lobulated hypointense T2 signal extra-axial mass (arrow). (**C**) Post-contrast T1-weighted axial MR image exhibits intense but heterogeneous enhancement of this lobulated right-sided extra-axial granulomatous mass. Patchy enhancement is also seen at the superior left cerebellar hemisphere and along the ventral and lateral surface of the pons. (**D**) Post-contrast T1-weighted sagittal MR image exhibits patchy and nodular post-contrast leptomeningeal enhancement (arrows) along the anterior surface of the third ventricle, the basal cistern, the ventral surface of pontomedullary neuraxis, and extending onto the proximal cervical cord.

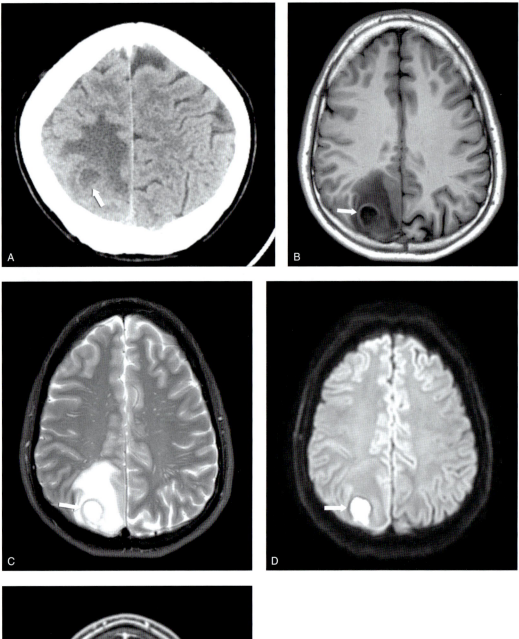

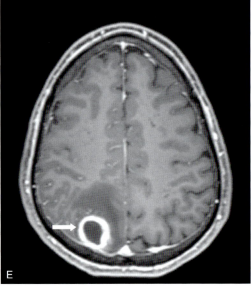

**Figure 38.7** Pyogenic abscess. (**A**) Non-contrast axial CT exhibits a right frontoparietal subcortical lesion (arrow) with mildly hyperdense peripheral capsule and central low attenuation, surrounded by extensive perilesional low-attenuating white matter edema. (**B**) T1-weighted axial MR image exhibits mildly hypointense T1 signal capsule (arrow) with central low T1 signal pus and surrounding irregular low T1 signal edema. (**C**) T2-weighted axial MR image exhibits hypointense T2 signal capsule of the abscess (arrow) with hyperintense T2 signal central pus as well as surrounding white matter edema. (**D**) Areas of diffusion restriction within the central pus (arrow) are seen on diffusion-weighted images. (**E**) Post-contrast T1-weighted axial MR image exhibits thick uniform ring enhancement of the peripheral capsule (arrow).

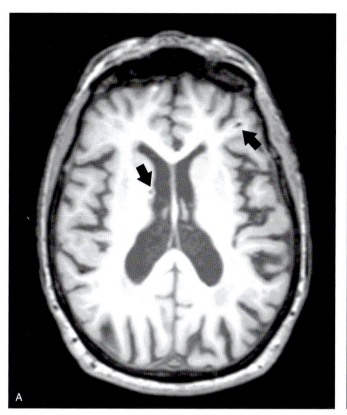

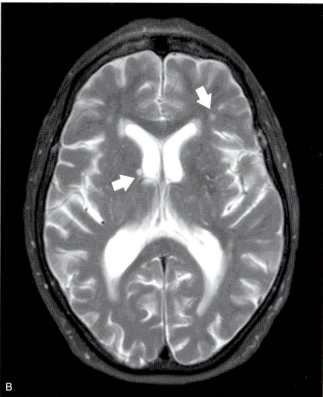

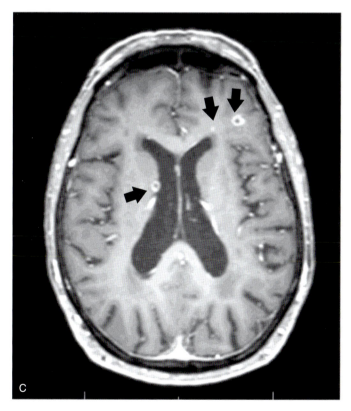

Figure 38.8 Metastatic deposits from lung carcinoma. (A) T1-weighted axial MR image in a patient presenting with seizures and having a known carcinoma of the lung exhibits presence of rounded CSF intensity lesions (short black arrows) at right periventricular region and left frontal lobe. (B) T2-weighted axial MR image exhibits hyperintense T2 signal of these lesions (short white arrows). There is no evidence for significant perilesional edema. (C) Post-contrast T1-weighted axial image exhibits peripheral rim enhancement of right periventricular and left frontal lesions with a punctate enhancing additional focus at left frontal lobe (short black arrows). On biopsy, these proved to be metastatic lung carcinoma.

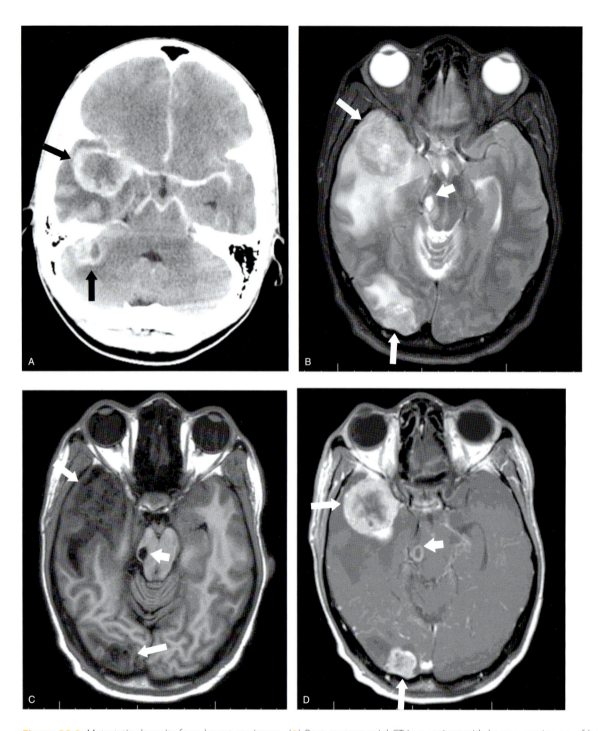

**Figure 38.9** Metastatic deposits from breast carcinoma. (**A**) Post-contrast axial CT in a patient with known carcinoma of breast exhibits multiple supratentorial and infratentorial enhancing masses (black arrows) with irregular peripheral rim enhancement and surrounding edema. (**B**) T2-weighted axial MR image exhibits heterogeneously hypointense to marginally hyperintense masses (arrows) at right temporal and occipital lobes with surrounding edema. A cystic right cerebral peduncular lesion (short arrow) with surrounding edema is also seen. (**C**) T1-weighted axial MR image exhibits heterogeneously hypointense T1 signal masses (arrows) at right temporal and occipital region with a CSF intensity hypointense T1 signal lesion at right cerebral peduncle (short arrow). (**D**) Post-contrast T1-weighted axial MR image exhibits heterogeneous but intense enhancement of right temporal and right occipital masses (arrows) with areas of non-enhancing central necrosis. Peripheral rim enhancement of right cerebral peduncular mass is seen (short arrow).

# 39 Creutzfeldt–Jakob disease

## Imaging description

Creutzfeldt–Jakob disease (CJD) is a rare prion-mediated disease with progressive and invariably fatal outcome. The imaging features differ according to the disease subtype (sporadic, variant, familial, and idiopathic). The most common form, sporadic CJD (sCJD), accounts for 85% of cases and has relatively characteristic imaging features [1,2]. High T2, FLAIR, and DWI signal in the striatum and cerebral cortex occurs classically (Figs. 39.1, 39.2), with thalamic involvement in a smaller number of cases. High-signal changes on DWI and FLAIR sequences have a very high sensitivity and accuracy for the detection of sCJD, exceeding 90% [2]. There is generally lack of enhancement with intravenous contrast, and T1-weighted images tend to be normal. Similarly, CT demonstrates cerebral atrophy but is otherwise normal. DWI imaging changes reflect true restriction of diffusion and are accompanied by apparent diffusion coefficient (ADC) changes. The DWI abnormalities precede FLAIR and T2 signal change and tend to persist for a long period of time.

A variant form of CJD (vCJD) has been described and linked to bovine spongiform encephalopathy (BSE). Symmetric areas of high signal in the pulvinar thalami are pathognomonic and termed the "pulvinar sign." This sign alone has a sensitivity of 78–90% and specificity of 100% for vCJD [2]. Similar to sCJD, these signal changes are seen on T2, FLAIR, and DWI sequences and there is no contrast enhancement. Although signal changes in pulvinar may be present in sCJD cases, these are less pronounced compared to signal change in the striatum.

## Importance

A correct diagnosis of CJD requires correlation of clinical, EEG, laboratory, and neuroimaging data. If a probable diagnosis of CJD is reached, special precautions become necessary in the performance of procedures on these patients.

## Typical clinical scenario

There are four different subsets of CJD. The most common, sporadic form accounts for 85% of cases and presents with rapidly progressive dementia and neurologic dysfunction. EEG changes suggestive of sCJD include generalized, triphasic,

sharp-wave complexes. CSF electrophoresis may reveal an increased level of 14-3-3 protein, and helps make a probable diagnosis of sCJD [1,2].

Variant CJD was first reported in the UK in 1996, and is causally related to BSE [1]. As compared to sCJD, vCJD predominantly affects younger patients (<30 years) and the clinical course is typically longer.

## Differential diagnosis

The imaging features of CJD are relatively classic and pathognomonic. Sporadic CJD should be differentiated from other conditions resulting in basal ganglia changes, including hypoxic injury, carbon monoxide (CO) poisoning, encephalitis, and Leigh's disease. The CO poisoning results in necrosis of the globus pallidus, unlike sCJD (Fig. 39.3). Leigh's disease and hypoxia may cause changes that are very similar to sCJD but the clinical picture is completely different (Fig. 39.4). As opposed to hypoxia and infarction, the diffusion restriction in sCJD persists for much longer periods.

Variant CJD can be readily diagnosed and differentiated from other disease entities owing to its pathognomonic pulvinar sign. However, disorders resulting in bilateral thalamic signal abnormality must be remembered and excluded, for example deep venous thrombosis and encephalitis.

## Teaching points

A combination of striatal and cortical FLAIR and diffusion signal abnormalities should raise a strong suspicion for sCJD, in the presence of a supportive history. The imaging appearance of the next most common type of CJD (vCJD) is also pathognomonic with bilateral, symmetrical pulvinar high signal.

REFERENCES

1. Collie DA, Sellar RJ, Zeidler M, Colchester AC, Knight R, Will RG. MRI of Creutzfeldt–Jakob disease: imaging features and recommended MRI protocol. *Clin Radiol* 2001; **56**(9): 726–39.
2. Tschampa HJ, Zerr I, Urbach H. Radiological assessment of Creutzfeldt–Jakob disease. *Eur Radiol* 2007; **17**(5): 1200–11.

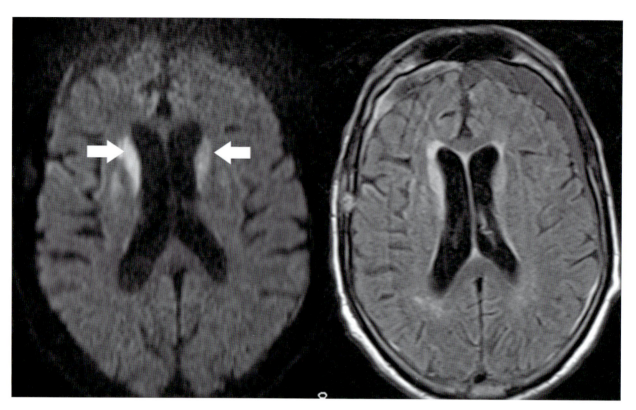

**Figure 39.1** Classic neuroimaging findings are noted in a patient with proven CJD. Axial diffusion and FLAIR images reveal symmetric areas of restricted diffusion (arrows) and high FLAIR signal in the caudate nuclei. Also noted is faint restricted diffusion in the right lentiform nucleus. The patient also has bilateral subdural hematomas in the frontal region from recent falls.

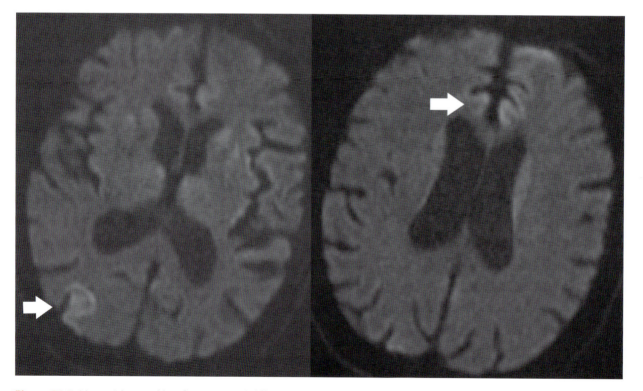

**Figure 39.2** More widespread but faint restricted diffusion is evident in the patient with rapidly progressive dementia. Note the involvement of the right occipital cortex (short arrow) and cingulate gyri (arrow) in addition to medial thalami and basal ganglia.

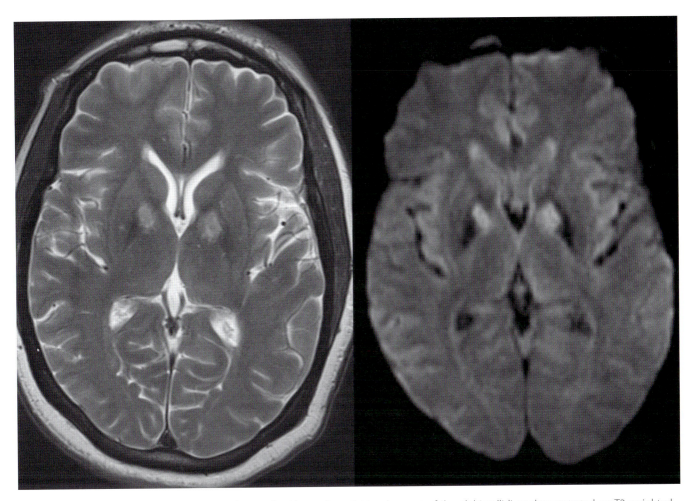

**Figure 39.3** Carbon monoxide poisoning is characterized by preferential involvement of the globi pallidi, as demonstrated on T2-weighted and DWI axial images. The caudate nuclei are spared.

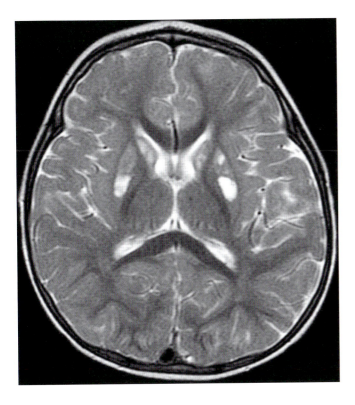

**Figure 39.4** Cystic areas of necrosis in bilateral caudate and lenticular nuclei are noted in this child with Leigh's disease on axial T2-weighted image.

# Herpes encephalitis

## Imaging description

Nearly 95% cases of herpes simplex encephalitis (HSE) are caused by herpes simplex virus 1 (HSV1), and it is the most common cause of fatal encephalitis [1,2]. Brain infection is likely a result of direct transmission of the virus from a peripheral site to the trigeminal or olfactory nerve, although other mechanisms include hematogenic transmission.

CT imaging in patients with HSE is frequently non-specific. It may reveal areas of hypodensity in the temporal or frontal lobes, but frank hemorrhage or enhancement is uncommonly seen. MRI should be obtained rapidly in patients suspected of harboring this diagnosis, since MRI can reveal the characteristic neuroanatomical pattern of involvement. Herpes encephalitis is generally unilateral in the initial phase, but there is progressive but asymmetric contralateral involvement in the later stages (Figs. 40.1, 40.2). The medial temporal and inferior frontal lobes are commonly affected, but most characteristically there is involvement of the insula (Fig. 40.1). HSE is frequently hemorrhagic, and enhancement is not a prominent feature in the early disease process. In later stages, patchy enhancement is frequently seen (Fig. 40.2C) [1]. The disease predominantly involves the cortex and subcortical white matter, and there is often extensive involvement of the limbic system.

DWI sequence is critical, and demonstrates patchy areas of restricted diffusion in the involved areas of the brain. Although the DWI restriction can mimic stroke, characteristic and non-vascular distribution is helpful to differentiate HSE from ischemic process. MRI is useful in the initial diagnosis, but also helpful in monitoring disease progression.

## Importance

Radiologists play a crucial part in the diagnosis and proper management of HSE. Recognition of the neuroanatomical distribution and characteristic pattern allows a presumptive diagnosis to be made.

## Typical clinical scenario

The clinical presentation is non-specific and consists of febrile illness, impairment of consciousness, altered sensorium, and seizures. Cerebrospinal fluid (CSF) shows a mild inflammatory pattern and polymerase chain reaction (PCR) analysis may allow a possibility of rapid diagnosis [2].

## Differential diagnosis

Differential considerations include other encephalitides, limbic encephalitis, seizures, and ischemic disease. Although differentiation from other types of infectious encephalitis may not always be possible, a particular distribution of involvement (insula, limbic system, inferior frontal and temporal lobe) favors HSE.

Limbic encephalitis (LE) and seizures may result in abnormalities, including restricted diffusion in the hippocampi (Fig. 40.3). However, standalone involvement of hippocampus, without other involvement of temporal or frontal lobe, argues against HSE and favors LE or manifestation of seizures.

As mentioned above, restricted diffusion in the context of HSE can mimic ischemic processes. The key differentiating points are non-vascular distribution of abnormalities in HSE and possibly demonstration of elevated cerebral blood volume (CBV) on perfusion MRI [2]. In comparison, the CBV is generally reduced in ischemic processes.

## Teaching points

Clinical features, supported by imaging findings, allow a presumptive diagnosis of HSE. When a suggestive pattern is noted on imaging, treatment with antiviral agents must be immediately instituted. Untreated HSE carries a significant mortality and morbidity, and outcomes can be improved with early institution of therapy.

REFERENCES
1. Core L. Spear PG. Infection with herpes simplex viruses. Part 1. *N Engl J Med* 1986; **314**: 686–91.
2. Cruz JCH, Domingues RC. Intracranial infections. In Atlas SW, ed., *Magnetic Resonance Imaging of the Brain and Spine*, 4th edn (ed. SW Atlas). Philadelphia, PA: Lippincott Williams & Wilkins; 2009; pp. 929–1025.

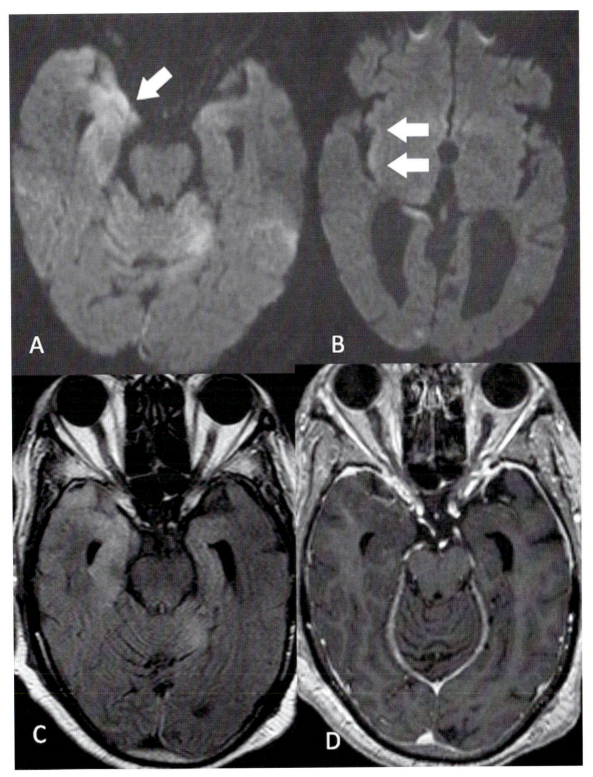

**Figure 40.1** Characteristic neuroimaging changes in HSE. (**A, B**) DWI, (**C**) FLAIR, and (**D**) enhanced T1-weighted images are shown. There is mildly restricted diffusion in right greater than left medial temporal lobe (arrow), right insula (double arrow), and left cerebellum. High signal is seen on the FLAIR image, and there is no enhancement.

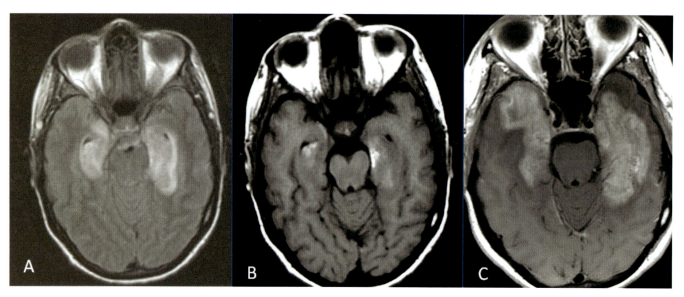

**Figure 40.2** Relatively more advanced changes are seen in another patient with proven HSE. Initial (**A**) FLAIR and (**B**) T1-weighted images suggest bilateral involvement of the medial temporal lobes. There are petechial hemorrhages bilaterally, seen as areas of T1 shortening. (**C**) A delayed follow-up post-contrast T1-weighted image after 2 weeks demonstrates confluent developing enhancement.

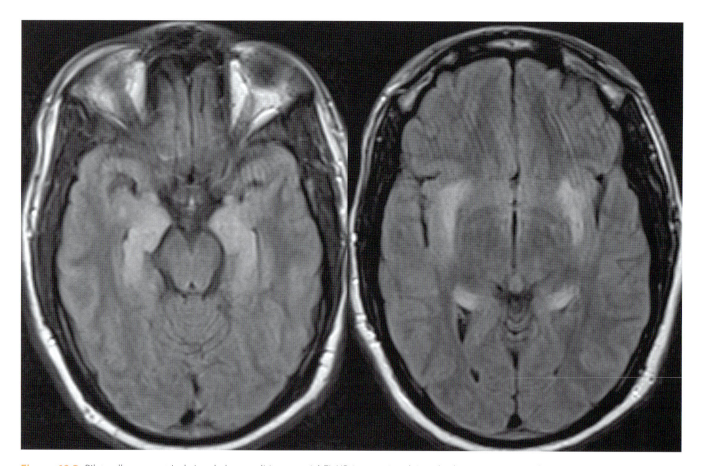

**Figure 40.3** Bilaterally symmetrical signal abnormalities on axial FLAIR images involving the hippocampi, para-hippocampal gyri, and insula, mimicking HSE. This patient with limbic encephalitis had gradual-onset confusion and mental status changes. Further evaluation revealed a lung carcinoma.

## Imaging description

Wernicke's encephalopathy (WE) is an acute neuropsychiatric syndrome that develops secondary to nutritional deficiency of thiamine (vitamin $B_1$), which is seen in alcoholics and non-alcoholics with nutritional deficiency as a result of a variety of gastrointestinal problems including anorexia nervosa, bariatric surgery, malabsorption, and hyperemesis.

Typical imaging findings include T2 signal increase in the medial and posterior thalami, mammillary bodies, tectal plate, and periaqueductal area (Fig. 41.1) [1]. Symmetric signal abnormality in the medial thalami is the most characteristic finding, seen in 80% of patients. Mammillary body involvement is seen in all patients in autopsy series but only in 50% of MRIs. Petechial hemorrhage within lesions has been reported to occur in autopsies but this is not a common finding on MRI.

Although there is no significant difference in their clinical presentation, alcoholic and non-alcoholic patients may have differences in their pattern of imaging abnormalities. Non-alcoholic patients show atypical MR imaging features including increased T2 signal in the cranial nerve nuclei, cerebellum dentate nuclei, vermis, red nuclei and caudate nuclei, splenium, cerebral cortex, and fornix [2,3]. These atypical findings are always seen with more typical findings. Depending on the timing of imaging and severity of damage the DWI signal is variable. Enhancement on post-contrast T1-weighted images is also seen in approximately half of the patients, and more frequently in alcoholic patients (Fig. 41.2) [2,4].

## Importance

If left untreated, damage to the mammillary bodies and thalamic nuclei, and interruption of the diencephalic–hippocampal circuits may result in Korsakoff psychosis, a form of severe amnesia characterized by memory loss and confabulation. Rapid thiamine substitution is associated with decreased mortality rates.

## Typical clinical scenario

Change in consciousness is the most common presenting symptom, seen in about 80% of the patients. Ocular symptoms such as nystagmus, conjugate gaze palsies, and ophthalmoplegia and ataxia are other common symptoms. More than half of the patients are malnourished alcoholics.

## Differential diagnosis

Symmetric increased T2 signal in medial thalami and mamillary bodies, with signal abnormalities in the periaqueductal gray matter and tectal plate, is virtually pathognomonic for WE. Bithalamic signal abnormalities can be seen with thrombosis of internal cerebral veins (Fig. 41.3), artery of Percheron territory infarcts (Fig. 41.4), encephalitis, Behcet's disease, extrapontine myelinolysis, mitochondrial disorders such as Leigh's disease, and variant Creutzfeldt–Jakob disease (Fig. 41.5).

---

### Teaching points

Nutritional thiamine deficiency in alcoholics and non-alcoholics may result in WE, which presents with characteristic T2 signal intensity increase in bilateral medial thalami, mammillary bodies, periaqueductal gray matter, and tectal plate.

---

REFERENCES

1. Geibprasert S, Gallucci M, Krings T. Alcohol-induced changes in the brain as assessed by MRI and CT. *Eur Radiol* 2010; **20**: 1492–501.
2. Sugai A, Kikugawa K. Atypical MRI findings of Wernicke encephalopathy in alcoholic patients. *AJR Am J Roentgenol* 2010; **195**: W372–3.
3. Zuccoli G, Santa Cruz D, Bertolini M, *et al.* MR imaging findings in 56 patients with Wernicke encephalopathy: nonalcoholics may differ from alcoholics. *AJNR Am J Neuroradiol* 2009; **30**: 171–6.
4. Unlu E, Cakir B, Asil T. MRI findings of Wernicke encephalopathy revisited due to hunger strike. *Eur J Radiol* 2006; **57**: 43–53.

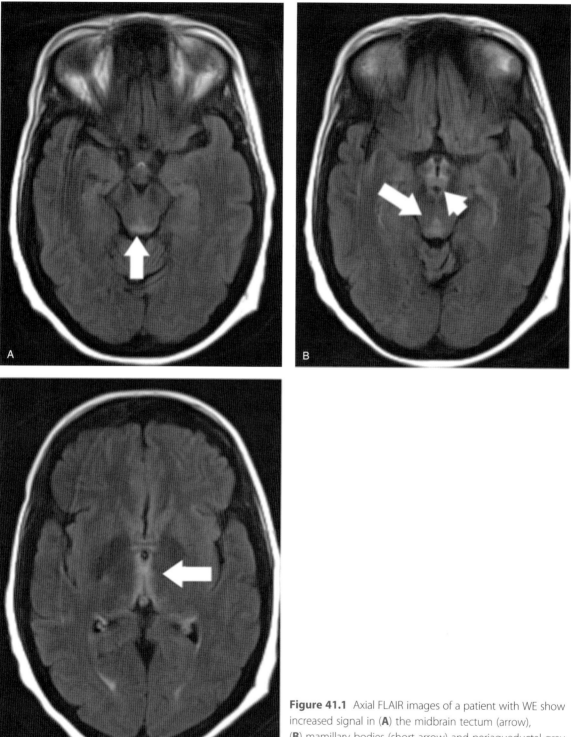

**Figure 41.1** Axial FLAIR images of a patient with WE show increased signal in (**A**) the midbrain tectum (arrow), (**B**) mamillary bodies (short arrow) and periaqueductal gray matter (arrow), and (**C**) medial thalami (arrow).

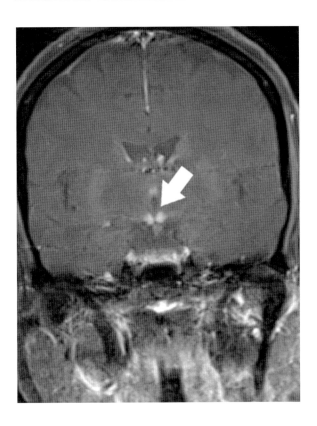

**Figure 41.2** Coronal post-contrast T1-weighted image shows enhancement of the mamillary bodies in a patient with WE, a pathognomonic finding.

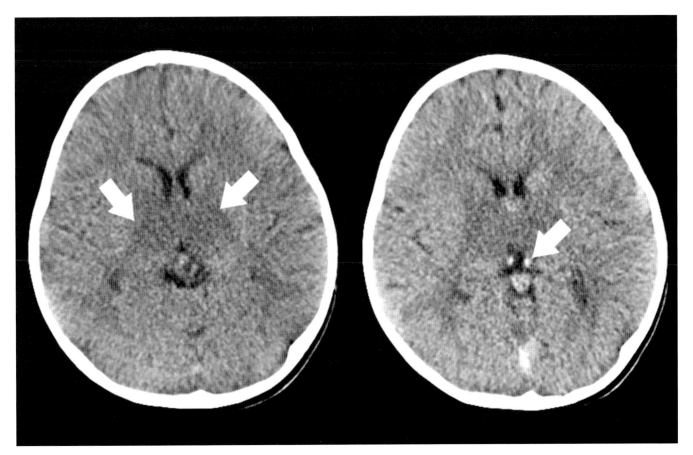

**Figure 41.3** Axial CT images show confluent hypoattenuation in bilateral thalami (arrows, left) and increased attenuation in the internal cerebral veins (arrow, right), reflecting venous thrombosis and venous infarct in the drainage area.

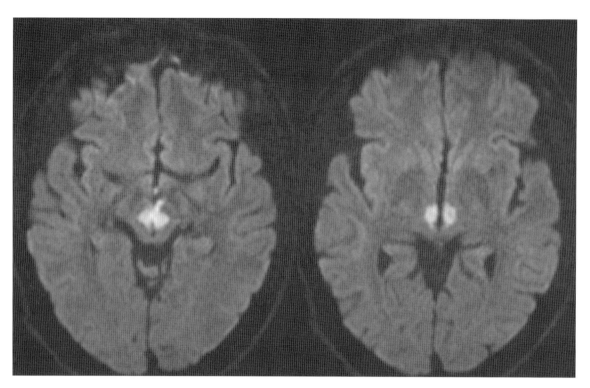

**Figure 41.4** Axial DWI images in a patient who acutely became comatose show symmetric areas of restricted diffusion in the medial aspects of the midbrain and thalami in the typical distribution of the artery of Percheron, compatible with acute infarction. The artery of Percheron is a single midline artery that arises from the top of the basilar artery and branches to supply these areas.

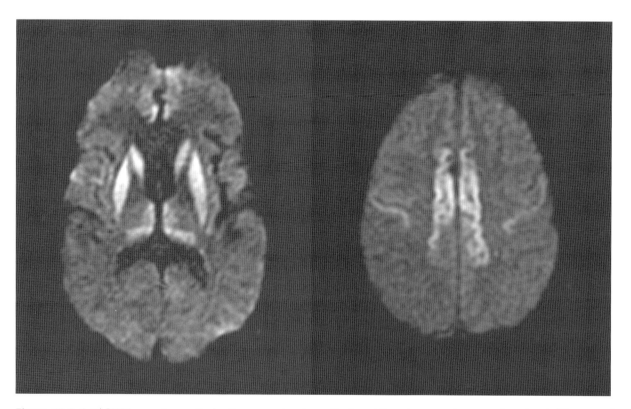

**Figure 41.5** Axial DWI images in a patient with progressive dementia show bilateral symmetric areas of restricted diffusion in the medial and posterior thalami, caudate nuclei, putamina, cingulated gyri, and perirolandic region compatible with Creutzfeldt–Jakob disease.

# Hypertrophic olivary degeneration

## Imaging description

Hypertrophic olivary degeneration (HOD) is a rarely encountered lesion that occurs secondary to focal lesions of the cerebellum or brainstem and results in trans-synaptic degeneration. HOD represents an end result of interruption of the dentatorubral–olivary pathway, the neuronal connections between the dentate nucleus of the cerebellum, the red nucleus, and the inferior olivary nucleus. HOD is considered a unique type of degeneration because it is associated with hypertrophy, rather than atrophy, of the inferior olivary neurons (Figs. 42.1, 42.2).

The dentatorubral–olivary pathway connects the dentate nucleus of the cerebellum, the contralateral red nucleus, and the ipsilateral inferior olivary nucleus. The dentatorubral tract connects the dentate nucleus to contralateral red nucleus via superior cerebellar peduncle, with fibers crossing in the decussation of the peduncle at the lower midbrain. The central tegmental tract connects the red nucleus to the ipsilateral inferior olivary nucleus. The dentatorubral–olivary pathway, also referred to as the "Guillain–Mollaret triangle," was described by Guillain and Mollaret in 1931 [1].

Interruption of the pathways comprising the Guillain–Mollaret triangle most commonly occurs from focal lesions of the brainstem. Brainstem insults that may lead to pathway interruption include ischemic infarction, demyelination, and hemorrhage, the last of these often related to hypertensive disease, cavernous malformations, or diffuse axonal injury.

Goto and coworkers performed postmortem studies in patients with primary pontine hemorrhages and documented the pathological changes of HOD [2]. Olivary hypertrophy is not seen immediately after the brainstem insult but typically appears in a delayed fashion, usually within 4–6 months. The pathologic process persists and is frequently visible after 10 months. Olivary hypertrophy typically resolves in 10–16 months, but olivary hyperintensity on T2-weighted images may persist even years after complete resolution of the hypertrophy [3].

HOD usually occurs unilaterally and located ipsilateral to the lesion if the lesion is in the brainstem, or contralateral to the lesion if the lesion is in the cerebellum as identified on MR images.

## Importance

HOD is a rare, degenerative disorder associated with a unique clinical presentation. This lesion should be differentiated from other, relatively more common causes of high signal in the medulla.

## Typical clinical scenario

The clinical hallmark of HOD is palatal myoclonus. However, other clinical findings may also include dentatorubral tremor and ocular myoclonus. As HOD presents some time after the first insult such as pontine hemorrhage, with new symptoms and new imaging findings, it may be confusing for both radiologists and clinicians.

## Differential diagnosis

High-intensity, focal signal alteration in the anterolateral part of the medulla is suggestive of HOD, but there are many other potential causes. HOD may be a result of such conditions as infarction, demyelination, tumor, cavernous malformation, and inflammatory or infectious processes. However, other than HOD, there are very few conditions where the high signal is restricted to the inferior olivary nucleus and there is accompanying focal enlargement.

Infarction in the inferior medulla may occur due to posterior inferior cerebellar artery (PICA) occlusion from embolus. Typically, the infarcts of medulla mainly involve the posterolateral rather than anterolateral medulla, and there is accompanying restricted diffusion. The infectious/inflammatory lesions and tumors are likely to enhance avidly with contrast, and they generally do not cause focal enlargement of the olive.

### Teaching points

HOD is a result of trans-synaptic degeneration of inferior olivary neurons due to a lesion in the Guillain–Mollaret triangle that results in characteristic palatal tremor. The hypertrophy is slow to develop and resolves in few months, but the high signal in the inferior olivary nucleus may persist for months to years.

REFERENCES

1. Guillain G, Mollaret P. Deux cas de myoclonies synchrones et rhythmes velopharyngo laryngo oculo diaphragmatiques. *Rev Neurol* 1931; **2**: 545–66.

2. Goto N, Kaneko M. Olivary enlargement: chronological and morphometric analyses. *Acta Neuropathol* 1981; **54**: 275–82

3. Uchino A, Hasuo K, Uchida S, *et al.* Olivary degeneration after cerebellar or brain stem hemorrhage: MRI. *Neuroradiology* 1993; **35**: 335–8.

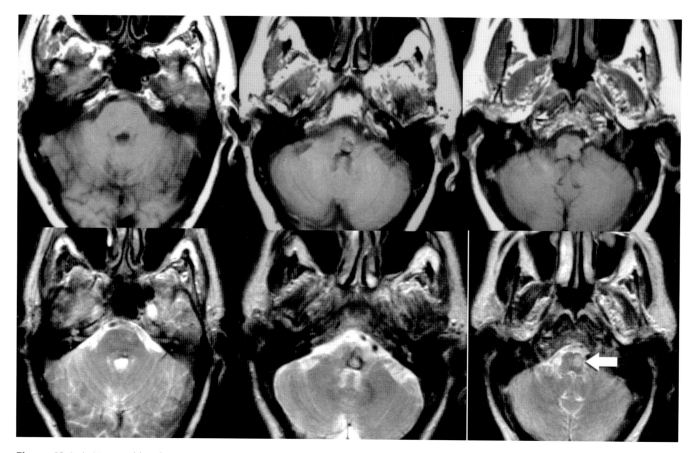

**Figure 42.1** A 65-year-old male presented with new-onset palatal tremor. A series of T1-weighted (top row) and T2-weighted (bottom row) images demonstrate presence of a cavernous malformation at the level of the pontomedullary junction on the left. There is a resultant ipsilateral high signal in the left medullary olive, consistent with HOD (arrow).

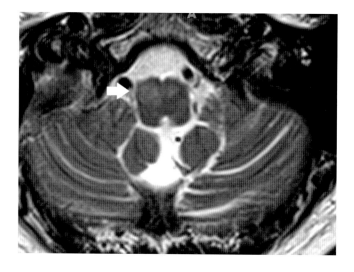

**Figure 42.2** HOD in a patient with pontine hemorrhage. Note the high signal and hypertrophy involving the right medullary olive (arrow). There is minimal high T2 signal in the left medullary olive as well, raising a suspicion of bilateral but asymmetric HOD.

# CASE 43 Adrenoleukodystrophy

## Imaging description

Inherited leukodystrophies (IL) comprise a broad group of progressive disorders caused by cellular enzyme deficiency, resulting in abnormal formation, metabolism, or destruction of myelin. The clinical and imaging features of IL are diverse, with overlapping features, often causing delay in diagnosis.

White matter signal abnormalities are the most common imaging findings in IL, which often help to confirm the clinical suspicion of IL but often lack specificity to establish the diagnosis [1,2]. One significant exception is adrenoleukodystrophy (ALD), in which MRI findings follow a distinctive pattern. The classic form, X-linked ALD, which accounts for 50–60% of the cases, can be a result of any of the 300 different mutations of the ABCD1 gene, mapped to chromosome Xq28. It presents between the ages of 2 and 12 years. The most common pattern of involvement in the initial stages is involvement of splenium of corpus callosum (Fig. 43.1). It then spreads to peritrigonal white matter, fornix, visual and auditory pathways, and corticospinal tracts. It typically spares the subcortical U-fibers (Fig. 43.2). The demyelination then spreads anteriorly and laterally, involving a large amount of cerebral white matter, especially in the most severe childhood phenotypes. When demyelination is active, the leading edge of demyelination enhances intensely. On MR spectroscopy, there is decreased NAA resonance, even in normal-appearing white matter, with increased choline and myoinositol resonances and lactate peak [2]. There may be diffusion restriction in the active inflammatory phase with decreased fractional anisotropy on diffusion tensor imaging, even in asymptomatic white matter.

## Importance

Adrenomyeloneuropathy (AMN), a milder adult-onset spinocerebellar form of ALD [3], predominantly affecting the corticospinal tracts (Fig. 43.3), spinocerebellar tracts, spinal cord, and cerebellum, and involving the cerebral white matter in only 20% of patients. Between 20% and 50% of heterozygous female carriers develop neurological disability that resembles AMN (Fig. 43.4), but the onset is later (mean age 35 years) and neurological symptoms somewhat milder than in males [4]. Clinical progression is slower in adults, and MR imaging abnormalities progress more slowly than those reported in childhood [5].

Loes *et al.* analyzed 206 boys and men with cerebral X-linked ALD, aged 2–74 years, with follow-up MRI in 140 subjects, and proposed five patterns based on the anatomic location of the initial T2 signal hyperintensity (Table 43.1). MRI progression in X-linked ALD depends on the patient's age, the initial MRI severity of scale score, and the anatomic location of the lesion [6]. The data can be utilized to predict the disease course and help in proper selection of patients for bone marrow transplant (BMT), which can stabilize demyelination, and hematopoietic stem cell transplantation

(HSCT), which can halt the progression of the disease in patients with inflammatory cerebral involvement [1].

**Table 43.1** Five patterns of X-linked ALD [6].

| | |
|---|---|
| Pattern 1 | Childhood: parieto-occipital white matter (rapid progression if contrast enhancement present and if the MRI abnormality manifested at an early age) |
| Pattern 2 | Adolescence: frontal white matter (rapid progression if MRI abnormality manifested at an early age) |
| Pattern 3 | Adults: corticospinal tract (MRI progression much slower) |
| Pattern 4 | Adolescence: cerebellar white matter (MRI progression much slower) |
| Pattern 5 | Childhood: concomitant parieto-occipital and frontal white matter (MRI progression much more rapid) |

## Typical clinical scenario

The classic X-linked ALD occurs exclusively in boys. Abnormal bronze pigmentation of skin due to adrenal insufficiency can precede neurological symptoms. The milder version presents with learning difficulties, attention deficit hyperactivity disorder (ADHD), gait disturbance, and visual impairment [1]. A more severe presentation with acute-onset seizures, encephalopathy, and adrenal crisis is also described. AMN typically presents in young adults with incontinence, progressive paraparesis, impotence, gait ataxia, and dysarthria [3].

## Differential diagnosis

AMN is a milder form of the disease. It presents clinically between the ages of 14 and 60 years and accounts for up to 20–25% of total cases of ALD (Fig. 43.3) [3]. A milder form of AMN afflicts 20–50% of heterozygous female carriers, who are clinically underrecognized, radiologically underdiagnosed, and medically undertreated [4]. The onset of symptoms is from 8 to 75 years of age, with mean presentation at 43 years. In a previous series of 76 subjects, MRI was positive in about 30% of the patients [7]. The MRI findings range from involvement of corticospinal tracts only (Fig. 43.4) to confluent diffuse T2 signal elevation with significant brain atrophy.

In early-onset peroxisomal disorders, such as Zellweger syndrome (ZS), neonatal adrenoleukodystrophy (NALD), and infantile Refsum disease (IRD), T2 signal abnormality can involve the dentate nucleus, superior cerebellar peduncles, brainstem, thalamus, and parieto-occipital white matter. Predominant involvement of frontal white matter is characteristic of Alexander's disease, whereas diffuse involvement of the supratentorial white matter is more compatible with metachromatic leukodystrophy.

219

## Teaching points

ALD, unlike many other ILs, exhibits a pattern of white matter involvement that helps in diagnosis and guiding treatment. The classic X-linked ALD presents with confluent high T2 and FLAIR signal spreading from splenium of corpus callosum to peritrigonal parietal occipital white matter. A contrast-enhanced study should always be performed in patients with leukodystrophy, to assess for possible advancing front of enhancement. Atypical forms of AMN, especially in adult males and less commonly in heterozygous female carriers, should be considered when symmetric corticospinal tract signal abnormalities are present.

REFERENCES

1. Cappa M, Bizzarri C, Vollono C, Petroni A, Banni S. Adrenoleukodystrophy. *Endocr Dev* 2011; **20**: 149–60.

2. Barker PB, Horská A. Neuroimaging in leukodystrophies. *J Child Neurol* 2004; **19**: 559–70.

3. Li JY, Hsu CC, Tsai CR. Spinocerebellar variant of adrenoleukodystrophy with a novel ABCD1 gene mutation. *J Neurol Sci* 2010; **290**: 163–5.

4. Jangouk P, Zackowski KM, Naidu S, Raymond GV. Adrenoleukodystrophy in female heterozygotes: underrecognized and undertreated. *Mol Genet Metab* 2012; **105**: 180–5.

5. Eichler F, Mahmood A, Loes D, et al. Magnetic resonance imaging detection of lesion progression in adult patients with X-linked adrenoleukodystrophy. *Arch Neurol* 2007; **64**: 659–64.

6. Loes DJ, Fatemi A, Melhem ER, et al. Analysis of MRI patterns aids prediction of progression in X-linked adrenoleukodystrophy. *Neurology* 2003; **61**: 369–74.

7. Fatemi A, Barker PB, Uluğ AM, et al. MRI and proton MRSI in women heterozygous for X-linked adrenoleukodystrophy. *Neurology* 2003; **60**: 1301–7.

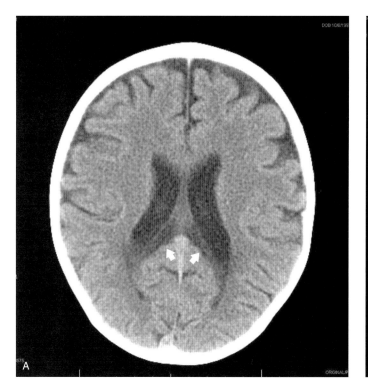
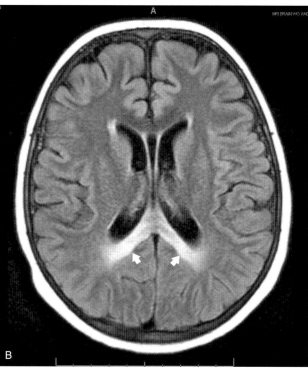

**Figure 43.1** X-linked ALD in a 12-year-old boy initially diagnosed with ADHD and learning difficulties. (**A**) Non-contrast axial CT reveals hypodense attenuation at the splenium of corpus callosum (short arrows). (**B**) Axial FLAIR image reveals hyperintense signal at the splenium of corpus callosum (short arrows).

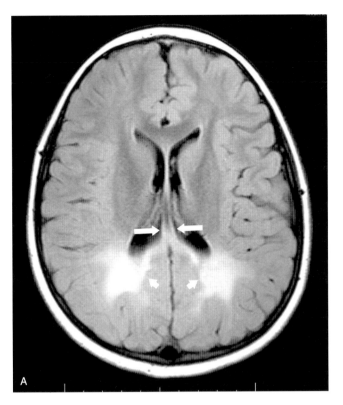

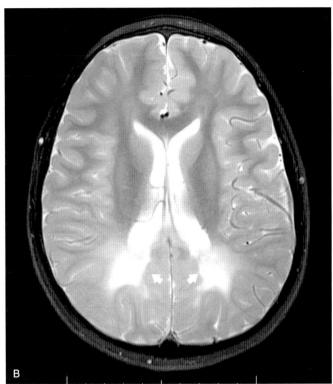

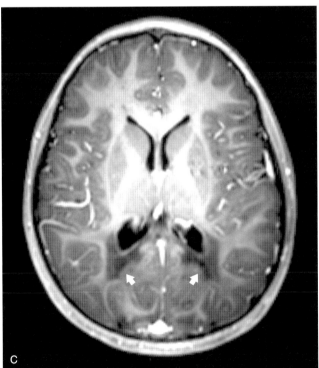

**Figure 43.2** X-linked ALD in an 8-year-old boy with seizures and visual impairment. (**A**) Axial FLAIR image reveals confluent hyperintense signal at bilateral peritrigonal parietal occipital white matter (short arrows), also involving the splenium of corpus callosum and columns of fornix (arrows). (**B**) Axial T2-weighted image reveals confluent hyperintense signal at bilateral parietal occipital white matter (short arrows), sparing the subcortical U-fibers. (**C**) Post-contrast T1-weighted image reveals confluent hyperintense signal at bilateral parietal occipital white matter (short arrows) with faint enhancement at the edge of the lesion.

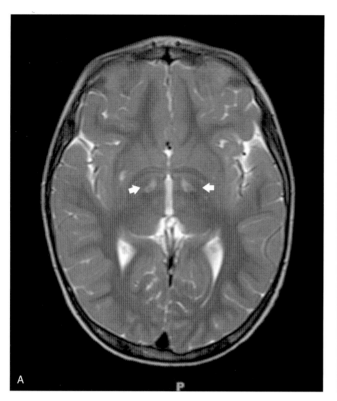

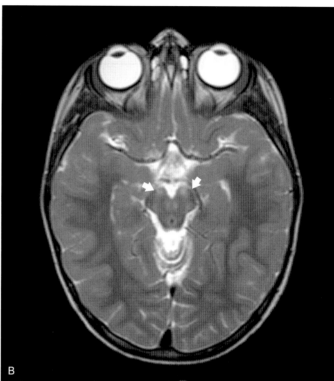

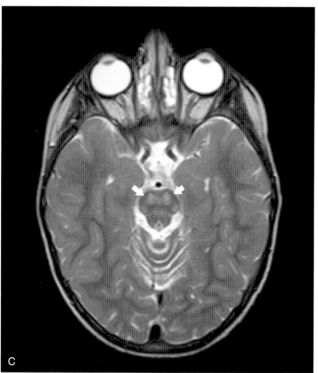

**Figure 43.3** AMN in a 14-year-old male with gait ataxia and bilateral motor weakness. (**A, B, C**) T2-weighted axial MR images reveal hyperintense signal abnormality involving bilateral posterior limb of internal capsule, cerebral peduncles, and midbrain along the expected course of corticospinal tracts (short arrows).

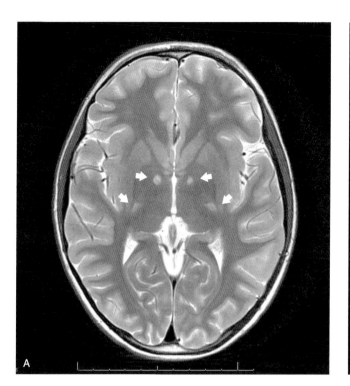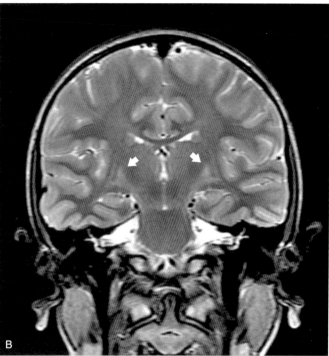

**Figure 43.4** AMN in a 24-year-old female with dysarthria and progressive quadriparesis. T2-weighted (**A**) axial and (**B**) coronal images exhibit bilateral symmetric high T2 signal abnormalities (short arrows) involving the genu and posterior limb of bilateral internal capsule, extending into cerebral peduncles.

## Imaging description

Traumatic brain injury (TBI) is the most common neurologic disorder. Approximately 1.5 million TBI cases are seen in the USA every year. About 80% of these are mild (mTBI) (a.k.a. concussion). The operative definition of mTBI is based on any period of observed or self-reported

- transient confusion, disorientation, or impaired consciousness; or
- dysfunction of memory around the time of injury; or
- loss of consciousness lasting < 30 minutes.

It is considered safe to discharge patients with mTBI from the emergency department if the head CT and the neurologic exam are normal. About 15–30% of patients with mTBI will develop long-term symptoms including headache, confusion, cognitive and/or memory problems, fatigue, changes in sleep patterns, mood changes, and/or sensory problems such as changes in vision or hearing (post-concussion syndrome) [1]. While the exact pathophysiology of these symptoms is not clear, MRI with diffusion-weighted and susceptibility-weighted imaging (DWI and SWI) can demonstrate lesions in the brain when CT is completely normal (Figs. 44.1, Fig. 44.2), and the number and extent of these lesions appear to correlate with long-term outcome in mTBI patients [2].

SWI and DWI have the highest sensitivities for hemorrhagic and non-hemorrhagic lesions, respectively, which are presumed to reflect diffuse axonal injury (DAI). CT-negative contusions affecting the cortical surfaces are better demonstrated on other pulse sequences, as both SWI and DWI have shortcomings in assessing areas of the brain in close proximity to the skull. Recently, diffusion tensor imaging with fractional anisotropy maps and MR spectroscopy demonstrated alterations in axonal integrity and cerebral metabolites in mTBI patients compared with controls [3].

## Importance

Until recently no link between post-concussion syndrome and brain lesions could be established. New MRI techniques will allow better characterization of this entity.

## Typical clinical scenario

While the majority of mTBI patients recover completely shortly after the incident, some suffer from significant morbidity (miserable minority). Post-traumatic stress disorder and depression-related symptoms may also be present and compound the evaluation and treatment of these patients.

## Differential diagnosis

The differential diagnosis of multiple hypointense foci on SWI includes hypertensive or amyloid angiopathy-related microhemorrhages, metastases, cavernous malformations, and fat emboli – but in the appropriate clinical setting no differential diagnosis is required for post-traumatic lesions.

## Teaching points

New MRI techniques such as SWI and DWI provide valuable information in patients with mTBI and post-concussion syndrome and should be a routine part of MRI trauma protocols.

REFERENCES

1. Shenton ME, Hamoda HM, Schneiderman JS, et al. A review of magnetic resonance imaging and diffusion tensor imaging findings in mild traumatic brain injury. Brain Imaging Behav 2012; 6: 137–92.

2. Yuh EL, Mukherjee P, Lingsma HF et al. Magnetic resonance imaging improves 3-month outcome prediction in mild traumatic brain injury. Ann Neurol 2012; doi: 10.1002/ana.23783.

3. Kasahara K, Hashimoto K, Abo M, Senoo A. Voxel- and atlas-based analysis of diffusion tensor imaging may reveal focal axonal injuries in mild traumatic braininjury – comparison with diffuse axonal injury. Magn Reson Imaging 2012; 30: 496–505.

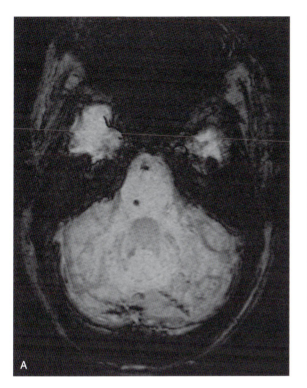

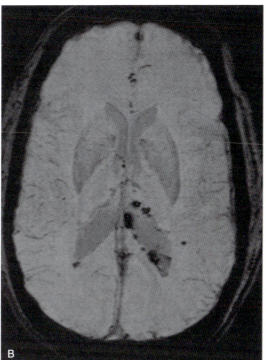

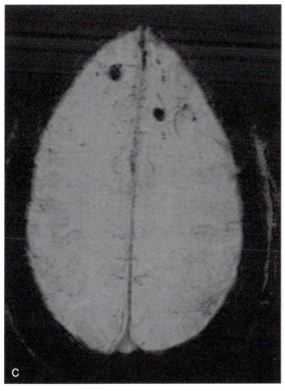

**Figure 44.1** (**A, B, C**) Axial SWI images show multiple small foci of susceptibility artifact secondary to blood products in the pons periventricular and subcortical regions which are not reliably seen on any other pulse sequence and initial CT.

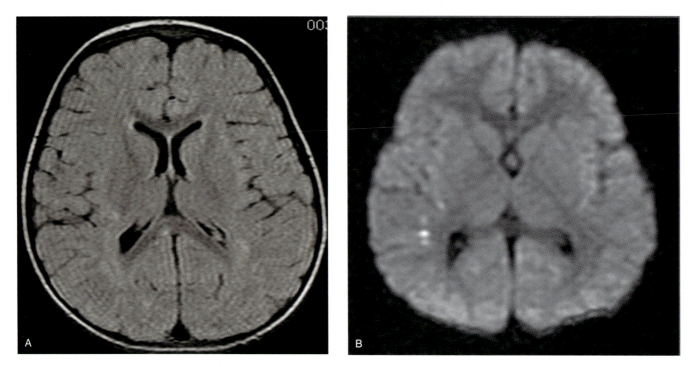

**Figure 44.2** (**A**) Axial FLAIR image shows no definite abnormality, whereas (**B**) DWI shows subcortical abnormal signal in the right temporal lobe compatible with non-hemorrhagic diffuse axonal injury.

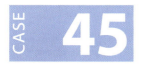

# CASE 45

# Isodense subdural hematoma

## Imaging description

Acute subdural hematomas (SDHs) are generally not difficult to detect on CT scans due to their typical crescentric shape and hyperdensity (65–90 HU) relative to the cerebral cortex (Fig. 45.1). However, recognition of subdural hematoma that has similar attenuation value to the gray matter may be challenging at times. The diagnosis is based on the "thickened cortex sign," where subdural hematoma overlies the cortex, as well as effacement of cortical sulci (Fig. 45.2). When the hematoma is relatively larger, secondary signs of mass effect may also be present such as inward buckling of the white matter, shift of midline structures, and compression of the lateral ventricles.

## Importance

Isodense subdural hematomas are likely to be missed unless the index of suspicion is high. This is especially true if the collections are bilateral and symmetrical, or unilateral but very small and with no associated mass effect. A missed diagnosis may result in improper management and possible discharge from the hospital. In some cases, an initially missed subdural hematoma may come to attention later with its expansion, increased mass effect, and possibly secondary brain injury.

## Typical clinical scenario

Acute subdural hematomas may appear isodense to the gray matter in the context of low hematocrit values (severe anemia), disseminated intravascular coagulation (DIC), or cerebrospinal fluid (CSF) dilution from associated arachnoid tear. Delayed presentation (2–3 weeks) after initial injury can also result in isodensity of the subdural blood products.

## Differential diagnosis

Awareness of this entity and a high degree of suspicion is all that is needed for the correct diagnosis of this condition. Use of thin-section images and "subdural window" setting may help identify relatively smaller collections. Intravenous contrast can also help delineate isodense SDH by highlighting the medially displaced cortical vessels and occasionally the subdural membrane around the SDH. An alternative is to obtain an MRI, which is almost always diagnostic.

## Teaching points

Detection of isodense subdural hematoma is based on the "thickened cortex sign" and inward buckling of white matter. In case of doubt, one should have a low threshold for recommending a contrast-enhanced CT or MRI to confirm this diagnosis.

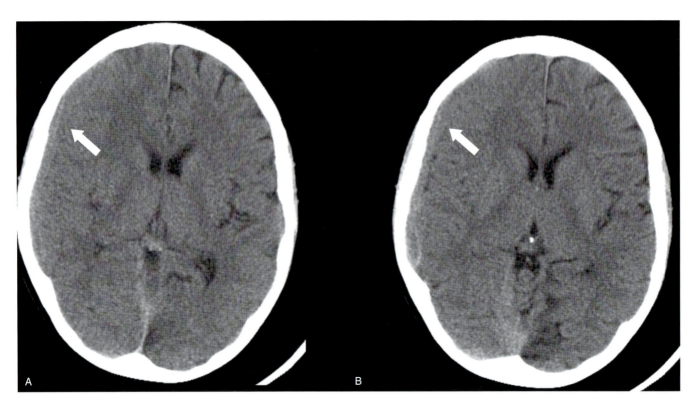

**Figure 45.1** (**A**) A thin crescentric isodense subdural hematoma is present along the right cerebral convexity (arrow). Note the apparent thickening of the cortex on the right side as well as effacement of sulci in comparison with the left side. (**B**) On a follow-up study after 5 days, the hematoma is slightly bigger and easier to detect, since it has become slightly hypodense in comparison to the gray matter.

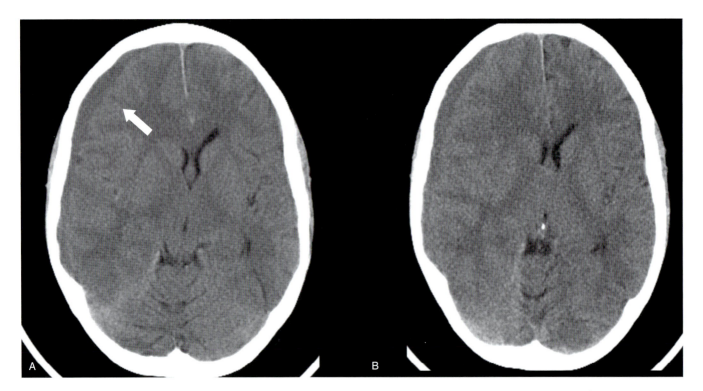

**Figure 45.2** (**A, B**) A larger, isodense subdural hematoma on CT. Note the thickened cortex sign as well as in-buckling of the gray–white junction (arrow).

# Posterior reversible encephalopathy syndrome

## Imaging description

Posterior reversible encephalopathy syndrome (PRES) is a clinicoradiological entity characterized by encephalopathy and symmetrical parieto-occipital edema. The most common imaging appearance of PRES is that of focal areas of symmetrical vasogenic edema [1]. The parietal and occipital lobes are affected most commonly, although involvement of frontal lobes, inferior temporo-occipital junction, and cerebellum may also be noted (Figs. 46.1, 46.2, 46.3). The involved areas demonstrate increased water content and there is T2 and FLAIR hyperintensity that typically reverses with resolution (Fig. 46.1). Diffusion-weighted imaging reveals that a vast majority of lesions do not display reduction in apparent diffusion coefficient (ADC) values, especially in the early stages. In fact, development of restricted diffusion (Fig. 46.2), which is encountered in 11–26% of patients, may signify an adverse outcome [2].

The distribution of PRES is reminiscent of involvement of watershed zones of the brain, with lesions favoring the cortex and subcortical white matter. Topographically, the lesions are often located between the MCA and ACA and MCA and PCA watersheds. Although symmetry of lesions and predominant supratentorial involvement are most common, other patterns do exist and may pose greater challenges to the diagnosis. The lesions may be asymmetric and could involve the deep gray matter (basal ganglia, thalamus) or white matter (internal/external capsules) or even the brainstem. Diffusion restriction may occur, signifying developing cytotoxic injury. Hemorrhagic manifestations (parenchymal hematoma, subarachnoid hemorrhage) have been reported in approximately 15% of patients (Fig. 46.3) [1].

The parenchymal changes of PRES may be accompanied by cerebral vascular abnormalities. Presence of vasoconstriction, beaded irregularity, and vessel pruning have all been described on MRA as well as catheter angiography. It is possible, however, that there is some clinical overlap between reversible vasoconstriction syndromes and PRES. The vascular abnormalities in PRES are reversible.

## Importance

PRES is usually reversible when treatment is instituted early. Since the clinical presentation is relatively non-specific, imaging plays a central role in the diagnosis. Delayed and missed diagnosis may delay appropriate therapy and result in chronic neurological sequelae.

## Typical clinical scenario

PRES has been recognized in the setting of a number of conditions including, but not restricted to, preeclampsia/eclampsia, allogeneic bone marrow transplantation, organ transplantation, autoimmune disease, high-dose chemotherapy, and triple-H therapy [1,2]. More recently, an association has also been described with infection, sepsis, and shock. Patients may present with a broad range of symptoms including headache, visual changes, paresis, alteration of mentation, and seizures. Generalized tonic–clonic seizures are relatively common. A common feature at the clinical exam is moderate to severe hypertension. However, nearly 20–30% of patients may not have significantly elevated pressures at presentation.

## Differential diagnosis

Differential diagnosis of PRES includes watershed or PCA territory ischemia (Fig. 46.4), venous thrombosis, demyelinating disorders, vasculitis, and encephalitis. The key to recognition of PRES is the symmetry of lesions, preferential involvement of cortex and subcortical white matter, and (generally) lack of restricted diffusion. In comparison, ischemic and inflammatory processes (encephalitis, vasculitis) will result in early restriction of diffusion.

## Teaching points

PRES is associated with a variety of conditions, and nearly 70% of patents have significantly elevated blood pressure at presentation. A bilateral vasogenic pattern of edema is classic, although other variations are commonly encountered. The diagnosis hinges on imaging manifestations, and rapid diagnosis can lead to early institution of therapy. With timely treatment, especially of elevated blood pressure and seizures, imaging manifestations often reverse.

REFERENCES

1. Bartynski WS. Posterior reversible encephalopathy syndrome, part 1: fundamental imaging and clinical features. *AJNR Am J Neuroradiol* 2008; **29**: 1036–42.

2. Ovarrubias DJ, Luetmer PH, Campeau NG. Posterior reversible encephalopathy syndrome: prognostic utility of quantitative diffusion-weighted MR images. *AJNR Am J Neuroradiol* 2002; **23**: 1038–48

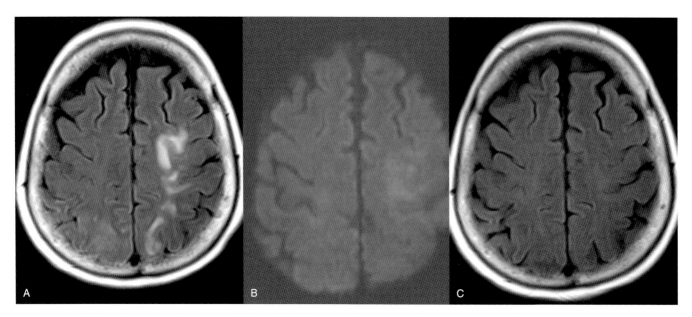

**Figure 46.1** PRES in the setting of acute renal failure. (**A**) FLAIR image demonstrates bilateral vasogenic edema (more advanced on the left) confined to subcortical and cortical regions. (**B**) Corresponding DWI image does not reveal restricted diffusion. (**C**) The abnormalities have reversed on this follow-up FLAIR image. The patient made an excellent recovery.

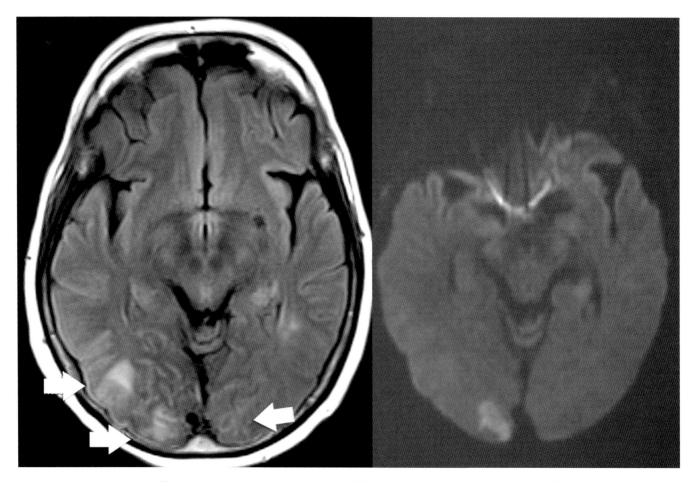

**Figure 46.2** Early restricted diffusion may be a poor prognostic sign in PRES. In this patient with bilateral high FLAIR/T2 signal lesions (arrows), the right occipital lesion shows restricted diffusion on b-1000 image.

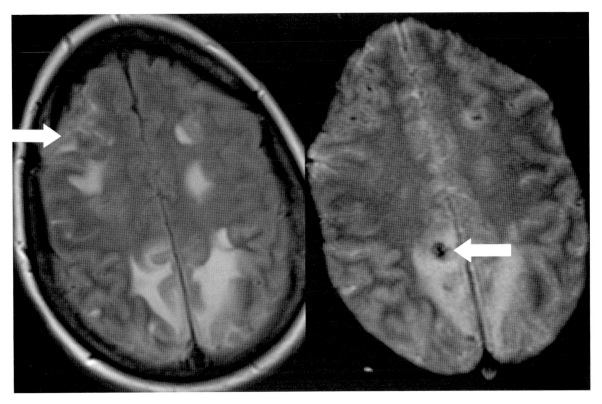

**Figure 46.3** FLAIR and GRE images demonstrate bilateral symmetrical frontoparietal lesions that are characteristic of PRES. Atypical signs include right frontal subarachnoid (thick arrow) and intraparenchymal foci of hemorrhage (arrow).

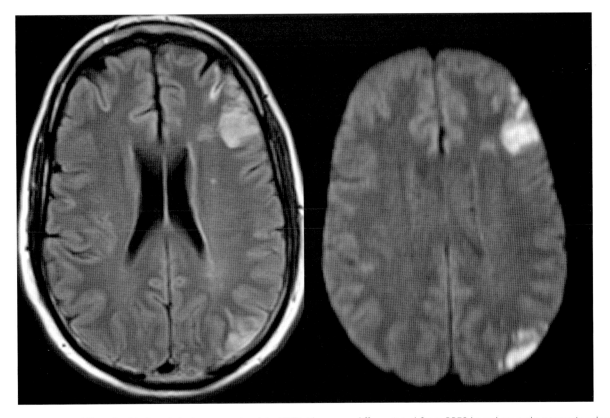

**Figure 46.4** Watershed ischemic lesions may simulate PRES. These are differentiated from PRES based on early cytotoxic edema and diffusion restriction, classic location, and clinical picture.

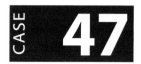

# Late-onset adult hydrocephalus secondary to aqueductal stenosis

## Imaging description

Hydrocephalus in adults is usually non-communicating secondary to obstruction of cerebrospinal fluid (CSF) pathways by tumor, mass effect, infection/inflammation, or blood by-products. Normal-pressure hydrocephalus (NPH) is a communicating form of hydrocephalus and usually seen in the elderly. Hydrocephalus secondary to aqueductal stenosis (AS) is a well-known entity in pediatric populations but it is not widely recognized in adults despite the fact that primary AS is responsible from 10% of the adult hydrocephalus cases [1]. The majority of adult-onset AS cases remain idiopathic, while X-linked recessive inheritance has been reported in some cases. It is not clear whether AS in adults exists since birth but symptoms are delayed, or if it develops later in life, although some evidence suggests that patients exhibit ventriculomegaly long before they develop symptoms.

Typically, a diagnosis of communicating hydrocephalus is suggested in an adult with ventriculomegaly and no obstructing lesion demonstrated on MRI. In this setting, standard MRI sequences show enlargement of the third and lateral ventricles with relative normal size of the fourth ventricle. Addition of a high-resolution T2-weighted sequence, such as CISS, FIESTA, or DRIVE, to standard imaging protocols, however, may allow positive demonstration of aqueductal webs and establish the diagnosis of non-communicating hydrocephalus (Fig. 47.1). Phase contrast CSF flow studies may demonstrate lack of flow through the cerebral aqueduct, but sensitivity and specificity of this technique are limited.

## Importance

Demonstration of AS will change the diagnosis from communicating to non-communicating hydrocephalus, which has significant implications for prognosis and treatment planning. Endoscopic third ventriculostomy is ideal for AS, whereas ventricular shunting may be preferred in communicating hydrocephalus.

## Typical clinical scenario

Adult-onset hydrocephalus secondary to AS usually presents with chronic symptoms of headache in relatively young patients, whereas in elderly patients symptoms resemble NPH (cognitive decline, gait apraxia, and incontinence) [2,3].

## Differential diagnosis

Ineffective CSF resorption with or without AS may be secondary to prior subarachnoid hemorrhage, meningeal infectious or inflammatory processes, and trauma. A detailed past medical history should be taken to exclude these possibilities. Potential small neoplastic or inflammatory masses obstructing CSF pathways should be carefully sought on high-quality MRI with contrast material. Tectal gliomas are low-grade tumors that may obstruct CSF flow at the aqueduct and may be difficult to see due to lack of enhancement and high T2 signal mimicking CSF (Fig. 47.2).

### Teaching points

Primary aqueductal stenosis presenting in adults is a relatively common cause of adult hydrocephalus. High-resolution T2-weighted MRI sequences are often the only way to positively identify septations in the cerebral aqueduct and should be a routine part of adult hydrocephalus imaging protocols.

REFERENCES

1) Tisell M. How should primary aqueductal stenosis in adults be treated? A review. *Acta Neurol Scand* 2005; **111**: 145–53.

2) Tisell M, Tullberg M, Hellström P, Blomsterwall E, Wikkelsø C. Neurological symptoms and signs in adult aqueductal stenosis. *Acta Neurol Scand* 2003; **107**: 311–17.

3) Fukuhara T, Luciano MG. Clinical features of late-onset idiopathic aqueductal stenosis. *Surg Neurol* 2001; **55**: 132–6.

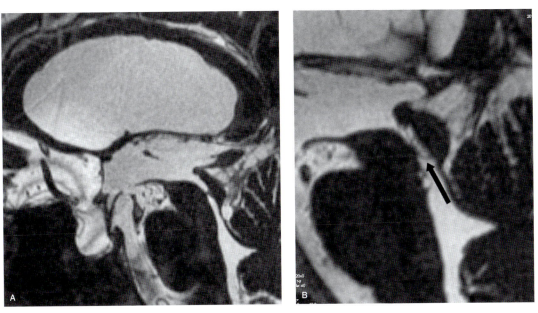

**Figure 47.1** Sagittal heavily T2-weighted images (CISS) of the brain of two different adult patients with supratentorial hydrocephalus demonstrate (**A**) simple and (**B**) complex webs (septa), accounting for non-communicating hydrocephalus. These webs were not visible on standard images. The first patient has a defect at the floor of the third ventricle due to endoscopic ventriculostomy.

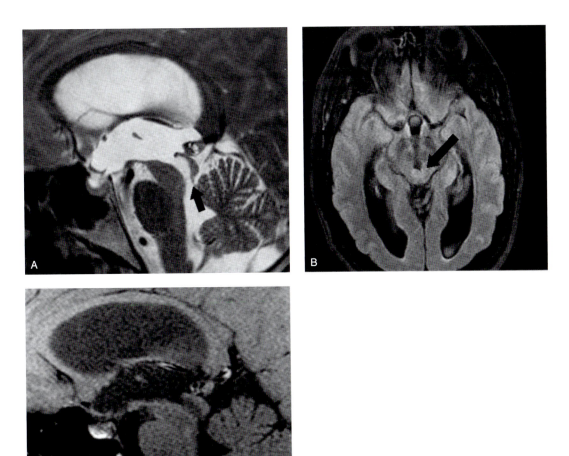

**Figure 47.2** Tectal glioma. (**A**) Sagittal T2-weighted image shows widening of the aqueduct (arrow), but it is difficult to see the mass located within the aqueduct, which shows (**B**) hyperintense signal on FLAIR and (**C**) slightly elevated T1 signal compared to CSF.

## Imaging description

Intracranial hypotension (IH) is characterized by cerebro-spinal fluid (CSF) hypovolemia induced by lumbar puncture, surgical CSF leaks, or spontaneously developing CSF leak (spontaneous intracranial hypotension, SIH). Irrespective of the causation, the imaging findings tend to be similar and rather pathognomonic. These imaging features have been best described in the context of SIH.

Characteristic imaging features include presence of diffuse pachymeningeal enhancement, subdural fluid collections, engorgement of venous structures, pituitary hyperemia, and sagging of the brain (pseudo-Chiari malformation). The subdural collections are generally thin, bilateral hygromas and seen over the convexities (Fig. 48.1). However, subdural hematomas with variable mass effect on the brain parenchyma may also be noted. Pachymeningeal enhancement is the best-known manifestation; it is typically diffuse and non-nodular, and spares the basal meninges. Sagging of the brain is quite specific and can be accompanied with downward bowing of the optic chiasm, effacement of the prepontine cistern, and descent of cerebellar tonsils (Fig. 48.2). Numerous findings have also been described on spinal imaging (Fig. 48.3), including diffuse dural enhancement, subdural CSF collections, dilated epidural veins, and retrospinal C1–C2 fluid collections. The localization of CSF leak may require CT myelography or MRI with intrathecal gadolinium administration.

## Importance

Although the imaging findings in SIH are characteristic, misdiagnosis is not uncommon and can result in improper management. For example, there are reports in the literature of unnecessary evacuation of subdural collections and suboccipital decompression for brain sagging. These imaging features are reported to resolve after treatment of underlying CSF leak by conservative management, epidural blood patch, or surgical repair.

## Typical clinical scenario

The clinical hallmark of intracranial hypotension is an orthostatic headache that generally occurs or worsens within 15 minutes of assuming the upright position. However, many variations are possible, and in some patients the headache may be chronic in nature. Signs of meningeal irritation (photophobia, neck stiffness) occur frequently.

## Differential diagnosis

The meningeal enhancement in this syndrome must be differentiated from infectious and neoplastic disorders. Infectious causes of meningeal enhancement frequently result in leptomeningeal involvement as well as preferential involvement of basal cisterns (Fig. 48.4), in distinction to SIH. Neoplastic processes result in distinct irregularity and nodularity, features that are typically absent in SIH. Brain sagging in SIH can be confused with Chiari I malformation. However, patients with Chiari malformation have a pointed or peg-shaped configuration of cerebellar tonsils, compared to the normal, rounded configuration of tonsils in SIH.

### Teaching points

The constellation of imaging features described above allows confident diagnosis of intracranial hypotension. Once a diagnosis is established, further management may be aided by accurate detection of the site of CSF leakage.

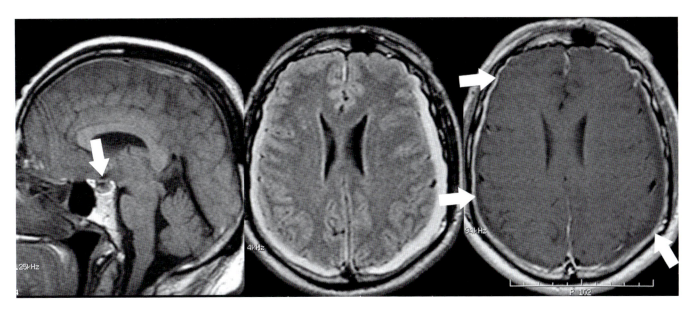

**Figure 48.1** MRI in a patient with severe spontaneous postural headache. Sagittal T1-weighted image reveals sagging appearance of the brainstem, distension of venous structures (straight sinus, superior sagittal sinus), and sagging of optic chiasm (arrow). Axial FLAIR image demonstrates bilateral subdural collections. Enhanced T1-weighted imaging helps to differentiate the thickened, enhancing dura (arrows) from underlying hypointense subdural effusions.

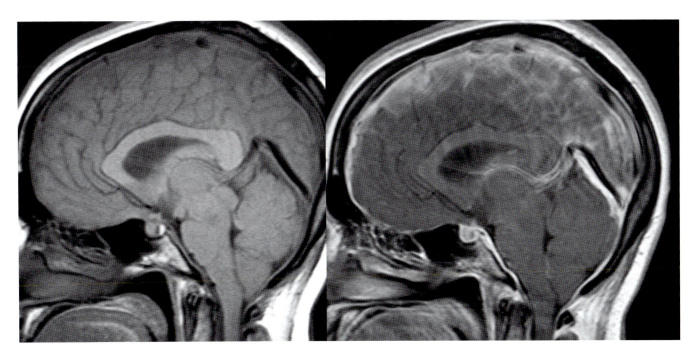

**Figure 48.2** Pre- and post-contrast T1-weighted images display enlarged pituitary gland, distended venous sinuses, and effaced prepontine cistern. Also note the low-lying tonsils and effacement of foramen magnum. This can easily be mistaken for Chiari I malformation (pseudo-Chiari malformation).

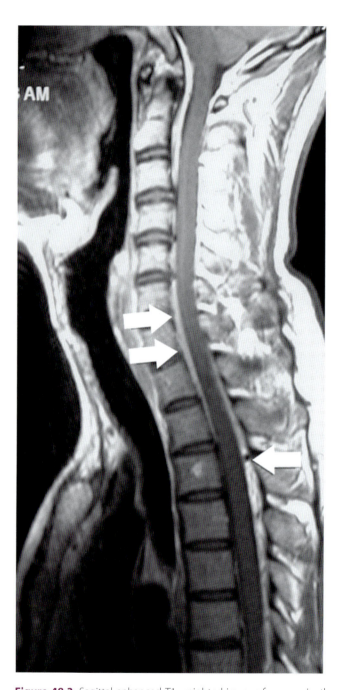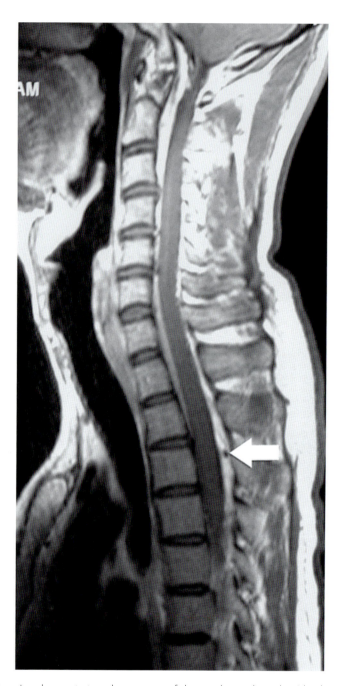

**Figure 48.3** Sagittal enhanced T1-weighted images from cervicothoracic spine demonstrate enhancement of dura and an enlarged epidural venous plexus (double arrows). Also note some prominent flow voids in the epidural space (arrow).

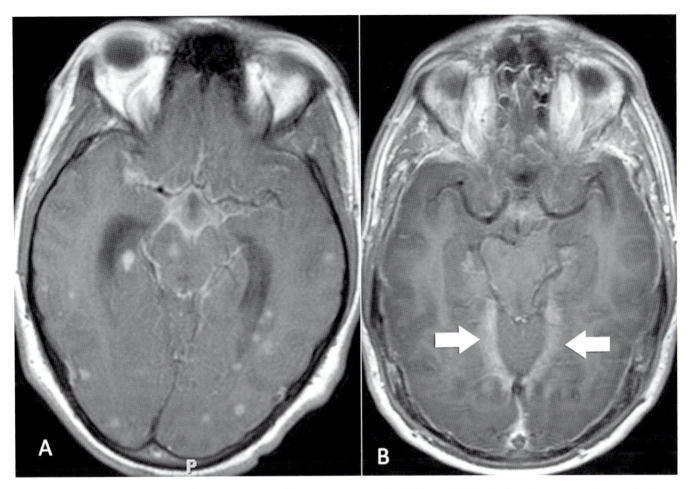

**Figure 48.4** Axial enhanced images from patients with (**A**) tubercular meningitis (TBM) and (**B**) SIH. Contrast the marked difference in the distribution and appearance of the meningeal thickening and enhancement. In the patient with TBM, multiple enhancing granulomas are present and the meningeal enhancement is limited to the basal leptomeninges. In contrast, the patient with SIH demonstrates smooth enhancement of dura over the convexities and along the tentorium (arrows) with sparing of the basal meninges.

# Idiopathic intracranial hypertension

## Imaging description

The main role of imaging in this condition historically focused on exclusion of other pathological lesions that resulted in elevated intracranial pressure (ICP). CT was often used as a screening study to exclude a mass lesion prior to the lumbar puncture. The advent and widespread use of MRI disclosed abnormalities that indicate or suggest idiopathic intracranial hypertension (IIH) itself.

A number of imaging features have been described in IIH, and they uniformly pertain to sequelae of elevated intracranial pressure and/or CSF volume. The "empty sella" sign may result from a downward herniation of an arachnocele through the diaphragma sella. The pituitary gland may be compressed or flattened against the sellar floor. Elevated ICP may be transmitted to the optic nerve sheath (ONS), resulting in prominence of ONS, flattening of the posterior globe, or even intraocular protrusion of the optic nerve head (Fig. 49.1). Other signs include optic nerve tortuosity and optic nerve enhancement due to venous congestion.

There is an increasing realization that patients with suspected IIH must also be imaged with MR venography (MRV), in addition to routine MRI. MRV helps to rule out sinovenous thrombosis as a secondary cause of IIH and commonly demonstrates sinovenous stenoses in patients with IIH (Figs. 49.2, 49.3). Farb et al. identified venous stenoses in as many as 90% of patients with IIH, with a reported sensitivity and specificity of 93% using a contrast-enhanced elliptic centric-ordered imaging (1). It should be noted that standard time-of-flight (TOF) techniques are frequently associated with artifactual loss of signal in the transverse and sigmoid sinuses, and are unreliable in the detection of sinovenous stenosis. Optimal evaluation for underlying sinovenous stenosis includes either contrast-enhanced MRV or CT venography (CTV).

Whether sinovenous abnormalities are the cause or effect of IIH is still under considerable debate. Several groups describe the use of sinovenous stenting to treat the regions of cerebrovenous stenosis, based on the presumption that venous outflow obstruction constitutes the underlying etiology in most cases of IIH. However, long-term outcomes are unclear and a prospective, randomized study is needed to address this very important issue.

## Importance

While IIH is a predominantly clinical diagnosis, supportive imaging features are helpful in confirming the diagnosis and excluding other causes of elevated ICP.

## Typical clinical scenario

IIH is an idiopathic disorder that presents with headache and, often, vision changes in women of childbearing age with obesity. Visual impairment may be either transient or progressive and can lead to tunnel vision or blindness. Diplopia may occur and can be related to cranial neuropathies, most frequently of the 6th nerve. Patients may complain of tinnitus that is generally pulse synchronous and ameliorated by jugular compression.

## Differential diagnosis

IIH-related stenotic lesions must be differentiated from sinovenous thrombosis (SVT) as well as developmentally hypoplastic sinuses (Fig. 49.3). The sinovenous stenoses are often bilateral and tapered in appearance. In comparison, discrete filling defects are noted in the sinuses in SVT. Careful attention to source images can help differentiate stenotic lesions from filling defects of intraluminal thrombi. The hypoplastic sinuses are generally unilateral, and typically associated with a small ipsilateral jugular bulb.

### Teaching points

MRV or CTV should be routinely considered in the assessment of IIH, and these imaging modalities frequently reveal sinovenous stenoses. It is however unclear at this time whether the stenoses are secondary to extrinsic compression on the dural leaflets of the sinuses from elevated CSF pressure, or may constitute an underlying abnormality that is causative in the syndrome of IIH.

REFERENCES

1. Farb RI, Vanek I, Scott JN, et al. Idiopathic intracranial hypertension: the prevalence and morphology of sinovenous stenosis. Neurology 2003; 60: 1418–24.

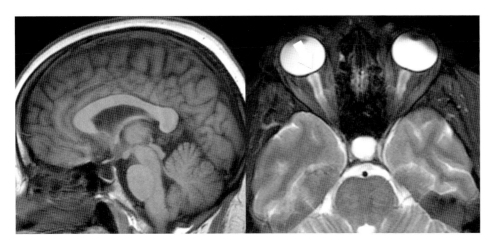

**Figure 49.1** Sagittal T1-weighted image reveals an empty sella, with pituitary gland flattened against the sellar floor. Axial T2-weighted image also demonstrates empty sella, prominent optic nerve sheaths, and flattening of the posterior globe (arrow).

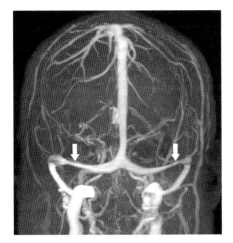

**Figure 49.2** Contrast-enhanced MRV in this patient with IIH demonstrates sinovenous stenosis involving the distal transverse sinuses (arrows). This appearance should not be confused with hypoplastic sinus, since the proximal transverse sinuses are normal in size and jugular bulbs are normally developed bilaterally.

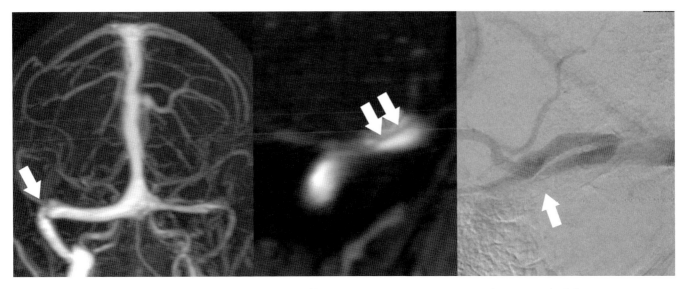

**Figure 49.3** The stenosis may be very focal and sometimes difficult to appreciate on MIP images. In this patient, the left transverse sinus is hypoplastic (note small jugular bulb) and short-segment right-sided distal transverse stenosis was overlooked initially. Careful review of sagittal reconstructed source images shows septations (double arrow) within the sinus and a focal stenosis distally. The stenosis is also confirmed on DSA imaging. Note the focal tapered appearance and marked flow limitation.

## Imaging description

Incidental sellar and suprasellar masses are common on MRI. The most common entity accounting for incidental sellar/suprasellar lesions is Rathke's cleft cyst (RCC), followed by non-functioning pituitary adenomas. RCCs are benign cysts arising from the remnants of the Rathke's pouch and are found in up to one-third of autopsy populations [1]. RCCs measuring >2 mm are found in 4% of an autopsy series [2]. They are most commonly located within the sella in the pars intermedia region in midline, although they can extend into the suprasellar region when they are large, and rarely occur in the suprasellar region without a sellar component (Figs. 50.1, 50.2).

The majority of RCCs will have increased T1 signal, with some showing isointense T1 signal and occasionally hypointense T1 signal. About 70% of RCCs will show markedly hyperintense T2 signal, but decreased T2 signal is characteristic of this entity and, when present, allows differentiation from other mass lesions (Fig. 50.3). Most asymptomatic lesions will not enhance. When enhancement is present it is thin, smooth, and limited to the cyst capsule. Enhancement of RCC may be secondary to rupture of the cyst causing inflammatory reaction, and it is more commonly seen in symptomatic patients. Occasionally, non-enhancing small nodule(s) may be present within the RCC, and these may move depending on the patient's position (Fig. 50.4).

## Importance

Although there are no reliable data on the natural history of RCC, it is believed that incidentally discovered RCCs, for the most part, remain asymptomatic and should not require surgery or other treatment. Differentiation of symptomatic RCCs from other mass lesions may have a significant impact on the preoperative work-up and surgical approach.

## Typical clinical scenario

RCCs are often found incidentally, although sometimes they can enlarge and compress the adjacent structures, presenting with headache, visual field deficit, and hypopituitarism. Rarely, RCCs may present with apoplexy symptoms including severe sudden-onset headache, decreased visual acuity, nausea, vomiting, and meningismus [3].

## Differential diagnosis

Pituitary adenomas are one of the most common sellar/suprasellar masses; they can be easily differentiated from RCC in most cases on the basis of their solid component. Rarely a pituitary adenoma may be completely cystic and mimic RCC (Fig. 50.5). Cystic adenomas often show irregularity and nodularity at their borders, a feature which is not common in RCC. Also, adenomas tend to be off midline whereas RCCs are almost always midline. Craniopharyngiomas are suprasellar masses that usually have thick irregular walls that enhance and show calcifications on CT, which allow differentiation in most cases (Fig. 50.6). Rarely, it may be difficult to differentiate an unusually thin-walled craniopharyngioma from an unusually thick-walled RCC. Small nodules that are occasionally seen in RCC do not enhance, whereas craniopharyngioma nodules always enhance. Arachnoid cysts can occasionally occur in the suprasellar region. Their signal follows that of the CSF on all pulse sequences and they do not enhance (Fig. 50.7) as compared to RCCs, which only occasionally show completely isointense signal with CSF on all sequences. Epidermoid tumors are rare, and high signal on DWI is characteristic (Fig. 50.8).

## Teaching points

RCCs are common cystic masses in the sellar/suprasellar region and should be differentiated from cystic adenomas, craniopharyngiomas, arachnoid cysts, and epidermoids. A cystic sellar/suprasellar mass in midline with variable T1 and T2 signal and no enhancement is indicative of RCC.

REFERENCES

1. Trifanescu R, Ansorge O, Wass JA, Grossman AB, Karavitaki N. Rathke's cleft cysts. *Clin Endocrinol (Oxf)* 2012; **76**: 151–60.
2. Teramoto, A., Hirakawa, K., Sanno, N., *et al.* Incidental pituitary lesions in 1,000 unselected autopsy specimens. *Radiology* 1994; **193**: 161–4.
3. Binning MJ, Liu JK, Gannon J, Osborn AG, Couldwell WT. Hemorrhagic and nonhemorrhagic Rathke cleft cysts mimicking pituitary apoplexy. *J Neurosurg* 2008; **108**: 3–8.

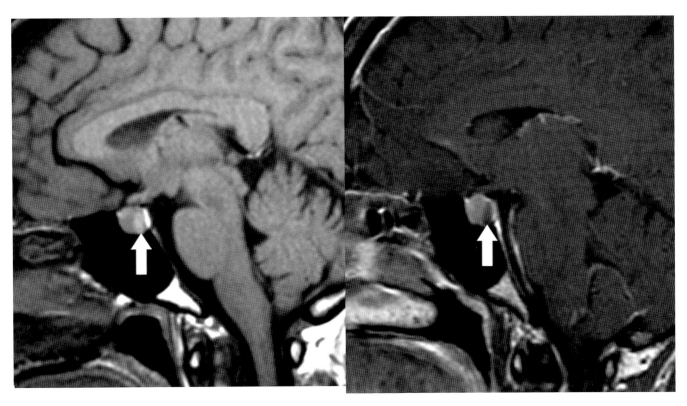

**Figure 50.1** Sagittal pre-contrast (left) and post-contrast (right) T1-weighted images show a typical Rathke's cleft cyst (RCC) in the pars intermedia region (between the anterior and posterior glands) (arrows). RCC is hyperintense on pre-contrast images but appears relatively hypointense on post-contrast images, compared to the intensely enhancing pituitary gland. This lesion was markedly hyperintense on T2-weighted imaging.

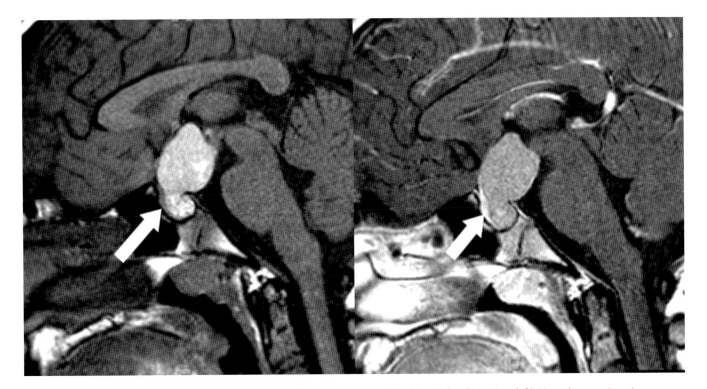

**Figure 50.2** A large sellar and suprasellar RCC that shows hyperintense signal on T1-weighted imaging (left). Note the prominently enhancing normal pituitary gland (arrows) compressed toward the anterior aspect of the sella by the RCC. Also note the absence of enhancement of the cyst on the post-contrast image (right).

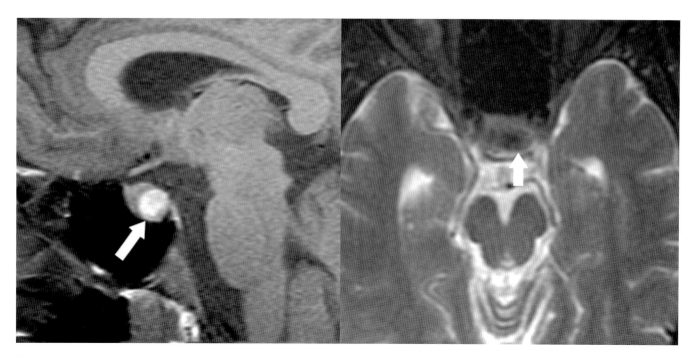

**Figure 50.3** An intrasellar RCC in its characteristic location with bright T1 signal (left) and dark T2 (right) signal secondary to its high protein content.

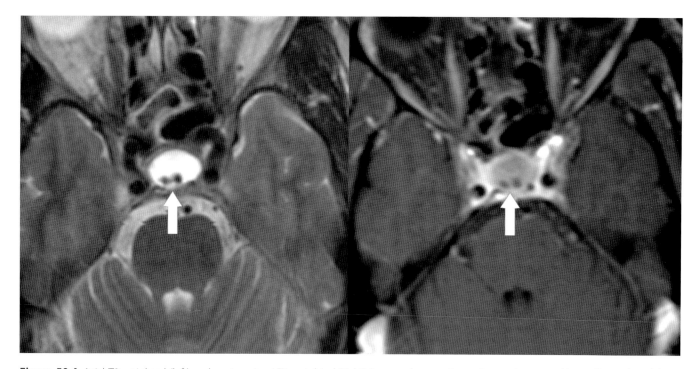

**Figure 50.4** Axial T2-weighted (left) and post-contrast T1-weighted (right) images show an intrasellar cystic mass with small mural nodules (arrows) that do not enhance with contrast compared to pre-contrast images. Although rarely seen, these nodules are characteristic of RCC and represent cellular debris. Enhancing nodules in a cystic suprasellar mass, on the other hand, would be characteristic of craniopharyngioma.

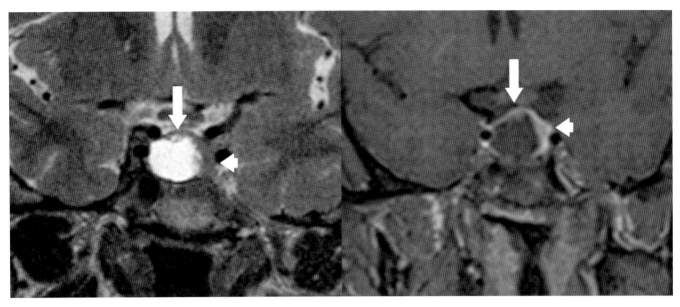

**Figure 50.5** Coronal T2-weighted (left) and post-contrast T1-weighted (right) images show a cystic mass in the sella with a tiny nodular component (arrows) along its superior margin that shows enhancement on post-contrast image. The pituitary gland is displaced to the left (short arrows). The enhancing nodule and off-midline location are features that favor cystic adenoma over RCC.

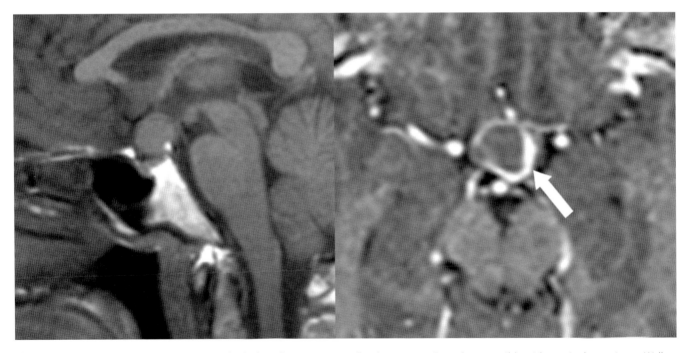

**Figure 50.6** A suprasellar cyst with a relatively thick and asymmetric wall enhancement (arrow), compatible with craniopharyngioma. Wall enhancement in RCC is rare, and when it occurs it is usually uniform.

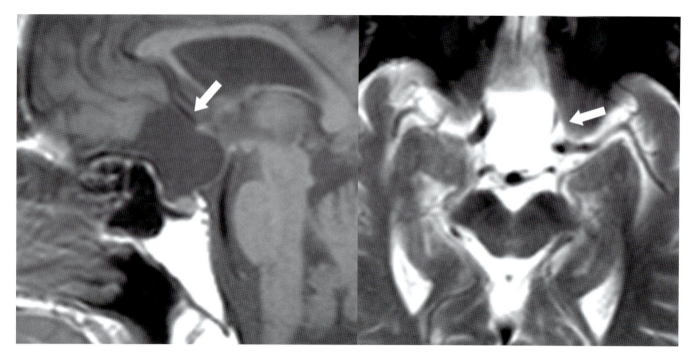

**Figure 50.7** A large suprasellar cyst that shows isointense signal to CSF on all pulse sequences, and that has no solid component or perceptible wall, compatible with arachnoid cyst. RCC signal is almost always different than CSF signal in at least one pulse sequence.

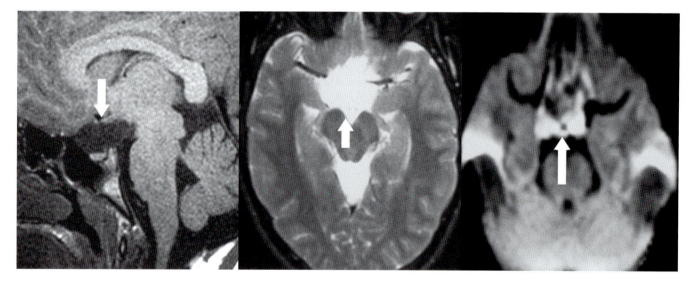

**Figure 50.8** A suprasellar cyst shows CSF signal on T1-weighted (left) and T2-weighted (middle) images. DWI (right) shows very high signal, which is diagnostic for epidermoid tumor.

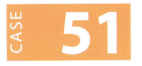

# CASE 51 FLAIR sulcal hyperintensity secondary to general anesthesia

## Imaging description

The FLAIR pulse sequence completely suppresses the bright signal from cerebrospinal fluid (CSF) due to a 180-degree inversion pulse followed by an excitation pulse applied at the null point for CSF. Dark CSF signal on a T2-weighted image increases the detection sensitivity of hyperintense lesions near the CSF surfaces, making FLAIR an indispensible sequence for brain imaging.

Non-suppression of CSF signal on FLAIR is generally attributed to increased protein concentration in the CSF, resulting in decreased T1 relaxation time, and this finding can be seen in a variety of conditions including acute and subacute subarachnoid hemorrhage (SAH), meningitis, leptomeningeal metastases and inflammation, vascular congestion secondary to venous occlusion or arterial collateral flow, and artifact from field inhomogeneity created by metal or other foreign material. Perhaps the most common reason for sulcal hyperintensity on FLAIR images in a hospital setting, however, is high concentrations of oxygen inhalation during MRI, which is a routine procedure for patients receiving general anesthesia for MRI scanning (Fig. 51.1). It has been shown that administration of a high fraction of inspired oxygen during general anesthesia correlates with increased CSF signal intensity on brain FLAIR MR images, and that patients receiving 100% oxygen almost invariably show sulcal hyperintensity, whereas under 50% oxygen this phenomena is unlikely to occur [1,2]. While the exact mechanism is not clear, increased oxygen concentration in CSF, coupled with the mild paramagnetic feature of oxygen, is believed to be responsible from T1 shortening of CSF.

## Importance

Sulcal hyperintensity on FLAIR is most commonly secondary to inhalation of 100% oxygen during MRI. Since some of the other possible causes of FLAIR sulcal hyperintensity include serious conditions that require extensive work-up (Table 51.1), radiologists should be aware whether a patient who exhibits this finding inhaled high-fraction oxygen during scanning.

## Typical clinical scenario

High concentration of oxygen inhalation during MRI is a common occurrence for anybody who is receiving sedation or general anesthesia regardless of the type of anesthetic used or the reason for anesthesia. There is no known adverse effect or neurotoxicity associated with increased oxygen concentration in CSF, which is reversible shortly after cessation of high-concentration oxygen inhalation.

## Differential diagnosis

The distribution of sulcal hyperintensity may be helpful in differential diagnosis. Oxygen-inhalation-related FLAIR hyperintensity uniformly involves the supratentorial and

**Table 51.1** Possible causes of FLAIR hyperintensity in the subarachnoid space.

Oxygen Inhalation during MRI scanning
CSF flow artifact in the basilar cisterns
Recent IV gadolinium- or iodine-based contrast administration hours (days in the setting of renal failure) before MRI
Artifact as a result of susceptibility from metal, e.g., aneurysm clips, shunt reservoirs
Subarachnoid hemorrhage
Meningitis
Meningeal carcinomatosis
Venous congestion/slow flow as seen in intracranial hypotension, compression by adjacent mass, and dural sinus thrombosis
Collateral vessels as seen in moyamoya disease
Recent seizure activity

infratentorial CSF spaces (but not the ventricles) whereas the disease processes mentioned usually involve one part more than the other (Figs. 51.2–51.6). Also, with oxygen-related hyperintensity, no abnormal enhancement is seen, if gadolinium is given, in contrast to neoplastic, infectious, and inflammatory conditions of the subarachnoid system, which almost always show some contrast enhancement.

## Teaching points

Sulcal hyperintensity on FLAIR may be observed secondary to high concentrations of oxygen inhalation during MRI scanning, in addition to a variety of conditions including SAH, meningitis, and carcinomatosis. Radiologists should not overinterpret this finding and embark on an extensive work-up if the patient received oxygen during scanning. However, it is not infrequent that patients with SAH, meningitis, meningeal carcinomatosis, etc. require anesthesia for MRI. In these patients controlling the amount of oxygen inhaled is important. CSF sulcal hyperintensity does not occur in patients receiving 50% oxygen [2].

REFERENCES

1. Frigon C, Jardine DS, Weinberger E, et al. Fraction of inspired oxygen in relation to cerebrospinal fluid hyperintensity on FLAIR MR imaging of the brain in children and young adults undergoing anesthesia. *AJR Am J Roentgenol* 2002; **179**: 791–6

2. Braga FT, da Rocha AJ, Hernandez Filho G, et al. Relationship between the concentration of supplemental oxygen and signal intensity of CSF depicted by fluid-attenuated inversion recovery imaging. *AJNR Am J Neuroradiol* 2003; **24**: 1863–8.

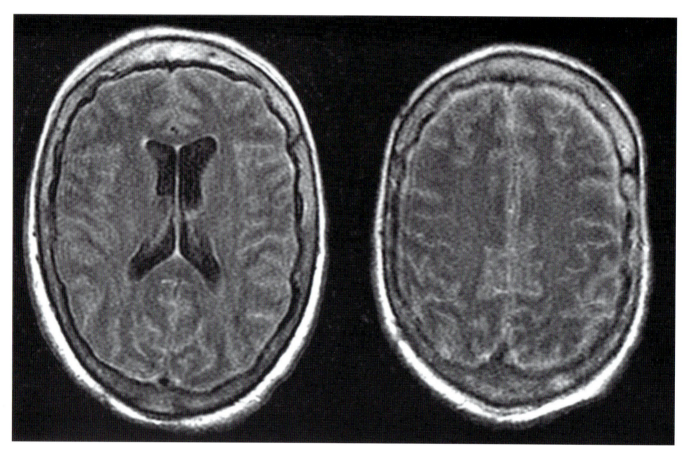

**Figure 51.1** Axial FLAIR images show diffusely increased signal in the sulci of the supratentrorial brain secondary to 100% oxygen inhalation during MRI scanning. Note that the CSF signal in the ventricles is normal.

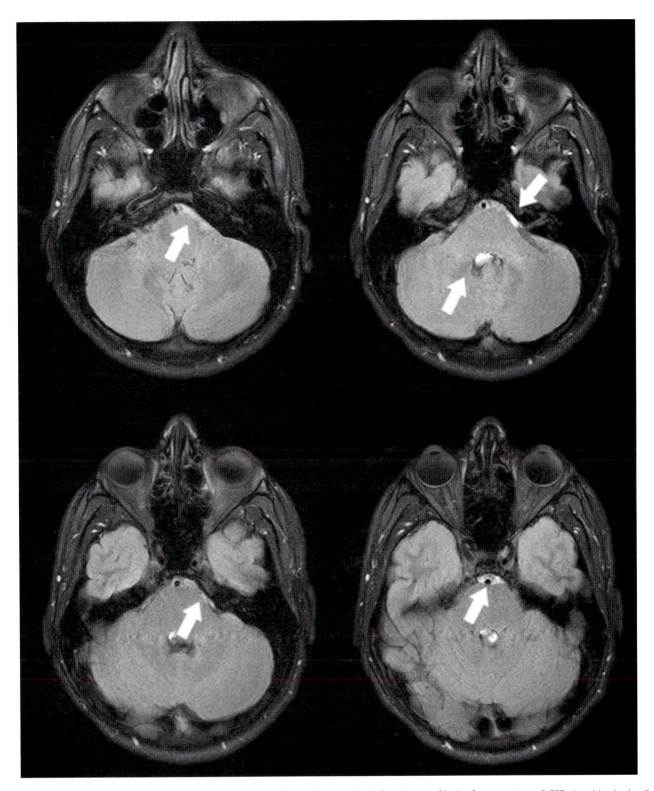

**Figure 51.2** Serial FLAIR images through the posterior fossa show multiple focal areas of lack of suppression of CSF signal in the basilar cisterns and the fourth ventricle secondary to CSF flow artifacts, which are very common in the basilar cisterns but should not happen in the supratentorial extraventricular CSF spaces.

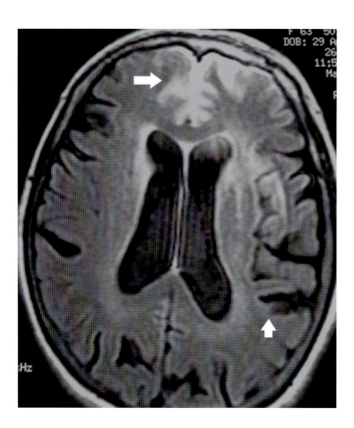

**Figure 51.3** Axial FLAIR image showing artifactually increased signal within the anterior frontal region sulci (arrow) secondary to field inhomogeneity created by the patient's metallic dental hardware. Note the normal suppressed CSF signal in the left parietal sulci (short arrow) and elsewhere.

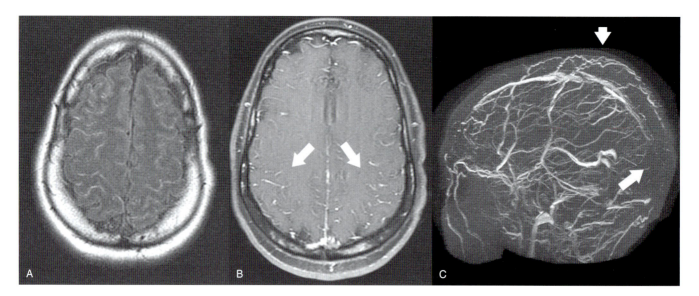

**Figure 51.4** Superior sagittal sinus thrombosis. (**A**) Axial FLAIR and (**B**) post-contrast T1-weighted MRI show extensive sulcal hyperintensity and corresponding contrast enhancement (arrows) in the cerebral sulci secondary to superior sinus thrombosis shown on (**C**) 2D time-of-flight (TOF) MRV (arrow). Note congested cerebral cortical veins (short arrow), which are presumably responsible from FLAIR hyperintensity. Arterial collateral vessels such as seen in moyamoya disease and angiomatous malformations as seen in Sturge–Weber syndrome can also cause a similar appearance.

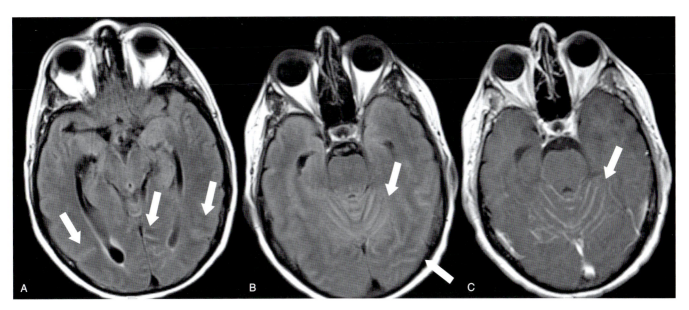

**Figure 51.5** Leptomeningeal carcinomatosis from breast cancer. (**A**, **B**) Axial FLAIR and (**C**) post-contrast T1-weighted images demonstrate abnormal increased signal in the cerebral and cerebellar sulci (arrows) on FLAIR with corresponding enhancement. Similar appearance can occur with infectious or granulomatous meningitis.

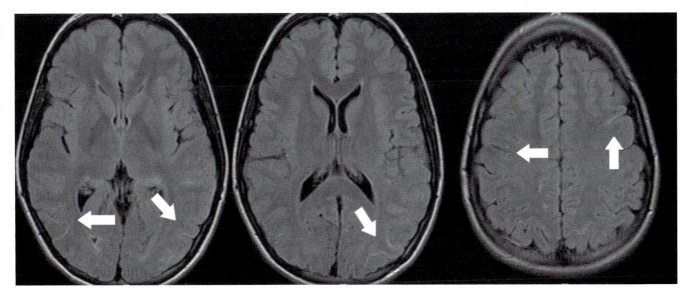

**Figure 51.6** Acute subarachnoid hemorrhage. Serial FLAIR images show several sulci that demonstrate increased signal (arrows) in this patient with acute-onset headache and subarachnoid hemorrhage confirmed with CT and lumbar puncture.

# Virchow–Robin spaces

## Imaging description

Virchow–Robin spaces (VRS) (a.k.a. perivascular spaces) are fluid spaces around arteries and veins that extend from the subarachnoid space through the brain parenchyma. VRS contain interstitial fluid, which cannot be differentiated from CSF on imaging studies [1]. VRS are routinely seen on MRI, particularly high-quality MRI, in all age groups and are considered to be a normal finding [2]. The most common locations of VRS include the basal ganglia, specifically the inferior portions of the putamen and globus pallidus, periventricular and subcortical regions of the supratentorial brain, and the brainstem, in particular the midbrain and pons.

VRS show identical signal to CSF on all pulse sequences and lack surrounding signal abnormalities and enhancement (Fig. 52.1). Particularly in the elderly, VRS can have a confluent appearance (Fig. 52.2). Rarely, dilated VRS can attain large sizes and bizarre shapes and mimic cystic mass lesions (Fig. 52.3) [3]. They may rarely be symptomatic from mass effect. The number and size of the VRS increase with age, but it is common to see VRS in young children. An association between dilated VRS and cerebral microvascular disease and Alzheimer disease has been reported, but no causal relationship has been established with these or other diseases [4,5].

## Importance

VRS is a normal imaging finding and should be differentiated from disease entities presenting with similar cysts.

## Typical clinical scenario

Incidental finding. Rarely, markedly enlarged VRS can cause mass effect and related symptoms.

## Differential diagnosis

Lacunar infarcts occur in the same locations as VRS and in the chronic stage show CSF signal lesion. Increased signal on FLAIR in the brain parenchyma surrounding chronic lacunar infarcts is almost always present, represents gliosis, and allows differentiation from VRS (Fig. 52.4). Cystic periventricular leukomalacia is usually a sequela of hypoxic injury in preterm babies, and like chronic lacunar infarcts it shows gliosis around the lesions. In immunocompromised patients, cryptococcosis should be considered in the differential diagnosis. The pseudocysts of cryptococcosis may closely mimic VRS but can be differentiated from VRS by their FLAIR signal, which is different than CSF (Fig. 52.5). Neurocysticercosis can present in its vesicular stage with cystic lesions that resemble VRS but the scolex is visualized eccentrically, located within the cyst as a punctate structure that has a signal different than CSF (Fig. 52.6). Mucopolysaccharidosis is a rare metabolic disease that can present with markedly dilated VRS; the patient's history and increased FLAIR signal surrounding the dilated VRS are helpful in differential diagnosis (Fig. 52.7).

## Teaching points

VRS is a normal finding seen in all age groups. VRS show CSF signal on all sequences and lack surrounding gliosis. Rarely, they can have bizarre shapes and large sizes.

REFERENCES

1. Kwee RM, Kwee TC. Virchow–Robin spaces at MR imaging. *Radiographics* 2007; **27**: 1071–86.
2. Groeschel S, Chong WK, Surtees R, Hanefeld F. Virchow–Robin spaces on magnetic resonance images: normative data, their dilatation, and a review of the literature. *Neuroradiology* 2006; **48**: 745–54.
3. Salzman KL, Osborn AG, House P, *et al.* Giant tumefactive perivascular spaces. *AJNR Am J Neuroradiol* 2005; **26**: 298–305.
4. Patankar TF, Mitra D, Varma A, *et al.* Dilatation of the Virchow–Robin space is a sensitive indicator of cerebral microvascular disease: study in elderly patients with dementia. *AJNR Am J Neuroradiol* 2005; **26**: 1512–20.
5. Chen W, Song X, Zhang Y. Assessment of the Virchow–Robin Spaces in Alzheimer disease, mild cognitive impairment, and normal aging, using high-field MR imaging. *AJNR Am J Neuroradiol* 2011; **32**: 1490–5.

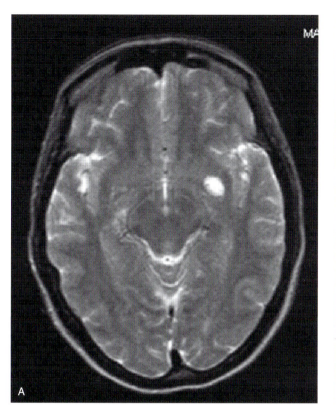

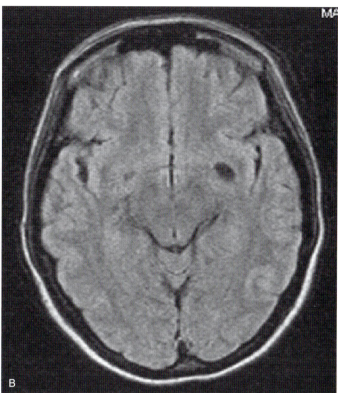

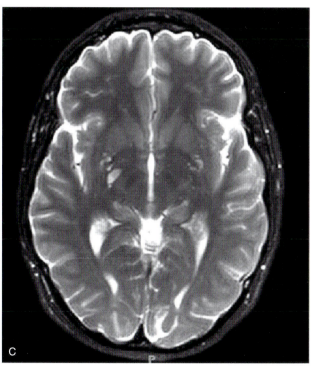

**Figure 52.1** (A) A well-defined ovoid structure in the inferior aspect of the left putamen on T2-weighted imaging shows complete suppression of signal on (B) FLAIR, with no abnormal signal in the surrounding parenchyma. These are characteristic features of VRS. (C) Axial T2-weighted image from another patient shows similar bilateral VRS of variable sizes in the characteristic locations.

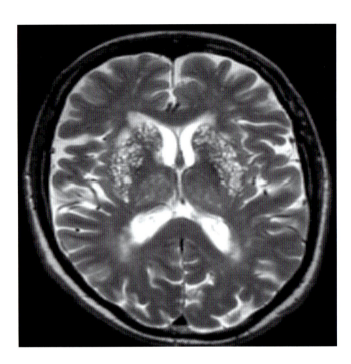

**Figure 52.2** Dilated VRS in bilateral basal ganglia regions in an elderly patient.

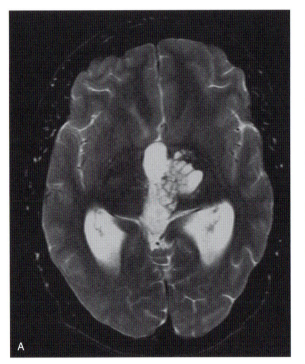

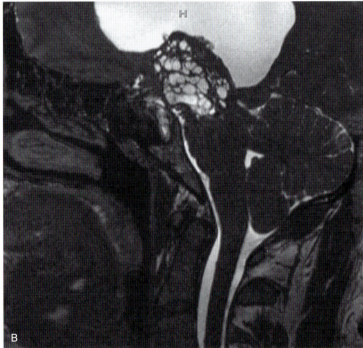

**Figure 52.3** (**A**) Markedly enlarged VRS in the left thalamic region compressing the third ventricle and causing hydrocephalus. (**B**) High-resolution CISS image shows the multiloculated nature of this much more clearly.

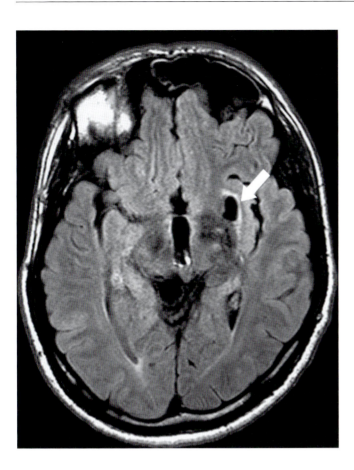

**Figure 52.4** Axial FLAIR image shows increased signal (arrow) surrounding a cystic lesion in the left putamen, indicating that this is an old lacunar infarct-related encephalomalacia rather than VRS.

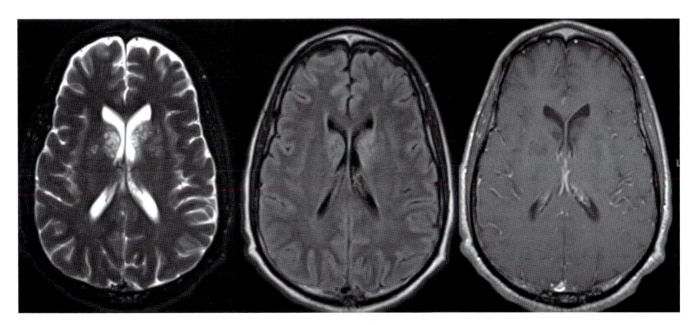

**Figure 52.5** A patient with HIV/AIDS and bilateral cystic spaces in the basal ganglia on T2-weighted images without complete suppression of fluid signal on FLAIR image, characteristic of cryptococcal pseudocysts. No enhancement is seen on post-contrast T1-weighted image.

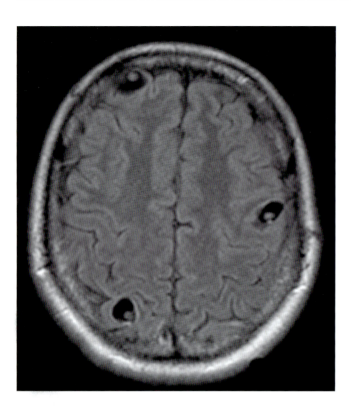

**Figure 52.6** Axial FLAIR image shows multiple cysts in the subcortical regions with a punctuate area of non-suppression of fluid signal eccentrically located within the cysts, representing the cysticercosis scolex.

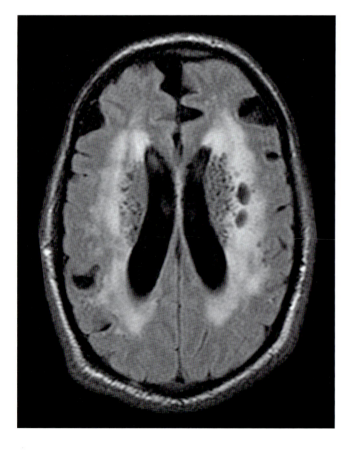

**Figure 52.7** Mucopolysaccharidosis. Numerous dilated VRS of varying size in the periventricular regions with extensive abnormal white matter signal.

# 53 Arachnoid granulations

## Imaging description

Arachnoid granulations (AG) are CSF-filled protrusions of arachnoid that extend into the dural venous sinuses via openings in the dura. AGs play a role in drainage of CSF into the venous sinuses. Typically, AGs are encountered in the superior sagittal, transverse, or sigmoid sinuses and range from 2 to 8mm in size [1]. They can be easily seen due to signal characteristics that mimic those of CSF, i.e., hypodense on CT, hypointense on T1-weighted images, and hyperintense on T2-weighted sequences (Figs. 53.1, 53.2, 53.3). The signal on FLAIR imaging may be either hypo- or hyperintense, and there is generally no enhancement with contrast.

Large AGs may present as filling defects in the sinuses and can be confused with thrombus or tumor (Figs. 53.1, 53.2). It is important to remember that although most AGs communicate with the dural venous sinuses, occasionally these may be located in the temporal bone and do not communicate directly with venous circulation [1]. The temporal bone AGs can enlarge with time in response to CSF pulsations. These can be causative of cephalocele formation and spontaneous CSF leaks (CSF otorrhoea).

## Importance

Large AGs may be mistaken for other entities and thereby prompt unnecessary and expensive work-up. On the other hand, these may be overlooked as a potential site of spontaneous CSF leaks if one is not familiar with the imaging pattern.

## Typical clinical scenario

AGs are often incidental findings on imaging. Very rarely, AGs may result in spontaneous CSF leaks. Enlarging AGs may erode through the bone and project into the temporal bone or across the anterior cranial fossa. These may provide a pathway for the spread of infectious agents to the meninges and result in meningitis.

## Differential diagnosis

Large AGs present as intradiploic masses and simulate lytic lesions on CT (Fig. 53.3). Lack of enhancement and CSF-like signal help differentiate these from primary or metastatic neoplasms.

AGs must also be considered in the differential diagnosis of intraluminal filling defects in the venous sinuses, such as thrombus or neoplasms. Rounded shape, well-defined margins, lobulated outline, as well as the CSF-like signal of AGs, are helpful in accurate diagnosis.

## Teaching points

AGs are often small (2–8mm), but they can be large or giant. Occurrence in predictable locations, CSF-like composition, and lack of enhancement are characteristic features on imaging studies.

REFERENCES

1. Trimble CR, Harnsberger HR, Castillo M, Brant-Zawadzki M, Osborn AG. "Giant" arachnoid granulations just like CSF?: NOT!! *AJNR Am J Neuroradiol* 2010; **31**: 1724–8.

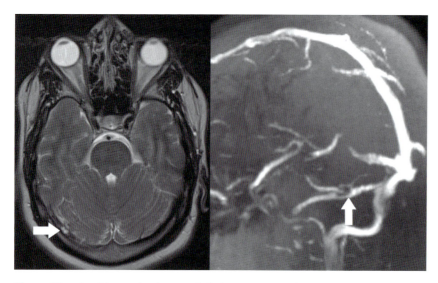

**Figure 53.1** Axial T2-weighted image (left) demonstrating a focal, high T2 lesion in the right transverse sinus, consistent with an arachnoid granulation. In this patient with suspected sinus thrombosis, a time-of-flight (TOF) MRV was also obtained (right). The focal, well-defined nature of the filling defect (arrow), the CSF-like signal on T2-weighted study, and the typical location favor an arachnoid granulation rather than a thrombus.

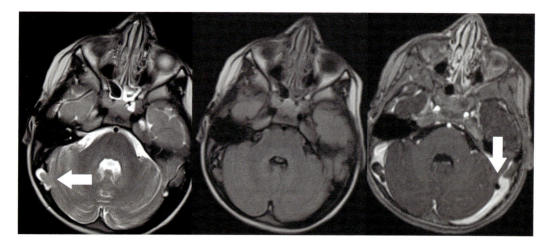

**Figure 53.2** A slightly more complicated case of arachnoid granulation projecting into the right transverse sinus. Axial T2-weighted, T1-weighted, and enhanced T1-weighted images are shown in succession. Note the presence of a small amount of brain tissue that was a part of the right occipital lobe projecting into the arachnoid granulation as well as the sinus (horizontal arrow). There was no enhancement of this lesion. Also note a tiny, left-sided arachnoid granulation (vertical arrow).

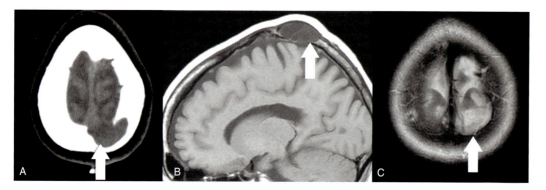

**Figure 53.3** (**A**) Axial CT was considered suspicious for a lytic lesion. (**B**, **C**) However, MRI demonstrates signal characteristics of this lesion that are similar to CSF, it has close proximity to the superior sagittal sinus, and there was no enhancement, thereby favoring a large arachnoid granulation (arrow).

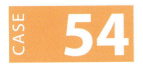

# CASE 54 Benign external hydrocephalus

## Imaging description

Benign external hydrocephalus (BEH) (a.k.a. benign extra-axial fluid collections of infancy) is a clinicoradiologic entity characterized by increased head circumference and enlargement of the CSF (subarachnoid) spaces in the frontal and interhemispheric regions (Fig. 54.1). The ventricular size is often normal, although mild prominence of the ventricles and basilar cisterns may be seen. The etiology is unknown, but ineffectual resorption of CSF by immature arachnoid villi is the most widely accepted theory (1).

This is considered to be a self-limiting condition, and it does not require specific treatment. BEH usually presents around the age of 6 months, and enlargement of the head usually stabilizes by the age of 18 months (1). Some patients exhibit gross motor delay, which is often transient. Long-term follow-up studies are lacking, but one such study reported mild psychomotor delay in some patients (2).

## Importance

Rapid increase in head size in infants is usually an alarming finding, which may indicate increased intracranial pressure secondary to tumor or hydrocephalus, although the most common reason is BEH. The exact incidence of BEH is not known. A review of incidental findings in a study reported that 0.6% of the children were found to have external hydrocephalus (3). Most infants with BEH are normal, although BEH is associated with increased incidence of subdural hematomas.

## Typical clinical scenario

The typical patient is an infant with a rapidly enlarging head circumference on well-child exam which leads to a CT scan. The head size is greater than the 95th percentile (macrocephaly). Two-thirds of the patients are male infants. A history of prematurity is common. Patients are otherwise normal, although some may have motor delay, torticollis, and abnormal head shape. Forty percent of patients have one or more close relatives with a history of macrocephaly.

## Differential diagnosis

The clinical differential diagnosis includes increased intracranial pressure secondary to tumors, hydrocephalus, etc., which can be easily eliminated by imaging. On imaging, brain atrophy preferentially involving the frontal lobes looks alike, although patients with atrophy have normal or decreased head circumference. Low-attenuation subdural collections such as hygroma and chronic subdural hematomas, as can be seen in non-accidental trauma cases, may mimic BEH when they are symmetric (Figs. 54.2, 54.3, 54.4). The cerebral sulci adjacent to the collections are normal or widened in BEH and effaced or compressed in chronic subdural collections. Cortical veins traverse the collection in BEH, and these are easily visualized on MRI and sometimes on CT. Non-visualization of the cortical veins adjacent to the fluid collection suggests subdural collection.

## Teaching points

Enlargement of frontal and interhemispheric subarachnoid spaces in infants with macrocephaly is related to BEH which is often a self limited condition and should be differentiated from subdural collections.

REFERENCES

1. Zahl SM, Egge A, Helseth E, Wester K. Benign external hydrocephalus: a review, with emphasis on management. *Neurosurg Rev* 2011; **34**: 417–32.
2. Yew AY, Maher CO, Muraszko KM, Garton HJ. Long-term health status in benign external hydrocephalus. *Pediatr Neurosurg* 2011; **47**: 1–6.
3. Gupta SN, Belay B. Intracranial incidental findings on brain MR images in a pediatric neurology practice: a retrospective study. *J Neurol Sci* 2008; **264**: 34–7.

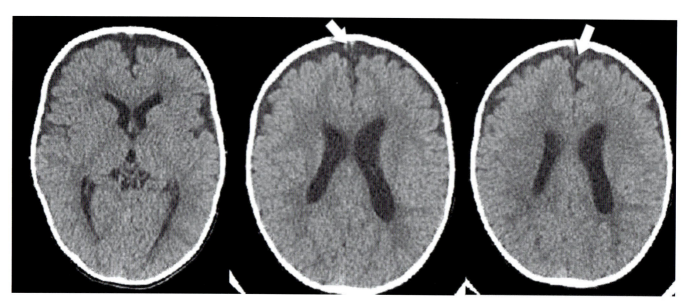

**Figure 54.1** A 4-month-old presented with macrocephaly. Axial CT images show fluid attenuation in the frontal regions bilaterally with dilatation of the anterior interhemispheric fissure. Note veins traversing the fluid collection (arrows), which excludes the possibility of subdural collections. Also note that the brain surface adjacent to the collections is not flattened. This constellation of findings indicates BEH. The same imaging features in a baby with microcephaly might indicate brain atrophy.

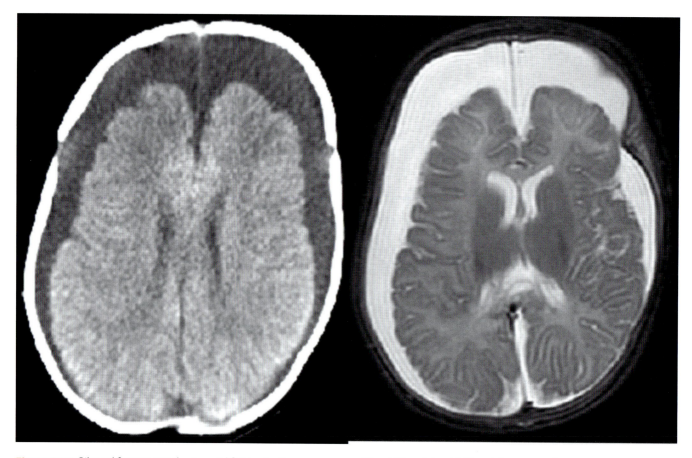

**Figure 54.2** Bilateral frontoparietal extra-axial fluid collections are seen on CT and T2-weighted MRI with flattening of the brain surface adjacent to the collections and lack of vessels traversing the collections, suggesting that these are located in the subdural space rather than the subarachnoid space. This patient was diagnosed with bilateral subdural hygromas and ultimately with non-accidental trauma.

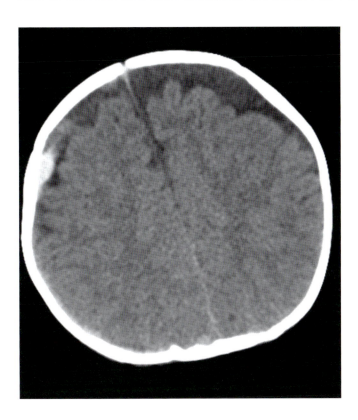

**Figure 54.3** Axial CT shows an acute subdural hematoma on the right and an enlarged extra-axial space on the left, suggesting the possiblitiy of different-age subdural collections and non-accidental trauma. Close inspection reveals that the left-sided collection is subarachnoid, given the lack of flattening of the adjacent brain surface. The trauma that led to the right acute subdural hematoma was witnessed, and the social services excluded non-accidental trauma.

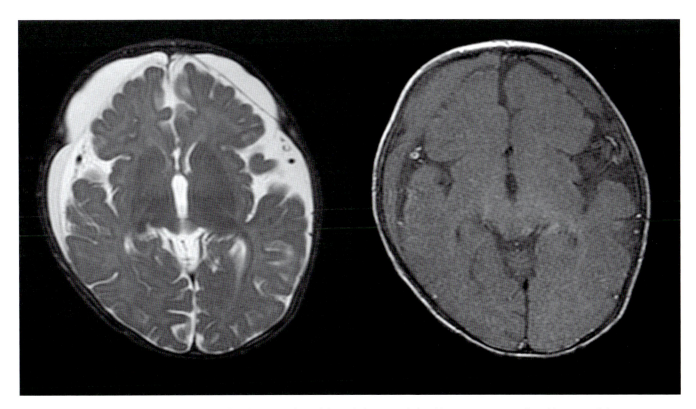

**Figure 54.4** Axial T2-weighted and T1-weighted images show bilateral chronic subdural hematomas as well as dilatation of the subarachnoid space particularly in the Sylvian fissures with multiple vessels identified within. This patient had a metabolic disease known as glutaric aciduria type I, which has a tendency for spontaneous subdural collection and brain atrophy.

# Pitfalls in CTA

## Imaging description

Computerized tomographic angiography (CTA) has become the most commonly used first-line imaging exam for detection and characterization of aneurysms of the circle of Willis, although MRA is also used for similar purposes and DSA remains the gold standard in many centers [1]. With its multiplanar reformatting, bone subtraction, and 3D volume rendering capabilities, CTA offers very high sensitivity for detection and accuracy for characterization of intracranial aneurysms, although there remain some limitations [2]. Small aneurysms and aneurysms that are in close proximity to bones can be missed by CTA. Also, venous contamination can pose interpretive difficulties by mimicking or hiding aneurysms and other abnormalities such as dissections or stenoses [3]. A less common problem is mistaking a dural-based mass for an aneurysm. This occurs when a meningioma or other extra-axial mass is in close proximity to the vessels and shows enhancement similar to vessels (Figs. 55.1, 55.2, 55.3). Many, but not all, of the missed findings on CTA can retrospectively be correctly identified, emphasizing the need for improving the interpretive skills of radiologists and the CTA techniques that would allow easier interpretation.

## Importance

Underdiagnosis or overdiagnosis of an intracranial aneurysm has significant implications for patient management and outcome.

## Typical clinical scenario

Most obvious reasons for a suspicion of an intracranial aneurysm are acute subarachnoid hemorrhage and/or acute-onset severe headache, although many other signs and symptoms may lead clinicians to suspect intracranial aneurysms. Also, intracranial aneurysms are frequently seen incidentally.

## Differential diagnosis

Veins, when opacified, can mimic aneurysms on CTA. Venous opacification is a unique problem for CTA, as in MRA and DSA arteries and veins are not visualized on the same image. Perfecting the CTA technique is important, but because of very short circulation time in the brain venous contamination is impossible to avoid completely. The most problematic anatomic sites for venous contamination include the cavernous carotid artery, the carotid terminus, and the basilar tip. Careful evaluation of venous structures in these regions is imperative. Because cortical bone and opacified arteries have very similar attenuation values, evaluation of vessels as they traverse the skull base requires extra caution. Bone removal algorithms are helpful but do not necessarily improve accuracy significantly.

Avidly enhancing mass lesions next to vessels often show a slight difference in attenuation compared to vessels, but this may not be readily apparent on standard window and level settings; using wider window settings usually allows one to see this subtle difference. Enhancing mass lesions may have a very large contact to the vessel but lack an obvious aneurysm neck, a feature that can be best appreciated on source images or multiplanar reformats. As a general rule, 2D source images and multiplanar reformats are much more helpful than 3D volume-rendered images in elucidating the features that help differentiating artifacts from real findings.

## Teaching points

Skull-base bones, venous contamination, and avidly enhancing masses may cause interpretive errors in CTAs. It is imperative to be aware of these potential problems and pay particular attention to these features, using the source images rather than volume-rendered images.

REFERENCES

1. McKinney AM, Palmer CS, Truwit CL, Karagulle A, Teksam M. Detection of aneurysms by 64-section multidetector CT angiography in patients acutely suspected of having an intracranial aneurysm and comparison with digital subtraction and 3D rotational angiography. *AJNR Am J Neuroradiol* 2008; **29**: 594–602.
2. Romijn M, Gratama van Andel HA, van Walderveen MA, *et al.* Diagnostic accuracy of CT angiography with matched mask bone elimination for detection of intracranial aneurysms: comparison with digital subtraction angiography and 3D rotational angiography. *AJNR Am J Neuroradiol* 2008; **29**: 134–9.
3. Teksam M, Casey S, McKinney A, Michel E, Truwit CL. Anatomy and frequency of large pontomesencephalic veins on 3D CT angiograms of the circle of Willis. *AJNR Am J Neuroradiol* 2003; **24**: 1598–601.

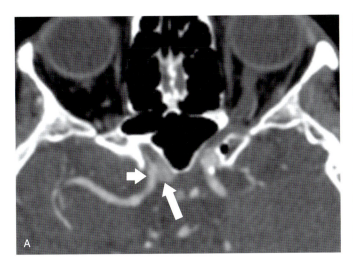

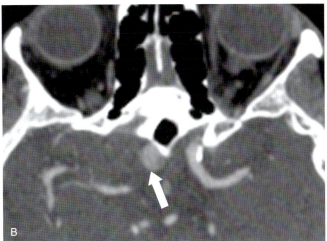

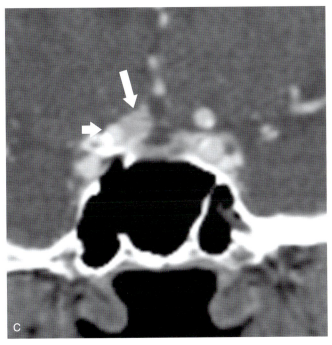

Figure 55.1 (A, B) Axial and (C) coronal CTA source images show a rounded structure (arrows) intimately associated with the supraclinoid internal carotid artery (short arrows), giving the impression of an aneurysm because this meningioma has the same degree of enhancement as the carotid artery.

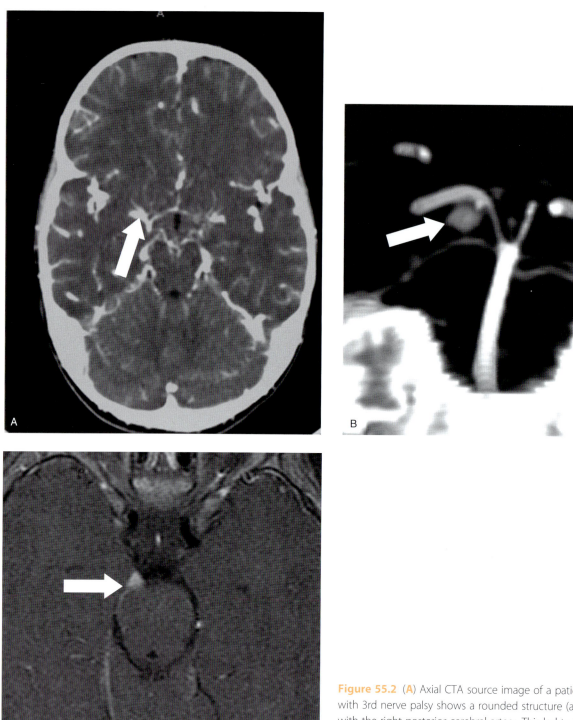

**Figure 55.2** (**A**) Axial CTA source image of a patient who presented with 3rd nerve palsy shows a rounded structure (arrow) associated with the right posterior cerebral artery. This led to the suspicion of an aneurysm, which was strengthened by (**B**) a volume-rendered image. A catheter angiogram was negative, and (**C**) MRI performed later showed an avidly enhancing schwannoma of the 3rd nerve.

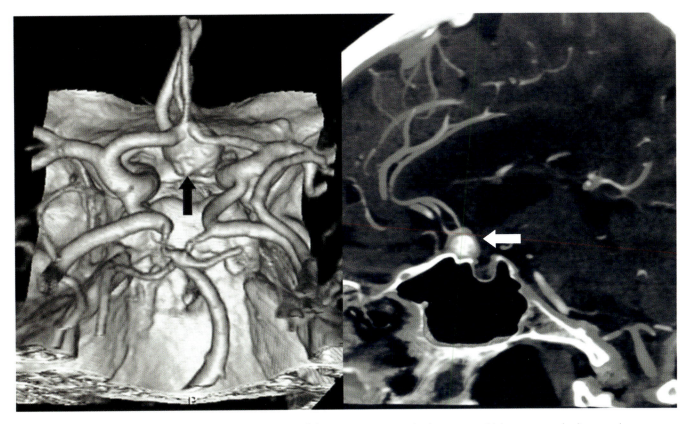

**Figure 55.3** Volume-rendered image shows an "aneurysm" of the anterior communicating artery, which was correctly diagnosed as a calcified and markedly enhancing planum sphenoidale meningioma on the source image.

# Asymmetric pneumatization of the anterior clinoid process

## Imaging description

Radiologists rely on symmetry of the paired anatomic structures when interpreting images of the brain and skull base. Pneumatization of the paranasal sinuses and mastoids is not always symmetric, however. While asymmetrically pneumatized cells are easy to characterize on CT, they may lead to diagnostic errors on MRI due to decreased conspicuity of bony landmarks (Figs. 56.1, 56.2). When a part of the skull base is not pneumatized it usually contains normal marrow (and surrounding cortical bone), which appears on MRI as a T1 hyperintense structure that may mimic an enhancing mass. Completely pneumatized cells are extremely hypointense on all pulse sequences and may mimic the flow void of an aneurysm when in close proximity to the vessels (Figs. 56.1, 56.3). Alternatively, a pneumatized air cell may develop mucosal inflammation that can create diagnostic confusion when asymmetric (Figs. 56.4, 56.5).

## Importance

Erroneous calls made on MRI as a result of asymmetrically pneumatized cells are usually reversed by additional work-up. There is usually no harm inflicted other than unnecessary anxiety and cost. The radiologist's reputation may be damaged irreversibly, however.

## Typical clinical scenario

Since asymmetric pneumatization of air cells is merely an anatomic variation, no specific clinical presentation can be ascribed. These are frequently misinterpreted as aneurysms or mass lesions.

## Differential diagnosis

The primary role of the radiologist in these cases is to make the diagnosis of a normal anatomic variant and not invoke a diagnostic work-up. The common locations for asymmetric pneumatization include the anterior clinoid and pterygoid processes of the sphenoid bone, and the petrous apices of the temporal bone. Non-pneumatized bone contains fatty marrow, which can be positively characterized by comparing the unenhanced T1-weighted images to the contrast-enhanced ones and making sure that the "lesion" follows the fat signal on all pulse sequences. Fat-suppressed images are not essential but very helpful in confirming the presence of fat. In differentiating an anterior clinoid process air cell from an aneurysm, knowledge of the precise location of this cell is important. When there is a true aneurysm one can also identify the anterior clinoid process next to it whether it is pneumatized or not.

## Teaching points

Asymmetric pneumatization of skull-base structures may mimic enhancing mass lesions or aneurysms if the presence of this anatomic variation is not recognized. The anterior clinoid processes and pterygoid processes of the sphenoid bone, and the petrous apices, are the most common sites of asymmetric pneumatization that can be confusing for radiologists. Recognizing the fat and air signal on all pulse sequences, along with a precise knowledge of the anatomy, is important in avoiding this error. If ambiguity still persists a non-contrast CT is often enough to clarify.

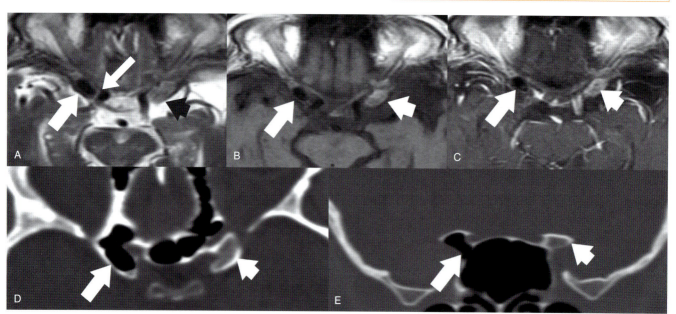

**Figure 56.1** (**A**) Axial T2-weighted, (**B**) T1-weighted, and (**C**) post-contrast T1-weighted images from a standard brain MRI show a pneumatized right anterior clinoid process (ACP) (arrows) and a non-pneumatized (marrow-filled) left ACP (short arrows), which is simply an

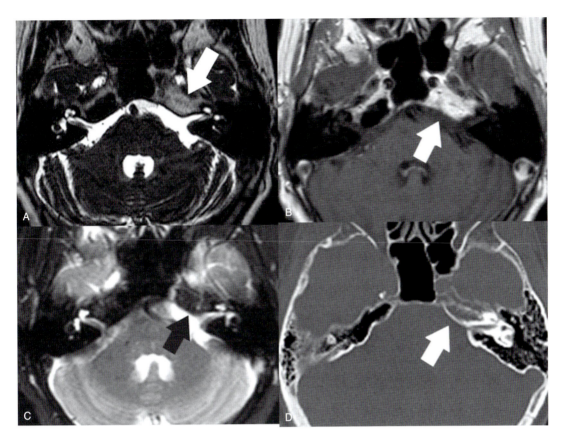

**Figure 56.2** (**A**) Axial T2-weighted and (**B**) post-contrast T1-weighted images of the posterior fossa show a hyperintense "lesion" in the left petrous apex, possibly representing an enhancing mass, and a pneumatized right petrous apex with signal void. (**C**) Fat-suppressed T2-weighted and (**D**) CT images from the same level prove that the lesion is actually the normal marrow in a non-pneumatized petrous apex.

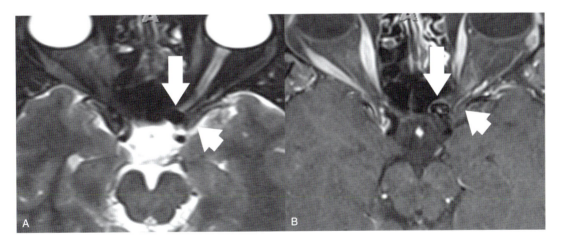

**Figure 56.3** Left ICA aneurysm. (**A**) Axial T2-weighted and (**B**) post-contrast T1-weighted MRI show an ovoid signal void (arrows) next to the left ACP (short arrows). The ACP can be seen as a separate marrow-containing structure next to the lesion. The possibility of an ethmoid air cell projecting into this region was ruled out by noting the small amount of enhancement in the center of the lesion seen on the post-contrast image. DSA confirmed a large ophthalmic segment aneurysm.

**Figure 56.1** (cont.) anatomic variation, although erroneous diagnoses of a right paraclinoid carotid aneurysm on the basis of apparent signal void next to the carotid artery (thin arrow) or a left clinoid mass such as meningioma on the basis of presumed enhancement may be offered. Note that the non-pneumatized left ACP shows a thin rim of dark signal, i.e., cortex, surrounding the marrow space on unenhanced images. (**D**) High-resolution axial and (**E**) coronal CT of the same patient clearly shows air in the right and bone in the left clinoid processes.

**265**

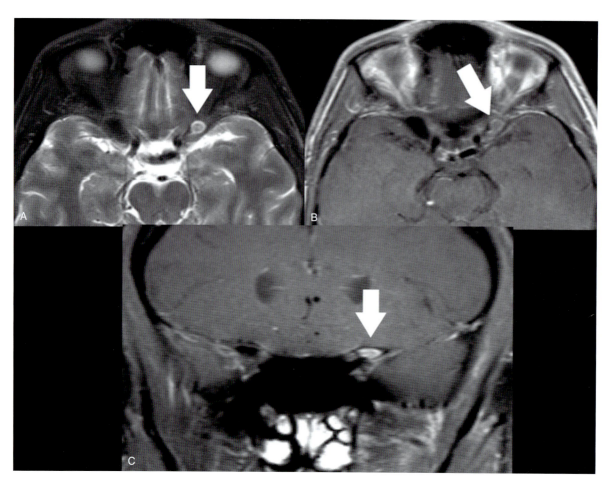

**Figure 56.4** (**A**) Axial T2-weighted, (**B**) axial post-contrast T1-weighted, and (**C**) coronal post-contrast T1-weighted images show bilateral pneumatized ACPs with mucosal inflammatory change in the left ACP that can potentially be mistaken for an intracranial lesion unless one notes the anatomic site and the thin rim of dark signal, i.e., cortex, surrounding the lesion.

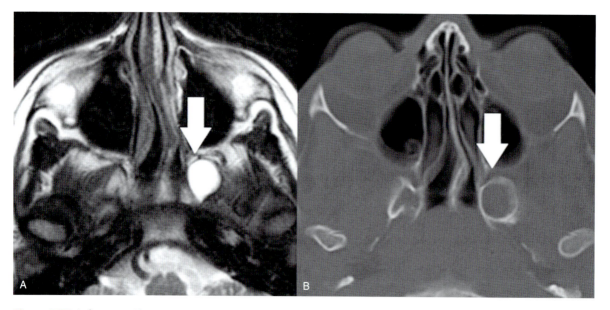

**Figure 56.5** Left pterygoid process asymmetric pneumatization and inflammatory change. (**A**) Axial T2-weighted image shows a hyperintense lesion at the skull base which represents sinus inflammatory change in a pneumatized pterygoid process of the sphenoid sinus. (**B**) This is easier to appreciate on axial CT. Note the non-pneumatized right pterygoid process.

# Fibrous dysplasia of skull base

## Imaging description

Primary bone disorders involving the skull base present with non-specific MRI appearances. While MRI is very helpful in delineating the extent of involvement it is not as helpful in providing a specific diagnosis. In primary osseous abnormalities of the skull base, combining MR with high-resolution bone CT is essential.

Fibrous dysplasia (FD) is a common benign bone disorder secondary to replacement of normal bone marrow by woven bone and fibrous tissue. It can be lytic or sclerotic or polyostotic and can involve any bone in the body [1]. The involvement of calvarium, skull base, and facial bones is seen in about 50% of the cases of polyostotic FD. There are three distinct imaging patterns based on CT findings. The most common is a mixed pagetoid pattern (Fig. 57.1) with areas of radiolucency and radiodensity and bone expansion. A sclerotic FD with ground-glass density (Fig. 57.2) and a predominantly cystic FD with central lucency and sclerotic borders (Fig. 57.3) are the other varieties. The MRI appearance of FD is variable, ranging from avidly enhancing lesions to no enhancement, and from markedly hyperintense T2 signal to markedly hypointense T2 signal [2].

## Importance

FD may mimic multiple other bony conditions of the skull base and can have a misleading appearance on MRI. As with other skull-base lesions, correlation with CT findings is essential.

## Typical clinical scenario

Many times, FD of skull base is an incidental imaging observation. However, hemifacial deformity, pain, facial swelling, or cranial nerve involvement may be a presenting feature. Almost 70% of FD cases are monostotic and are found in young adults. Involvement of maxilla and mandible is more common than ethmoidal bone, sphenoidal bone, frontal bone, or temporal bone. About 25% of FD cases are polyostotic, and these are more commonly diagnosed in the pediatric age group, more often between the ages of 8 and 10 years. The skull and facial bones are involved in about 50%, presenting with craniofacial asymmetry, focal pain, and tenderness. McCune–Albright syndrome is seen in about 5% of all FD cases.

## Differential diagnosis

Paget's disease is the most common differential diagnosis. It usually presents in the elderly population, involves the temporal bone and calvarium, and spares the craniofacial area. Expansile bone lesion with mixed lytic and sclerotic appearance and a "cottonwool" lesion within the affected bones are characteristics of Paget's disease (Fig. 57.4). Ossifying fibroma can mimic FD, with sclerotic margins and relatively low-density predominantly fibrous center. However, it tends to be more focal, mass-like, and predominantly within the sinonasal region (Fig. 57.5). Intraosseous meningioma in the skull base is relatively rare. However, there is usually adjacent dural thickening or an enhancing en plaque soft tissue mass. Chondrosarcoma is generally centered at the petroclival fissure, exhibits chondroid matrix on CT scan, and displays high T2 signal on MRI. Mixed lytic and sclerotic metastatic secondary deposits from carcinoma of breast and prostate is also an important differential diagnosis.

### Teaching points

As with any skull-base lesion, imaging with both CT and MRI is essential. However, bone CT is more specific than MRI. In complicated cases with cranial nerve palsies, a T1-weighted fat-saturated MRI sequence is very helpful.

REFERENCES

1. Amit M, Fliss DM, Gil Z. Fibrous dysplasia of the sphenoid and skull base. *Otolaryngol Clin North Am* 2011; **44**: 891–902.
2. Laine FJ, Nadel L, Braun IF. CT and MR imaging of the central skull base. Part 2. Pathologic spectrum. *Radiographics* 1990; **10**: 797–821.

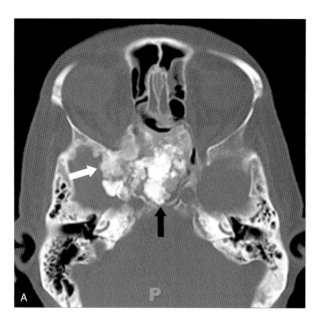
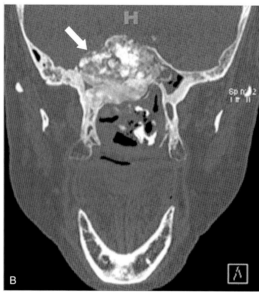

**Figure 57.1** Pagetoid fibrous dysplasia. (**A**, **B**) Mixed expansile sclerotic and lytic lesion of basisphenoid (white arrows) with "cottonwool" sclerotic bone lesions in the center (black arrow).

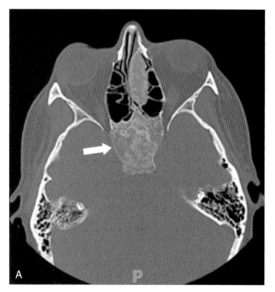
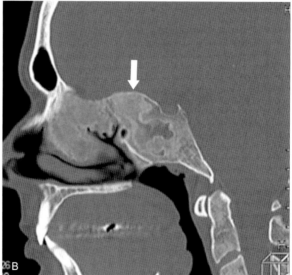
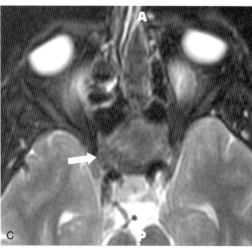

**Figure 57.2** Sclerotic fibrous dysplasia. (**A**) Axial and (**B**) reconstructed sagittal CT imaging reveals expansile predominantly sclerotic bone lesion of the basisphenoid and ethmoidal bone with ground-glass appearance (arrow). (**C**) Axial T2-weighted imaging reveals low T2 signal of corresponding bone (arrow). This alone can be confounding, if not combined with CT findings to diagnose fibrous dysplasia.

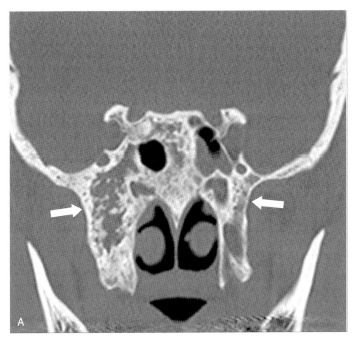

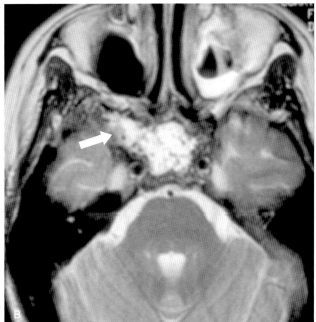

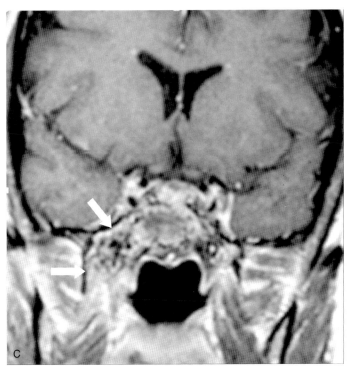

**Figure 57.3** Cystic fibrous dysplasia. (**A**) Coronal non-contrast CT exhibits expansile brain lesion involving the basisphenoid and pterygoid plates with sclerotic rim and lytic central areas (arrows). (**B**) Axial T2-weighted imaging reveals areas of high T2 signal (arrow) within low T2 signal rim. (**C**) Coronal post-contrast T1-weighted imaging reveals diffuse heterogeneous enhancement (arrow).

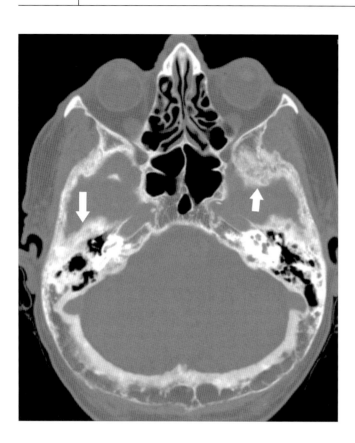

**Figure 57.4** Paget's disease. Mixed, expansile, lytic and sclerotic lesions of calvarium are seen, including basisphenoid, greater wing of sphenoid bone (arrow), temporal bone (arrow), and occipital bone.

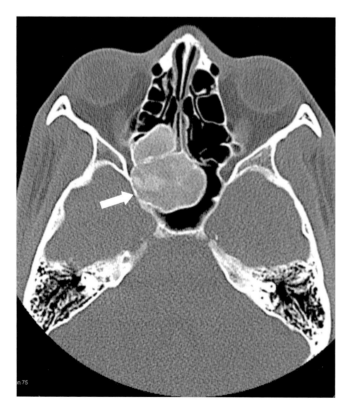

**Figure 57.5** Ossifying fibroma. Well-demarcated expansile spheno-ethmoidal sinus mass with relatively lower-density center is seen surrounded by ossific rim (arrow).

# Sphenoid bone pseudolesion

## Imaging description

Incidentally identified bone lesions in the sphenoid are common in the area of liberal CT imaging for common conditions such as sinusitis and headache. Incidental sphenoid bone lesions are rarely malignant. The most common intrinsic benign bone lesions of the sphenoid include fibrous dysplasia (FD) and ossifying fibromas, with rare lesions including giant cell tumors, giant cell reparative granulomas, osteoblastomas, lipomas, and hemangiomas. Although benign, these lesions can become symptomatic secondary to bone expansion and obstruction of sinus drainage or compression of adjacent structures such as cranial nerves and extraocular muscles. Because of this potential many of these lesions require clinical work-up, imaging follow-up and surgery if the symptoms warrant.

Separate from these benign tumors and much more common is a condition called pseudolesion or arrested pneumatization of the sphenoid bone, which is incompletely understood but presumably a developmental condition with no growth potential. These lesions are always asymptomatic; they show a well-defined sclerotic margin, internal curvilinear calcifications intermixed with fat, and lack of bone expansion (Figs. 58.1–58.4). They are almost always associated with underdevelopment of the ipsilateral sphenoid sinus and are thought to occur as a result of premature arrest of pneumatization of the sphenoid sinus.

## Importance

Pseudolesion of the sphenoid (a.k.a. arrested pneumatization) is benign and does not require extensive work-up or surgical intervention.

## Typical clinical scenario

Asymptomatic "lesions" incidentally seen on CT or MRI.

## Differential diagnosis

The most important radiological finding in differential diagnosis is bone expansion. Pseudolesion does not expand the bone, whereas most other conditions do. The most common lesion of the sphenoid bone is FD, which usually exhibits a ground-glass density and bone expansion on CT (Fig. 58.5). The curvilinear calcifications and fat seen in pseudolesion are different than the matrix mineralization seen in FD. On MRI, FD signal is variable and often heterogeneous, with foci of avid enhancement frequently seen. Pseudolesion should not show enhancement, or more than minimal enhancement. Ossifying fibroma exhibits some overlapping characteristics with pseudolesion but they are commonly expansile, in contrast to pseudolesions. Remodeling or erosion of the cortex adjacent to a bone lesion on CT, significant enhancement, and lack of fat on MRI should always prompt diagnosis of a more aggressive process than pseudolesion (Fig. 58.6).

## Teaching points

Pseudolesion or arrested pneumatization of the sphenoid is a benign process which is characterized by a non-expansile lucency with well-defined sclerotic margins, internal fat, curvilinear internal calcifications, and underpneumatized ipsilateral sphenoid sinus. Bone expansion or cortical erosion should prompt a different diagnosis.

REFERENCES

1. Efune G, Perez CL, Tong L, Rihani J, Batra PS. Paranasal sinus and skull base fibro-osseous lesions: when is biopsy indicated for diagnosis? *Int Forum Allergy Rhinol* 2012; **2**: 160–5.

2. Welker KM, DeLone DR, Lane JI, Gilbertson JR. Arrested pneumatization of the skull base: imaging characteristics. *AJR Am J Roentgenol* 2008; **190**: 1691–6.

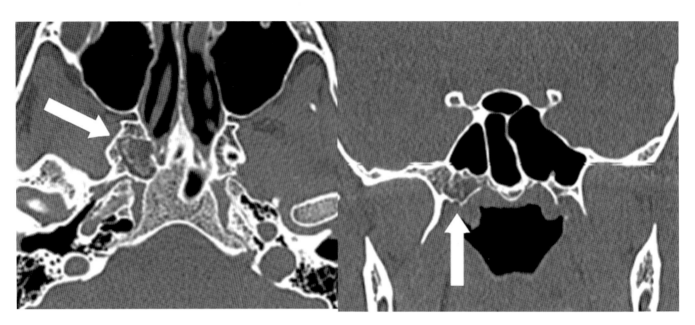

**Figure 58.1** Axial and coronal CT show a well-defined sphenoid bone lesion (arrow) with slightly sclerotic margins, internal linear calcifications, and fat density. Note that there is no bone expansion and the ipsilateral sphenoid sinus is hypoplastic as compared to the other side.

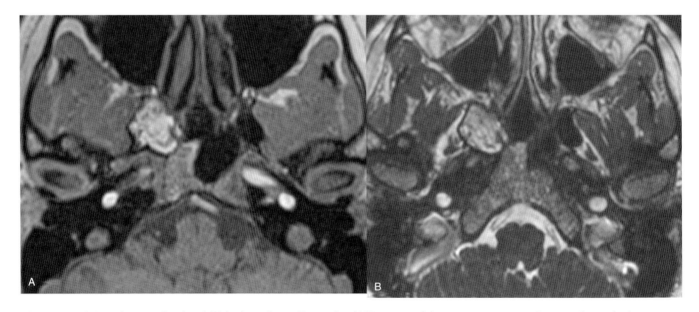

**Figure 58.2** (**A**) Axial T1-weighted and (**B**) high-resolution T2-weighted MR images of the same patient as in Fig. 58.1 shows the lesion to be of fat signal. The sclerotic rim is defined as a hypointense line around the lesion on both images.

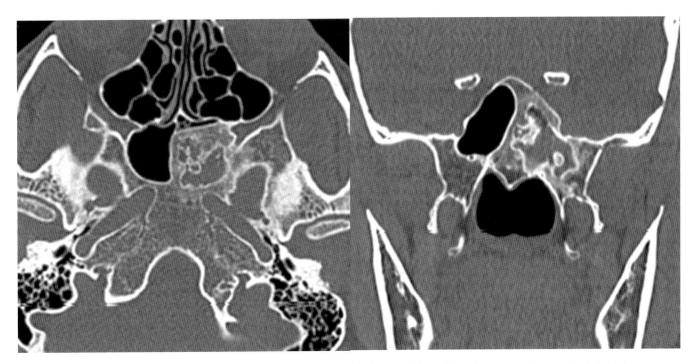

**Figure 58.3** A larger pseudolesion of the sphenoid bone displays similar characteristics, with no bone expansion and ipsilateral sinus non-pneumatization.

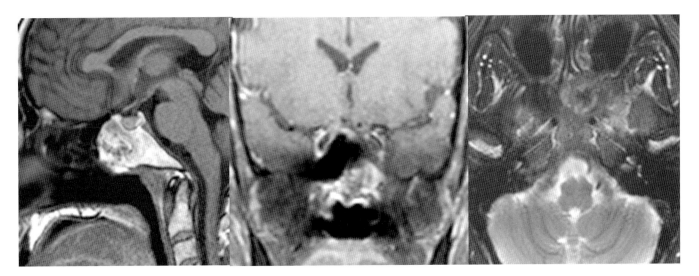

**Figure 58.4** The same lesion as in Fig. 58.3 shows heterogeneously bright T1 signal (left), no significant contrast enhancement (middle), and minimally increased T2 signal (right) on MRI.

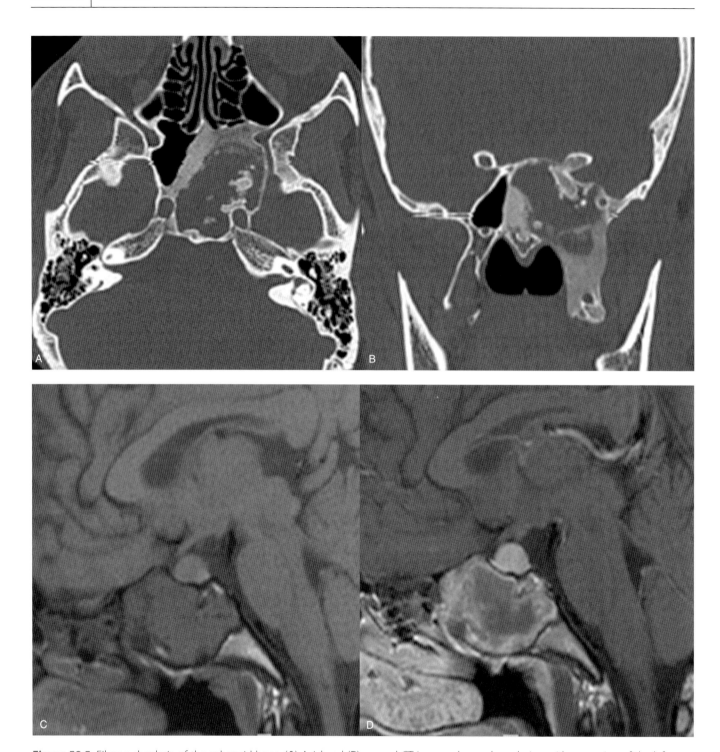

**Figure 58.5** Fibrous dysplasia of the sphenoid bone. (**A**) Axial and (**B**) coronal CT images show a large lesion with expansion of the left pterygoid process (compare to the normal right side) and ground-glass density in the marrow cavity, which are characteristic of FD. (**C**) Sagittal pre-contrast and (**D**) post-contrast MR images show prominent enhancement in FD. FDs have a wide range of contrast enhancement features, ranging from avid enhancement to no enhancement.

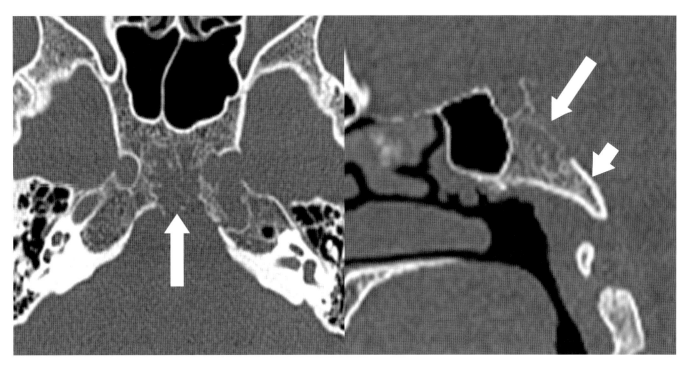

**Figure 58.6** Ill-defined lytic-appearing lesion in the clivus with erosion of the posterior cortex (arrows) is suspicious of a more aggressive lesion. Contrast the normal cortex (short arrow) with the eroded cortex. MR imaging showed an associated soft tissue mass, and biopsy revealed chordoma.

# 59 Clival lesions

## Imaging description

Literally meaning a slope, the clivus is the part of the central skull base sloping upward from the foramen magnum to the dorsum sellae. It is composed of basisphenoid and basiocciput and thus forms an important boundary of the posterior skull base, but is easily accessible from the middle skull base.

Lesions of the clivus are predominantly osseous and mainly neoplastic [1]. It may be a primary mass arising from clivus such as chordoma [2]; secondary involvement from an adjacent primary such as invasive pituitary macroadenoma, chondrosarcoma, or nasopharyngeal carcinoma; part of a multicentric systemic process such as multiple myeloma and plasmacytoma; metastatic secondary deposits from a primary elsewhere in the body; or a metabolic bone process such as fibrous dysplasia or Paget's disease. Imaging with MRI and CT can help to differentiate amongst these conditions and arrive at a narrow and focused diagnostic possibility.

## Importance

A diverse spectrum of conditions can involve clivus. Benign conditions such as fibrous dysplasia and Paget's disease do not need any active treatment, multiple myeloma may require specific medical therapy, plasmacytoma may require radiation therapy, and chordoma and chondrosarcoma require surgical resection. A biopsy procedure is highly invasive, with associated morbidity, although endoscopic methods have improved the accessibility of many clival lesions. A comprehensive diagnosis with MRI and CT imaging can help determine the next step in treatment.

## Typical clinical scenario

Most clival lesions may present with headaches and cranial neuropathies, especially of cranial nerve VI. If the cavernous sinus is involved, cranial nerves III and IV may be additionally affected, leading to visual complaints and ophthalmoplegia. Involvement of cranial nerve V2 can lead to facial pain. In case of more inferior lesions, cranial nerves IX–XII may be affected with involvement of the jugular foramen and hypoglossal canal.

## Differential diagnosis

The clivus is the second most common location for chordoma, after the sacrum. It is a locally aggressive neoplasm arising from primitive notochord remnant. It commonly arises from the spheno-occipital synchondrosis, and is more likely a midline mass, although it can be eccentric [2]. It is an expansile mass with high T2 signal, intermediate to low T1 signal, and moderate to marked post-contrast enhancement (Fig. 59.1), although occasionally chordomas do not show enhancement on post-contrast imaging. Bone window CT scan exhibits lytic bone destruction.

A pituitary macroadenoma originates in the sella, involving the pituitary gland, and it may extend into the sphenoid sinus and central skull base. Sagittal MR sequence exhibits a central skull base mass contiguous with pituitary mass with sellar expansion and breach of the floor. Inability to visualize the normal pituitary gland on a sagittal image separate from a clival lesion strongly suggests the possibility of invasive pituitary macroadenoma (Fig. 59.2). Most of these locally aggressive giant pituitary adenomas are gonadotropin-secreting adenomas or prolactinomas in man [3]. MMP-9, a zinc-containing endopeptidase, is suggested to be a biomarker for invasive pituitary macroadenoma [4].

Fibrous dysplasia can have a deceptive appearance on MRI. It can have high T2 signal, low T2 signal, or a heterogeneous appearance. The diagnosis is suggested by a typical ground-glass appearance on CT scan (Fig. 59.3).

Plasmacytoma can be solitary or part of multiple myeloma. It presents as a lytic destructive mass on CT scan with its epicenter in the marrow space, and it can have a significant extraosseous soft tissue component. On MRI, it exhibits iso- to hypointense T1 signal and homogeneous low T2 signal that is isointense to grey matter (Fig. 59.4).

When a primary nasopharyngeal carcinoma invades the clivus, it is considered a T3 disease. T1-weighted sagittal MRI reveals the extent of bone marrow infiltration. The mass reveals low T2 signal with patchy but intense post-contrast enhancement (Fig. 59.5).

Chondrosarcoma arises in the petroclival synchondrosis and usually presents with cranial nerve V and VI palsy [5]. On CT scan, a lytic destructive soft tissue mass in the petroclival region also exhibits typical chondroid matrix and calcification. On MRI, a low T1 signal mass reveals very high T2 signal, like chordoma, and intense post-contrast enhancement (Fig. 59.6).

Non-Hodgkin's lymphoma and metastases are also important and pertinent differential diagnoses for a clival lesion that present as decreased T1 signal on MRI; presence of additional marrow-replacing lesions in the skull and spine would be helpful in the differential diagnosis.

---

### Teaching points

With its multiplanar imaging capabilities, MRI is the best modality to detect and characterize clival lesions. Sagittal T1-weighted sequence is highly sensitive to detect low T1 signal lesion, contrasted against high T1 signal of fatty clival bone marrow. High T2 signal favors chordoma and chondrosarcoma. If the epicenter of the lesion is within the nasopharynx, lymphoma and nasopharyngeal carcinoma are quite likely. Eccentric, petroclival origin favors chondrosarcoma. Involvement of sella turcica and pituitary gland with suprasellar extension favors invasive pituitary macroadenoma. CT scan is a complementary investigation and shows bone destruction. It is helpful in the evaluation of fibrous dysplasia, Paget's disease, and bone tumors.

REFERENCES

1. Laine FJ, Nadel L, Braun IF. CT and MR imaging of the central skull base. Part 2. Pathologic spectrum. *Radiographics* 1990: **10**: 797–821.

2. Erdem E, Angtuaco EC, Van Hemert R, Park JS, Al-Mefty O. Comprehensive review of intracranial chordoma. *Radiographics* 2003; **23**: 995–1009

3. Madsen H, Borges TM, Knox AJ, *et al.* Giant pituitary adenomas: pathologic–radiographic correlations and lack of role for p53 and MIB-1 labeling. *Am J Surg Pathol* 2011; **35**: 1204–13

4. Gong J, Zhao Y, Abdel-Fattah R, *et al.* Matrix metalloproteinase-9, a potential biological marker in invasive pituitary adenomas. *Pituitary* 2008; **11**: 37–48.

5. Hong P, Taylor SM, Trites JR, *et al.* Chondrosarcoma of the head and neck: report of 11 cases and literature review. *J Otolaryngol Head Neck Surg* 2009; **38**: 279–85.

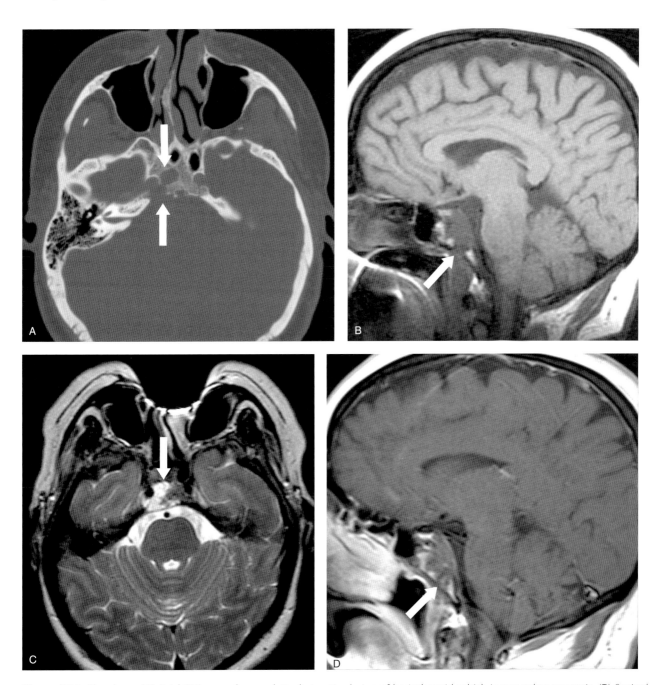

**Figure 59.1** Chordoma. (**A**) Axial CT image shows a lytic destructive lesion of basisphenoid, which is somewhat eccentric. (**B**) Sagittal T1-weighted MR image exhibits an intermediate T1 signal clival mass with its epicenter at the spheno-occipital synchondrosis. (**C**) Axial T2-weighted MR image exhibits high T2 signal eccentric mass of the basisphenoid. (**D**) Sagittal post-contrast T1-weighted MR image exhibits patchy post-contrast enhancement. Note that elevation of dura dorsal to clivus, which can give rise to headaches.

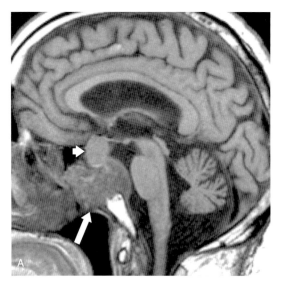

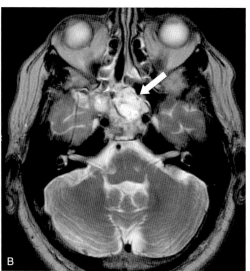

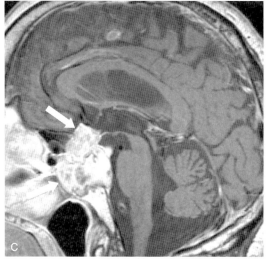

**Figure 59.2** Invasive pituitary macroadenoma. (**A**) Sagittal T1-weighted MR image exhibits an enlarged pituitary gland (short arrow) isointense to gray matter with suprasellar extension. It is contiguous with a soft tissue mass within the sphenoidal sinus with exophytic extension into the prepontine cistern and destruction of the superior part of the clivus (arrow). (**B**) Axial T2-weighted MR image exhibits intermediate to high T2 signal of the irregular sphenoidal and clival mass. (**C**) Sagittal post-contrast T1-weighted MR image exhibits heterogeneous but intense post-contrast enhancement. A misleading dural tail is seen at the inferior extent of the mass.

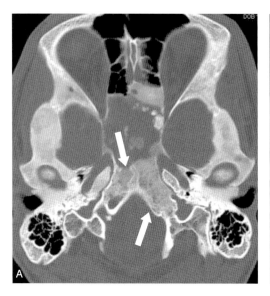

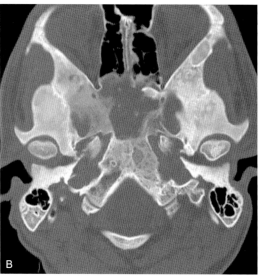

**Figure 59.3** Fibrous dysplasia. (**A**, **B**) Axial CT with bone window reveals lytic sclerotic ground-glass appearance of basiocciput with expansile ground-glass appearance of the squamous temporal bone. There is preservation of cortex.

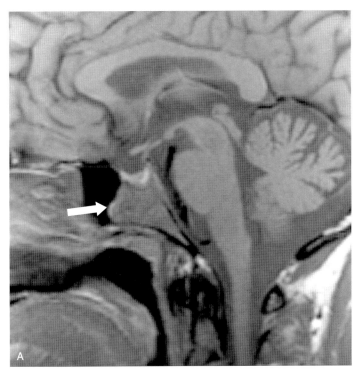

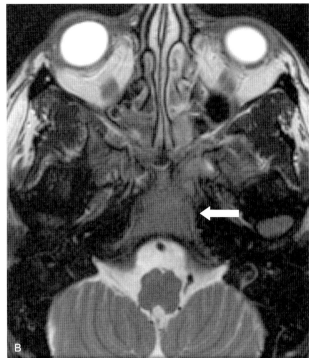

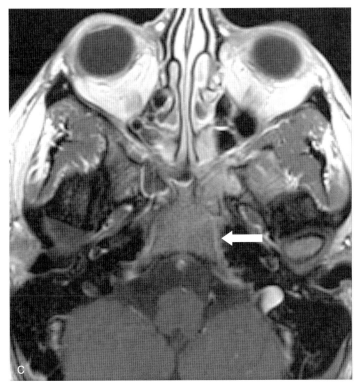

**Figure 59.4** Plasmacytoma. (**A**) Sagittal T1-weighted MR image reveals replacement of normal high T1 signal fat with intermediate T1 signal in clivus. (**B**) Axial T2-weighted MR image reveals homogeneous low T2 signal isointense to gray matter. (**C**) Axial post-contrast T1-weighted MR image reveals moderate patchy post-contrast enhancement.

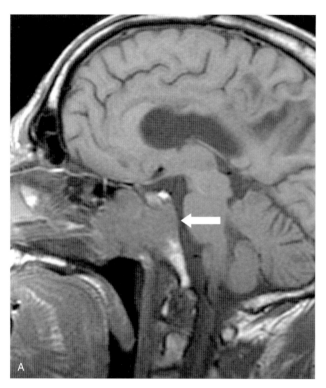

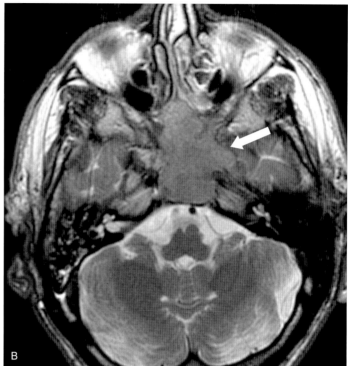

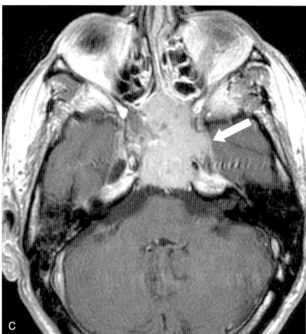

**Figure 59.5** Nasopharyngeal carcinoma. (**A**) Sagittal T1-weighted MR image reveals infiltrating right nasopharyngeal soft tissue mass invading the sphenoidal sinus and clivus. (**B**) Axial T2-weighted MR image reveals low T2 signal expansion of clivus with extension into sphenoidal and ethmoidal sinus and infiltration of skull base. (**C**) Axial post-contrast T1-weighted MR image exhibits patchy post-contrast enhancement of the mass, which also extends into medial left middle cranial fossa.

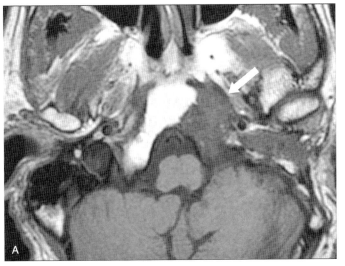

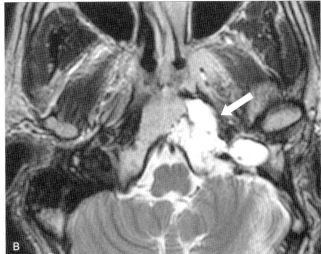

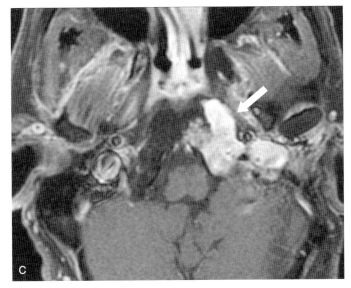

**Figure 59.6** Chondrosarcoma. (**A**) Axial T1-weighted MR imaging reveals a low T1 signal mass along the left petroclival region, lateral to clivus. (**B**) Axial T2-weighted MR imaging reveals a very high T2 signal mass with presence of low T2 signal foci, likely areas of calcification. (**C**) Axial post-contrast fat-saturated T1-weighted MR imaging reveals intense but somewhat heterogeneous post-contrast enhancement.

## Imaging description

Perineural spread (PNS) is a mechanism whereby tumor, or another pathological condition, spreads along loose connective tissue of the perineurium. It is a common complication of head and neck cancers [1]. Although any cranial nerve can be involved by PNS, it is most commonly observed along the branches of cranial nerves V and VII and their anastomotic branches.

Direct imaging signs include enlargement, irregularity, and excessive enhancement of the cranial nerves and their branches (Figs. 60.1, 60.2). With high-resolution MR imaging, the nerve itself can frequently be visualized (Fig. 60.1B). Within the neural foramina and bony canals, the nerve is normally seen surrounded by a small perineural venous plexus. Care should be taken to avoid mistaking this normal plexus for perineural enhancing tumor. After the nerve exits the neural foramen or canal, it is generally seen surrounded by fat. It is important to pay close attention to normally observed fat pads along the neural foramina on unenhanced T1-weighted images. Presence of tumor along the cranial nerves obliterates the normally observed high T1 signal of these fat pads (Table 60.1). In advanced cases, enlargement or destruction of neural foramina and canals can be seen. Continued retrograde tumor spread can involve the cisternal segments of the cranial nerves and, ultimately, the brainstem.

Occasionally, indirect finding of denervation of muscles can bring the attention of the radiologist to otherwise unsuspected perineural tumor spread. For example, mandibular nerve involvement can result in denervation of the muscles of mastication, anterior belly of digastric muscle, and mylohyoid; and hypoglossal nerve involvement can produce denervation of the tongue muscles.

## Importance

Failure to recognize PNS can have considerable implications for treatment planning of head and neck carcinomas. A missed diagnosis of PNS may contribute to distant tumor recurrence because of inadequate total tumor volume treatment or failure to target all involved areas.

## Typical clinical scenario

Common symptoms include pain, paresthesia, burning sensation in the nerve distribution, diplopia, blurred vision, and weakness in the distribution of the nerve. The onset of clinical symptoms is often delayed, and as many as 40% of patients are clinically asymptomatic [1].

## Differential diagnosis of PNS

Perineural spread has been rarely reported with rhinocerebral mucormycosis, *Aspergillus* infection, and sinonasal sarcoidosis. Other causes of enlarged and enhancing cranial nerves also include viral neuritis, histiocytosis, meningeal carcinomatosis, leukemia, and lymphoma (Fig. 60.3).

**Table 60.1** Important spaces/foramina to be scrutinized on imaging in the assessment of head and neck tumors [1].

| Cranial nerve (or branch) | Important space(s)/foramina |
|---|---|
| Ophthalmic division of trigeminal nerve (V1) | Supraorbital foramen |
| Maxillary division of trigeminal nerve (V2) | Foramen rotundum, pterygopalatine fossa, canal and foramen for the infraorbital nerve, vidian canal, palatine foramen |
| Mandibular division of trigeminal nerve (V3) | Foramen ovale, and mandibular foramen for the inferior alveolar nerve |
| Facial nerve (VII) | Stylomastoid foramen and descending facial nerve canal |

> ### Teaching points
>
> Detection of tumor spread along the nerves can often alter the treatment plan significantly. PNS has been shown to be associated with an increased risk of local recurrence, nodal metastasis, and decreased patient survival.

REFERENCES

1. Gandhi D, Gujar S, Mukherji SK. MR imaging of perineural spread of head and neck tumors. *Top Mag Res* 2004; **15**: 79–85.

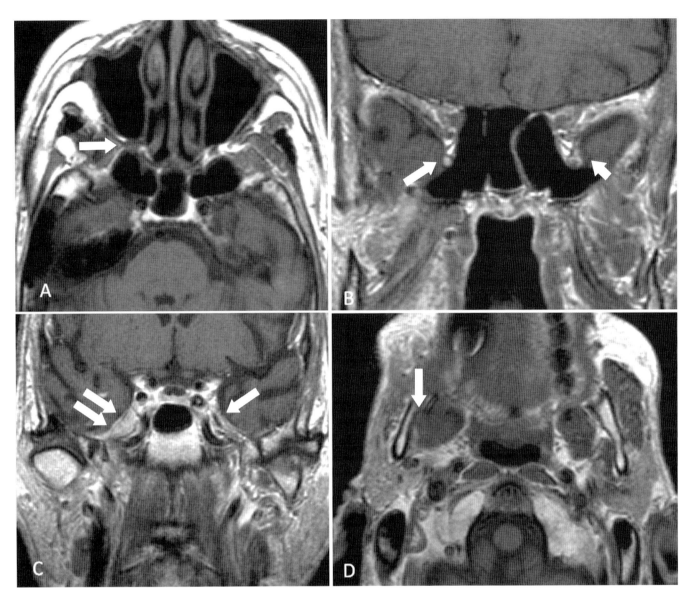

**Figure 60.1** Retrograde perineural spread along V2 in a setting of right lower eyelid squamous cell carcinoma. There is also gross antegrade tumor spread along the V3 division. (**A**) Axial T1-weighted image shows a subtle mass in the right pterygopalatine fossa replacing the normal fat (arrow). (**B**) Coronal T1-weighted enhanced image demonstrates enhancement of right V2 in the foramen rotundum (long arrow). Compare with normal perineural venous plexus of V2 on the left (short arrow). (**C**) The tumor reached the Meckel's cave on the right side and then spread antegradely along the V3 (double arrow). The single arrow shows the normal left Meckel's cave. (**D**) Axial T1-weighted image demonstrates downward extension of the tumor into the masticator space and along the inferior alveolar nerve (arrow). Note the enlarged foramen for the inferior alveolar nerve and denervation atrophy of the masseter muscle.

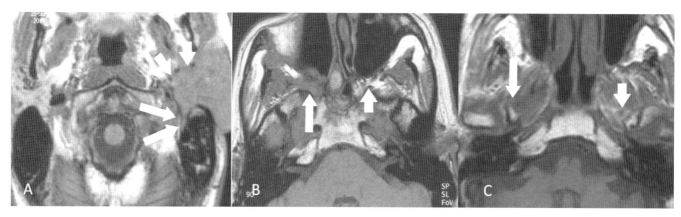

**Figure 60.2** The importance of scrutinizing the fat pads adjacent to skull base foramina in the early detection of perineural spread. (**A**) Axial T1-weighted image reveals a hypointense mass (short arrows) in the left parotid gland that extends into the left stylomastoid foramen (arrows). This is the most frequent pathway for involvement of the facial nerve by perineural spread. (**B**) Axial T1-weighted image in a patient with adenoid cystic carcinoma of the soft palate shows the presence of a mass in the right pterygopalatine fossa (arrow). The tumor ascended in perineural fashion along the palatine nerves. Note the presence of normal fat in the left pterygopalatine fossa (short arrow). (**C**) Antegrade spread of squamous cell carcinoma along the V3 (same patient as in Fig. 60.1). Note replacement of normal fat pad medial to the lateral pterygoid muscle by the perineural tumor (arrow), and the normal left V3 below the foramen ovale (short arrow).

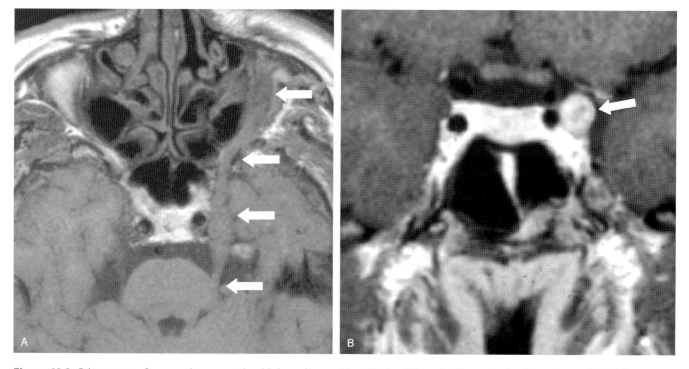

**Figure 60.3** Other causes of nerve enlargement should always be considered in the differential diagnosis of perineural spread. (**A**) Schwannoma of the trigeminal nerve with extension along the V2 (arrows). (**B**) Sacroidosis of left nerve III.

# Cochlear dysplasia

## Imaging description

The spectrum of congenital cochlear and vestibular anomalies is very wide, ranging from complete absence of the inner ear structures to minimal dysplastic chances that are difficult to visualize. Essentially all of these present with bilateral congenital sensorineural hearing loss, however [1].

The most severe variety is known as labyrinthine aplasia (Michel's anomaly), where there is no cochlea, vestibule, or semicircular canal development at all. Common cavity is lesser in severity and refers to a single "cystic" space that represents a combination of dysplastic vestibule and cochlea that does not closely resemble either [2]. When the developmental arrest occurs around week 7 of gestation the cochlea is better formed and may present as incomplete partition type I (IP-I) (Fig. 61.1), where there is incomplete development of all turns of the cochlea, with lack of modiolus. When there is normal differentiation of the basilar turn of the cochlea with incomplete partition between middle and apical cochlear turns and a large vestibular aqueduct (LVA), it is known as incomplete partition type II (IP-II) anomaly (Figs. 61.2, 61.3). This is also known as the classic Mondini type of anomaly, although in the literature the term Mondini is commonly used, erroneously, to refer to a wide spectrum of inner ear anomalies [3]. An even milder form of cochlear dysplasia is due to incomplete development of the apical turn of the cochlea, which occurs at week 8 of gestation (Fig. 61.4). It results in modiolus deficiency with mild asymmetry of the scalar vestibuli and scala tympani. It is often associated with LVA.

## Importance

Diagnosis of the type of cochlear dysplasia provides crucial information for the surgical planning of cochlear implantation. The only absolute contraindication for cochlear implantation is cochlear aplasia. Patients with common cavity deformity, cochlear hypoplasia, incomplete partition deformities, lateral semicircular canal dysplasia, and enlarged vestibular aqueduct may potentially undergo cochlear implantation. However, knowledge of these deformities preoperatively is critical to success in implantation because the presence of the deformities governs electrode array choice and necessitates alterations in operative technique. Radiologically, it is important to be able to differentiate between cochlear aplasia, which cannot be implanted, and common cavity, which is amenable to implantation. For presurgical work-up, information about aberrant facial nerve, labyrinthitis ossificans, otomastoiditis, high riding jugular bulb, and possible aberrant internal carotid artery is very important [4]. All of this information can be provided with high-resolution temporal bone CT with < 1 mm slice thickness. A properly placed stimulator wire enters the cochlea at the round window and is seen in the basal and the second turn of the cochlea (Fig. 61.5).

## Typical clinical scenario

Congenital sensorineural hearing loss (SNHL) is the most common clinical presentation. Audiologic testing in pediatric age group is necessary for early diagnosis of SNHL.

## Differential diagnosis

Only about 20% of the congenital SNHL cases will demonstrate one of the anomalies described. The majority of these patients have lesions below the resolution of current imaging techniques.

## Teaching points

In evaluation of patients with congenital sensorineural deafness for cochlear implant candidacy it is important to be able to differentiate common cavity from cochlear aplasia. Most cochlear hypoplasia cases are implantable, although the choice of implant and surgical technique is dependent on the type and degree of labyrinthine anomaly.

REFERENCES

1. Lowe LH, Vézina LG. Sensorineural hearing loss in children. *Radiographics* 1997; **17**: 1079–93.

2. Shah LM, Wiggins RH. Imaging of hearing loss. *Neuroimaging Clin N Am* 2009; **19**: 287–306.

3. Davidson HC, Harnsberger HR, Lemmerling MM, *et al*. MR evaluation of vestibulocochlear anomalies associated with large endolymphatic duct and sac. *AJNR Am J Neuroradiol* 1999; **20**: 1435–41.

4. Witte RJ, Lane JI, Driscoll CL, *et al*. Pediatric and adult cochlear implantation. *Radiographics* 2003; **23**: 1185–200.

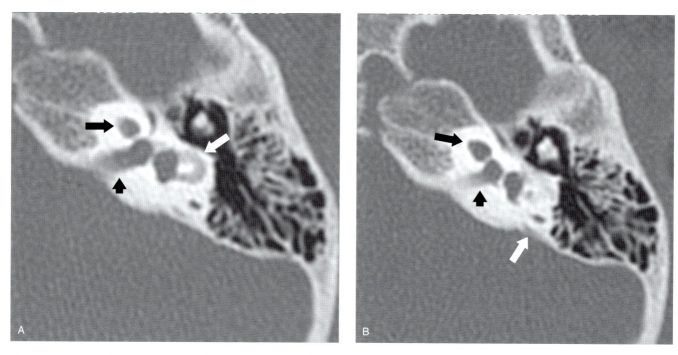

**Figure 61.1** Incomplete partition type I (cystic cochlea). (**A**) A dysmorphic small cochlear cavity without internal architecture is seen (black arrow) with normal size and shape of vestibule and semicircular canal (white arrow). A smaller internal acoustic canal (short black arrow) likely represents cochlear nerve hypoplasia, which should be confirmed by MRI. (**B**) The vestibular aqueduct exhibits normal caliber (white arrow).

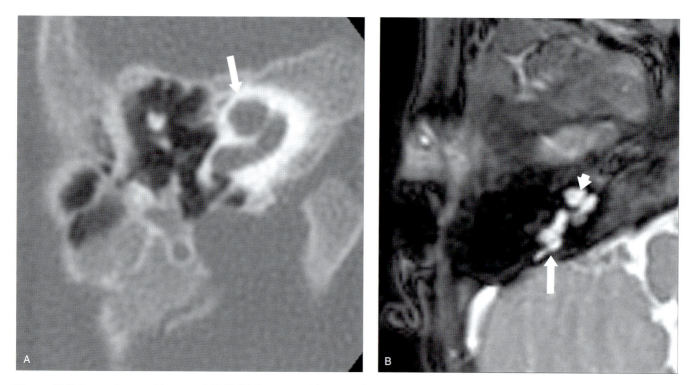

**Figure 61.2** Incomplete partition type II (IP-II). (**A**) On temporal bone CT, there is lack of partition between the second and apical turn of the cochlea, which appears bulbous (arrow). The basilar turn is well developed, however. (**B**) 3D FIESTA T2-weighted MRI shows lack of partition between the apical and second turn of the cochlea (short arrow). The vestibular aqueduct exhibits normal caliber (arrow).

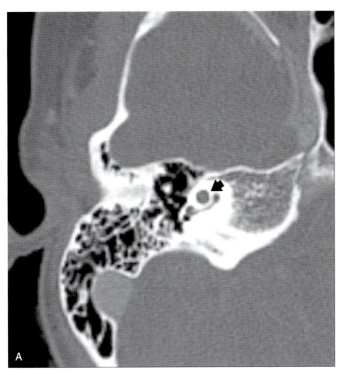

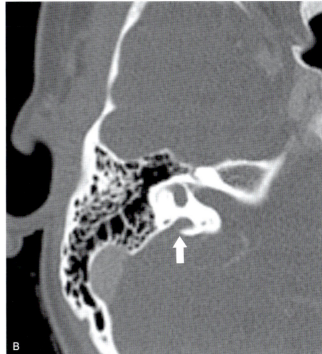

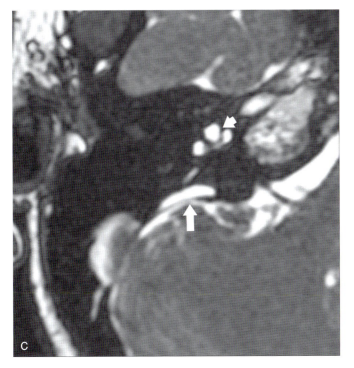

**Figure 61.3** Classic Mondini malformation. (**A, B**) Temporal bone CT exhibits bulbous second and apical turn of the cochlea with lack of partition (short black arrow). The basilar turn of the cochlea appears normal. The vestibular aqueduct is enlarged (white arrow). (**C**) 3D FIESTA T2-weighted MRI shows lack of partition between the second and apical turn of the cochlea (short white arrow) with dilated vestibular aqueduct (white arrow).

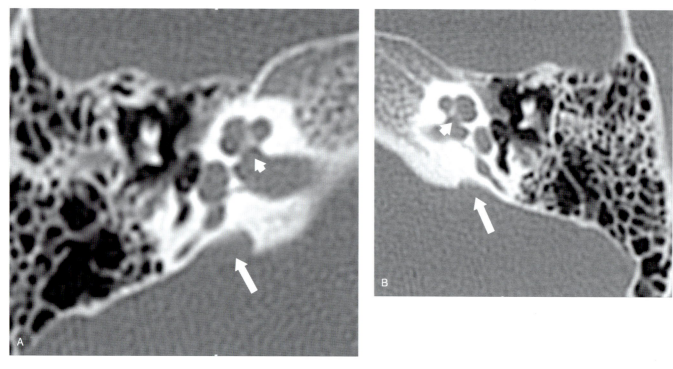

**Figure 61.4** Mild dysplasia. Modiolar deficiency. (**A, B**) The modiolus (short arrow) appears attenuated and flattened. The region of endolymphatic duct and sac (long arrow) is markedly enlarged.

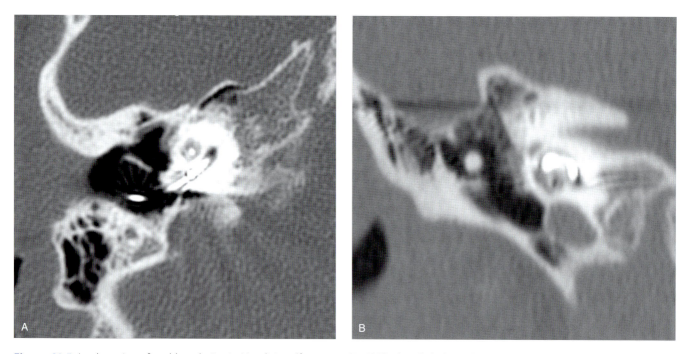

**Figure 61.5** Implantation of cochlear device in Mondini malformation. (**A, B**) The beaded electrode wire enters the round window, extends into the basal turn of the cochlea, reaching up to the second turn. There is no evidence for kinking or breaking.

# Labyrinthitis ossificans

## Imaging description

Labyrinthitis ossificans (LO) is a disease process that is most often a sequela of purulent inflammation of the inner ear that results from bacterial meningitis. Pathologic ossification of spaces ensues within the lumen of the bony labyrinth and cochlea that can progress to new bone formation. The cochlea is most commonly involved, and early changes are often observed in the scala tympani of the basal turn. The ossification then spreads to the cochlear apical turn.

The course of progression has been divided into three characteristic stages: acute, fibrous, and ossification [1]. The acute stage is characterized by purulent inflammatory exudate that fills the perilymphatic spaces (Fig. 62.1). The second stage, or stage of fibrosis, consists of fibroblast proliferation within the perilymphatic spaces. The third stage, of ossification, is characterized by osteogenesis (Fig. 62.2).

In the early stages, CT is generally unrevealing and can be false negative. However, MRI may be able to demonstrate early changes within the membranous labyrinth that are not appreciated on CT. High-resolution, fast spin-echo, T2-weighted MRI can demonstrate the loss of normal hyperintensity of membranous labyrinth even in the early stages of LO (Fig. 62.3) [2].

In the later stages of LO, high-resolution temporal bone CT (HRCT) is extremely valuable in demonstrating the extent of ossification and for treatment planning. On occasion, a very extensive ossification can result in virtually complete obliteration of the membranous labyrinth and can be confused with congenital otic dysplasia (Fig. 62.4).

## Importance

The advent of cochlear implantation has greatly increased the clinical significance and importance of diagnosing LO correctly. In the presence of LO, the surgeon needs to have a very good understanding of the extent of disease in order to plan appropriate modifications to cochlear implantation procedure.

## Typical clinical scenario

Bacterial meningitis is the most common cause of acquired sensorineural hearing loss (SNHL) in childhood, and LO. Deafness results from spread of the infection to the labyrinth and consequent end-organ damage. Rarely, LO may be seen after viral labyrinthitis, trauma to inner ear, labyrinthine infarction, or tumors.

## Differential diagnosis

The differential diagnosis includes all other causes of sensorineural hearing loss. Usually, a history of meningitis is forthcoming and helps point towards the correct diagnosis. In advanced cases of LO, the membranous labyrinth may be completely obliterated due to extensive ossification. In such cases, it must be differentiated from otic dysplasia, for example Michel's anomaly. The key feature differentiating the two is the width and contour of the otic capsule, which is reduced in otic dysplasias but normal in LO.

### Teaching points

LO is an important cause of acquired SNHL. Although in itself not a contraindication for cochlear implant, the presence of LO induces surgical difficulty and requires the use of modified techniques. Very extensive ossification or calcification is associated with reduction in the residual spiral ganglion cells, and cochlear implantation is less effective in these cases.

REFERENCES
1. Paparella MM, Sugiura S. The pathology of suppurative labyrinthitis. *Ann Otol Rhinol Laryngol* 1967; **76**: 554–86.
2. Arriaga MA, Carrier D. MRI and clinical decisions in cochlear implantation. *Am J Otol* 1996; **17**: 547–53.

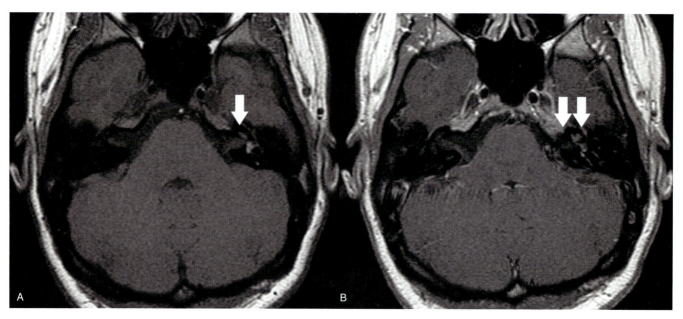

**Figure 62.1** Acute hemorrhagic labyrinthitis in a patient presenting with dysequilibrium and left-sided sensorineural hearing loss. (**A**) Axial T1-weighted MR images reveal high signal intensity (arrow) within the left membranous labyrinth signifying proteinaceous fluid or hemorrhage. Compare with the normal right side. (**B**) Cochlear enhancement (double arrows) is noted following the administration of gadolinium.

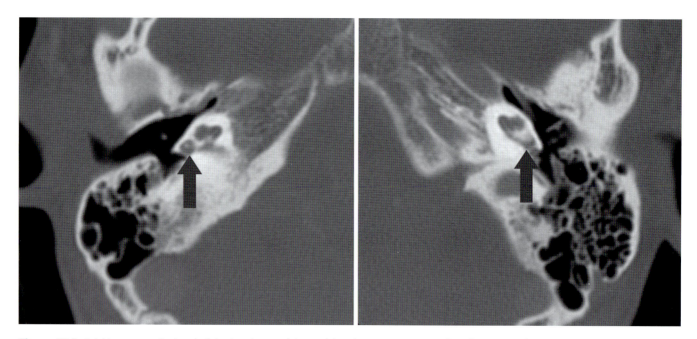

**Figure 62.2** Axial images at the level of the basal turn of the cochlea demonstrate areas of ossification involving the basal turns of bilateral cochleae (arrows: note greater involvement of left cochlea). The etiology of labyrinthitis ossificans in this case was antenatal exposure to maternal rubella.

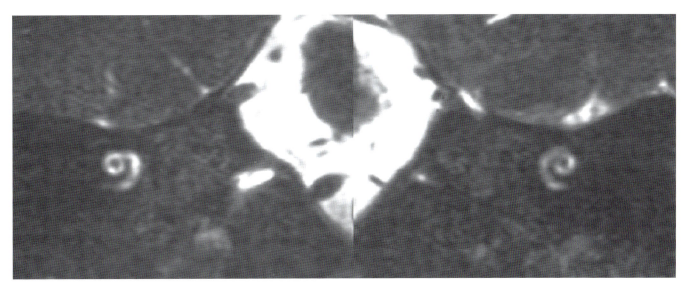

**Figure 62.3** Patient with a remote history of meningitis and bilateral sensorineural hearing loss. CT scan of the temporal bone was negative. Coronal oblique CISS (T2*-weighted 3D) sequence shows reduced intensity of the fluid signal in the left cochlea and an irregular outline on the right side. A preoperative diagnosis of labyrinthine fibrosis was made. The surgeons chose to implant the right side, in view of its less severe involvement.

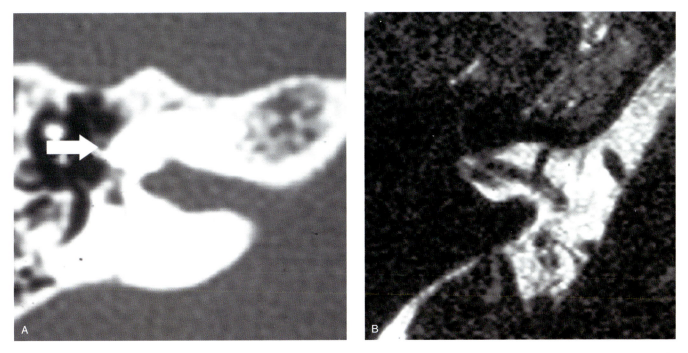

**Figure 62.4** (A) Advanced labyrinthitis ossificans demonstrated on thin-section CT. (B) MR image at an approximately similar anatomic level reveals complete obliteration of cochlear and vestibular fluid signal. MRI is advantageous in the preoperative evaluation of such patients to confirm the presence of the cochlear nerve. Also in (A), note that the convexity subtended by the basal turn of the cochlea is intact (arrow). In comparison, patients with cochlear aplasia will demonstrate a very small otic capsule and essentially flat medial wall of the middle ear.

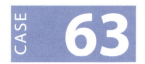

# Superior semicircular canal dehiscence

## Imaging description

Superior semicircular canal dehiscence (SSCD) is a recently described entity that is characterized by vestibular symptoms elicited by sound or pressure. Minor was the first to associate this clinical phenomenon with an anatomical defect of the superior semicircular canal detected with high-resolution computed tomography (HRCT) [1]. When the bone over the canal becomes thin or dehiscent, it acts as an additional window for the vestibular system, thereby allowing pressure and noise changes to induce vestibular activity. Over the last decade, this entity has been increasingly diagnosed and treated, although it is still not entirely clear whether the bony defect is congenital or acquired.

The sound is normally transmitted via stapes through the oval window into the cochlea. The round window dissipates the pressure, transmitting it back into the middle ear. Under normal conditions, the pressure in the semicircular canal remains constant. In the presence of a dehiscent roof, the superior semicircular canal (SSC) acts as another window and allows transmission of pressure to the vestibular apparatus, resulting in vertigo.

HRCT is diagnostic of this condition in the appropriate clinical setting by demonstrating dehiscence or uncovering at the roof of the SSC. It is usually unilateral (Fig. 63.1) but may be bilateral. Thin-section coronal images are generally diagnostic, but in case of doubt, radial reformats along the plane of the SSC or thin-section reformats perpendicular to the SSC orientation may be helpful (Fig. 63.2). It is important to correlate imaging findings with the clinical information, as the resolution of CT may not be sufficient to show a very thin layer of bone. Asymptomatic SSCD is common and should not be overdiagnosed. The role of MRI in evaluating SSCD is under investigation.

## Importance

SSCD may be associated with disabling vertigo and dizziness. More widespread knowledge of this condition is needed amongst radiologists. When evaluating the HRCT of temporal bones, the search pattern should always include assessment of the SSC and its roof.

## Typical clinical scenario

Patients with SSCD usually present with symptoms of sound-induced vertigo, nystagmus, or both (Tullio's phenomenon). Some patients may complain of chronic imbalance. Hyperacusis is defined as an unusual sensitivity to normal everyday sounds and may be a part of this syndrome.

## Differential diagnosis

Clinically, the differential diagnosis includes benign paroxysmal positional vertigo, perilymph fistula, and otosclerosis. However, the imaging appearance is characteristic and pathognomonic.

## Teaching points

SSCD is an important cause of vertigo and associated with characteristic clinical signs and imaging features. HRCT is diagnostic and generally sufficient for treatment planning. The treatment consists of conservative therapy in cases of lesser severity, or surgical approaches for covering the defect or plugging the semicircular canal [2].

REFERENCES

1. Minor LB. Superior canal dehiscence syndrome. *Am J Otol* 2000; **21**: 9–19.
2. Carey JP, Migliaccio AA, Minor LB. Semicircular canal function before and after surgery for superior canal dehiscence. *Otol Neurotol* 2007; **28**: 356–64.

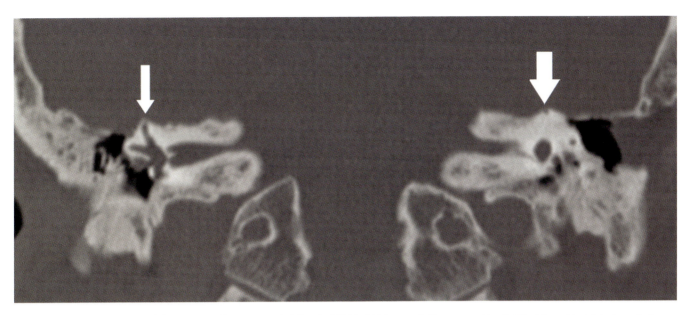

**Figure 63.1** Coronal HRCT of the temporal bones reveals left-sided SSCD (thick arrow). Compare with slightly thinned but intact roof of semicircular canal on the right (thin arrow).

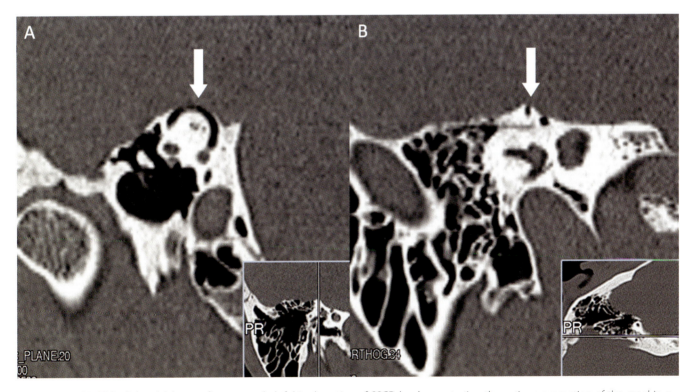

**Figure 63.2** (**A, B**) Radial multiplanar reformats are helpful in detection of SSCD by demonstrating the entire cross-section of the canal in a single image. Note the wide dehiscence (arrow) in this case.

# Fluid entrapment in the petrous apex cells

## Imaging description

The petrous apex (PA) is a part of the petrous bone that extends medial to the inner ear structures and contributes to the central skull base. It is not amenable to otoscopic examination, and the disease processes that involve the PA often generate symptoms that are very non-specific such as headache, tinnitus, and hearing loss, making imaging the most important part of diagnosis.

PA cells are normally pneumatized in a symmetric fashion, but asymmetric pneumatization occurs in about 30% of the population and may lead to diagnostic errors, particularly on MRI (see Case 56). The most common abnormality in the PA is fluid entrapment (a.k.a. effusion). Fluid entrapment does not require surgical intervention in most cases and should be differentiated from the "surgical" lesions of the PA such as cholesterol granulomas (CG) and cholesteatomas [1].

Fluid entrapment presents as opacified air cells on CT without expansion and preservation of bony septations between air cells. On MRI, increased T2 signal is seen almost invariably and mildly elevated T1 signal is not infrequent, which may lead to confusion with CG, which is always T1 bright (Fig. 64.1). On post-contrast imaging there is no significant enhancement associated with entrapped fluid other than mild lacy enhancement around the cells. Fluid entrapment is seen at least 10 times more commonly than the most frequent lesions such as CG.

Entrapped fluid is sometimes referred to as mucoceles in the literature, which is a misnomer. Mucoceles develop secondary to obstruction of the drainage of a sinus and are characterized by expansion of sinus cavity and bone erosion. True mucoceles of the PA are very rare; unlike trapped fluid, they require surgical drainage.

## Importance

Because the clinical assessment of PA abnormalities is limited, imaging evaluation of the PA has a central role in diagnosis and radiologists should strive to provide a specific diagnosis rather than a list of differential diagnoses that require different treatments.

## Typical clinical scenario

Fluid entrapment is usually seen on imaging studies performed for headache, tinnitus, vertigo, or hearing loss, and mistaken for CG or cholesteatomas.

## Differential diagnosis

CG is the most common lesion of the PA after fluid entrapment, although it is 10 times less frequent than fluid entrapment. CG is an inflammatory process that develops as a reaction to the presence of blood by-product within the PA cell and shows very characteristic imaging features such as very bright T1 signal (secondary to methemoglobin), variable but often bright T2 signal, expansion of the PA, and erosion of bony septa (Figs. 64.2, 64.3). The bright T1 signal does not suppress with fat-suppression techniques.

Cholesteatomas consist of keratin debris generated by squamous epithelium. The characteristic feature of cholesteatomas is bone erosion and expansion. On MRI, bright DWI signal is specific for cholesteatomas, which exhibit decreased T1, increased T2 signal, and no enhancement with contrast material (Fig. 64.4).

Meningoceles emanating from the Meckel's cave region and extending into the PA pose a significant problem, as the surgical approach to these is different because of CSF leak. These lesions show identical signal to CSF on all pulse sequences and do not enhance; high-resolution images usually reveal a neck between the Meckel's cave and the meningocele (Fig. 64.5).

Petrous apicitis is a severe acute infection of the PA, and because of its proximity to the brain it should be treated as an emergency. The clinical context is different in that these patients are usually acutely ill and have draining ears secondary to accompanying otomastoiditis. CT shows opacification of the PA with erosion of the septa and the cortex but no significant bone expansion.

Chondrosarcoma, plasmocytoma, Langerhans cell histiocytosis, and metastasis of the petrous apex usually present with lytic bone lesions associated with an enhancing soft tissue mass, and should not be confused with CG, cholesteatomas, meningocele, or fluid entrapment (Fig. 64.6).

## Teaching points

Entrapped fluid in the petrous apex air cells is common and should be differentiated from more significant disease processes such as cholesterol granulomas, cholesteatomas, meningoceles, and tumors.

REFERENCES

1. Moore KR, Harnsberger HR, Shelton C, Davidson HC. "Leave me alone" lesions of the petrous apex. *AJNR Am J Neuroradiol* 1998; **19**: 733–8.

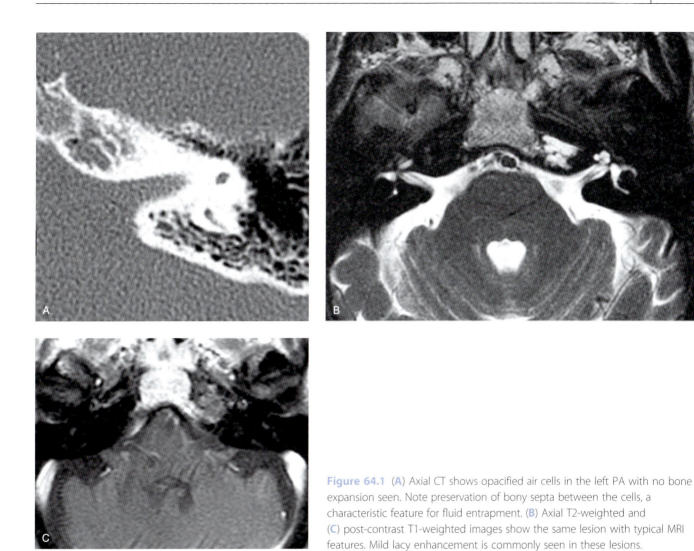

**Figure 64.1** (**A**) Axial CT shows opacified air cells in the left PA with no bone expansion seen. Note preservation of bony septa between the cells, a characteristic feature for fluid entrapment. (**B**) Axial T2-weighted and (**C**) post-contrast T1-weighted images show the same lesion with typical MRI features. Mild lacy enhancement is commonly seen in these lesions.

**Figure 64.2** Cholesterol granuloma. (**A**) Axial T1-weighted, (**B**) T2-weighted, and (**C**) CT images show a slightly expansile lobulated lesion that shows markedly elevated T1 signal and mixed but mostly elevated T2 signal. Scalloped bone margins are noted on CT.

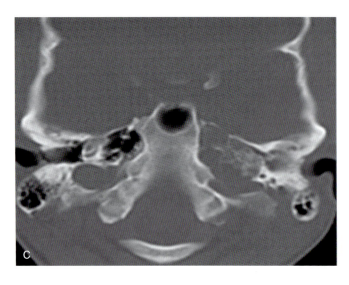

Figure 64.2 (cont.)

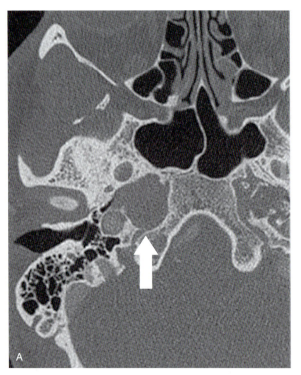

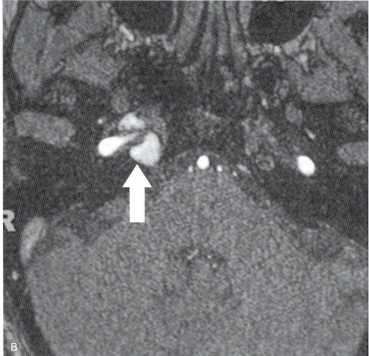

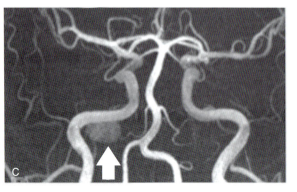

Figure 64.3 Cholesterol granulomas. (A) Axial CT shows a lytic expansile lesion in the right PA (arrow). (B) Axial source and (C) MIP images from MRA show that the CG surrounds the petrous carotid canal and mimics an aneurysm because of its markedly increased T1 signal projection into the MIP images.

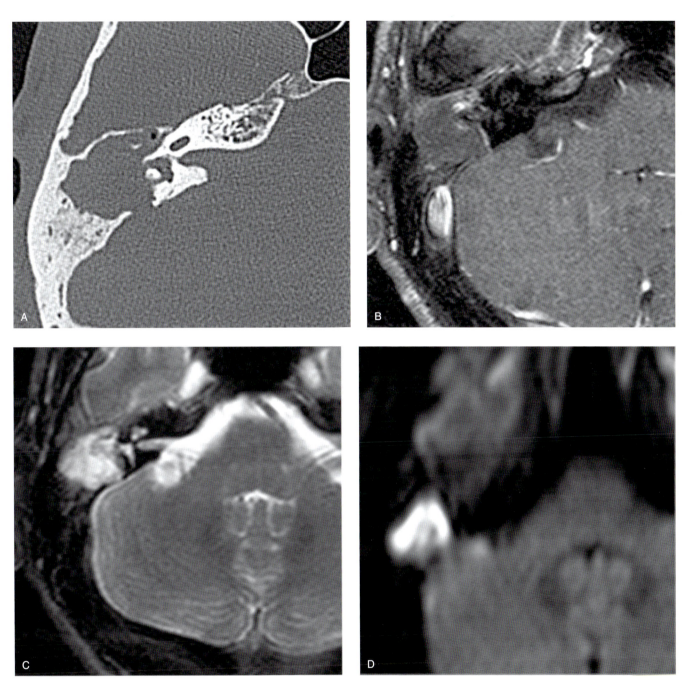

**Figure 64.4** (**A**) Axial CT image shows a lytic expansile lesion in the right middle ear and mastoids that erodes into the lateral semicircular canal. The lesion shows (**B**) decreased T1 signal and no enhancement, (**C**) increased T2 signal, and (**D**) markedly increased DWI signal, compatible with cholesteatoma.

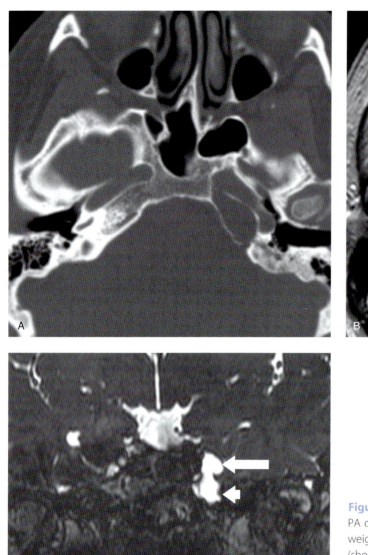

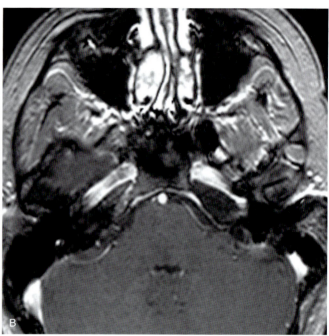

Figure 64.5 (A) A lytic-appearing expansile lesion is seen in the left PA on axial CT. It shows CSF signal on (B) T1-weighted and (C) T2-weighted images without enhancement. Note extension of the lesion (short arrow) into the intracranial compartment (long arrow) next to the Meckel's cave. This was a meningocele.

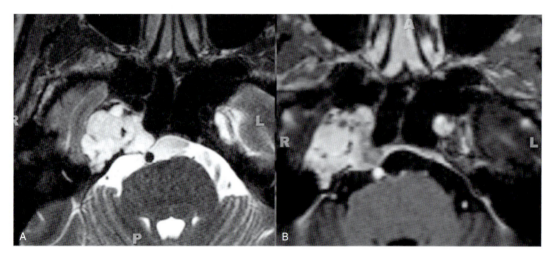

Figure 64.6 (A) Axial T2-weighted and (B) post-contrast T1-weighted images show an expansile mass in the right PA with bright T2 signal and enhancement. This was a chondrosarcoma.

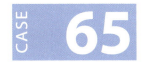
## Imaging description

Cholesteatoma is a unique, mass-like, destructive and expansile soft tissue lesion of the middle ear, which is a sequela of the reparative process of a perforated tympanic membrane. The stratified squamous epithelial tissue, while attempting to heal the perforation, leads to a ball of exfoliated keratin material surrounded by granulation tissue with lytic enzymes [1].

Pars flaccida cholesteatoma is considered primary cholesteatoma. It begins in the posterosuperior portion of the tympanic membrane, which is more susceptible to infections, and is situated superior to the lateral process of malleus. Pars flaccida accounts for about 80% of all acquired cholesteatomas. It is usually seen in Prussak's space, associated with blunting of scutum, and extends medially to the posterior part of epitympanum and mesotympanum (Fig. 65.1).

Pars tensa cholesteatoma accounts for 10–20% of all acquired middle ear cholesteatomas and is considered secondary acquired cholesteatoma. It is generally seen in relation to the lower two-thirds of the tympanic membrane, at the site of perforation or retraction pocket at the pars tensa portion of the tympanic membrane. It is seen as a soft tissue mass in the posterior mesotympanum, situated medial to the ossicles, and may involve the region of sinus tympani, facial nerve recess, and aditus ad antrum (Fig. 65.2). Erosion of auditory ossicles, especially the long process of incus and superstructure of stapes, is common. It is locally aggressive, and erosion of the adjoining bony structures and auditory ossicles is both characteristic and diagnostic [2].

Cholesteatoma involving the epitympanic attic is quite common, also involving the mastoid cavity and petrous temporal bone in varying degrees. There may be invasion of the semicircular canals, most commonly the lateral semicircular canal and cochlea, most likely the basal turn, leading to labyrinthine fistula and a more complicated clinical presentation (Fig. 65.3). If erosion of the facial nerve canal or extension into the sinus tympani is present, it is important that the otologist should be informed.

## Importance

Cholesteatoma is one of the more common radiological diagnoses in clinical practice. Once diagnosed, the treatment involves extensive surgery with mastoidectomy, ossicular reconstruction, and formation of a common cavity between the external auditory canal (EAC) and the mastoid antrum. It is important to include a detailed description of the extent of the lesion and possible ossicular and bony erosion, to help the otologist make the appropriate choice of the type of surgery.

## Typical clinical scenario

The commonest presenting symptom is unilateral conductive hearing loss. It is more common in males and is associated with a history of recurrent or chronic middle ear infections.

Foul-smelling but painless otorrhea with a history of perforation or retraction of the tympanic membrane is very common. Advanced and aggressive cholesteatomas can erode into the semicircular canals or cochlea, resulting in additional symptoms such as vertigo or sensorineural hearing loss.

## Differential diagnosis

Chronic inflammatory disease with possible bony and ossicular erosion is a radiological challenge and sometimes indistinguishable. The bony erosion, however, is more diffuse in the case of inflammatory process. Chronic granulomatous tissue can be more focal, but it does not have the typical location preference (Figs. 65.4, 65.5). Congenital cholesteatoma presents with a small focal mass medial to an intact tympanic membrane, without history of recurrent infections and without evidence for ossicular or bony erosion.

Cholesterol granuloma of the middle ear can exhibit bony involvement, blunting of the scutum, and ossicular erosion. However, there is no history of perforation of tympanic membrane, and it exhibits a typical blue eardrum and has a common clinical presentation of tinnitus. On MRI, high T1 signal is characteristic.

Glomus tympanicum paraganglioma is seen as a focal soft tissue mass overlying the cochlear promontory but without significant bony erosion.

## Teaching points

Temporal bone CT without contrast is the preferred imaging examination in a patient suspected of having cholesteatoma. Coronal plane imaging can optimally visualize involvement of Prussak's space, epitympanic recess, and tympanic antrum. Possible erosion of the tegmen tympani, facial nerve canal, semicircular canals, and cochlea is best evaluated on CT. Post-contrast T1-weighted imaging can help differentiate a non-enhancing cholesteatoma from avidly enhancing inflammatory tissue. Impeded diffusion on diffusion-weighted images can confirm the presence of cholesteatoma [3].

REFERENCES

1. Karmody CS, Northrop C. The pathogenesis of acquired cholesteatoma of the human middle ear: support for the migration hypothesis. *Otol Neurotol* 2012; **33**: 42–7.
2. Lemmerling MM, De Foer B, Verbist BM, VandeVyver V. Imaging of inflammatory and infectious diseases in the temporal bone. *Neuroimaging Clin N Am* 2009; **19**: 321–37.
3. Yamashita K, Yoshiura T, Hiwatashi A, *et al*. Detection of middle ear cholesteatoma by diffusion-weighted MR imaging: multishot echo-planar imaging compared with single-shot echo-planar imaging. *AJNR Am J Neuroradiol* 2011; **32**: 1915–18.

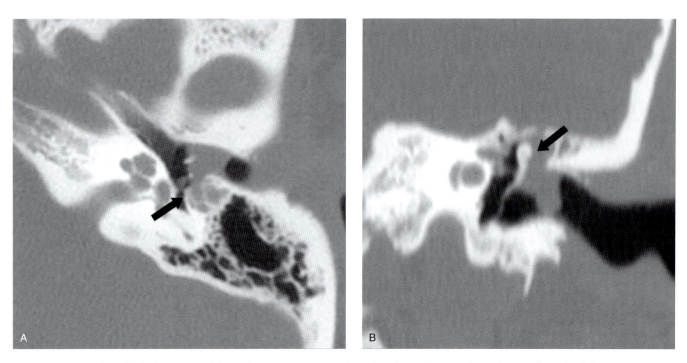

**Figure 65.1** Pars flaccida cholesteatoma. (**A**) A soft tissue mass is seen lateral to the malleus involving the pars flaccida of the tympanic membrane, extending into the epitympanum and also the mastoid antrum with bony erosion (arrow). (**B**) The malleus is displaced medially (arrow) with the mass extending into the external auditory canal.

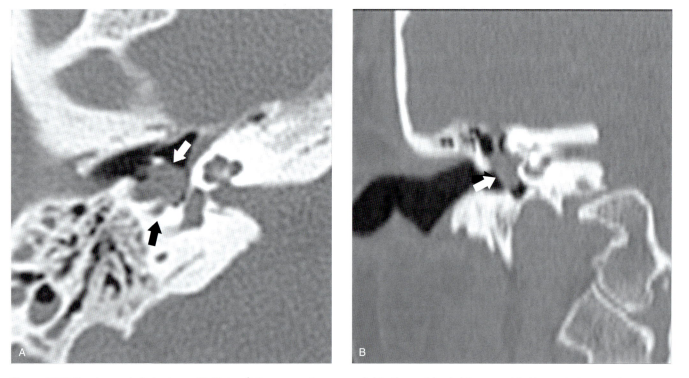

**Figure 65.2** Pars tensa cholesteatoma. (**A, B**) A soft tissue mass is seen medial to the ossicles (white arrows) in the posterior mesotympanum, involving the sinus tympani (black arrow) and facial nerve recess with erosion of the long process of the incus. (**C, D**) Areas of restricted diffusion (short arrow) with decreased apparent diffusion coefficient (arrow) are visualized within the mass-like lesion.

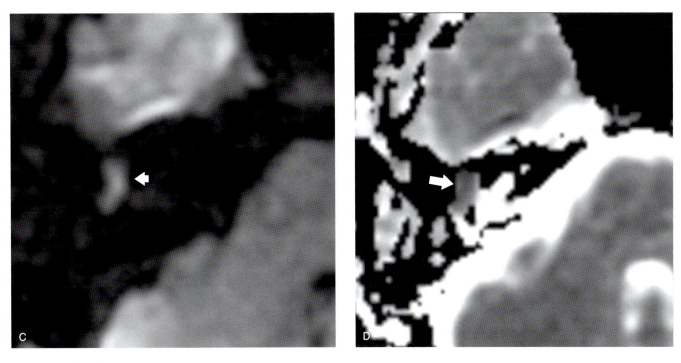

**Figure 65.2** (cont.)

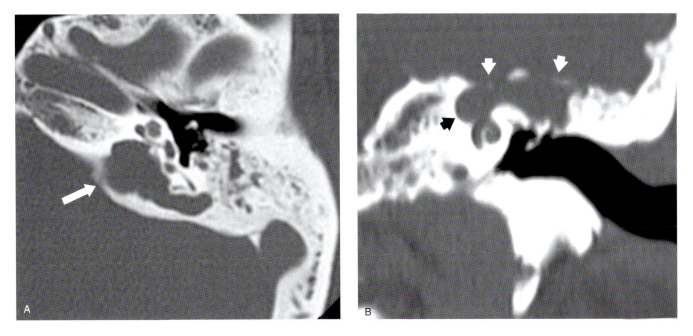

**Figure 65.3** Attic cholesteatoma. (**A, B**) A large soft tissue mass involving the epitympanic recess and tympanic antrum (short arrows) erodes the basal turn of the cochlea, creating a labyrinthine fistula. (**C, D**) The mass exhibits iso to low T1 and T2 signal with retained secretions of mastoid air cells exhibiting high T2 signal. (**E**) On fat-saturated T1-weighted post-contrast axial imaging, the cholesteatoma does not enhance. However, there is peripheral rim enhancement along the margin of the cavity (arrow), where there is likely persistence of granulation tissue. (**F**) Hyperintense restricted diffusion (arrow) is visualized on diffusion-weighted images.

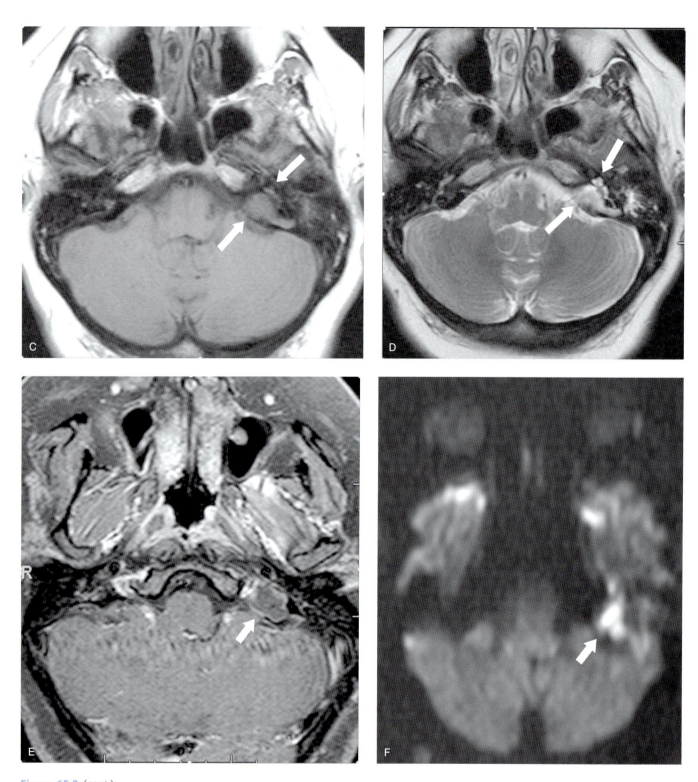

**Figure 65.3** (cont.)

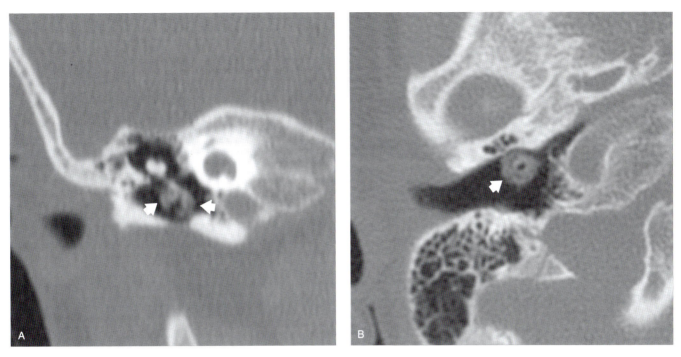

**Figure 65.4** Chronic granulation of middle ear. (**A, B**) Irregular soft tissue visualized around the myringotomy tube (short arrows) within a centrally perforated tympanic membrane. The non-dependent mass-like soft tissue is not seen within Prussak's space and is not medial to the ossicles. There is lack of ossicular erosion or bony involvement.

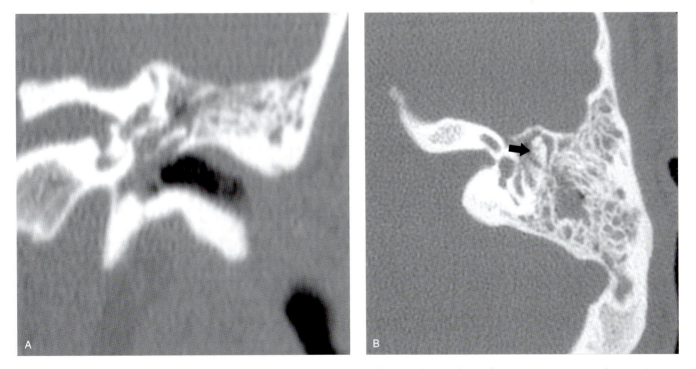

**Figure 65.5** Chronic otomastoiditis with otitis media. (**A, B**) Extensive opacification of mastoid air cells, tympanic antrum, and tympanic cavity is seen with mild erosion of the short process of the incus (arrow). However, there is no blunting of the scutum, erosion of the long process of the incus, or aggressive mass-like behavior within the mastoid antrum.

## Imaging description

Malignant otitis externa (MOE) is an uncommon infection of the external auditory canal (EAC) that has a propensity to spread outside the temporal bone. MOE is seen in elderly diabetic patients, and *Pseudomonas aeruginosa* is the most common organism responsible. Infection from the EAC spreads through the small perforations along the floor of the cartilaginous portion of the EAC and extends medially to the skull base including the jugular canal and stylomastoid foramen, nasopharynx, parapharyngeal space, parotid space, and infratemporal fossa. More medial and superior extension results in involvement of the petrous apex, dural sinuses, meninges, and brain [1]. Involvement of the stylomastoid foramen leads to facial nerve paralysis, and this is the most commonly involved cranial nerve in MOE. Involvement of the jugular foramen causes deficits of cranial nerves IX, X, and XI, and petrous apex involvement may result in trigeminal and abducens nerve palsies.

The diagnosis of MOE is difficult and requires the presence of clinical, radiologic, and microbiologic findings. Demonstration of bone involvement in the mastoid and soft tissue involvement outside the EAC is diagnostic of MOE in the appropriate clinical setting (Figs. 66.1, 66.2). CT is usually the first imaging study obtained, and it is very accurate in demonstrating bone erosion, which is present in about 70% of cases [2]. Often, cortical bone erosion is very subtle and requires careful scrutiny of all cortical margins of the mastoid bone. Tc-99m MDP bone scan is much more sensitive than CT and is positive in essentially all cases of MOE, although its specificity is quite poor. Soft tissue involvement outside the EAC can be seen on CT, although findings are often subtle. MRI is much more accurate in the assessment of the extent of disease because of its superior contrast resolution and multiplanar capability (Fig. 66.1).

Evaluation of response to treatment with imaging is problematic. MRI and CT continue to be abnormal even after successful treatment. Ga-67 citrate scintigraphy may be useful, as it becomes negative after treatment.

## Importance

EOM is a potentially fatal disease. Imaging findings may be subtle, particularly in the early stages. Establishing the diagnosis early improves outcomes.

## Typical clinical scenario

Great majority of patients have diabetes and present with severe otalgia, aural fullness, otorrhea, and conductive hearing loss. Immunocompromised patients are at risk for developing MOE.

## Differential diagnosis

Carcinoma of the ear canal may have similar clinical and radiologic findings, and biopsy is necessary to rule out neoplastic processes.

### Teaching points

In elderly patients with external otitis subtle CT findings of loss of cortical integrity of the mastoid bone may help in establishing the diagnosis of MEO. MRI is necessary for the assessment of full extent of the disease.

REFERENCES

1. Carfrae MJ, Kesser BW. Malignant otitis externa. *Otolaryngol Clin North Am* 2008; **41**: 537–49, viii–ix.
2. Sudhoff H, Rajagopal S, Mani N, *et al.* Usefulness of CT scans in malignant external otitis: effective tool for the diagnosis, but of limited value in predicting outcome. *Eur Arch Otorhinolaryngol* 2008; **265**: 53–6.

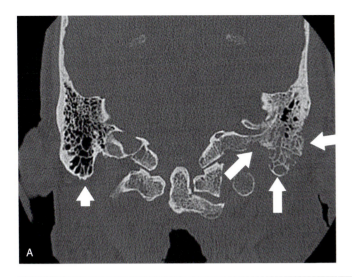

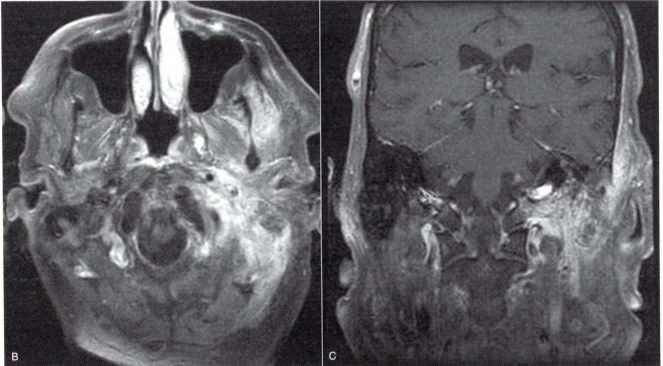

Figure 66.1 (A) Coronal CT shows some mastoid opacification in this patient with ear pain and external otitis. Note erosion of the cortex around the mastoid (arrows) and compare it to the normal side (short arrow), which is a clue that the process extended beyond the temporal bone. (B) Axial and (C) coronal post-contrast T1-weighted MR images reveal the true extent of disease, which involved the skull base and infratemporal fossa and surrounded the carotid artery.

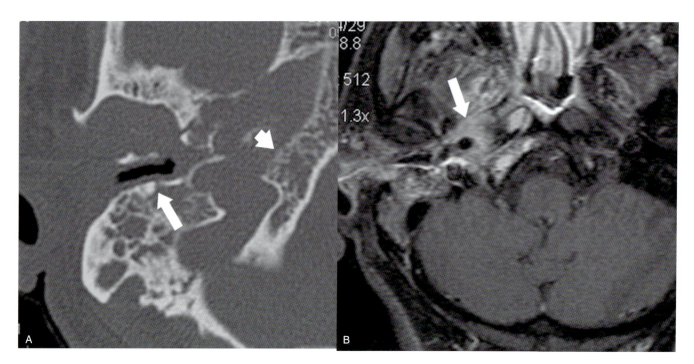

**Figure 66.2** (**A**) Axial CT shows some soft tissue thickening in the EAC and mastoid opacification. Subtle bone erosion is present in the posterior wall of the EAC (arrow) and the lateral portion of the clivus (short arrow). (**B**) On post-contrast axial T1-weighted MR imaging there is abnormal soft tissue enhancement surrounding the carotid canal (arrow) and in the clivus.

# Temporal bone fractures

## Imaging description

Patients with temporal bone fractures usually have severe intracranial injuries as well, and temporal bone fractures may be difficult to diagnose on head CT due to insufficient resolution provided. Free air in the posterior fossa, middle cranial fossa adjacent to the mastoid, infratemporal fossa, and temporomandibular joint should prompt a search for temporal bone fracture.

The temporal bone region is anatomically complex, containing many important and vital vascular, nervous, and sensorineural structures including internal carotid artery, middle meningeal artery, sigmoid sinus, jugular bulb, cranial nerves V, VI, VII, and VIII, and the otic capsule containing sensitive sensorineural organelles and the membranous inner ear [1].

The traditional classification of temporal bone fractures indicates the relationship of the fracture line with the long axis of the petrous portion of the temporal bone. A newer classification describes temporal bone fractures on the basis of whether the otic capsule is involved or spared [2]. Otic-capsule-violating fractures involve the labyrinth, causing injury to the cochlea, vestibule, or semicircular canals, and are more commonly associated with complications such as sensorineural hearing loss, CSF otorrhea, and facial nerve injury. Otic-capsule-sparing fractures are more commonly associated with intracranial injuries such as epidural hematoma and subarachnoid hemorrhage. However, this classification was not considered significantly better than the traditional system in predicting the likelihood of sustaining specific injuries from fracture of the temporal bone [3].

## Importance

It is important to identify temporal bone injuries, as they can cause devastating complications such as sensorineural hearing loss, conductive hearing loss, balance disturbance, perilymphatic fistula, CSF leak, vascular injury, or facial nerve paralysis which may escape clinical detection because of distracting injuries in polytrauma patients. Many temporal bone fractures are identified at routine cervical, maxillofacial, or head CT scans by radiologists and brought to the attention of referring physicians. A high index of suspicion is required for timely diagnosis of temporal bone fractures on initial imaging studies. High-resolution temporal bone CT is required for comprehensive assessment of these injuries.

## Typical clinical scenario

It requires a high-energy blunt head trauma to cause a temporal bone fracture. Motor vehicle accidents, sports injuries, home and work accidents, assault, gunshot wounds, and falls are common causes [2]. About 18% of patients with skull fracture have temporal bone fractures. Swelling and ecchymosis around the external ear present as a classic "Battle sign." Hemotympanum and hemorrhage of external auditory canal is commonly seen. A high-energy trauma may also cause damage to other intracranial structures, and CT scan is positive in up to 85% of the patients for other intracranial findings such as extra-axial or parenchymal hemorrhages. Depending on injuries to the vital structures contained within it, the symptoms may include vertigo, conductive hearing loss, facial nerve paralysis, sensorineural hearing loss, and CSF leak, which may be masked by other injuries sustained by the patient.

## Differential diagnosis

Longitudinal fractures account for 70–90% of temporal bone fractures and occur secondary to lateral impact causing a fracture line running parallel to the petrous ridge. They are often associated with fractures of squamous temporal bone and parietal bone, involving the external auditory canal, tympanic membrane, and middle ear cavity, but they usually spare the otic capsule. Involvement of auditory ossicles, however, is common. The injury occurs in a two-step process. A crush injury to the temporal bone is followed by massive fissuration of the petrous bone [4]. The facial nerve canal is more often involved at the tympanic segment or in the region of the geniculate ganglion. On temporal bone CT, a fracture line parallel to the long axis of the petrous temporal bone is seen (Fig. 67.1). The commonest complications of longitudinal fracture are ossicular injury, tympanic membrane rupture, hemotympanum, and conductive hearing loss.

Transverse fractures are secondary to occipital or frontal impact and account for 10–30% of temporal bone fractures. They typically result from trauma to the occipital, frontal, or craniocervical region with the line of force extending from anterior to posterior [1]. The fracture line is perpendicular to the long axis of the petrous temporal bone (Fig. 67.2). A lateral subtype extends from the posterior petrous surface to the otic capsule, while a medial subtype extends from the posterior petrous surface through IAC to the region of the geniculate ganglion of the facial nerve canal. It more commonly involves the otic capsule, with injury to the labyrinthine structures, cochlear nerve, or the footplate of stapes. The fracture line generally originates in the vicinity of the jugular foramen or foramen magnum. Common complications include sensorineural hearing loss, perilymphatic fistula, and facial nerve paralysis [5]. When the fracture line involves the carotid canal the likelihood of carotid artery injury increases, although lack of involvement does not exclude this possibility.

Mixed fracture in polytrauma includes both the longitudinal and transverse components (Fig. 67.3), often causing injury to both otic capsule and auditory ossicles.

## Teaching points

Free air in the infratemporal fossa, temporomandibular joint, and posterior fossa seen on head CT should be regarded with suspicion for temporal bone fracture. Dedicated temporal bone multidetector CT should be performed if there is a high degree of suspicion for temporal bone fractures. Systematic assessment of the clinically most important structures, including middle ear ossicles, facial nerve canal, otic capsule, tegmen, and carotid canal must be performed and mentioned in the report. It is also important to look for intracranial injuries.

REFERENCES

1. Zayas JO, Feliciano YZ, Hadley CR, et al. Temporal bone trauma and the role of multidetector CT in the emergency department. Radiographics 2011; 31: 1741–55.

2. Little SC, Kesser BW. Radiographic classification of temporal bone fractures clinical predictability using a new system. Arch Otolaryngol Head Neck Surg 2006; 132: 1300–4.

3. Rafferty MA, Mc Conn Walsh R, Walsh MA. A comparison of temporal bone fracture classification systems. Clin Otolaryngol 2006; 31: 287–91.

4. Montava M, Deveze A, Arnoux PJ, et al. Petrous bone fracture: a virtual trauma analysis. Otol Neurotol 2012; 33: 651–4.

5. Ulug T, Arif Ulubil S. Management of facial paralysis in temporal bone fractures: a prospective study analyzing 11 operated fractures. Am J Otolaryngol 2005; 26: 230–8.

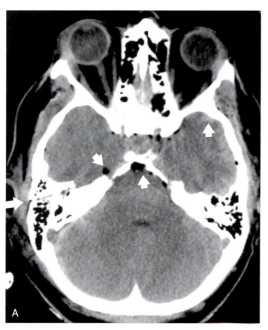

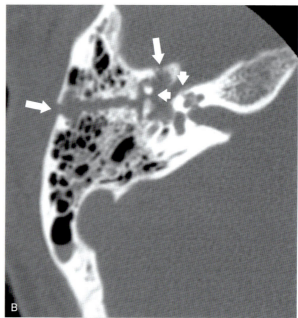

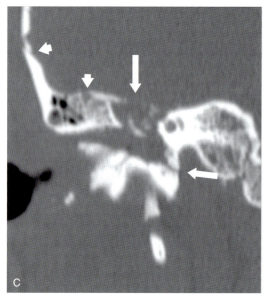

**Figure 67.1** Longitudinal fracture of temporal bone. (**A**) Non-contrast head CT reveals a fracture line parallel to the long axis of the right petrous temporal bone (arrow). Numerous foci of pneumocephalus are seen (short arrow). Left temporal hemorrhagic contusion is identified (short arrow). (**B**) Multidetector temporal bone axial CT reveals a fracture line parallel to the long axis of the petrous temporal bone (arrow), involving the middle ear cavity and resulting in incudomalleolar separation (short arrow). There is also mild dehiscence of the geniculate facial nerve canal (short arrow). (**C**) Coronal reconstruction CT of temporal bone reveals fracture of tegmen tympani (long arrow) and medial wall of hypotympanum (arrow). There are fractures of the lateral floor of the middle cranial fossa (short arrow) and the parietal bone (short arrow).

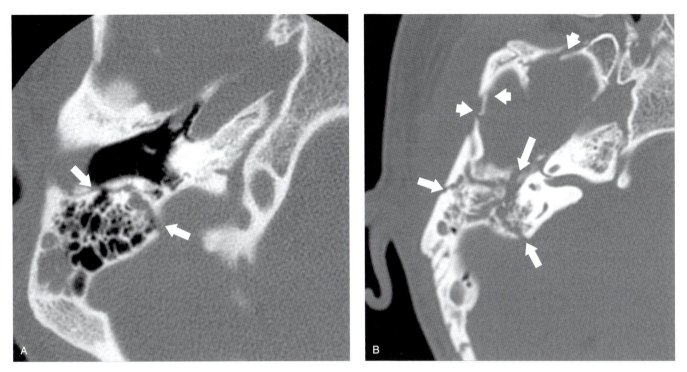

**Figure 67.2** Transverse fracture of temporal bone. (**A**) Multidetector temporal bone axial CT reveals a fracture line perpendicular to the long axis of the petrous temporal bone originating from the jugular fossa (arrows). (**B**) Axial CT at a higher level reveals posterior subtype of the transverse fracture across the otic capsule (arrows) involving the facial nerve canal (long arrow). Comminuted fracture of squamous temporal bone is also seen (short arrows).

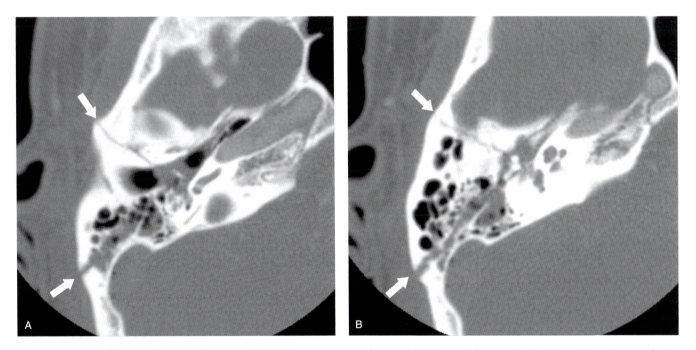

**Figure 67.3** Mixed fracture of temporal bone. (**A, B**) Multidetector temporal bone axial CT reveals fracture lines both parallel and perpendicular to the long axis of petrous temporal bone (arrows) involving the external auditory canal and middle ear cavity.

# 68 Allergic fungal sinusitis

## Imaging description

The spectrum of chronic sinusitis is wide and includes diverse etiologies such as pyogenic, allergic, and fungal. In patients with a known history of allergies and with sinonasal polyposis, the body's immune system responds to the presence of fungal elements within the paranasal sinus infection, leading to over-production of eosinophilic mucin [1]. This is generally seen in immunocompetent, non-diabetic, and otherwise healthy populations. It is most commonly seen in young male adults in warm and humid climates.

On CT, there is opacification and expansion of multiple paranasal sinuses containing a centrally high-attenuating dense material (Fig. 68.1). On MRI, a central variable T1 and low T2 signal representing eosinophilic mucous is surrounded by low T1 and high T2 signal of the thickened mucosa (Fig. 68.2) [2,3]. The signal may be so low on T2-weighted images that it can mimic air (Fig. 68.2B).

## Importance

The clinical spectrum of chronic rhinosinusitis represents diverse etiologies. Making the correct diagnosis of allergic fungal sinusitis allows for more accurate treatment options for this condition, including surgical resection and debridement.

## Typical clinical scenario

The presence of chronic rhinosinusitis with nasal discharge and congestion, headaches, fever, and facial pain and pressure is common. The maxillary sinus is the most commonly involved sinus. The pain may be infraorbital or periauricular. Involvement of frontal sinus results in headache of forehead and supraorbital region. A history of allergies and underlying nasal polyp is common in these patients. In severe cases with bony remodeling and orbital complications, facial deformity, proptosis, and diplopia can be seen.

## Differential diagnosis

The clinical spectrum of rhinosinusitis includes acute sinusitis, chronic purulent sinusitis, aspergilloma, and invasive fungal sinusitis. Acute sinusitis shows areas of sinus opacification with fluid levels. In cases of large pus collection, restricted diffusion may be seen. In chronic sinusitis, soft tissue opacification with thickening and sclerosis of sinus walls is seen. Acute invasive fungal sinusitis is seen in an immuno-compromised patient with bone destruction and soft tissue invasion of deep face, orbit, and skull base. Chronic invasive fungal sinusitis is common in patients with diabetes and is associated with adjoining soft tissue invasion.

Radiologically, benign paranasal sinus masses such as inverted papilloma, sinonasal polyposis, mucoceles, and ossifying fibroma should be ruled out. Mucocele tends to have low attenuation density on CT with high T2 signal on MRI (Fig. 68.3). An expansile mass with osseous periphery and soft tissue fibrous center is seen in ossifying fibroma (Fig. 68.4). Inverted papilloma arises in the middle meatus with secondary involvement of maxillary sinus, is usually non-calcified, and results in bony remodeling (Fig. 68.5). Sinonasal polyposis may be bilateral or unilateral, display low attenuation density on CT, and extend from the maxillary antrum into the nasal cavity (Fig. 68.6). In allergic fungal sinusitis, central high-density material is surrounded by a low-attenuating rim of thickened mucosa. Extremely low T2 signal, which looks like air, surrounded by high T2 signal thickened mucosa, is characteristic on T2-weighted MRI. Invasion of the retroantral fat, maxillary ridge, and adjoining orbital structures can also be seen and may mimic more aggressive disease processes.

## Teaching points

Expansile sinonasal mass with high-density center surrounded by low-density rim on CT, and low T2 signal center surrounded by high T2 signal rim on MRI, is the characteristic imaging appearance of allergic fungal sinusitis. There may be bone expansion and invasion. It is usually seen in patients with atopy.

REFERENCES

1. Hutcheson PS, Schubert MS, Slavin RG. Distinctions between allergic fungal rhinosinusitis and chronic rhinosinusitis. *Am J Rhinol Allergy* 2010; **24**: 405–8.
2. Aribandi M, McCoy VA, Bazan C. Imaging features of invasive and noninvasive fungal sinusitis: a review. *Radiographics* 2007; **27**: 1283–96.
3. Zinreich SJ, Kennedy DW, Malat J, *et al.* Fungal sinusitis: diagnosis with CT and MR imaging. *Radiology* 1988; **169**: 439–44.

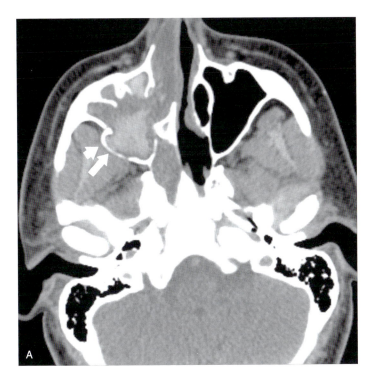 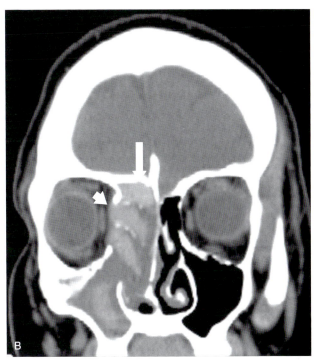

**Figure 68.1** Non-contrast CT scan of maxillofacial region. (**A**) Axial CT shows complete opacification of right maxillary sinus and right nasal passage with central high-density structure surrounded by low-attenuating rim (arrow). There is remodeling of the posterior wall of the right maxillary sinus, extending into the retroantral pad of fat (short arrow). (**B**) Coronal CT shows lobulated areas of high attenuation (arrow) within low-attenuating opacification of maxillary and ethmoidal sinuses extending into the right nasal passage. There is erosion of right lamina papyracea with extension of the mass into the medial orbital cavity (short arrow).

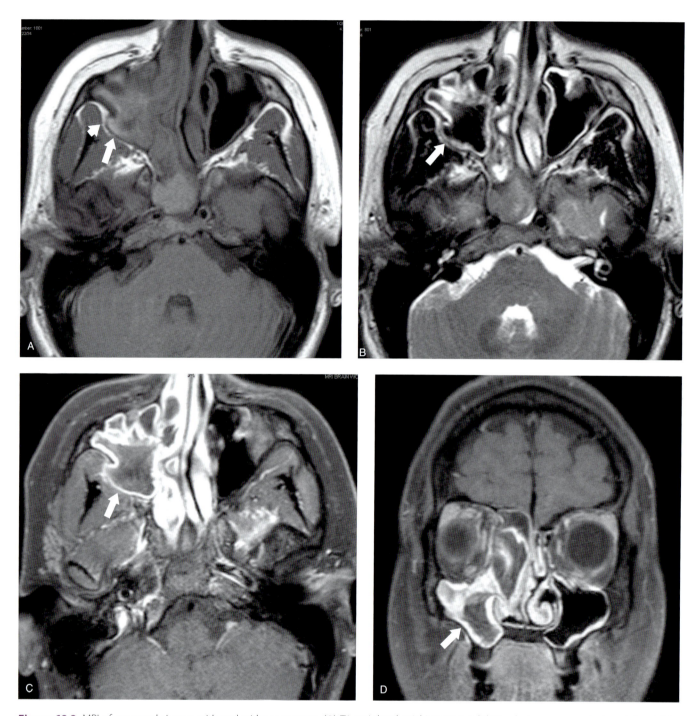

**Figure 68.2** MRI of paranasal sinuses with and without contrast. (**A**) T1-weighted axial imaging exhibits a heterogeneous lesion at the right maxillary sinus (arrow) with expansile posterior wall extending into retromaxillary pad of fat (short arrow). The cortical margins are intact. The fungal mass displays high T1 signal. (**B**) T2-weighted axial imaging exhibits a markedly low T2 signal mass surrounded by high T2 signal mucosal thickening. The signal intensities of right maxillary fungal infection (arrow) and left maxillary air appear almost similar.
(**C**, **D**) Fat-saturated post-contrast T1-weighted axial and coronal imaging reveals intense enhancement of the thickened mucosa (arrow).

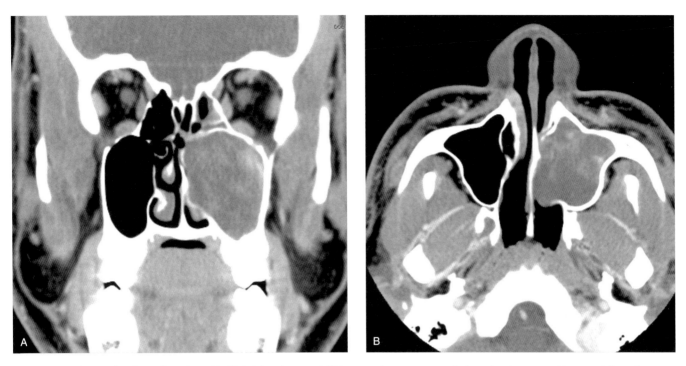

**Figure 68.3** Mucocele of maxillary sinus. (**A**, **B**) Axial and coronal CT images show an expansile low-density mass with remodeling of maxillary sinus.

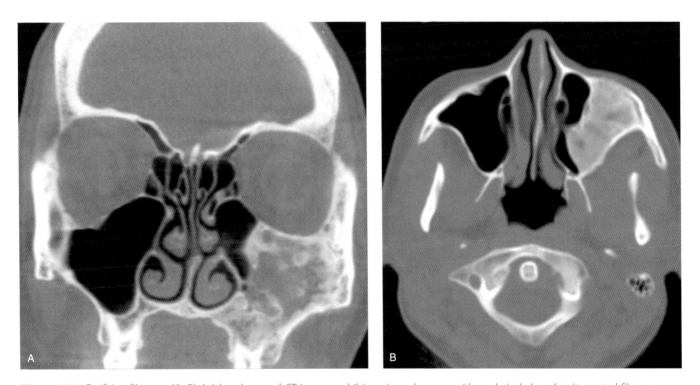

**Figure 68.4** Ossifying fibroma. (**A**, **B**) Axial and coronal CT images exhibit an irregular mass with a relatively low-density central fibrous component surrounded by a calcific rim.

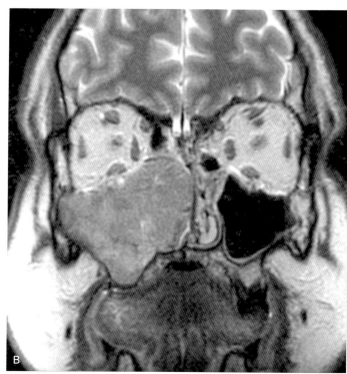

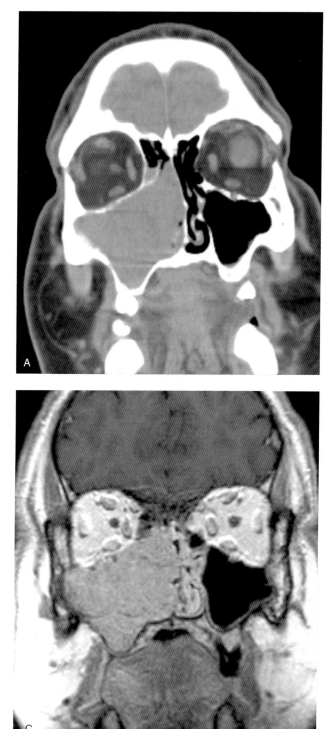

**Figure 68.5** Inverted papilloma. (**A**) Soft tissue attenuation density mass exhibits (**B**) low T2 signal and (**C**) heterogencous post-contrast enhancement on MRI.

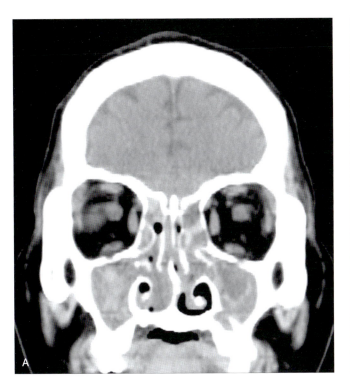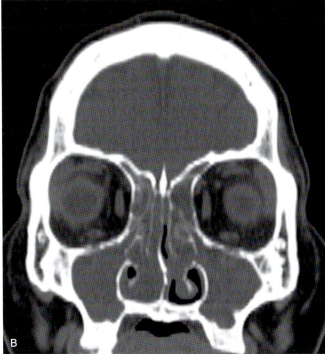

**Figure 68.6** Sinonasal polyposis. (**A**, **B**) Non-neoplastic swelling of sinonasal mucosa is a chronic inflammatory condition, often with allergic etiology. Soft tissue density with polypoid outline contains areas of high attenuation that likely represents inspissated mucus. Also note marked thickening of the sinus walls.

## Imaging description

Invasive fungal sinusitis occurs predominantly in immuno-compromised patients or patients who are on chronic steroid therapy or have diabetes. The most dreaded acute invasive form is seen in severely immunocompromised patients, while the chronic form is more common in diabetics.

In acute invasive fungal sinusitis, there is rapid invasion of mucosa, submucosa, and blood vessels with neutrophilic infiltrates. On CT, there is complete or partial soft tissue opacification of the paranasal sinus with mucosal thickening. Areas of bone erosion are common, with infiltration of adjacent fat and soft tissues (Fig. 69.1), but can be subtle. Intraorbital and intracranial extension takes place along the perivascular or perineural spread [1] or through direct bony invasion (Fig. 69.2). On MRI, the sinus secretions exhibit low T1 and high T2 signal [2]; however, high T1 signal may suggest proteinaceous content or fungal aggregation [3]. Fungal elements may also cause low T2 signal, which can look analogous to air within the sinuses (Fig. 69.3). When the sphenoid sinus is involved, there is a high incidence of cavernous sinus thrombosis and obliteration of the internal carotid artery (Fig. 69.2). Intracranial extension through cribriform plate and orbital invasion is common when ethmoidal sinuses are involved. Involvement of the maxillary sinus results in encroachment of retroantral fat or premaxillary soft tissue. Mucormycosis is more commonly associated with acute invasive fungal sinusitis, while in more than 50% of cases with chronic invasive fungal sinusitis *Aspergillus fumigatus* is the culprit.

## Importance

Acute invasive fungal sinusitis is associated with a very high, up to 80%, mortality without appropriate medical and surgical treatment. Rapid orbital involvement, cavernous sinus thrombosis, carotid occlusion, and cerebral infarction and hemorrhage are some of the morbid complications. Radical surgical resection and debridement with systemic antifungal therapy is the treatment of choice.

## Typical clinical scenario

Rapidly progressive fever, congestion, nasal discharge with headaches and orbital pain in an immunocompromised patient is the most common clinical presentation for acute invasive fungal sinusitis. Chronic invasive fungal sinusitis is more common in patients with diabetes, chronic steroid therapy, or AIDS and develops over a period of months to years. Chronic sinus pain, nasal discharge, fever, and epistaxis are more common presenting symptoms.

## Differential diagnosis

In general, acute invasive fugal sinusitis mimics infiltrative infectious and inflammatory conditions, whereas chronic invasive fungal sinusitis should be differentiated from sinonasal neoplasms. Sinonasal squamous cell carcinoma is typically seen in immunocompetent patients and exhibits an aggressive antral soft tissue mass with secondary bone destruction of sinus walls and extension into multiple adjacent neck and orbital compartments (Fig. 69.4). Wegener's granulomatosis (Fig. 69.5) is a destructive process centered on the nasal cavity that can result in extensive bony erosion, but the amount of abnormal soft tissue is much less. It usually involves the nasal septum and turbinates and rarely involves the sphenoidal sinus. Acute inflammation of sinonasal mucus is more common within the maxillary and ethmoidal sinuses, with presence of air-fluid levels containing bubbly or frothy secretions (Fig. 69.6). There may be mucosal thickening or opacification of sinuses, but no associated perisinus soft tissue infiltration or bone erosion should be present.

Aggressive sinonasal masses such as non-Hodgkin's lymphoma or melanoma are predominantly solid lobulated masses. Melanotic melanoma displays low T2 signal and mildly high T1 signal due to the presence of melanin, free radicals, metal ions, and hemorrhage (Fig. 69.7). Inflammation of sinuses and nasal cavity for more than 12 consecutive weeks is considered as chronic rhinosinusitis. There is thickening of mucosal lining with or without soft tissue opacification due to chronic inflammation (Fig. 69.7). The retained secretions can exhibit high T1 and low T2 signal due to chronic inspissation and increased protein content (Fig. 69.7). Aggressive pyogenic sinusitis can result in subperiosteal and postseptal abscess, cavernous sinus thrombosis, or meningitis. However, the patients are generally immunocompetent. Air-fluid levels are common, with areas of mucosal thickening, and bony erosion is less common.

### Teaching points

High index of suspicion is essential for the diagnosis of invasive fungal sinusitis. Non-specific changes of sinusitis in immunocompromised patients with subtle bone erosion or infiltration of perisinus soft tissue is an important diagnostic clue which can be easily missed if specific attention is not directed to these findings. Even subtle periorbital or leptomeningeal enhancement indicates extension of disease outside the paranasal sinus and requires prompt and aggressive intervention. Specific attention should be directed to the cavernous sinus and internal carotid artery in cases where the sphenoid sinus is involved.

REFERENCES

1. Chan L, Singh S, Jones D, Diaz EM, Ginsberg LE. Imaging of mucormycosis skull base osteomyelitis. *AJNR Am J Neuroradiol* 2000 **21**: 828–31.

2. Aribandi M, McCoy VA, Bazan C. Imaging features of invasive and noninvasive fungal sinusitis: a review. *Radiographics* 2007; **27**: 1283–96.

3. Groppo ER, El-Sayed IH, Aiken AH, Glastonbury CM. Computed tomography and magnetic resonance imaging characteristics of acute invasive fungal sinusitis. *Arch Otolaryngol Head Neck Surg* 2011; **137**: 1005–10.

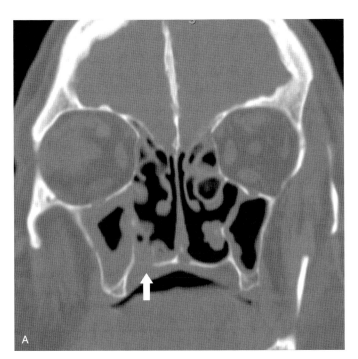

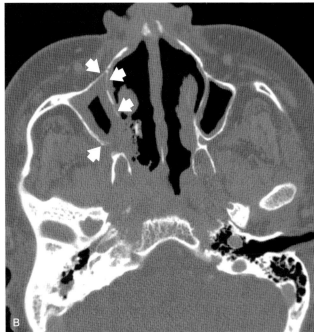

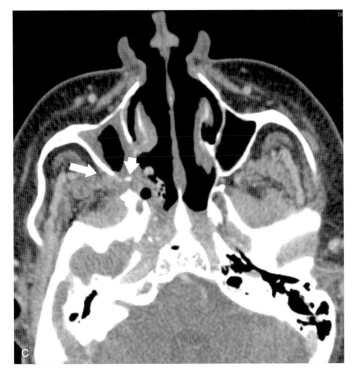

**Figure 69.1** Acute invasive fungal sinusitis. (**A**, **B**) Nodular soft tissue mass centered in the nasal cavity with demineralization of nasal septum and erosion of the hard palate on the right (arrow). Punctate foci of bone demineralization and erosion are seen along the anterior and medial wall of the right maxillary sinus (short arrows). There is permeative destruction of the medial and posterior lateral wall of the maxillary sinus (short arrows). (**C**) Soft tissue window exhibits destruction of posterior wall of right maxillary sinus (short arrow), with the soft tissue extending into right pterygopalatine fossa (arrow).

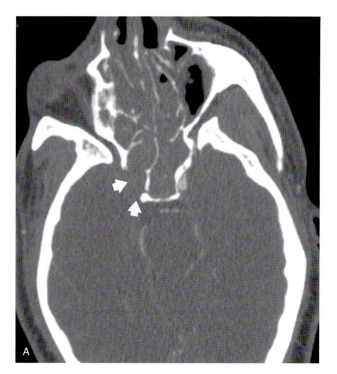

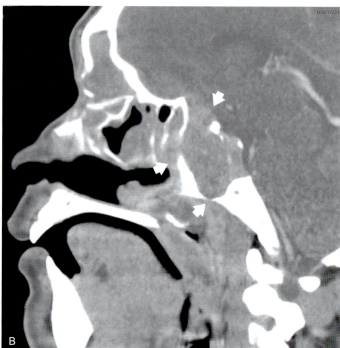

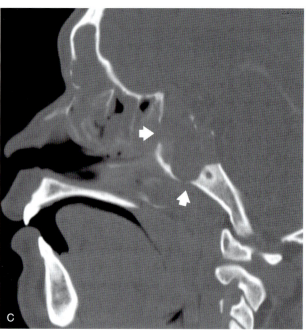

**Figure 69.2** Chronic invasive fungal sinusitis: CT imaging. (**A**) Axial CT images displays an irregular sinonasal soft tissue mass with intracranial extension along bony erosion of the right lateral wall of the sphenoid sinus (short arrow), with invasion of cavernous sinus and obliteration of right internal carotid artery (short arrow). (**B**) Sagittal reconstruction shows patchily enhancing aggressive sphenoid sinus mass resulting in bony destruction of clivus (short arrow) and sella turcica (short arrow) with intracranial extension (short arrow). Soft tissue mass is also seen in the frontal sinus. (**C**) Bone window of sagittal reconstruction exhibits extensive bony erosion (short arrows).

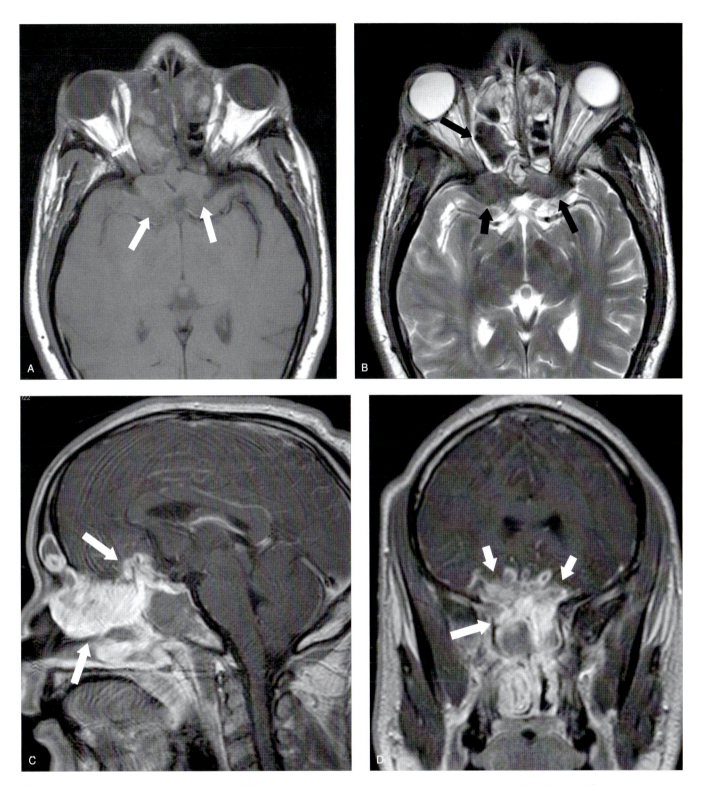

**Figure 69.3** Chronic invasive fungal sinusitis: MR imaging. (**A**) T1-weighted axial imaging exhibits a mildly high T1 signal fungal masses within right posterior and left anterior ethmoidal air cells (arrow). The intracranial extension of fungal granuloma exhibits iso to mildly high T1 signal (arrow). (**B**) T2-weighted axial imaging exhibits a low T2 signal intracranial extension of the sinonasal mass (arrow). Low T2 signal fungal mass at posterior right ethmoidal (arrow) and anterior left ethmoidal air cells exhibit signal intensity similar to air within the posterior left ethmoidal air cells. There is remodeling of right lamina papyracea with extension of invasive sinusitis into the medial right orbit (arrow). (**C**) Post-contrast T1-weighted sagittal image shows an enhancing mass at ethmoid sinus and anterior skull base (arrow) with intracranial extension (arrow). Erosion and invasion of sphenoid sinus and clivus is seen. (**D**) Post-contrast T1-weighted coronal image shows enhancing intracranial extension of aggressive sinonasal mass (arrows) with mild leptomeningeal enhancement.

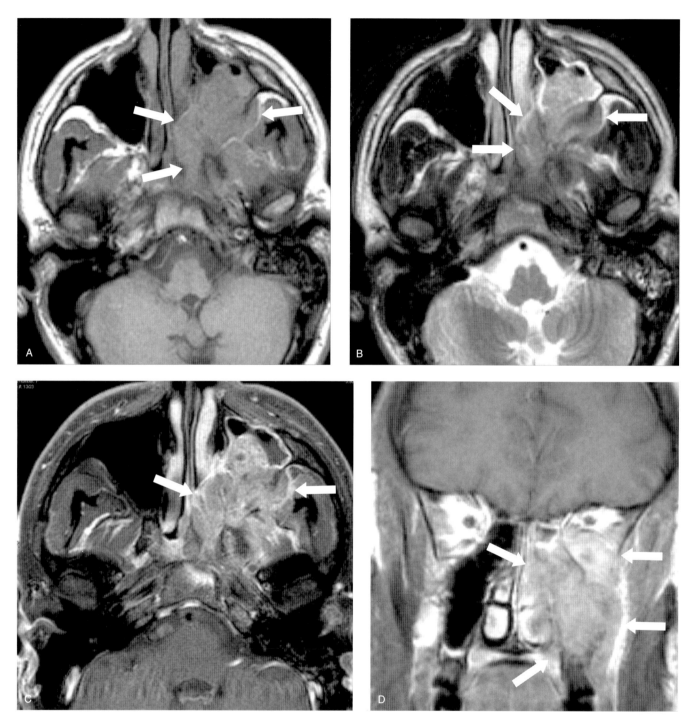

**Figure 69.4** Sinonasal squamous cell carcinoma. (**A**) T1-weighted axial image exhibits mildly high T1 signal left maxillary sinus mass extending to the left side of the nasal cavity (arrow), also involving the nasopharynx (arrow), the retroantral pad of fat (arrow), the pterygopalatine fossa, and the masticator space. (**B**) T2-weighted axial imaging exhibits heterogeneously low T2 signal of the sinonasal mass in extending into nasopharynx, pterygopalatine fossa, pterygomaxillary fissure, and masticator space. (**C**) Post-contrast fat-saturated T1-weighted axial image exhibits patchy moderate enhancement of the solid sinonasal mass extending into the nasopharynx and adjoining neck spaces. Intense enhancement of mildly thickened left maxillary sinus mucosa is seen. Note enhancement within the left side of the clivus and the right side of the nasopharynx. (**D**) Post-contrast T1-weighted coronal image exhibits a moderately enhancing left sinonasal mass infiltrating into the inferior part of the left orbit (arrow), laterally extending into the masticator space (arrow) with infiltration of the left side of the hard palate (arrow).

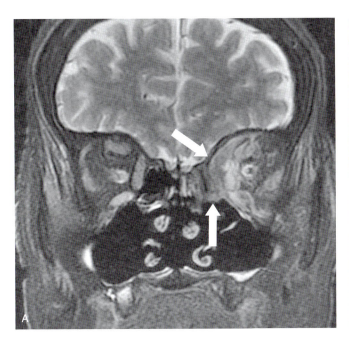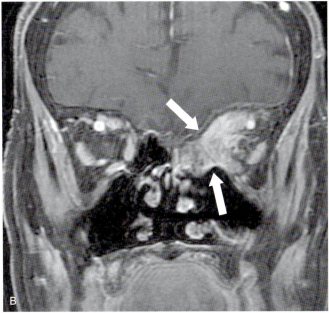

**Figure 69.5** Wegener's granulomatosis. (**A**) T2-weighted coronal imaging exhibits a low T2 signal nodular mass at the left ethmoidal sinus (arrows) extending into the left medial orbital compartment. The nasal septum is eroded. (**B**) Post-contrast fat-saturated T1-weighted image exhibits patchy intense post-contrast enhancement of the mass-like granuloma (arrows).

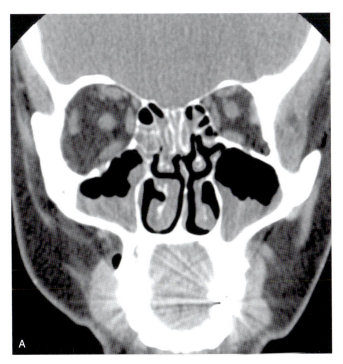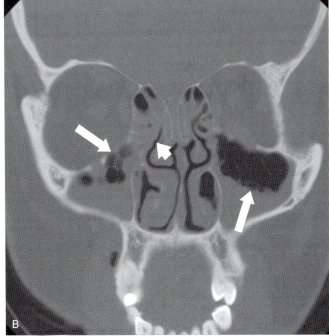

**Figure 69.6** Acute rhinosinusitis. (**A**, **B**) Coronal non-contrast CT exhibits air-fluid levels at bilateral maxillary sinuses with frothy and bubbly secretions (arrows). There is presence of inflammatory tissue obstructing the right ostiomeatal complex (short arrow).

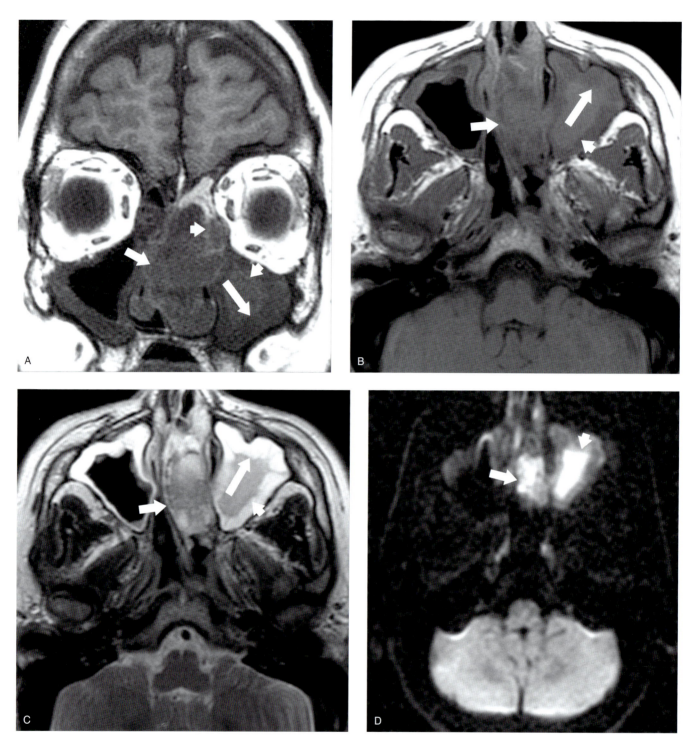

**Figure 69.7** Sinonasal melanoma with chronic rhinosinusitis. (**A**, **B**) T1-weighted axial and coronal images exhibit mildly high T1 signal lobulated left nasal mass (arrow), also involving the nasal septum, lateral wall, and middle turbinate. Low T1 signal polypoid mucosal thickening is seen at bilateral maxillary sinuses (long arrow). High T1 signal retained secretions are seen at left maxillary sinus (short arows).
(**C**) T2-weighted axial image exhibits low T2 signal, expansile, lobulated, left nasal cavity mass (arrow). High T2 signal polypoid mucosal thickening is seen at bilateral maxillary sinuses (long arrow). Low T2 signal retained secretions are seen at left maxillary sinus (short arrow).
(**D**) Restricted diffusion is seen at malignant left nasal cavity mass (arrow) and also at left maxillary sinus pyogenic secretions (short arrow).
(**E**, **F**) Post-contrast T1-weighted axial and coronal images exhibit avid enhancement of the malignant left nasal cavity mass (arrow). Enhancement of the mucosal edges of polypoid thickened maxillary sinus mucosal lining with water content is seen (long arrow). The retained secretions exhibit little post-contrast enhancement (short arrows).

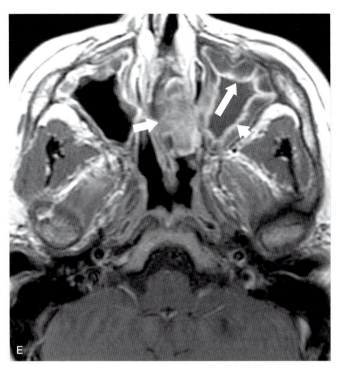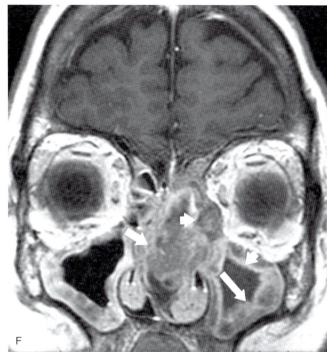

**Figure 69.7** (cont.)

## Imaging description

Cerebrospinal fluid (CSF) leak from the skull base is most commonly secondary to bony defects occurring after blunt head trauma or surgery. The most common location for post-traumatic CSF leak is the cribriform plate. Patients presenting with CSF leak who have no history of prior trauma or surgery are said to have spontaneous CSF leak. The most common site for spontaneous CSF leak at the skull base is the sphenoid sinus, more specifically the lateral wall of the sphenoid sinus, which may be weaker than the other sites due the incomplete fusion of the greater wings of the sphenoid bone with the basisphenoid, a.k.a. the Sternberg's canal [1,2]. The second most common site is the ethmoid roof and cribriform plate. Multiple sites of leak may be seen in up to 30% of patients.

Unenhanced high-resolution CT is usually performed first, and this shows the defect in the majority of cases. Well-defined soft tissue and fluid attenuation structures can be seen in the sinuses adjacent to the bone defect and represent meningoceles or encephaloceles (collectively known as cephaloceles). Cephaloceles mimic inflammatory sinus disease such as mucoceles or lytic bone lesions on CT (Figs. 70.1, 70.3). High-resolution MRI is helpful in identifying cephaloces, revealing their content and differentiating them from inflammatory mucosal changes (Figs. 70.2, 70.4). CT cisternogram is performed in cases where non-invasive methods are equivocal or show multiple potential sites of leak to pinpoint the exact location of the skull-base defect.

Spontaneous CSF leak patients have a high incidence of idiopathic intracranial hypertension (IIH), also known as pseudotumor cerebri, which is probably the underlying cause for CSF leak in at least some of the patients [3,4]. No single specific imaging sign of IIH exists, although these patients have a high incidence of the empty sella sign, enlargement of the optic nerve sheaths, and flattening of the globe at the optic nerve heads on their MRI studies, as well as stenoses of the transverse venous sinuses (Fig. 70.5). Multiple focal areas of bony thinning of the skull base, referred to as arachnoid pits, are frequently seen in patients with spontaneous CSF leak and may be etiologically related to the leak, although this finding may also be present in individuals without CSF leak (Fig. 70.6) [5].

## Importance

Identifying the site of CSF leak is critically important for treatment planning. Mistaking cephaloceles for inflammatory mucosal change can have catastrophic consequences. Recognizing the association between spontaneous CSF leaks and IIH is critical; the recurrence rate of CSF leak in patients whose IIH is not addressed appears to be higher.

## Typical clinical scenario

Patients are generally obese middle-aged women who present with spontaneous clear rhinorrhea. Significant overlap exists in the characteristics of patients with spontaneous CSF leak and IIH. Patients with IIH classically present with headache, pulsatile tinnitus, and visual changes.

## Differential diagnosis

Mucoceles or sinus mucosal inflammatory changes can mimic cephaloceles, particularly on CT. MRI is helpful in differentiating these.

---

**Teaching points**

The lateral wall of the sphenoid sinus is the most common site of leak in patients with spontaneous CSF rhinorrhea, and is often associated with cephaloceles protruding into the sphenoid sinus. IIH may be the underlying cause for CSF leak.

---

REFERENCES

1. Tomazic PV, Stammberger H. Spontaneous CSF-leaks and meningoencephaloceles in sphenoid sinus by persisting Sternberg's canal. *Rhinology* 2009; **47**: 369–74.

2. Barañano CF, Curé J, Palmer JN, Woodworth BA. Sternberg's canal: fact or fiction? *Am J Rhinol Allergy* 2009; **23**: 167–71.

3. Woodworth BA, Prince A, Chiu AG, *et al.* Spontaneous CSF leaks: a paradigm for definitive repair and management of intracranial hypertension. *Otolaryngol Head Neck Surg* 2008; **138**: 715–20.

4. Schlosser RJ, Bolger WE. Significance of empty sella in cerebrospinal fluid leaks. *Otolaryngol Head Neck Surg* 2003; **128**: 32–8.

5. Shetty PG, Shroff MM, Fatterpekar GM, *et al.* A retrospective analysis of spontaneous sphenoid sinus fistula: MR and CT findings. *AJNR Am J Neuroradiol* 2000; **21**: 337–42.

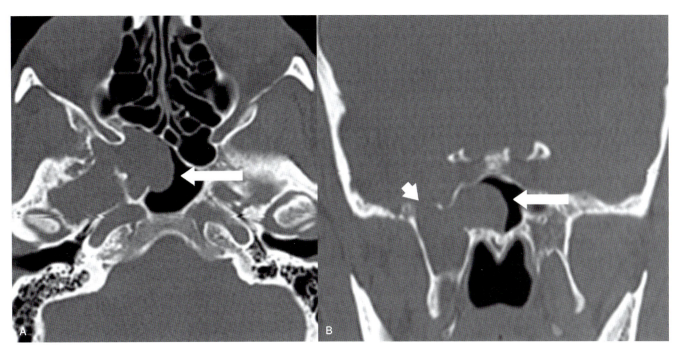

**Figure 70.1** (**A**) Axial and (**B**) coronal CT images show a well-defined soft tissue mass (arrows) in the sphenoid sinus that may be misinterpreted as a mucous retention cyst if the bony defect along the lateral wall of the sinus (short arrow) is not recognized.

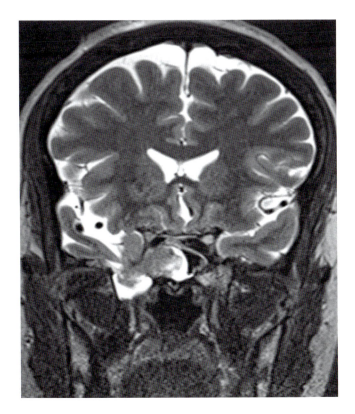

**Figure 70.2** Coronal T2-weighted MRI of the same patient as in Fig. 70.1 shows a large cephalocele with brain parenchyma as well as CSF within.

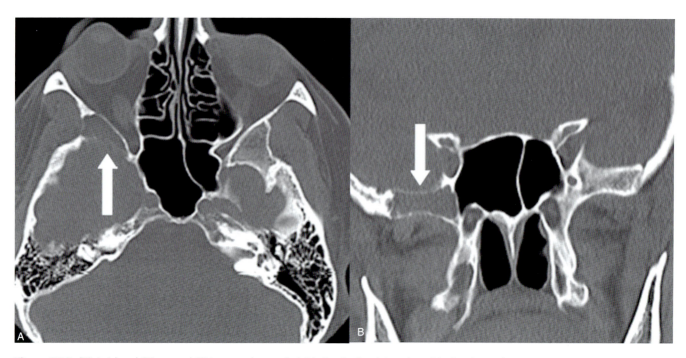

**Figure 70.3** (**A**) Axial and (**B**) coronal CT images show a "lytic" lesion in the right sphenoid wing (arrows).

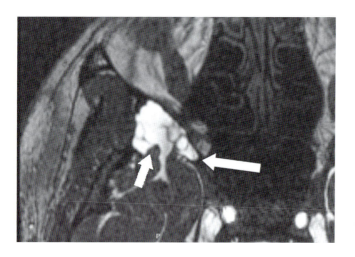

**Figure 70.4** Axial heavily T2-weighted high-resolution MRI of the same patient as in Fig. 70.3 shows that the brain parenchyma and CFS spaces extend into the bone lesion (arrow), compatible with a cephalocele that opens to the sphenoid sinus (long arrow), which is responsible for the clinical presentation of CSF rhinorrhea.

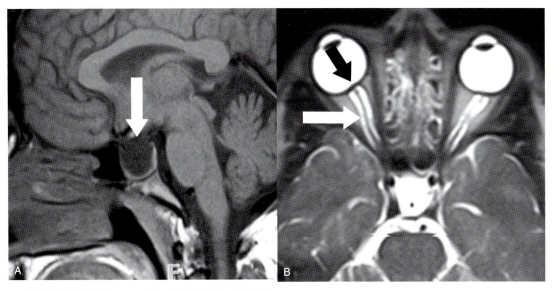

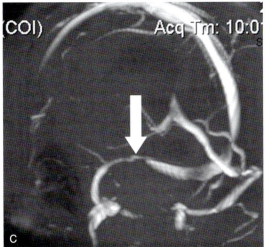

Figure 70.5 All the imaging signs of pseudotumor cerebri (IIH) are shown on the MRI/MRV of the same patient: (**A**) empty sella sign (arrow), (**B**) dilatation of CSF spaces around the optic nerves (arrow), bulging of optic nerve heads into the globes (papilledema) (black arrow), and (**C**) stenosis of the right transverse sinus (arrow). These signs are non-specific in isolation but should be highly suspicious for IIH when present together.

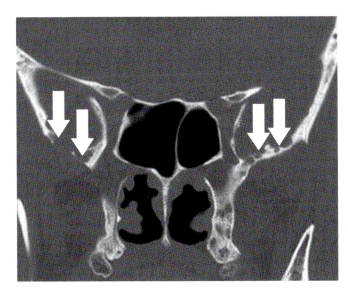

Figure 70.6 Multiple arachnoid pits (arrows) are shown on this coronal CT. Arachnoid pits are more frequently present in cases of cephaloceles than in normal individuals.

## Imaging description

Juvenile nasal angiofibromas (JNAs) are benign, fibrovascular tumors that are locally invasive and infiltrative [1]. Malignant conversion has been reported, but it is rare in tumors that have not been irradiated [2].

CT and MRI play a vital and often complementary role in assessment of these tumors. Axial and coronal CT images with bone windows best demonstrate the degree of bone remodeling and erosion. High-resolution, contrast-enhanced MRI is very useful in demonstrating the soft tissue extent, and to evaluate possible intracranial or cavernous sinus extension. Larger and more vascular tumors display obvious flow voids within the mass, representing intratumoral vessels. The mass typically enhances briskly with contrast, both on MRI and on CT. Differentiation of obstructed sinus secretions versus soft tissue mass from sinus invasion is difficult on CT but easily assessed by MRI.

The tumor is thought to arise from the lateral margin of the posterior nasal cavity, adjacent to the sphenopalatine foramen (Fig. 71.1). Large tumors are dumbbell-shaped or bilobed, with one portion of the tumor bulging into the nasopharynx and the other extending towards the pterygopalatine fossa. These tumors can demonstrate extensive locoregional spread along natural tissue planes. Superiorly, the mass can erode into the sphenoid sinus, cavernous sinus, sella, and middle cranial fossa. Laterally, the tumor may spread into the pterygomaxillary and sphenopalatine fossae. Larger tumors cause a characteristic bowing of the posterior wall of the maxillary sinus (Fig. 71.2). Occasionally the mass can erode through the greater wing of the sphenoid bone, thereby exposing the dura of the middle cranial fossa.

Angiography is usually performed in the same sitting as preoperative embolization. Typical angiographic features include hypertrophy of the arteries supplying the tumor. The predominant blood supply is from the ECA (terminal branches of the internal maxillary artery and anterior division of the ascending pharyngeal artery) (Fig. 71.3), but supply from ICA may arise in the tumors that erode through the skull base or have an intracranial component [1]. There is typically an early-appearing, intense, inhomogeneous vascular blush that persists until late in the venous phase.

## Importance

It is important to realize the vascular nature of this neoplasm on imaging, so as to avoid unnecessary biopsy and the potential for severe bleeding during the procedure.

## Typical clinical scenario

JNA classically occurs in adolescent males, with a peak incidence at 14–17 years of age [1]. The most common presentation is with nasal obstruction and recurrent epistaxis. If drainage is impeded by a large tumor, sinusitis or otitis may develop. Anosmia, proptosis, facial or temporal swelling, and extraocular muscle palsies may be seen, depending on the size and the direction of the tumor spread. A lobulated reddish-gray mass can be observed in the nasal cavity on endoscopy.

## Differential diagnosis

JNAs should be differentiated from other masses that occur in the nasopharynx and posterior nasal cavity, including nasopharyngeal carcinoma (NPC), rhabdomyosarcoma (RMS) (Fig. 71.4), and anterochoanal polyp. Nasopharyngeal carcinomas arise in the mucosal space of the nasopharynx and can result in erosion of the skull base. These (and other masses mentioned in the differential) generally do not present with severe episodic epistaxis and do not result in enlargement of the sphenopalatine foramen. NPC and RMS can enhance with contrast, although to a much lesser degree than JNA, and these masses do not demonstrate any flow voids on MRI.

---

### Teaching points

Adolescent males presenting with epistaxis and/or nasal obstruction should be evaluated for the possibility of harboring a JNA. Location in the lateral aspect of the nasal cavity, expansion of the sphenopalatine foramen, bowing of the posterior wall of the maxillary sinus, and extremely vascular nature of the neoplasm all point towards a diagnosis of JNA.

---

REFERENCES

1. Gemmete JJ, Ansari SA, McHugh J, Gandhi D. Embolization of vascular tumors of the head and neck. *Neuroimaging Clin N Am* 2009; **19**: 181–98.
2. Batsakis J, KloppC, Newman W. Fibrosarcoma arising in a juvenile nasopharyngeal angiofibroma following extensive radiation therapy. *Am Surg* 1955; **21**: 786–93.

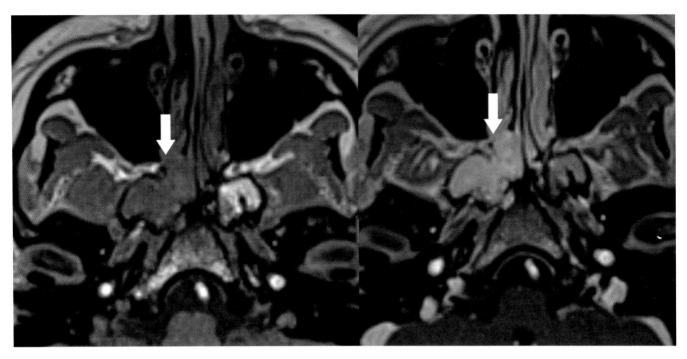

**Figure 71.1** Small, right-sided avidly enhancing JNA demonstrated on T1-weighted images without and with contrast. Note the characteristic involvement of the right sphenopalatine foramen (arrow).

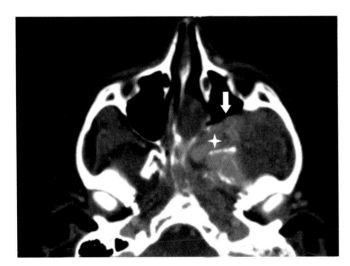

**Figure 71.2** An infiltrative, large left-sided JNA is seen on this enhanced CT of the neck. Note the widening of the sphenopalatine foramen (star) and characteristic bowing of the posterior wall of the maxillary sinus (arrow).

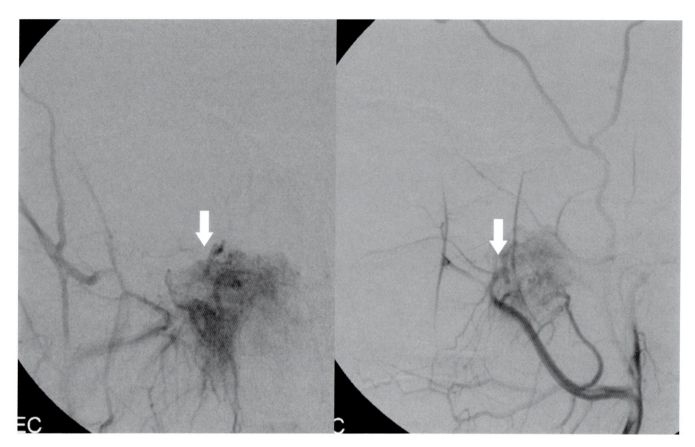

**Figure 71.3** Anteroposterior and lateral external carotid angiography displays a vascular blush associated with JNA (arrows). The mass is mainly supplied by internal maxillary artery and its sphenopalatine branches.

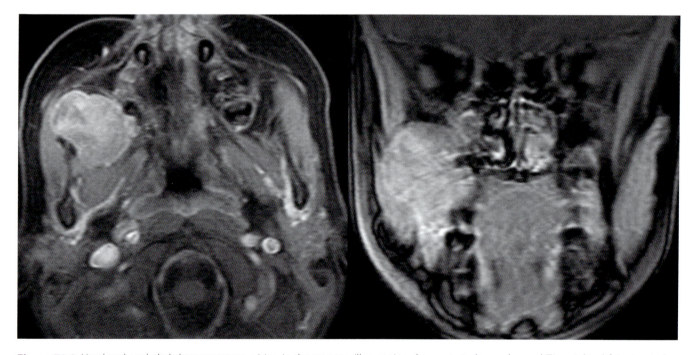

**Figure 71.4** Head and neck rhabdomyosarcoma arising in the retromaxillary region demonstrated on enhanced T1-weighted fat-saturated images. The epicenter of this mass is lateral to the sphenopalatine foramen.

# Idiopathic orbital pseudotumor

## Imaging description

Lesions of the orbit can have diverse etiologies and imaging appearances. The old classification based on intraconal or extraconal location is not helpful for specific diagnosis in most cases.

Idiopathic inflammatory pseudotumor of orbit is a quasi-neoplastic lesion that accounts for 5–10% of all orbital lesions and is the third most common orbital disorder following thyroid orbitopathy and lymphoproliferative conditions [1,2]. Mixed inflammatory infiltrate of pseudotumor can be seen in any area of the orbit, but most commonly involves the retro-bulbar compartment and takes the form of a mass. This is known as tumefactive pseudotumor; it accounts for about two-thirds of all cases (Fig. 72.1) and usually presents with prop-tosis, limitation of eye movements, and decreased vision.

Myositic type is the second most common, usually unilateral, involving single or multiple muscles, including the ten-dinous insertions (Fig. 72.2). Diplopia and limitation of ocular movements are common. Lacrimal gland pseudotumor is commonly associated with systemic disease and presents with enlarged and tender gland and proptosis of the orbital globe (Fig. 72.3). It can be associated with extraorbital extension [3]. Tolosa–Hunt syndrome is considered to be a form of pseudo-tumor involving the cavernous sinus.

Post-contrast imaging with CT scan should include a cor-onal acquisition [4]. MRI better delineates the soft tissue involvement and possible extension to the orbital apex, includ-ing involvement of the optic nerves. There are no specific signal characteristics for pseudotumor, although almost all cases show abnormal enhancement. While most lesions are hyperintense on T2-weighted images, some pseudotumor cases, particularly those that are subacute to chronic, may show decreased T2 signal.

## Importance

Imaging findings for a variety of orbital lesions tend to be non-specific. Orbital pseudotumor is an important differential diagnosis in lesions involving the retrobulbar intraconal region, extraorbital muscles, and lacrimal glands, especially when associated with pain. However, it is also possible to have this condition without orbital pain [3]. When it does not respond to steroid therapy, a biopsy for confirmation is indicated.

## Typical clinical scenario

The commonest presentation is in a middle-aged male or female with acute to subacute onset of orbital pain, inflam-mation, and swelling. The eye movements are restricted, with proptosis and possible diplopia. In a younger population, a waxing and waning pattern is more likely. Orbital pain was

formerly considered to be the hallmark of clinical diagnosis, but it is possible to have this condition without orbital pain [3].

## Differential diagnosis

Lymphoproliferative lesions of the orbit, especially non-Hodgkin's lymphoma, may be primarily orbital or secondary to systemic disease. It is the most common orbital mass lesion and accounts for more than 50% of cases of orbital pathology. It presents as a malleable mass that can involve the orbital fat, lacrimal gland (Fig. 72.4), or extraocular muscle; it can be indistinguishable from orbital pseudotumor but is often bilateral.

Thyroid ophthalmopathy characteristically affects the belly of the extraocular muscles and spares the tendinous insertions. When isolated, inferior rectus muscle is more commonly affected (Fig. 72.5). Clinically, thyroid dysfunction is often obvious, but orbital involvement may precede endocrine abnormalities in a small group of patients.

Wegener's granulomatosis is an autoimmune condition with necrotizing vasculitis, primarily involving the paranasal sinus and orbits (Fig. 72.6) with bone destruction. It is com-monly bilateral.

Systemic sarcoidosis can affect the orbit, most often the lacrimal gland. There is patchy enhancement of multiple orbital structures with granulomatous spread.

Phlegmonous orbital cellulitis can represent secondary spread from adjacent paranasal sinuses and is often associated with subperiosteal abscess.

## Teaching points

Pseudotumor of the orbit may present with well-defined mass lesions, muscular involvement, and diffuse infiltration of orbital tissues and may mimic lymphoproliferative dis-eases as well as thyroid ophthalmopathy. Presence of pain is an important clue to this diagnosis.

REFERENCES

1. Narla LD, Newman B, Spottswood SS, *et al*. Inflammatory pseudotumor. *Radiographics* 2003; **23**: 719–29,
2. Weber AL, Romo LV, Sabates NR. Pseudotumor of the orbit: clinical, pathologic, and radiologic evaluation. *Radiol Clin North Am* 1999; **37**: 151–68.
3. Mahr MA, Salomao DR, Garrity JA. Inflammatory orbital pseudotumor with extension beyond the orbit. *Am J Ophthalmol* 2004; **138**: 396–400.
4. LeBedis CA, Sakai O. Nontraumatic orbital conditions: diagnosis with CT and MR imaging in the emergent setting. *Radiographics* 2008; **28**: 1741–53.

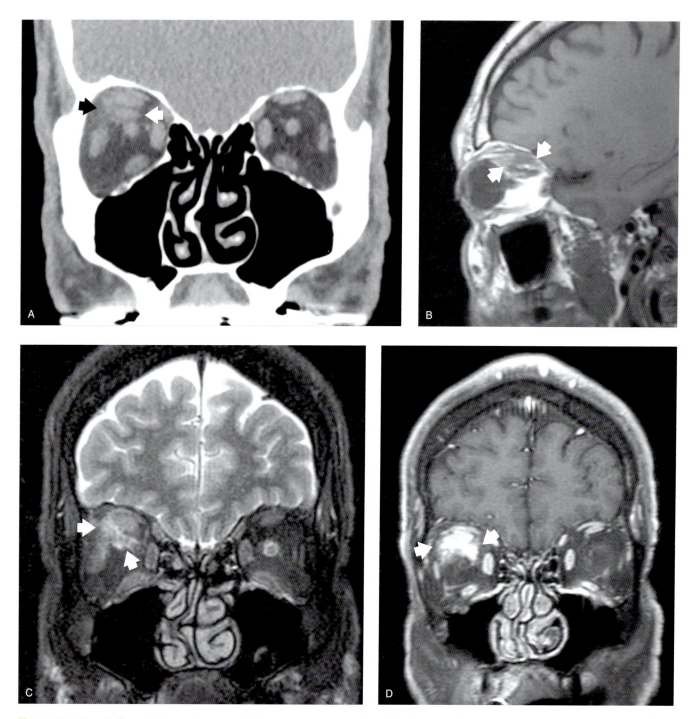

**Figure 72.1** Retrobulbar orbital pseudotumor. (**A**) Non-contrast coronal CT exhibits irregular soft tissue stranding in the superior retrobulbar intraconal compartment (short arrows). (**B**) T1-weighted sagittal MRI exhibits hypo- to isointense soft tissue stranding inferior to superior rectus muscle and superior to the optic nerve, with involvement of superior rectus muscle (short arrows). (**C**) T2-weighted coronal MRI exhibits patchy high T2 signal irregular soft tissue in intraconal compartment (short arrows), also infiltrating the superior rectus muscle, which also exhibits patchy high T2 signal. (**D**) T1-weighted fat-saturated post-contrast coronal MRI shows intense post-contrast enhancement of the irregular lesion.

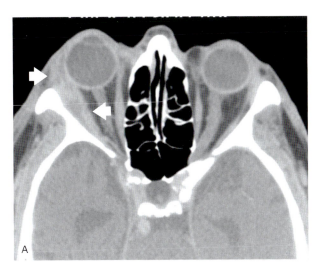 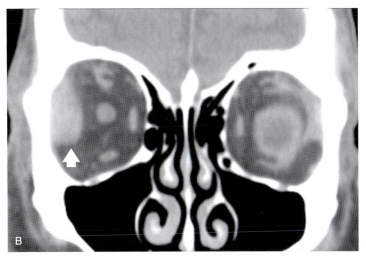

**Figure 72.2** Myositic orbital pseudotumor. (**A**) Post-contrast axial CT shows a patchily enhancing soft tissue mass in the lateral extraconal compartment of the right orbital cavity, also infiltrating the lateral rectus muscle and lacrimal gland (short arrows). (**B**) Post-contrast coronal CT exhibits infiltration and enlargement of the right lateral rectus muscle (short arrow) with infiltration of the adjoining lateral extraconal compartment.

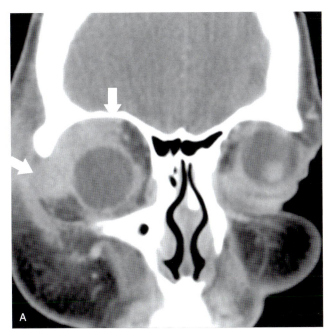 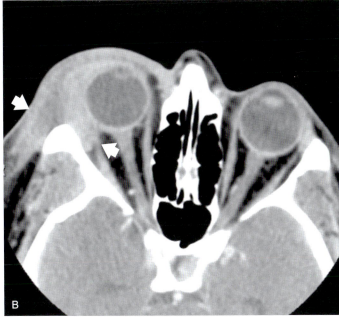

**Figure 72.3** Lacrimal gland orbital pseudotumor. (**A**) Post-contrast coronal CT exhibits marked infiltration and enlargement of right lacrimal gland, also extending into preseptal region, contiguous with orbital sclera, and resultant proptosis (arrows). (**B**) Post-contrast axial CT exhibits patchily enhancing enlarged right lacrimal gland with infiltrating soft tissue extending into extraorbital compartment (short arrows).

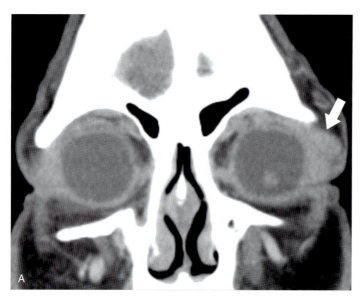

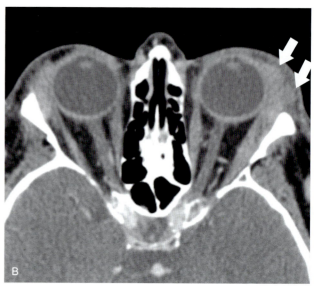

**Figure 72.4** Non-Hodgkin's lymphoma. (**A, B**) Post-contrast coronal and axial images exhibit enlargement and infiltration of the left lacrimal gland (arrow) extending into the preseptal region and posteriorly into the lateral extraconal compartment (arrows). Based only on imaging, it is not possible to differentiate this condition from orbital pseudotumor.

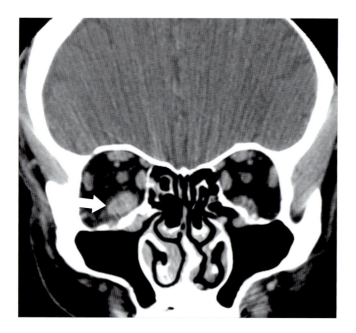

**Figure 72.5** Thyroid ophthalmopathy. Post-contrast coronal image exhibits enhancement and thickening of the belly of the inferior rectus muscle of right (arrow) more than left orbital cavity.

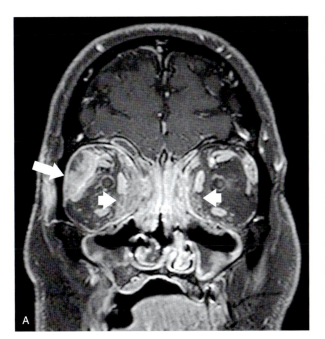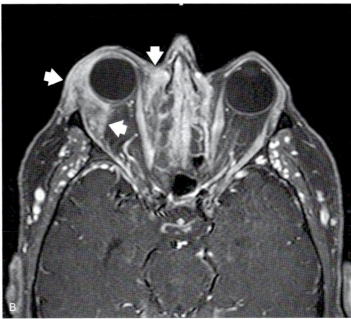

**Figure 72.6** Wegener's granulomatosis. (**A**) Post-contrast fat-saturated T1-weighted coronal image reveals a patchily enhancing sinonasal soft tissue mass, and extending and infiltrating medial extraconal compartment bilaterally (short arrows). There is also infiltration and involvement of the right lacrimal gland (arrow). The inferior part of the nasal septum is absent. (**B**) Post-contrast fat-saturated T1-weighted axial image reveals patchily enhancing soft tissue at the medial extraconal compartment, involving the lacrimal gland and extending into the preseptal region of the right orbit (short arrows).

## Imaging description

Optic neuritis (ON) is an acute inflammatory process of presumed autoimmune etiology in the majority of the cases. Although it can have diverse etiology, the most common reason is multiple sclerosis (MS). ON can be the first manifestation of MS [1], or could represent neuromyelitis optica (NMO), acute disseminated encephalomyelitis (ADEM), and less likely isolated pediatric ON, which tends to be post-viral, post-vaccination, or due to ADEM. Depending on the geographic cohort, 14% (Japan) to 77% (UK) of patients with ON are subsequently found to have multiple sclerosis [2]. ON is the initial presentation of MS in 15–25% of the patients, while about 70–90% of MS patients develop ON at some point.

The diagnosis of ON is made clinically and confirmed with MRI by demonstrating focal or segmental high T2 signal within a diffusely enlarged optic nerve [3]. On post-contrast imaging, diffuse or central enhancement of optic nerve is seen in about 90% of patients (Fig. 73.1). On diffusion-weighted imaging, there may be decreased diffusivity in the acute stage and increased diffusivity in chronic ON [3,4]. Presence of high T2 and FLAIR signal white matter lesions within the brain is a strong predictor for MS in the setting of ON.

NMO is a disabling inflammatory condition that targets astrocytes in the optic nerves and spinal cord. Clinically, it can be easily confused with MS because it is characterized by relapses leading to incremental deficits [5].

## Importance

It is important to confirm the clinical suspicion of ON with a properly performed MRI, which includes high-resolution STIR and post-contrast images of the orbits, as compressive optic neuropathy such as seen in optic nerve sheath meningioma and ischemic optic neuropathy may clinically mimic ON. It is also important to simultaneously image the brain and the spinal cord, as directed by symptoms, because of the strong association between ON and MS.

## Typical clinical scenario

The most common presentation is acute mono-ocular loss of visual acuity and eye pain over a few days. Other symptoms include impairment of vision in bright light, light flashes, impaired color vision, globe tenderness, and afferent pupillary defect. There is a 2:1 female predominance, presenting from 15 to 50 years of age, with an average of the early thirties. There is a greater prevalence in white Caucasian ancestry, with low prevalence in African or Asian ancestry.

## Differential diagnosis

Radiation-induced optic neuropathy generally tends to be bilateral and occurs about 1–3 years following radiation therapy for maxillofacial, anterior skull-base, pituitary, or parasellar masses. The MRI appearance is similar to ON (Fig. 73.2), but a history of previous radiation therapy for skull-base or brain tumor is always present.

Chronic relapsing inflammatory optic neuropathy may not be associated with demyelinating disorders or connective tissue diseases and presents with recurrent episodes of painful visual loss. MRI may be normal or may exhibit loss of volume at optic nerve with enlargement of optic nerve sheath (Fig. 73.3). There is a lack of significant post-contrast enhancement.

Granulomatous optic neuropathy is a manifestation of neurosarcoidosis or systemic sarcoidosis. The MRI appearance of the optic nerve is similar to that of ON (Fig. 73.4). However, there is evidence for intracranial neurosarcoidosis with leptomeningeal enhancement. Involvement of the lacrimal gland and extraorbital muscles may also be seen.

Optic nerve glioma is more often seen in pediatric patients with neurofibromatosis type 1. There is a tubular enlargement with moderate enhancement of optic nerve (Fig. 73.5). Rarely, it is also seen in adults, as a malignant optic nerve glioma.

Meningioma of optic nerve presents with painless progressive vision loss without any remissions. On MRI, there is thickening of the optic nerve sheath with isointense T1 and T2 signal to cerebral gray matter and intense post-contrast enhancement (Fig. 73.6). Tram-track calcification on CT scan may also be seen in some cases.

Ischemic optic neuropathy usually has no imaging correlate, although restricted diffusion on DWI can be seen in some cases.

---

### Teaching points

The imaging findings of ON are often subtle, and diagnosis hinges on proper imaging. A suggested protocol for MRI of the orbits includes axial fat-saturated FSE T2-weighted sequence (3 mm thickness, no skip), STIR coronal sequence (3 mm, no skip), and T1-weighted fat-saturated post-contrast sequence (3 mm, no skip). Additional T1-weighted pre-contrast coronal imaging may help evaluate possible soft tissue lesion of the orbit. Including axial and/or sagittal FLAIR image of the brain to look for plaques of demyelination is helpful.

---

REFERENCES

1. Swanton JK, Fernando KT, Dalton CM, *et al*. Early MRI in optic neuritis: the risk for clinically definite multiple sclerosis. *Mult Scler* 2010; **16**: 156–65.

2. Swanton JK, Fernando K, Dalton CM, *et al*. Is the frequency of abnormalities on magnetic resonance imaging in isolated optic neuritis related to the prevalence of multiple sclerosis? A global comparison. *J Neurol Neurosurg Psychiatry* 2006; **77**: 1070–2.

3. Hickman SJ, Wheeler-Kingshott CAM, Jones SJ, *et al.* Optic nerve diffusion measurement from diffusion-weighted imaging in optic neuritis. *AJNR Am J Neuroradiol* 2005; **26**: 951–6.

4. Fatima Z, Motosugi U, Muhi A, *et al.* Diffusion-weighted imaging in optic neuritis. *Can Assoc Radiol J* 2013; **64**: 51–5.

5. Morrow MJ, Wingerchuk D. Neuromyelitis optica. *J Neuroophthalmol* 2012; **32**: 154–66.

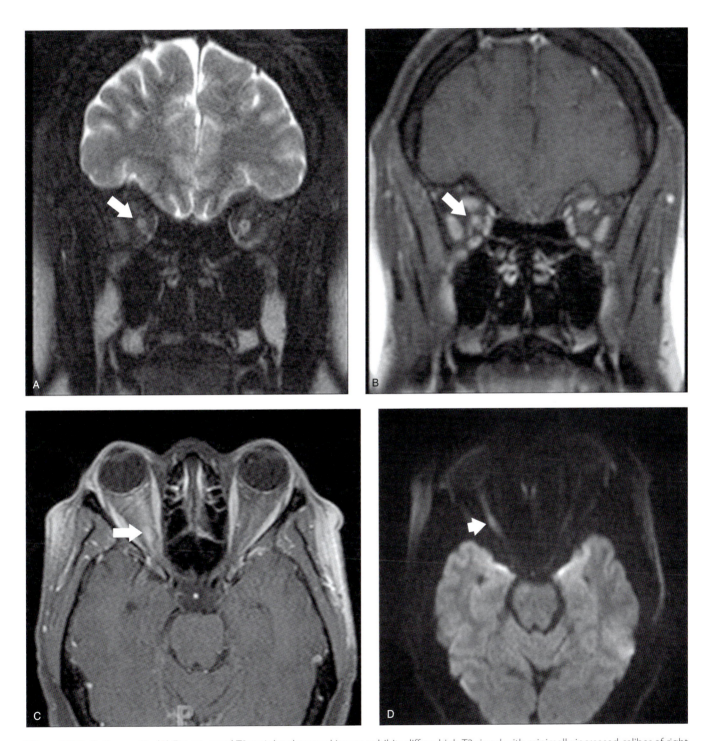

**Figure 73.1** Optic neuritis. (**A**) Fat-saturated T2-weighted coronal image exhibits diffuse high T2 signal with minimally increased caliber of right optic nerve (arrow). (**B**) Post-contrast fat-saturated T1-weighted coronal image exhibits intense enhancement of right optic nerve (arrow). (**C**) Post-contrast fat-saturated T1-weighted axial image exhibits focal enhancement of posterior part of intraorbital right optic nerve (arrow). (**D**) Diffusion-weighted axial image exhibits a focal area of impeded diffusion at the level of abnormal contrast enhancement (short arrow). (**E**) Sagittal FLAIR image shows an oblong high signal plaque of demyelination in the pericallosal area (short arrow).

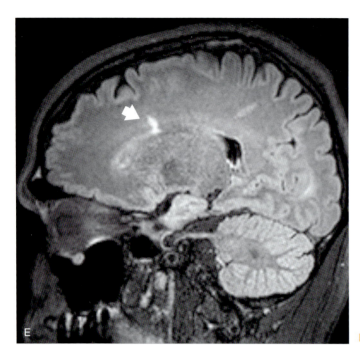

E

**Figure 73.1** (cont.)

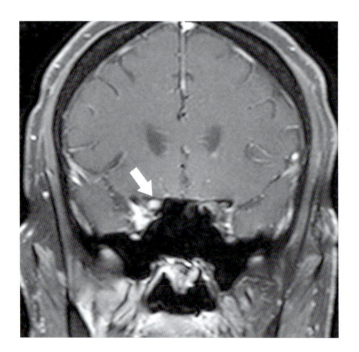

**Figure 73.2** Radiation-induced optic neuropathy. Post-contrast fat-saturated T1-weighted coronal image exhibits intense post-contrast enhancement and enlargement of right optic nerve (arrow) with faint enhancement of left optic nerve.

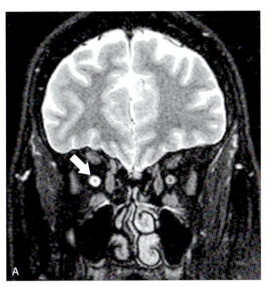
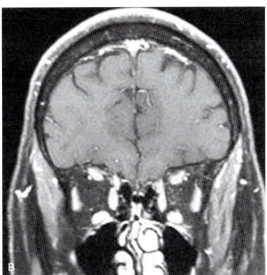

**Figure 73.3** Chronic inflammatory optic neuropathy. (**A**) Fat-saturated T2-weighted coronal image exhibits smaller caliber of right optic nerve (arrow) as compared to the left. (**B**) Post-contrast fat-saturated T1-weighted coronal image exhibits lack of significant post-contrast enhancement.

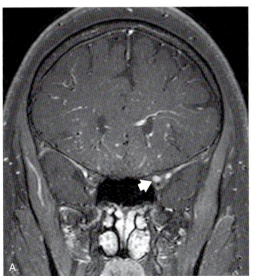
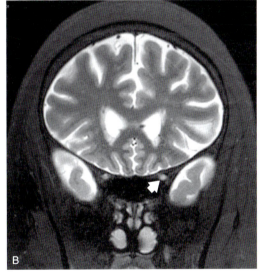

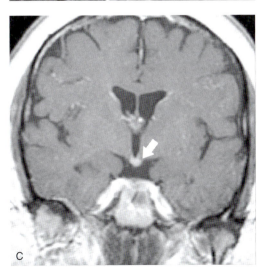

**Figure 73.4** Granulomatous optic neuropathy (orbital sarcoid). (**A**) Post-contrast fat-saturated T1-weighted coronal image exhibits intense enhancement of enlarged left optic nerve (short arrow). (**B**) Fat-saturated T2-weighted coronal image exhibits hyperintense on T2 signal of an enlarged left optic nerve (short arrow). (**C**) Post-contrast T1-weighted coronal image of brain exhibits patchy leptomeningeal enhancement of the floor of third ventricle (arrow).

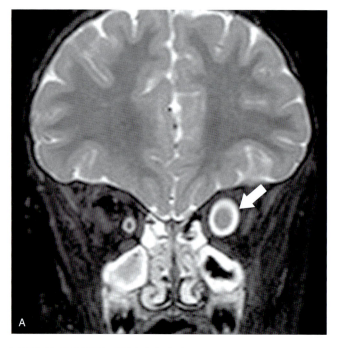

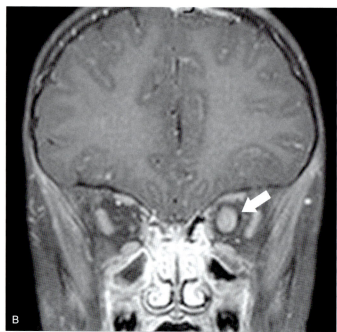

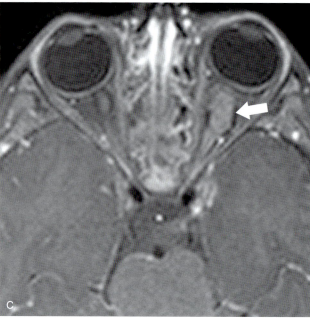

**Figure 73.5** Optic nerve glioma. (**A**) Fat-saturated T2-weighted coronal image exhibits marked enlargement of left optic nerve, including enlargement of optic nerve sheath (arrow). (**B**) Post-contrast fat-saturated T1-weighted coronal image exhibits moderate enhancement of enlarged left optic nerve (arrow). (**C**) Post-contrast fat-saturated T1-weighted axial image exhibits abnormal enhancement with tubular enlargement of left optic nerve (arrow).

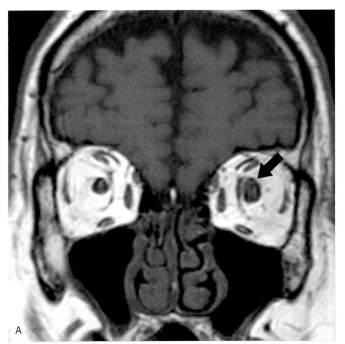

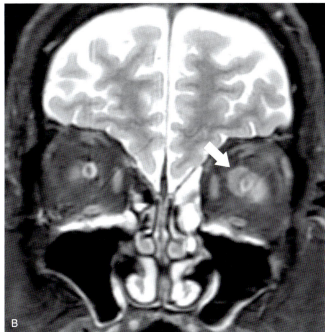

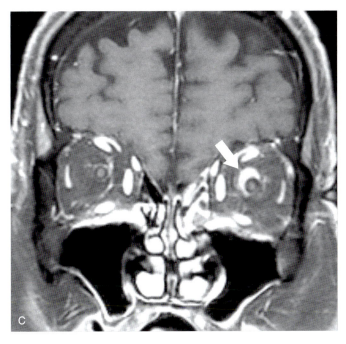

**Figure 73.6** Optic nerve sheath meningioma. (**A**) T1-weighted coronal image exhibits eccentric enlargement of left optic nerve (black arrow). (**B**) Fat-saturated T2-weighted coronal image exhibits eccentric thickening of nerve sheath of left optic nerve, which appears isointense to gray matter (arrow). (**C**) Post-contrast fat-saturated T1-weighted coronal image exhibits intense homogeneous enhancement of eccentric left optic nerve sheath meningioma (arrow).

# Intraparotid lymph nodes

## Imaging description

Most parotid masses are either benign or less likely malignant primary salivary gland tumors. The parotid glands arise from the oropharyngeal ectoderm and encapsulate late in embryologic development, entrapping lymphatic tissue within the parotid capsule and parenchyma. Anatomic studies confirm the presence of 4–7 lymph nodes in the superficial and 1–2 nodes in the deep parotid lobes [1].

It is common to see small normal intraparotid lymph nodes (IPLNs) on imaging studies, particularly on MRI (Fig. 74.1). Occasionally, reactive enlargement of IPLNs occurs, similar to reactive enlargement of neck nodes as seen in upper respiratory infections etc., mimicking parotid tumors [2]. The reactively enlarged IPLNs have a very homogeneous appearance, with attenuation values on CT and signal characteristics on MRI similar to neck lymph nodes outside the parotid, and should not be mistaken for tumor (Fig. 74.2). The reactive hyperplasia of IPLNs usually involves multiple nodes and is associated with extraparotid nodal hyperplasia. Warthin's tumor can be multifocal and involve the extraparotid tissues, but it is more heterogeneous, showing areas of cysts, nodules, and intense enhancement in most cases that can be readily differentiated from lymph nodes.

Beyond reactive hypertrophy, IPLNs can be affected by many diseases that regularly involve the neck nodes, including metastases, and present as if a primary salivary tumor. IPLN is the primary nodal drainage site for the frontal, temporal, and malar skin, pinna and external acoustic meatus, upper lip, eyelids, and root of the nose, and squamous cell carcinoma (SCC) or melanoma of the skin arising from these regions can present for the first time with a "parotid mass" (Fig. 74.3). Although quite uncommon, SCC of the oral cavity and oropharynx may metastasize to the parotid gland [3].

## Importance

The lymphoid tissue normally present within the parotid gland may give rise to benign and malignant diseases of the lymphoid tissue and masquerade as salivary tumors. Keeping in mind the possibility of lymphoid pathology in the differential diagnosis of parotid tumors is important.

## Typical clinical scenario

The most common scenario is incidental visualization of reactive hypertrophy of IPLNs, leading radiologists to consider parotid "masses." Occasionally, reactively enlarged IPLNs may be palpable and prompt a CT or MRI.

## Differential diagnosis

The differential diagnosis of multiple IPLN includes reactive hypertrophy, HIV-related lymphadenopathy, Kimura's disease, Castleman's disease, sarcoidosis, and lymphoma, as well as metastases from skin SCC.

## Teaching points

Reactively enlarged IPLNs are often mistaken for parotid tumors. Multiple unilateral or bilateral homogeneous intraparotid nodules most frequently represent reactive lymphoid hyperplasia and do not require further work-up in the absence of a systemic inflammatory or lymphoproliferative disease or head and neck malignancy.

REFERENCES

1. Pisani P, Ramponi A, Pia F. The deep parotid lymph nodes: an anatomical and oncological study. *J Laryngol Otol* 1996; **110**: 148–50.

2. Terada T. Hyperplastic intraparotid lymph nodes with incipient Warthin's tumor presenting as a parotid tumor. *Pathol Res Pract* 2008; **204**: 863–6.

3. Olsen SM, Moore EJ, Koch CA, Kasperbauer JL, Olsen KD. Oral cavity and oropharynx squamous cell carcinoma with metastasis to the parotid lymph nodes. *Oral Oncol* 2011; **47**: 142–4.

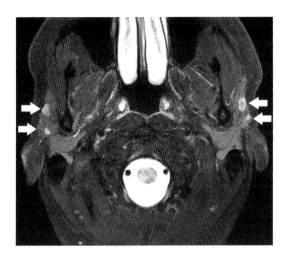

**Figure 74.1** Multiple small intraparotid lymph nodes (arrows) are seen on an axial fat-suppressed T2-weighted image.

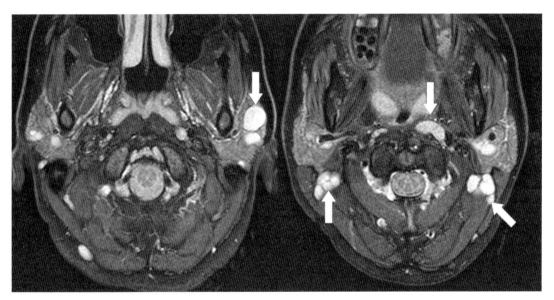

**Figure 74.2** Patient referred for palpable parotid mass. Axial T2-weighted MR images show a prominent left intraparotid lymph node which is homogeneous. Also note multiple prominent cervical and left retropharyngeal nodes (arrows). Clinical follow-up confirmed these to be reactively enlarged lymph nodes.

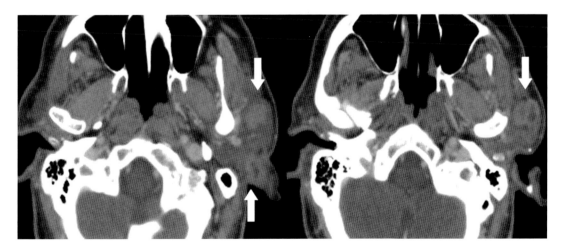

**Figure 74.3** Axial CT images of a patient who presented with a left parotid mass reveal multiple intraparotid enlarged lymph nodes, which turned out to be metastases from left frontal scalp squamous cell carcinoma.

# Benign mixed tumor

## Imaging description

Benign mixed tumor (BMT), also known as pleomorphic adenoma, is the most common primary neoplasm of the parotid gland, and accounts for about 80% of parotid masses. It presents as a relatively smoothly marginated and homogeneously enhancing ovoid mass which is slow-growing and clinically silent (Fig. 75.1) [1]. When involving the deep lobe, it has a characteristic pear shape when extending through the stylomandibular notch and may cause its widening (Fig. 75.2).

BMT is the only parotid neoplasm to have dystrophic calcification, if present. On MRI, it presents as relatively well-circumscribed or lobulated intraparotid mass with very high T2 signal and may exhibit a peripheral low T2 signal capsule [2]. High T2 signal is a very important differentiating feature, as most malignant tumors will show a relatively diminished T2 signal. High apparent diffusion coefficient (ADC) values in BMT compared to other benign and malignant lesions as well as normal parotid parenchyma is characteristic; however, this finding is not so specific as to avoid biopsy (Fig. 75.2) [3]. On dynamic contrast-enhanced imaging, a sharp uptake curve is seen followed by a plateau due to contrast retention, again not specific enough to avoid biopsy.

## Importance

BMT is the most common intraparotid mass and has fairly characteristic clinical and MRI features that allow an accurate diagnosis without biopsy in most cases, although many surgeons would want to have a definitive histopathological diagnosis before surgery for better surgical planning and patient counseling, as malignant tumors require a different surgical approach and have a different surgical risk profile. Fine-needle aspiration biopsy is safe and not associated with increased risk of recurrence, which occurs in about 10% of patients. It is also important for surgical planning to define the plane of facial nerve by drawing a line through the stylomastoid foramen to the lateral margin of the retromandibular vein.

## Typical clinical scenario

A painless mass palpated by the patient at the cheek or the angle of mandible is the most common presentation when BMT arises from the superficial lobe or the tail. However, it is quite common for BMT to involve the deep lobe and be non-palpable. In that case, difficulty in breathing, snoring, or ear pain are common symptoms. BMT is more common in middle-aged males and rare in African-Americans.

## Differential diagnosis

Low T2 signal, irregular and infiltrative margins, and multicentricity are hallmarks of malignant neoplasm of the parotid gland. Adenoid cystic carcinoma is a malignant primary neoplasm of the parotid gland and presents as an enhancing infiltrating mass, often presenting with facial nerve paralysis as perineural spread along the facial nerve is common (Fig. 75.3). Mucoepidermoid carcinoma is the most common primary malignant neoplasm of the parotid gland, and presents as a heterogeneous infiltrating parotid mass with irregular margins. On CT scan, it presents as a mixed attenuation density mass, while on MRI it exhibits low T2 signal (Fig. 75.4). Warthin's tumor is more commonly seen in elderly male smokers, and presents as well-circumscribed intraparotid masses, which may be solid or inhomogeneous. About a fifth of Warthin's tumors are multicentric. It also has the confounding distinction of being positive on PET and Tc-99m pertechnetate scan, as opposed to BMT, which is cold on both (Fig. 75.5). Intraparotid lymph node enlargement due to systemic or regional nodal metastasis can present as multiple intraparotid masses, with or without central necrosis.

## Teaching points

On CT, a smoothly marginated and homogeneously enhancing ovoid or pear-shaped mass arising within the parotid space, with or without dystrophic calcification is characteristic. On MRI, the high T2 signal is characteristic of BMT. When present, ADC values higher than normal parotid parenchyma is characteristic of BMT. A large asymptomatic mass arising from the deep lobe of parotid gland is almost always BMT, however for surgical planning, it is important to distinguish deep lobe parotid BMT from true parapharyngeal BMT by looking for a fat plane between the parotid gland and BMT.

REFERENCES

1. Shah GV. MR imaging of salivary glands. *Neuroimaging Clin N Am* 2004; **14**: 777–808.

2. Christe A, Waldherr C, Hallett R, *et al.* Imaging of parotid tumors: typical lesion characteristics in MR imaging improve discrimination between benign and malignant disease. *AJNR Am J Neuroradiol* 2011 **32**: 1202–7.

3. Habermann CR, Arndt C, Graessner J, *et al.* Diffusion-weighted echo-planar MR imaging of primary parotid gland tumors: is a prediction of different histologic subtypes possible? *AJNR Am J Neuroradiol* 2009 **30**: 591–6.

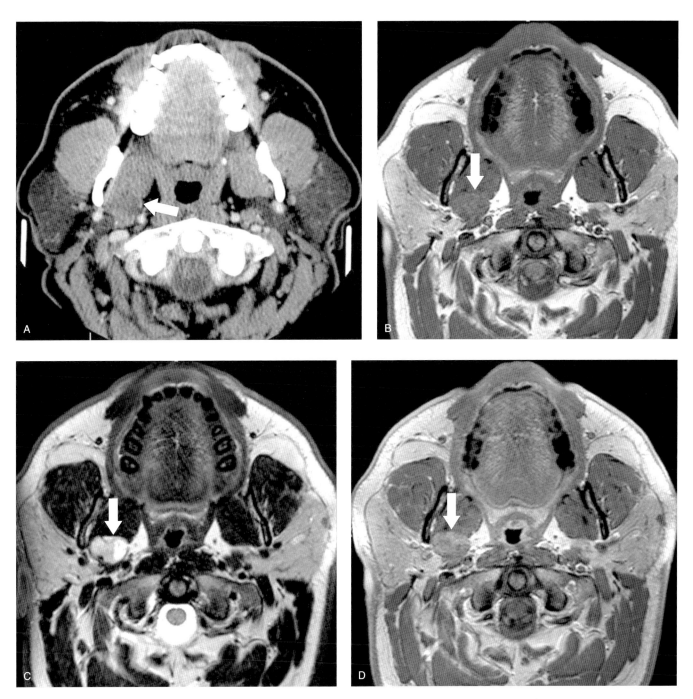

**Figure 75.1** BMT of deep lobe of parotid gland. (**A**) Contrast-enhanced axial CT exhibits a patchily enhancing heterogeneous mass in the deep lobe of the right parotid gland (arrow). (**B**) T1-weighted axial imaging exhibits a mass isointense to muscle (arrow). (**C**) T2-weighted axial imaging shows a heterogeneously high T2 signal mass (arrow). (**D**) Post-contrast T2-weighted axial imaging exhibits patchy enhancement (arrow).

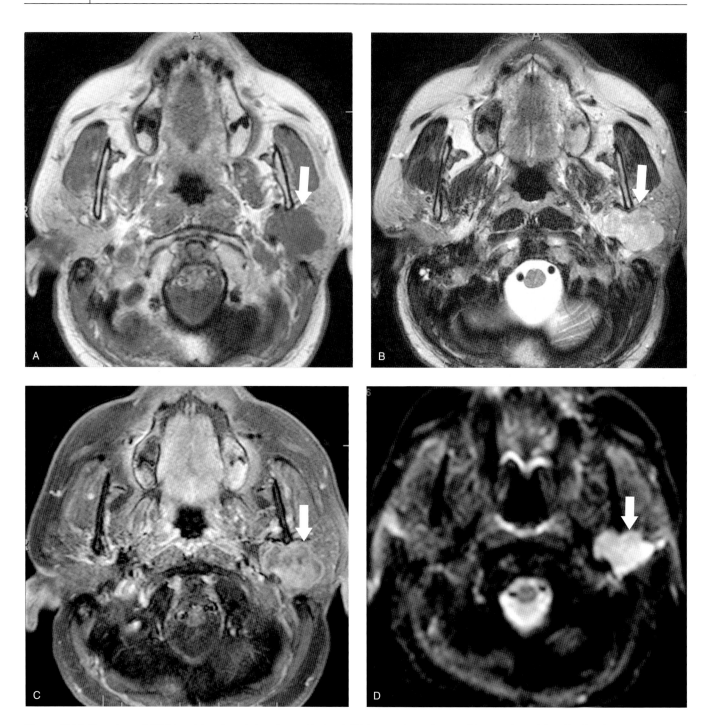

**Figure 75.2** Pear-shaped BMT involving deep lobe of parotid gland. (**A**) A pear-shaped, smoothly marginated, low T1 signal mass is seen extending from superficial to deep lobe of the left parotid gland through the stylomandibular notch (arrow). (**B**) A characteristic pear-shaped, smoothly marginated, high T2 signal mass with low T2 signal capsule (arrow) is seen extending through the stylomandibular notch from superficial to deep lobe. (**C**) Post-contrast fat-saturated T1-weighted axial image exhibits patchy post-contrast enhancement of the mass (arrow). (**D**) Hyperintense signal is seen on diffusion-weighted imaging (arrow). (**E**) The mass exhibits higher diffusion coefficient (arrow) than normal parotid parenchyma (short arrow).

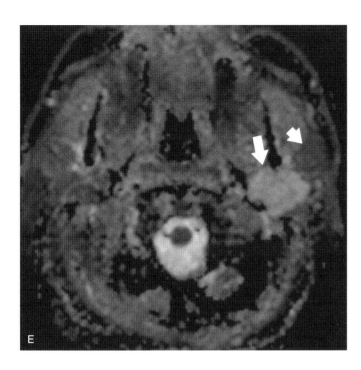

**Figure 75.2** (cont.)

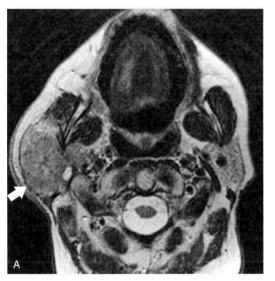

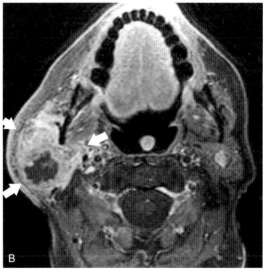

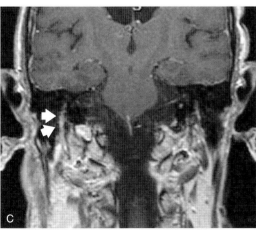

**Figure 75.3** Adenoid cystic carcinoma of parotid gland. (**A**) An expansile low T2 signal mass is seen at the superficial and deep lobe of right parotid gland without characteristic pear shape (arrow). (**B**) On fat-saturated post-contrast T1-weighted axial image, intense heterogeneous post-contrast enhancement with irregular tumor margins and central area of necrosis is seen (arrow). (**C**) Post-contrast T1-weighted coronal image exhibits perineural enhancement along the mastoid portion of the right facial nerve (short arrows).

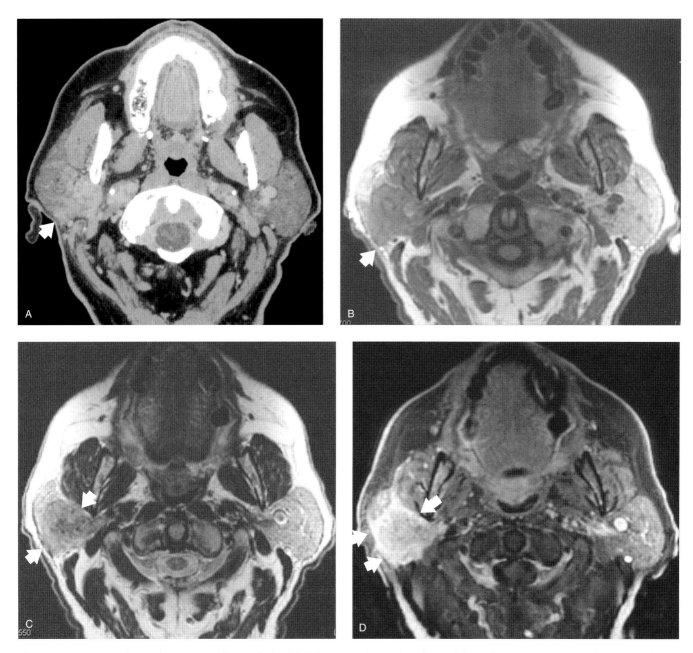

**Figure 75.4** Mucoepidermoid carcinoma of parotid gland. (**A**) Contrast-enhanced axial CT exhibits a heterogeneous, irregular mass at the superficial lobe of the right parotid gland (short arrow). (**B**) T1-weighted axial image exhibits low T1 signal mass at the superficial lobe (short arrow). (**C**) T2-weighted axial image shows irregular low T2 signal mass (short arrows). (**D**) Post-contrast fat-saturated T1-weighted axial imaging exhibits an intensely enhancing mass with irregular margins, with possible pericapsular spread (short arrows).

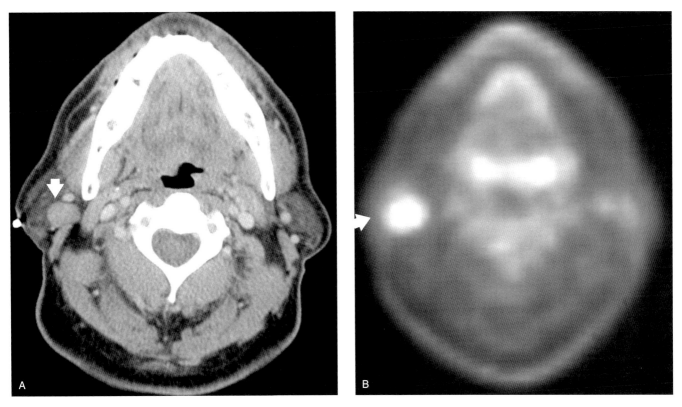

**Figure 75.5** Warthin's tumor. (**A**) Contrast-enhanced axial CT exhibits a patchily enhancing solid mass at the superficial lobe of the right parotid gland (short arrow). (**B**) FDG-PET imaging shows metabolic activity at the right parotid tumor.

## Imaging description

Repeated otorrhea and recurrent parotid swelling in infancy and childhood should prompt further cross-sectional imaging. One of the most important causes for this condition is infected first branchial cleft cyst. The branchial anomalies occur as a result of persistence of vestigial remnants of first branchial apparatus [1,2]. They are rare lesions. The first branchial cleft cyst accounts for only 8–10% of branchial cleft anomalies. They are divided into two major types [3]. Type I first branchial cleft cyst occurs in the preauricular area and lies parallel to the external artery canal (EAC) and lateral to the facial nerve (Fig. 76.1). Type II first branchial cysts are located posterior or inferior to the angle of the mandible and are intimately associated with the parotid gland and facial nerve (Fig. 76.2). There is generally presence of a sinus track reaching up to the junction of the membranous and bony portion of the external auditory canal and in close proximity to the facial nerve [2,3].

## Importance

The first branchial cleft anomalies are relatively rare. A high index of suspicion in patients with a cyst or sinus around EAC and within the parotid gland is important. Incision and drainage of suppurative fluid collection can result in repeated recurrence. Definitive total surgical excision, achieved with a superficial parotidectomy approach with facial nerve identification and facial nerve exposure, results in excellent outcomes [4].

## Typical clinical scenario

A compressible mass in the parotid or periparotid area in infancy and childhood is more common; however, the initial diagnosis can be made in patients of any age. Recurrent pre- or postauricular swelling, sometimes seen with respiratory tract infections with or without discharge from the external auditory canal, is a more typical clinical history. Recurrence in a patient with a history of abscess drainage in the parotid gland should raise suspicion of a first branchial cleft cyst [5].

## Differential diagnosis

A benign cystic mass of the parotid gland, such as obstructive or traumatic retention cyst, exhibits low T1 and high T2 signal without post-contrast enhancement (Fig. 76.3). Lymphatic malformation, formerly known as cystic hygroma (Fig. 76.4), is more commonly a multilocular infiltrating serpiginous mass with low T1 and high T2 signal on MRI. However, if unilocular, it may be difficult to differentiate from first branchial cleft cyst. A neck abscess appears as a thick-walled lobulated mass with peripheral ring enhancement. It is commonly seen in lymph-node-bearing submandibular or retropharyngeal space, rarely within the parotid gland (Fig. 76.5). However, it is associated with cellulitis and pericapsular involvement and is clinically associated with rapid onset with marked fever and tenderness. A necrotic or suppurative intraparotid lymph node can present as an ovoid and cystic mass within the parotid gland. If single, it is difficult to differentiate from infected first branchial cleft cyst.

## Teaching points

An ovoid, non-enhancing, cystic mass in the area around the EAC or within the parotid gland should raise the suspicion for first branchial cleft cyst. When infected, it can exhibit peripheral contrast enhancement with inflammatory changes within the parotid gland and surrounding soft tissue.

REFERENCES

1. Benson MT, Dalen K, Mancuso AA, et al. Congenital anomalies of the branchial apparatus: embryology and pathologic anatomy. *Radiographics* 1992; **12**: 943–60.
2. Ankur G, Bhalla AS, Sharma R. First branchial cleft cyst (type II). *Ear Nose Throat J* 2009; **88**: 1194–5.
3. Work WP. Newer concepts of first branchial cleft defects. *Laryngoscope* 1972; **82**: 1581–93.
4. Bajaj Y, Tweedie D, Ifeacho S, Hewitt R, Hartley BE. Surgical technique for excision of first branchial cleft anomalies: how we do it. *Clin Otolaryngol* 2011; **36**: 371–4.
5. Triglia JM, Nicollas R, Ducroz V, Koltai PJ, Garabedian EN. First branchial cleft anomalies: A study of 39 cases and a review of the literature. *Arch Otolaryngol Head Neck Surg* 1998; **124**: 291–5.

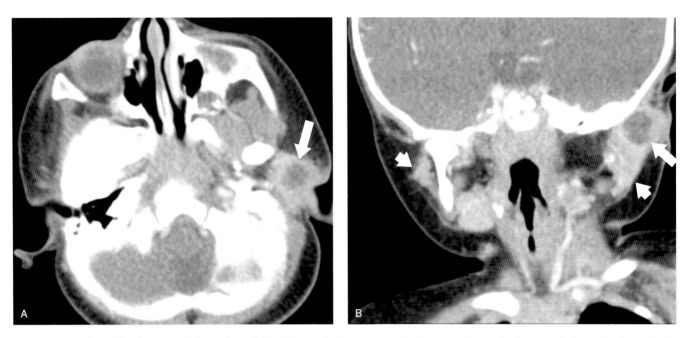

**Figure 76.1** Infected first branchial cleft cyst (type I). (**A, B**) A rounded low-attenuating intraparotid mass in the preauricular region (arrow) with peripheral rim enhancement is seen, with a patchily enhancing and enlarged parotid gland (left small arrow). It lies in a plane parallel to the external auditory canal and lateral to the expected course of the facial nerve.

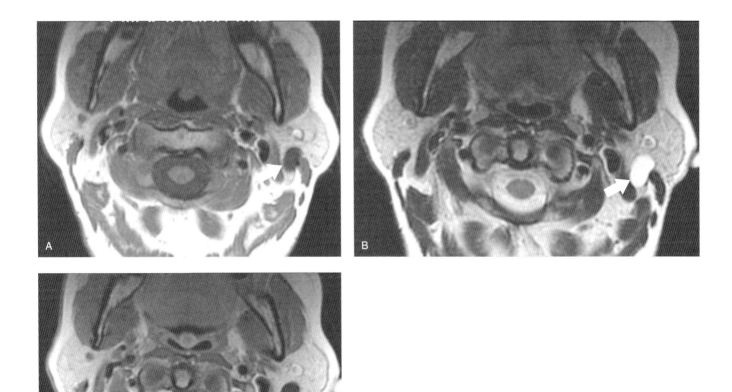

**Figure 76.2** First branchial cleft cyst (type II). (**A**) An oval, low T1 signal and marginated lesion is seen within the parotid gland posterior and inferior to the angle of the mandible (arrow). (**B**) The lesion exhibits high T2 signal with thin wall, compatible with a benign cyst (arrow). (**C**) On post-contrast imaging, there is no significant enhancement of the lesion (arrow).

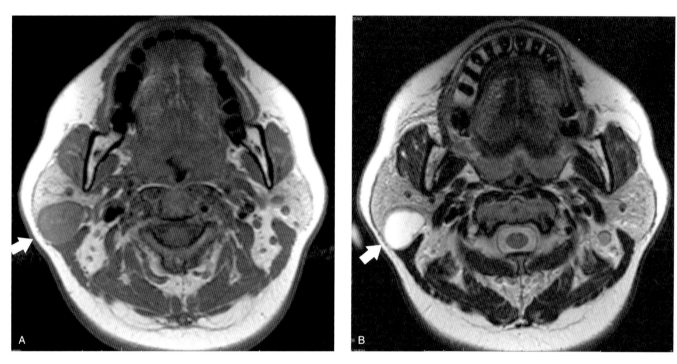

**Figure 76.3** Obstructive or traumatic retention cyst. (**A**, **B**) A rounded, well-defined low T1 and high T2 signal mass within the superficial lobe of the parotid gland (arrow). No discernible tissue characteristics were seen on postsurgical histopathologic examination.

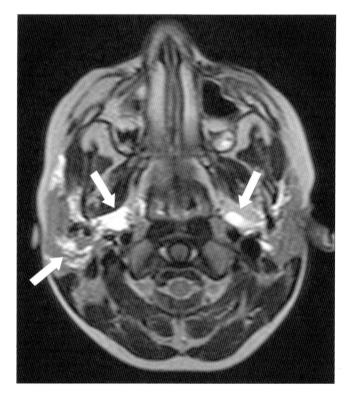

**Figure 76.4** Lymphatic malformation. Serpiginous multilocular high T2 signal channels are seen bilaterally within the suprahyoid neck spaces, including parapharyngeal, masticator, and parotid space.

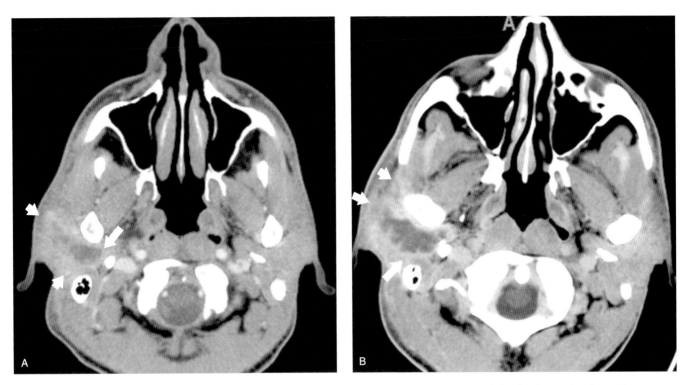

**Figure 76.5** Parotid abscess. (**A**, **B**) An elongated low-attenuating lesion is seen within the right parotid gland with peripheral rim enhancement (arrow). There is patchy enhancement and enlargement of the right parotid gland with pericapsular and subcutaneous stranding (short arrows).

# Nasopharyngeal cysts

## Imaging description

Cystic mass lesions of the nasopharynx are common and often encountered incidentally on CTs and MRIs done for other reasons. The most common cystic masses seen in the nasopharynx are mucous retention cysts (MRC), which are often asymptomatic. MRC can occur anywhere in the upper aerodigestive system, but the nasopharynx is the most frequent site, followed by the valleculae. MRC wall has a pseudostratified ciliated epithelium and the cyst contains fluid that appears hypoattenuating on CT, hypointense on T1-weighted MRI, and markedly hyperintense on T2-weighted MRI, although cysts with a high protein content can demonstrate increased T1 and decreased T2 signal (Fig. 77.1) [1].

MRCs can be found anywhere in the nasopharynx but most commonly involve the lateral recesses and occasionally obstruct the Eustachian canals. They range from a few millimeters up to 20 mm in size. MRCs are covered with intact mucosa on endoscopic exam and may only be appreciated if they create a bulge on the nasopharyngeal wall.

Tornwaldt's cysts result from obstruction of the pharyngeal bursa, which is a persistent embryonic communication between the roof of the nasopharynx and the notochord. These cysts may be found in about 3% of the adult population. They are characteristically located in midline and show similar imaging characteristics to the MRC except for their location (Figs. 77.2, 77.3). They are often asymptomatic; although early reports of associated occipital headache exist, this has not been substantiated [2].

A third type of cyst seen in the nasopharynx is a tonsillar crypt cyst. These are usually smaller in size, in the order of a few millimeters, and located within the lymphoid tissue (Fig. 77.4).

## Importance

Nasopharyngeal cysts are common and often asymptomatic. They are only visible on imaging studies in most cases, and the radiologist should recognize them for what they are and avoid unnecessary work-up. When these cysts interfere with the Eustachian canal they can cause mastoiditis.

## Typical clinical scenario

These are almost always incidental findings.

## Differential diagnosis

Nasopharyngeal mass lesions should be considered in the differential diagnosis. On good-quality contrast-enhanced CT and MRI it is easy to recognize the typical imaging features, although non-contrast exams may show a soft tissue "fullness" that may mimic other mass lesions.

> ## Teaching points
>
> Various forms of benign nasopharyngeal cysts are commonly seen as incidental finding on CT and MRI of the brain, sinuses, and cervical spine. They are well-defined lesions with fluid signal/attenuation and should be separated from solid nasopharyngeal masses.

REFERENCES

1. Ben Salem D, Duvillard C, Assous D, *et al.* Imaging of nasopharyngeal cysts and bursae. *Eur Radiol* 2006; **16**: 2249–58.
2. Goodwin RW. Tornwaldt's disease: characteristic headaches syndrome and etiology. *Laryngoscope* 1944; **54**: 66–75.

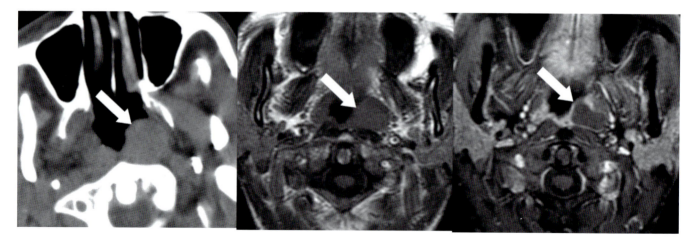

**Figure 77.1** Axial CT and MRI exam of the nasopharynx show some soft tissue fullness in the left fossa of Rosenmuller (arrows) which is difficult to differentiate from a mass, although the post-contrast T1-weighted image (right) reveals a very well-defined mucous retention cyst covered by intact mucosa.

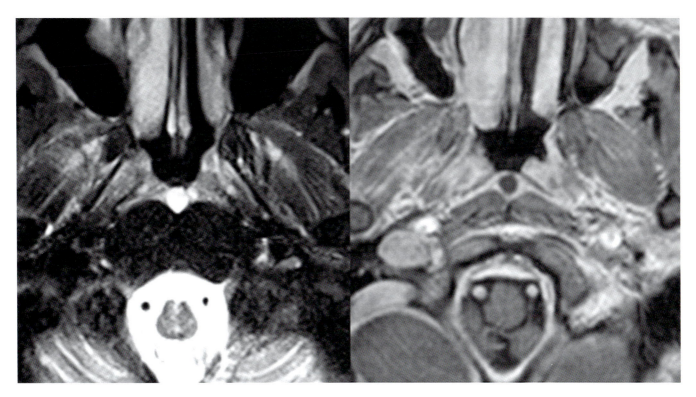

**Figure 77.2** Typical Tornwaldt's cyst with midline location, T2 hyperintensity, and no enhancement.

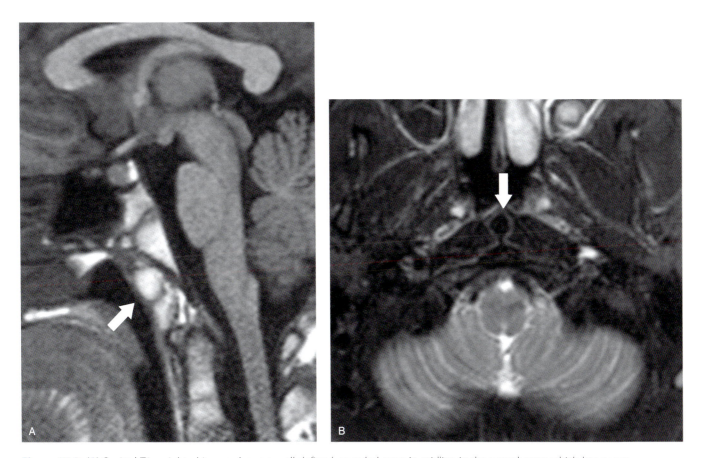

**Figure 77.3** (**A**) Sagittal T1-weighted image shows a well-defined, rounded mass in midline in the nasopharynx which has a very hypointense signal on (**B**) T2-weighted image, compatible with a Tornwaldt's cyst with high protein content.

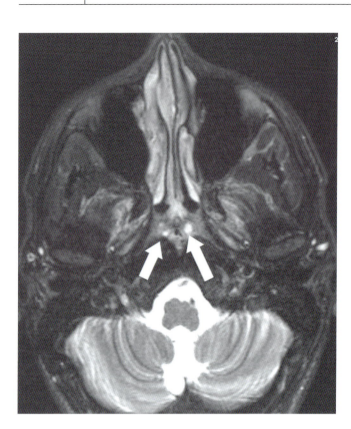

**Figure 77.4** Axial T2-weighted image shows multiple small cysts within the crypts of nasopharyngeal lymphoid tissue.

# CASE 78 Cystic nodal metastasis

## Imaging description

Squamous cell cancer (SCC) arising from the upper aerodigestive tract is common, and the first clinical presentation of SCC is a palpable neck mass in more than 30% of the cases as a result of metastatic nodes. Palpable neck mass often leads to CT or MRI, which show enlarged lymph node(s) and sometimes the primary mass in the pharynx or larynx. Most metastatic nodes are solid and show varying degrees of central fluid attenuation or signal due to necrosis, particularly when they are larger than 3 cm.

A nodal metastasis that is completely or mostly cystic is a phenomenon seen with increasing frequency secondary to increase in human papilloma virus (HPV)-related SCC of the neck (Figs. 78.1, 78.2) [1]. HPV-related SCC has a tendency to involve the oropharynx, and currently the majority of oropharyngeal SCC is secondary not to smoking but to HPV infection, which occurs in younger individuals who often lack the typical history associated with SCC of the neck, i.e., smoking and alcohol abuse. Clinicians and radiologists who are less familiar with this phenomenon may not be as concerned with the possibility of cancer in patients presenting with a cystic neck mass, and may consider congenital cystic masses such as branchial cleft cysts or lymphatic malformations as the likely etiology. To compound matters further, these cystic metastatic nodes may not have any appreciable FDG uptake on PET studies due to their cystic nature. Adult patients presenting with cystic neck masses should appropriately be worked up for the presumptive diagnosis of SCC of the pharynx.

## Importance

The incidence of HPV-related SCC of the neck is increasing, while the classic tobacco-related SCC is decreasing, and this has resulted in a change in patient demographics. Currently most oropharyngeal SCC patients have HPV DNA in their tumor tissue and are younger. In some series HPV-related SCC makes up 80% of all oropharyngeal cancers. Cystic nodal metastases can occur in HPV-related SCC, and should not be mistaken for benign cysts.

## Typical clinical scenario

A young male non-smoker presenting with a painless neck mass that did not resolve with antibiotic treatment is a common scenario. Depending on the primary site, patients may have variable symptoms, but oropharyngeal primaries in particular tend to be asymptomatic unless they are large.

## Differential diagnosis

Although second branchial cleft cysts (BCC) and cystic lymphatic malformations are traditionally considered in the differential diagnosis for a patient with a cystic lateral neck mass, all patients over the age of 35 with a cystic mass in nodal basins should undergo needle biopsy and/or surgical resection and endoscopic evaluation of the pharynx. Statistically it is very unlikely for congenital cysts to present in adulthood, with the notable exception of thyroglossal duct cysts, which occur in a classic midline location and should not be confused with a nodal mass. Thyroid cancer nodal metastases can also be cystic and should be considered in the differential diagnosis (Fig. 78.3). Acutely infected lymph nodes (lymphadenitis or suppurated lymph nodes) can have cystic appearance, but these are tender to touch and associated with erythema, fever, and leukocytosis (Fig. 78.4).

> ## Teaching points
>
> A cystic mass in nodal basins in adult patients is much more likely to be a manifestation of HPV-related SCC of the pharynx than a benign cyst.

REFERENCES

1. Goldenberg D, Begum S, Westra WH, *et al.* Cystic lymph node metastasis in patients with head and neck cancer: an HPV-associated phenomenon. *Head Neck* 2008; **30**: 898–903.

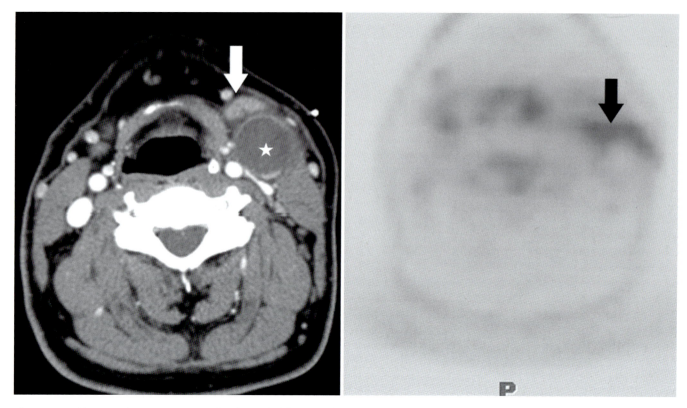

**Figure 78.1** Young male patient presented with a palpable mass which was cystic on CT and did not pick up FDG on subsequent PET. This was proven to be a metastatic lymph node. Arrow points to the submandibular gland, which shows enhancement and FDG uptake.

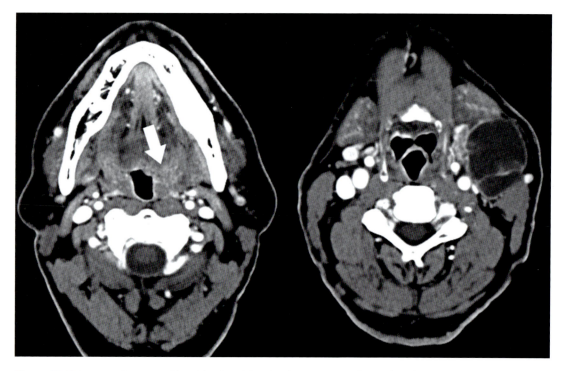

**Figure 78.2** Large cystic mass with minimal peripheral enhancement and an enhancing septum was a metastatic node from a small left tonsil SCC (arrow).

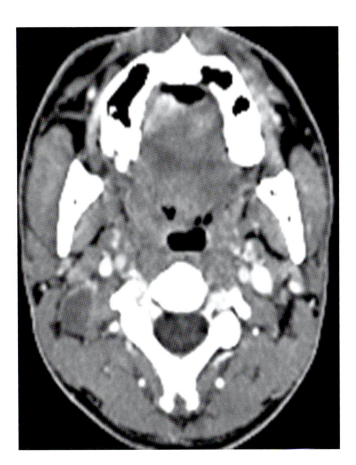

Figure 78.3 Cystic nodal mass in the right level II was proven to be metastasis from papillary thyroid carcinoma.

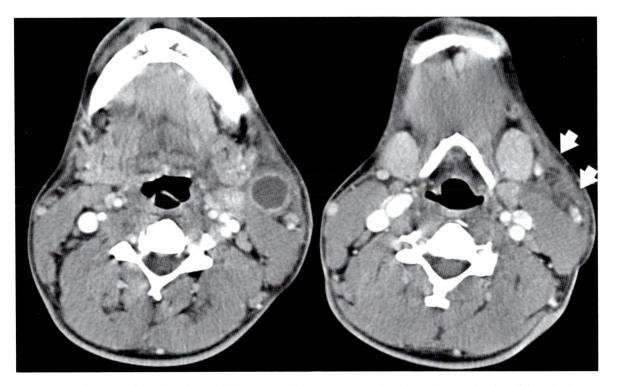

Figure 78.4 Cystic nodal mass in left level II in a patient with tenderness and erythema. Note induration of the subcutaneous tissue (arrows) adjacent to the mass, compatible with suppurative adenitis.

# Low-flow vascular malformations

## Imaging description

Mulliken and Glowacki's seminal work resulted in a widely accepted biologic classification of congenital vascular anomalies into vascular tumors (hemangiomas) and vascular malformations, based on their endothelial characteristics [1]. Hemangioma is a vascular tumor characterized by rapid endothelial proliferation shortly after birth. The lesion is typically absent at birth, demonstrates growth in early infancy, followed by a spontaneous resolution in childhood.

On the other hand, vascular malformations are structural anomalies that have a normal growth rate and endothelial turnover. These are congenital, have an equal gender incidence, and almost never involute spontaneously. These lesions can be divided into low-flow vascular malformations (LFVMs) (capillary, venous, lymphatic, and mixed) and high-flow vascular malformations (arteriovenous malformations and fistulas).

The capillary malformations (e.g., port-wine stains) are well-demarcated lesions, typically pink in infancy. Imaging is typically done to exclude associated deeper lesions and associated CNS or ocular abnormalities, rather than to assess the capillary malformation itself. Venous and lymphatic malformations of the head and neck may present with a mass or facial deformity and may coexist.

Both venous and lymphatic malformations typically demonstrate a bright signal on T2 imaging. For this reason, T2-weighted sequences, preferably with fat suppression, are quite useful in delineating the entire extent of the lesion. Venous malformations (VMs) enhance avidly, but the enhancement pattern is heterogeneous. VMs may also display adjacent enhancing tubular or serpentine channels (Figs. 79.1, 79.2). Presence of phleboliths is virtually pathognomonic of VMs. Phleboliths are hypointense on all T1- and T2-weighted sequences (Fig. 79.1), and hyperdense, lamellated in appearance on CT.

The enhancement pattern of lymphatic malformations (LMs) is more variable. Circumferential, mild rim enhancement is common with macrocystic LMs (Fig. 79.3). The microcystic lesions can enhance markedly and mimic other mass lesions. On MRI, macrocysts are T2 hyperintense and T1 hypointense, while on CT they are hypodense. On both MRI and CT, the imaging characteristics may be altered by intracystic hemorrhage. There is variable enhancement of cyst septations on both MRI and CT. However, LMs may enhance briskly, in the setting of super-infection and inflammation.

## Importance

Accurate diagnosis is important, since the treatment is multidisciplinary and varies according to the type of malformation.

## Typical clinical scenario

VMs in the head and neck can present as superficial masses, resulting in cosmetic issues, swelling, skin discoloration, and pain. Lesions occurring in deep compartment may result in difficulty in swallowing or chewing, or bleeding. LMs present early in life and have a strong predilection for head and neck. Sudden enlargement may follow infection or intralesional hemorrhage.

## Differential diagnosis

Lymphangiomas and VMs must be differentiated from high-flow lesions and hemangiomas. The high-flow arteriovenous malformations (AVMs) display a cluster of flow voids on MRI (Fig. 79.4). A CTA or dynamic MRA will establish a firm diagnosis, although DSA may be necessary in some cases. Differentiating hemangiomas from VMs may be difficult; hemangiomas can have vessels within the lesion that are helpful in the differential diagnosis when present (Fig. 79.5). These vessels show arterial flow spectra on Doppler and flow voids on MRI.

> ## Teaching points
>
> LFVMs commonly occur in the head and neck region. Phleboliths are a characteristic feature of VMs. Flow voids in and around the lesion are suggestive of high-flow AVMs. Small flow voids within the lesion are characteristic of hemangiomas.

REFERENCES

1. Mulliken JB, Glowacki J. Hemangiomas and vascular malformations in infants and children: a classification based on endothelial characteristics. *Plast Reconstr Surg* 1982; **69**: 412–22.

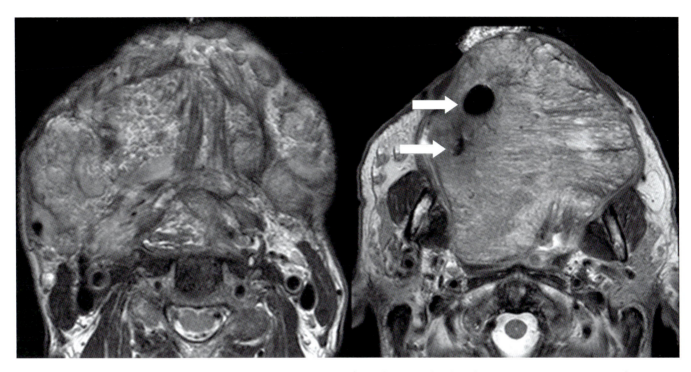

**Figure 79.1** Extensive venous malformation of the tongue and base of mouth. T2-weighted axial images demonstrate a large, infiltrative, trans-spatial mass with tubular and rounded channels as well as phleboliths (arrows). These findings are characteristic of venous malformations.

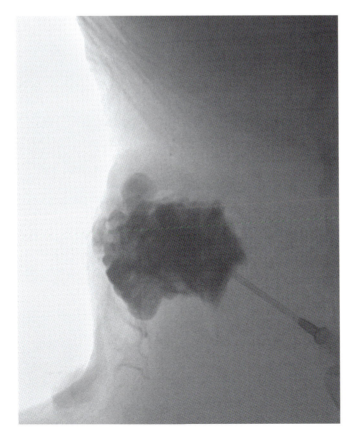

**Figure 79.2** A direct puncture of venous malformation of the neck demonstrates a typical channel consisting of stagnant, venous spaces. This patient was treated with sclerotherapy.

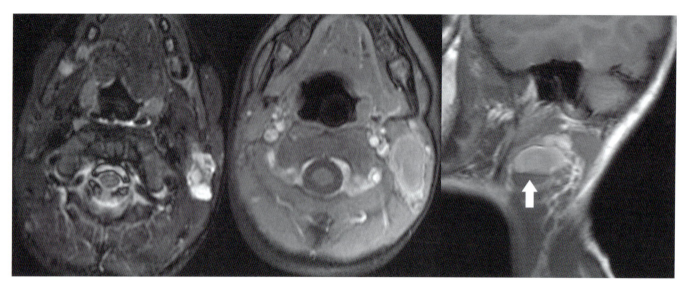

**Figure 79.3** Axial T2-weighted, enhanced fat-suppressed T1-weighted, and sagittal T1-weighted images demonstrate a presumed infected lymphangioma of the neck. Note a heterogeneous appearance on T2-weighted imaging, mild circumferential enhancement and a fluid-fluid level.

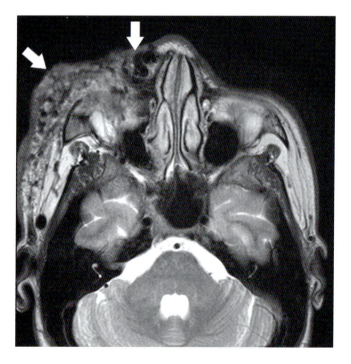

**Figure 79.4** Large, high-flow AVM of the face. Presence of extensive, tubular flow voids is suggestive of high-flow vascularity associated with these lesions (arrows).

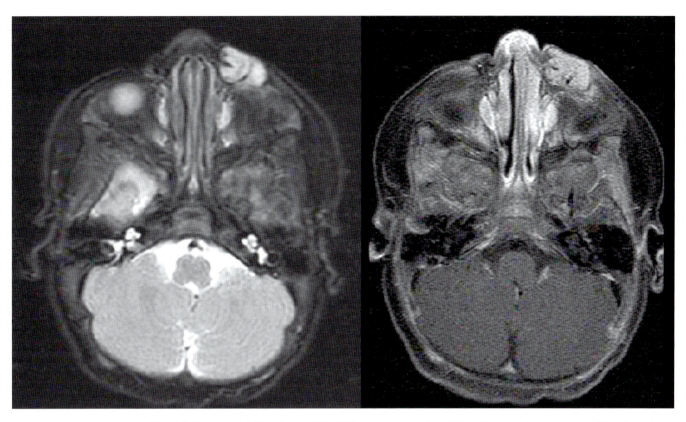

**Figure 79.5** Hemangioma of the left lower eyelid. Note flow voids within the mass on both T2-weighted and post-contrast T1-weighted images, which helps to differentiate this from a VM.

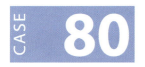 

## Imaging description

The parapharyngeal space (PPS) is the central space of the suprahyoid neck, which is in close relationship with multiple other neck spaces. It extends as an inverted pyramid from the base of the skull down to the junction of the posterior belly of the digastric muscle and the hyoid bone. Apart from fat, it contains only vessels, and no other content such as mucosa, muscle, lymph nodes, or bones, although ectopic minor salivary glands can occur in this space [1].

PPS tumors are rare, accounting for 0.5% of all head and neck neoplasms. However, with its conspicuity on CT and MRI, the PPS serves as an important landmark to identify the space of origin of a mass within the suprahyoid neck [2]. Between 70% and 80% of intrinsic lesions within the PPS are benign in nature, with salivary gland neoplasm being the commonest, accounting for about 50% of the benign masses [3]. This is followed by neurogenic tumors and paraganglioma, in descending order [4]. The commonest malignant neoplasm within the PPS is mucoepidermoid carcinoma arising from salivary tissue.

## Importance

Due to its deep location within the neck and its anatomic complexity, a PPS lesion is difficult and often impossible to diagnose clinically. Unless the mass is more than 2–3 cm in size, it is often clinically undetectable. The fat within the PPS serves as a natural contrast outlining a PPS mass on both CT and MRI. Depending on the direction in which the parapharyngeal fat is displaced by a mass, the space of origin for that mass can be determined.

## Typical clinical scenario

The most common presentation for a PPS mass is a painless parotid, oropharyngeal, or neck mass. Other symptoms include change in voice, abnormal pharyngeal sensation, dysphagia, dyspnea, otalgia, or facial pain [3]. Small lesions are often incidental findings on CT or MR imaging. Most masses are slow-growing and present in the adult age group, peaking in the fifth decade.

## Differential diagnosis

Benign mixed tumor (BMT) arises from the salivary gland and rests in the PPS. It appears as a well-defined and rounded soft tissue mass within the PPS, surrounded on all the sides by fat and separate from the parotid gland. When large, however, it appears contiguous with the deep lobe of the parotid gland. On CT, a well-defined but heterogeneous mass within PPS fat may exhibit foci of calcification. On MRI, iso- to hypointense T1 signal and hyperintense T2 signal and marked heterogeneous post-contrast enhancement is visualized (Fig. 80.1).

A neurogenic tumor, most likely schwannoma, appears to be a well-defined oval soft tissue mass with intermediate to hyperintense T2 signal and homogeneous post-contrast enhancement (Fig. 80.2).

A paraganglioma appears as an avidly enhancing soft tissue mass on CT scan. On T1-weighted MR imaging, it may exhibit high T1 signal, secondary to subacute haemorrhage, giving the matrix a "salt-like" appearance (Fig. 80.3). If larger, it may show presence of curvilinear and serpentine flow-void areas within it that appear like "pepper." On post-contrast imaging, there is rapid, dynamic, intense, post-contrast enhancement.

Venolymphatic malformations generally span across multiple compartments within the neck, and may sometimes be seen predominantly at the PPS. They appear as fluid-filled non-enhancing tubular channels with low attenuation on CT scan and hyperintense T2 signal on MRI (Fig. 80.4). The T1 signal is variable, with some of the hemorrhagic channels exhibiting hyperintense T1 signal, while predominantly lymphatic channels appear hyperintense.

A peritonsillar abscess within PPS displays high T2 signal and peripheral ring enhancement (Fig. 80.5). There is generally a history of previous tonsillar infection or abscess.

Large soft tissue masses from adjoining masticator space, parotid space, visceral space, carotid space, and even nasopharynx can extend within the PPS (Fig. 80.6).

---

### Teaching points

The most common intrinsic lesion of PPS is BMT. All primary PPS lesions should be entirely surrounded by fat, although when they are larger this is difficult to establish. More often, masses from surrounding spaces may encroach upon the PPS. The pharyngeal mucosal space mass pushes the PPS laterally, a parotid space mass pushes the PPS medially, a carotid space mass pushes the PPS anteriorly, and a masticator space mass pushes the PPS posteriorly.

---

REFERENCES

1. Shin JH, Lee HK, Kim SY, Choi CG, Suh DC. Imaging of parapharyngeal space lesions: focus on the prestyloid compartment. *AJR Am J Roentgenol* 2001; **177**: 1465–70.
2. Stambuk HE, Patel SG. Imaging of the parapharyngeal space. *Otolaryngol Clin North Am* 2008; **41**: 77–101.
3. Grosskopf CC, Kuperstein AS, O'Malley BW, Sollecito TP. Parapharyngeal space tumors: another consideration for otalgia and temporomandibular disorders. *Head Neck* 2013; **35**: E.153–6.
4. Gangopadhyay M, Bandopadhyay A, Sinha S, Chakroborty S. Clinicopathologic study of parapharyngeal tumors. *J Cytol* 2012; **29**: 26–9.

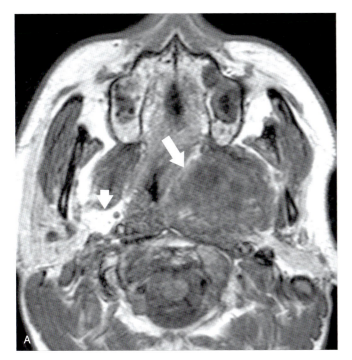

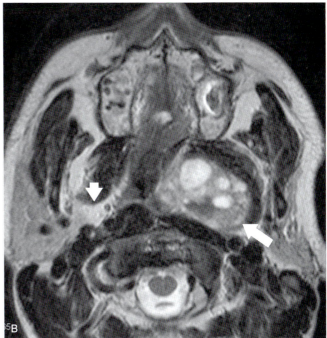

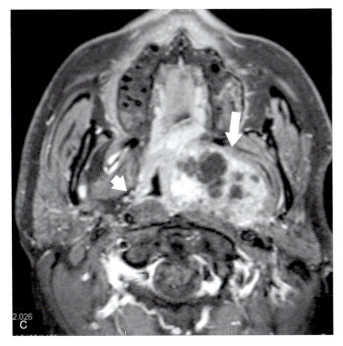

Figure 80.1 PPS benign mixed tumor (BMT). (A) T1-weighted axial MR imaging exhibits a rounded heterogeneous mass that exhibits isointense to hypointense T1 signal to muscle (arrow). The pharyngeal mucosal space is displaced medially, while the pterygoid muscles in the masticator space are displaced laterally. Note normal high T1 signal fat-filled PPS on the right (short arrow). (B) Fast spin-echo T2-weighted axial image exhibits a well-capsulated, heterogeneous left PPS mass with rounded areas of high T2 signal within a moderately high T2 signal matrix. There is presence of normal fat separating the lateral margin of the mass from the left parotid gland (arrow). Note normal mildly high T2 signal fat at right PPS (short arrow). (C) Post-contrast fat-saturated T1-weighted axial image exhibits intensely enhancing heterogeneous mass in the left PPS (arrow) with rounded non-enhancing areas of central fluid collection. Note enhancing veins of pterygoid plexus within the right PPS (short arrow).

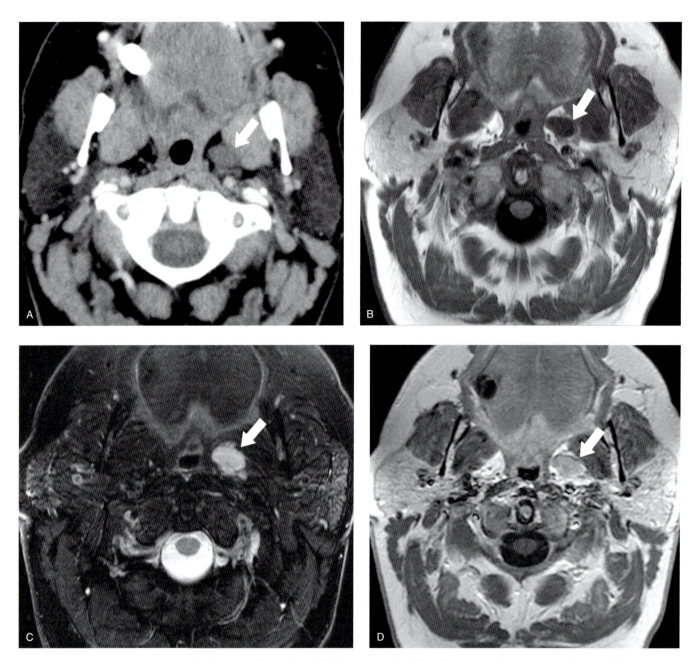

**Figure 80.2** PPS neurogenic tumor. (**A**) Contrast-enhanced axial CT shows an oval mildly enhancing soft tissue mass within the left PPS (arrow). (**B**) T1-weighted axial MR image exhibits an oval hypointense T1 signal mass within the left PPS, surrounded by high T1 signal fat (arrow). (**C**) Fat-saturated T2-weighted axial MR image shows that the mass exhibits hyperintense T2 signal (arrow). (**D**) Post-contrast T1-weighted axial MR image shows moderate enhancement of the mass (arrow).

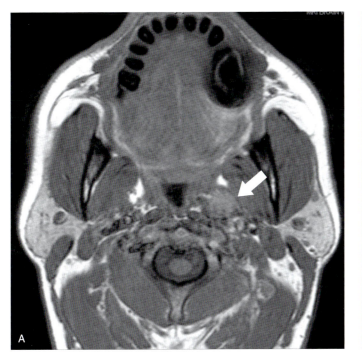

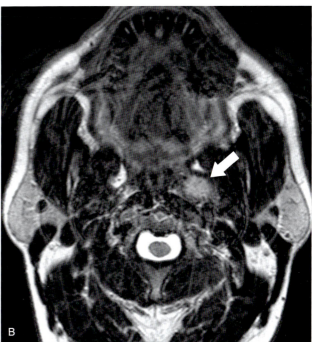

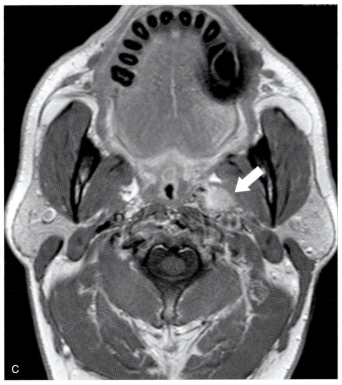

Figure 80.3 PPS paraganglioma. (A) T1-weighted axial MR image shows rounded left PPS mass with mildly hyperintense T1 signal matrix with a few curvilinear low T1 signal areas, giving a salt and pepper appearance (arrow). (B) T2-weighted axial MR image shows a heterogeneously hyperintense T2 signal rounded mass with presence of a few curvilinear flow voids (arrow). (C) Post-contrast T1-weighted axial MR image shows intense post-contrast enhancement (arrow).

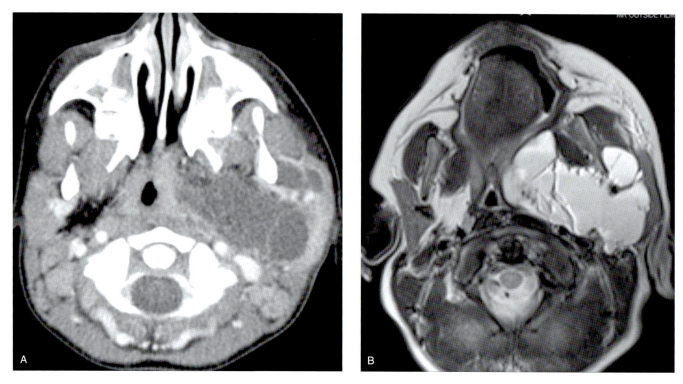

**Figure 80.4** Venolymphatic malformation. (**A**) Post-contrast axial CT exhibits large tubular low-attenuating lesion at left PPS, also seen at left parotid space and masticator space. Note normal low-attenuating fat-filled right PPS. (**B**) Fast spin-echo T2-weighted axial MR image exhibits fluid-filled tubular channels at left PPS, left masticator space, and left parotid space. Note normal high T2 signal fat-filled right PPS.

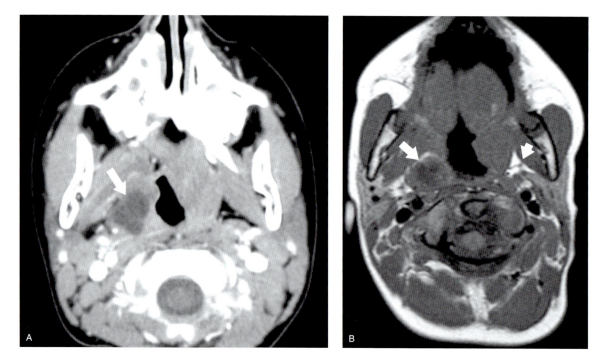

**Figure 80.5** Peritonsillar abscess. (**A**) Post-contrast axial CT reveals an irregular low-attenuating lesion at the right tonsillar pillar and palatine tonsil (arrow). This was found to be an abscess and was subsequently drained. (**B**) T1-weighted axial MRI, performed after 2 weeks of persistent symptoms, exhibits a right PPS heterogeneously hypointense T1 signal mass (arrow). Note normal high T1 signal fat-filled left PPS (short arrow). (**C**) Fast spin-echo T2-weighted axial MRI reveals loculated high T2 signal fluid collection at right PPS (arrow). Note normal high T2 signal fat-filled left PPS (short arrow). (**D**) Post-contrast fat-saturated T1-weighted axial MR image reveals patchy enhancement of the residual right tonsillar inflammatory phlegmon with peripheral enhancement of the right peritonsillar abscess (arrow).

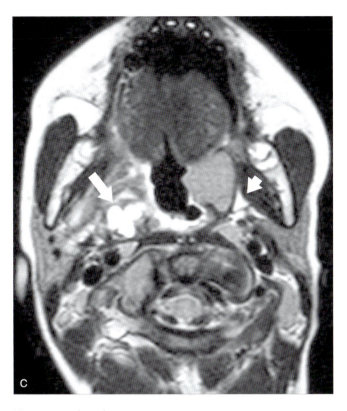

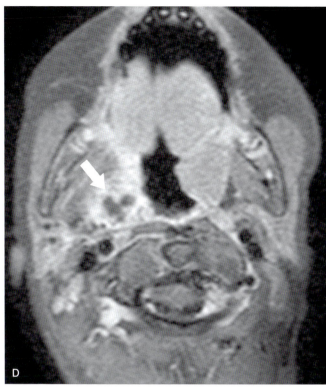

**Figure 80.5** (cont.)

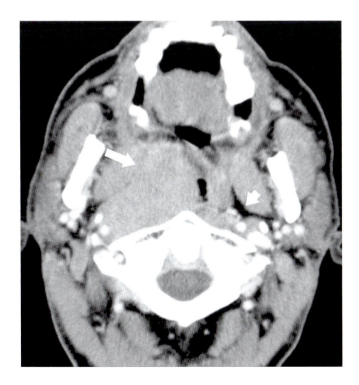

**Figure 80.6** HPV-positive nasopharyngeal carcinoma. Post-contrast axial CT reveals replacement of normal right PPS fat with a patchily enhancing large soft tissue mass originating from the right side of nasopharynx (arrow). Low-attenuating fat denotes left PPS (short arrow).

## Imaging description

Acute infections and abscesses of the neck are most commonly odontogenic in origin and occur in the vicinity of the oral cavity, and they may spread in some cases from there into the deep neck spaces. Acute infections of the salivary glands and lymph nodes (suppurative adenitis) account for the majority of the remaining cases. An abscess occurring within or in the vicinity of the thyroid is rare and should raise the suspicion of an underlying third branchial pouch anomaly, particularly in the pediatric population [1]. A sinus tract connecting the piriform sinus to the thyroid lobe has been recognized as the cause of childhood thyroid/perithyroid abscesses, and it may lead to recurrent infections if left untreated [1,2].

CT is the most commonly performed initial exam for a suspicion of neck abscess, and it shows a loculated fluid collection with variable rim enhancement in the region of the thyroid gland (Fig. 81.1). The overwhelming majority of cases occur in the left neck. Demonstration of a sinus tract emanating from the apex of the piriform sinus is diagnostic, and can be accomplished by barium swallow pharyngogram, CT with oral contrast, or endoscopic exam. However, exams performed during the acute inflammatory phase may be false negative [2]. It is believed that the sinuses or fistulas of the third or fourth branchial pouches are responsible, although there is a scarcity of thoroughly documented cases, and more recent studies have implicated the thymopharyngeal duct of the third branchial pouch as the more likely culprit [3,4].

## Importance

Most branchial anomalies arise from the second branchial pouch. Third branchial pouch anomalies account for only 3–10% of all branchial anomalies. The strong association between a left-sided intra/perithyroid abscess and third branchial pouch sinus is important to recognize, and should lead to a search for the underlying sinus tract to prevent recurrent abscesses.

## Typical clinical scenario

Third branchial pouch anomalies usually present with neck abscesses or acute suppurative thyroiditis in the pediatric age group. Clinical signs and symptoms include pain, tenderness, redness, fever, and leukocytosis. In newborns, they may present as a cystic mass.

## Differential diagnosis

In the proper clinical setting a loculated rim enhancing collection in the neck should be diagnosed as abscess and requires no differential diagnosis.

## Teaching points

Left-sided neck abscess in the vicinity of the thyroid and acute suppurative thyroiditis in children should prompt an investigation for a sinus tract arising from the piriform sinus.

REFERENCES

1. Pereira KD, Losh GG, Oliver D, Poole MD. Management of anomalies of the third and fourth branchial pouches. *Int J Pediatr Otorhinolaryngol* 2004; **68**: 43–50.

2. Stone ME, Link DT, Egelhoff JC, Myer CM. A new role for computed tomography in the diagnosis and treatment of pyriform sinus fistula. *Am J Otolaryngol* 2000; **21**: 323–5.

3. Thomas B, Shroff M, Forte V, Blaser S, James A. Revisiting imaging features and the embryologic basis of third and fourth branchial anomalies. *AJNR Am J Neuroradiol* 2010; **31**: 755–60.

4. James A, Stewart C, Warrick P, Tzifa C, Forte V. Branchial sinus of the piriform fossa: reappraisal of third and fourth branchial anomalies. *Laryngoscope* 2007; **117**: 1920–4.

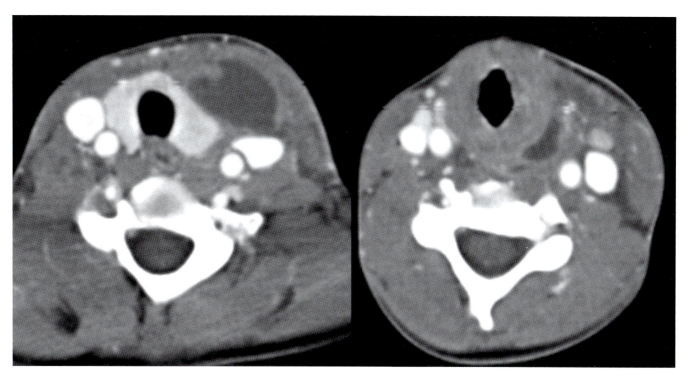

**Figure 81.1** Axial CT images of the neck demonstrate a fluid collection with an enhancing wall compatible with abscess adjacent to the left lobe of the thyroid. A sinus tract emanating from the apex of the left piriform sinus was found on endoscopy and cauterized.

## Imaging description

Classically, the parathyroid glands are situated posterior to the thyroid gland at the mid-superior and inferior pole bilaterally, and they are not easily detectable on cross-sectional imaging when they are normal. Up to 35% of lower parathyroid glands are ectopic, however, and may be present anywhere from the angle of the mandible to the lower anterior mediastinum.

A parathyroid adenoma is a benign neoplasm that secretes excessive parathyroid hormone (PTH), resulting in hypercalcemia. Due to its unpredictable location and hypermetabolic activity, Tc-99m sestamibi scintigraphy is considered to be the most specific technique to detect a parathyroid adenoma, although its sensitivity may be limited in small adenomas [1]. Ultrasound, CT, or MRI are used for anatomic correlation [2]. Recently, multiphasic contrast-enhanced CT, which can demonstrate contrast wash-in and wash-out characteristics of adenomas, has gained popularity, as it appears to have greater sensitivity and specificity compared to other techniques. Selective venous sampling of PTH for localization of parathyroid adenoma is reserved for complex postoperative cases where cross-sectional imaging and nuclear scintigraphy are inconclusive.

## Importance

Surgical excision is the most definite of treatment for parathyroid adenoma. However without preoperative imaging, it requires bilateral neck exploration for an acceptable cure rate. Decreased morbidity and improved success can be achieved with unilateral neck exploration following precise preoperative imaging [3,4].

## Typical clinical scenario

Patients with mild but prolonged hypercalcemia may have no or mild symptoms. These patients usually come to clinical attention by an abnormal serum calcium level detected during routine health care. Common presenting signs and symptoms include kidney stones, muscle cramps, bone pain, abdominal pain, psychiatric symptoms, syncope, and cardiac arrhythmias.

## Differential diagnosis

A parathyroid adenoma exhibits focal uptake of sestamibi on nuclear scintigraphy with about 90% sensitivity and specificity. On early scan, intense uptake by parotid, submandibular, thyroid, and parathyroid glands is seen. However, on delayed images, the parathyroid adenoma retains focal increased sestamibi uptake, while it washes out from thyroid gland and normal parathyroid glands (Fig. 82.1). On ultrasound, it appears to be a well-defined, rounded, hypoechoic but solid mass. On color Doppler, it exhibits hypervascularity. On CT scan, it appears as a well-circumscribed soft tissue mass with early and intense contrast enhancement. On MRI, it shows iso- to hypointense signal on T1-weighted images and hyperintense T2 signal (Fig. 82.1), with intense post-contrast enhancement.

A hypermetabolic thyroid gland can exhibit mildly persistent sestamibi activity and false positive scan (Fig. 82.2). A reactive lymph node in the paratracheal region or tracheoesophageal groove can mimic a parathyroid adenoma on cross-sectional imaging. However, it would not reveal hypervascularity on Doppler ultrasound or uptake on nuclear scintigraphy (Fig. 82.2).

Nuclear scintigraphy with Tc-99m sestamibi is more accurate for ectopic parathyroid adenomas (Fig. 82.3). Sometimes a thyroid adenoma can be exophytic and extend into the tracheoesophageal groove. On cross-sectional imaging and ultrasound, it may be misinterpreted as a parathyroid adenoma (Fig. 82.4). Conversely, an intrathyroid parathyroid adenoma may be misinterpreted as thyroid adenoma on cross-sectional imaging. However, nuclear scintigraphy is often able to differentiate between these two conditions. The most common reason for false negative scintigraphy is small adenomas (Fig. 82.5). Multiple adenomas and multigland hyperplasia are other sources of false negative and false positive results.

---

## Teaching points

Preoperative imaging of parathyroid adenomas provides precise anatomic localization and leads to minimally invasive surgeries and higher success rates. Nuclear scintigraphy has the highest specificity but lacks anatomic precision for minimally invasive surgery. Multiphasic CT provides the best road map for surgery and has a higher specificity than other anatomic imaging modalities. In difficult cases a combination of these two modalities is necessary. On CT, exophytic thyroid masses or enhancing paratracheal lymph nodes can mimic parathyroid adenoma, whereas intrathyroid parathyroid adenomas can be missed. Nuclear scintigraphy's sensitivity for small adenomas is less than satisfactory.

---

REFERENCES

1. Eslamy HK, Ziessman HA. Parathyroid scintigraphy in patients with primary hyperparathyroidism: 99m Tc sestamibi SPECT and SPECT/CT. *Radiographics* 2008; **28**: 1461–76.

2. Phillips CD, Shatzkes DR. Imaging of the parathyroid glands. *Semin Ultrasound CT MR* 2012; **33**: 123–9.

3. Rubello D, Casara D, Giannini S, *et al.* Importance of radio-guided minimally invasive parathyroidectomy using hand-held gamma probe and low (99m)Tc-MIBI dose. Technical considerations and long-term clinical results. *Q J Nucl Med* 2003; **47**: 129–38.

4. Casara D, Rubello D, Pelizzo MR, Shapiro B. Clinical role of 99mTcO4/MIBI scan, ultrasound and intra-operative gamma probe in the performance of unilateral and minimally invasive surgery in primary hyperparathyroidism. *Eur J Nucl Med* 2001; **28**: 1351–9.

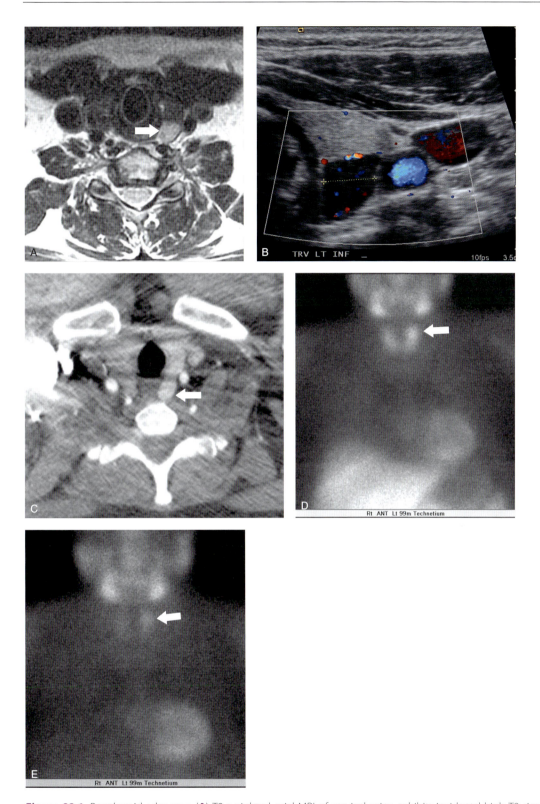

**Figure 82.1** Parathyroid adenoma. (**A**) T2-weighted axial MRI of cervical spine exhibits incidental high T2 signal nodule with relation to the posterior surface of superior pole of left thyroid gland (arrow). (**B**) Color Doppler ultrasound reveals a hypoechoic and hypervascular nodule posterior to superior pole of left lobe of thyroid gland, medial to the carotid artery and jugular vein. (**C**) Contrast-enhanced CT scan exhibits well-circumscribed enhancing soft tissue nodule posterior to the left lobe of thyroid gland (arrow). (**D**) Tc-99m sestamibi scan at 20 minutes exhibits normal tracer uptake within the parotid, submandibular, and thyroid glands with mildly high asymmetric activity at the superior pole of left lobe of thyroid (arrow). (**E**) Tc-99m sestamibi scan after 2 hours exhibits normal wash-out from thyroid glands with a focus of persistent sestamibi activity posterior to left superior thyroid lobe.

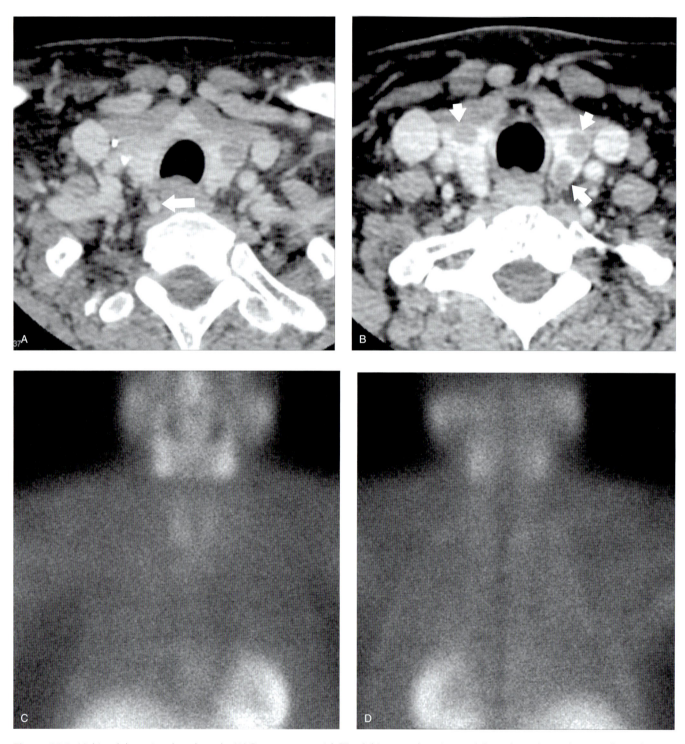

**Figure 82.2** Multinodular goiter, lymph node. (**A**) Post-contrast axial CT exhibits an enhancing nodule in the right tracheo-esophageal groove (arrow). (**B**) Post-contrast axial CT, more inferiorly, exhibits multiple rounded non-enhancing nodules (short arrows), compatible with known multinodular goiter. (**C**) Tc-99m sestamibi scan in anterior projection after 2 hours exhibits mildly persistent uptake at bilateral thyroid lobes. This is compatible with mildly hypermetabolic thyroid disease. (**D**) Tc-99m sestamibi scan in posterior projection up to 2 hours does not exhibit any significant tracer activity. Fine-needle aspiration cytology (FNAC) of the enhancing nodule seen on CT scan revealed an enhancing lymph node.

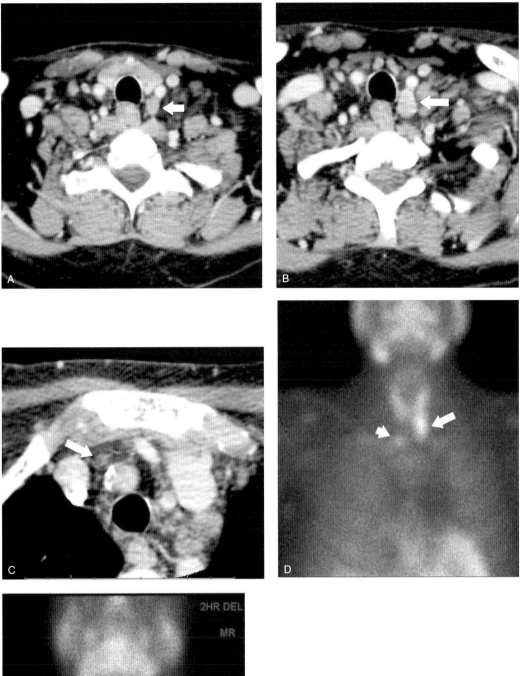

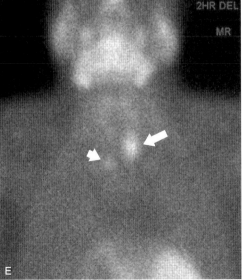

**Figure 82.3** Ectopic parathyroid adenoma. (**A**, **B**) Post-contrast CT in contiguous axial sections reveals a rounded enhancing nodule posterior to the inferior pole of left lobe of thyroid gland (arrow). (**C**) Post-contrast axial CT also reveals a smaller soft tissue nodule posterior to right sternoclavicular joint (arrow). (**D**) Tc-99m sestamibi scan after 20 minutes reveals more intense uptake at the inferior pole of left thyroid gland (arrow) with smaller uptake at the level of right sternoclavicular joint (short arrow). (**E**) Tc-99m sestamibi scan after 2 hours reveals persistent radiotracer activity at the inferior pole of left thyroid gland (arrow) and right sternoclavicular joint (short arrow), corresponding to enhancing soft tissue nodules seen on CT scan.

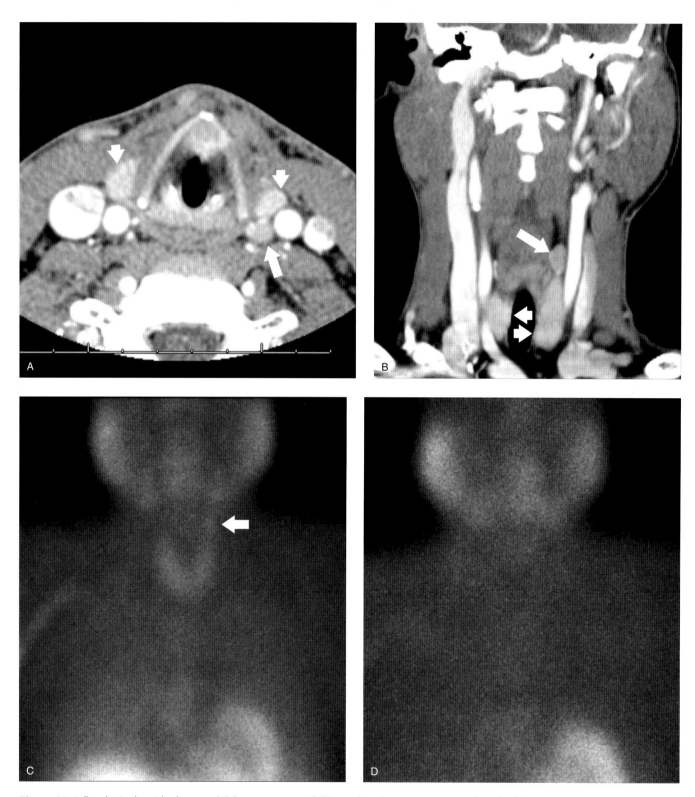

**Figure 82.4** Exophytic thyroid adenoma. (**A**) Post-contrast axial CT reveals enhancing superior poles of mildly prominent bilateral thyroid lobes (short arrows). There is an additional intensely enhancing nodule located posterior to the superior pole of left lobe of thyroid gland (arrow). (**B**) Post-contrast CT with coronal reconstruction exhibits the left-sided enhancing nodule (arrow) with mildly enlarged bilateral lobes of thyroid gland (short arrows) in the same anatomic plane. (**C**) Tc-99m sestamibi scan after 20 minutes reveals tracer uptake at bilateral thyroid lobes and at a nodule at the superior pole of left thyroid lobe (arrow). (**D**) Tc-99m sestamibi scan after 2 hours reveals wash-out of tracer activity.

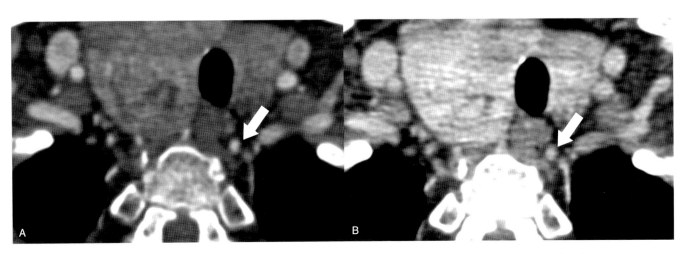

**Figure 82.5** Small adenoma. (**A**) Arterial and (**B**) venous phase images from a multiphasic CT exam show an intensely enhancing tiny adenoma posterior to the thyroid with decreasing enhancement on the venous phase due to rapid wash-out. Nuclear scintigraphy was negative.

## Imaging description

One of the popular measures for calculating the degree of stenosis uses ratio calculations to determine the percentage stenosis of the carotid bulb, as in the North American Symptomatic Carotid Endarterectomy Trial (NASCET) [1]. The formula for this calculation is: 1 − diameter of the stenotic segment of carotid/diameter of normal distal carotid × 100. The NASCET trial has shown that carotid endarterectomy is highly beneficial in symptomatic patients with ≥70% stenosis.

A particular subset of patients with high-grade stenosis have "near-occlusive" stenosis. When such a high degree of stenosis occurs, there is invariably a collapse of the lumen of the internal carotid artery (ICA) distal to the lesion. A collapsed ICA lumen may appear threadlike, and is referred to as the "string sign" on angiography [1]. These patients may later progress to complete carotid occlusion. Traditionally, patients with near-occlusive stenoses were treated with emergency revascularization, but it is now apparent that these patients actually have a lower risk of stroke under medical therapy than patients with marked (but not near-occlusive) stenosis, which is likely related to the presence of a better developed collateral vascular network.

MRA has been extensively utilized for evaluation of atherosclerotic disease. 2D TOF MRA provides a higher degree of flow contrast and is more resistant to saturation effects from slow flow, and is therefore more appropriate for distinguishing high-grade stenosis from occlusion. The anatomic correlate of TOF MRA in severe stenosis is "flow gap" or "flow void." Regardless of the TOF technique, the MRA overestimates the degree of stenosis. However, its strength lies in determining which patients do not have significant disease, and will therefore not require further examination. Because contrast in TOF techniques depends on flow, signal desaturation occurs in places where there is slow flow or turbulence. Contrast-enhanced 3D MRA is resistant to such effects, as it depends on the use of paramagnetic contrast and thereby uses T1 contrast rather than inflow effects (Fig. 83.1). Another technique that has gained popularity is "time-resolved" 2D or 3D contrast-enhanced MRA. Contrast-enhanced MRA is superior to TOF methods in distinguishing cases of near-occlusive stenosis from complete occlusion.

CTA is a non-invasive and widely available technique that produces images with high spatial resolution. CTA has also proven a valuable tool in correctly diagnosing near-occlusion from total occlusion (Fig. 83.2). Criteria for diagnosis of near-occlusion on CTA include a notable stenosis of the carotid bulb and the presence of distal ICA caliber reduction.

## Importance

Correct identification of near-occlusion has implications for management decisions. The management of carotid stenosis includes medical therapy, carotid endarterectomy, or stenting. It is important to understand that cases of near-occlusion of ICA may have a reduced risk of ipsilateral stroke compared to patients with severe stenosis of ICA.

## Typical clinical scenario

No specific clinical scenario is ascribed to near-occlusive stenosis. Symptomatic patients can present with transient ischemic attack (TIA) or stroke in the distribution of the affected carotid artery.

## Differential diagnosis

An important condition to be considered in the differential diagnosis is hypertrophied vasa vasorum in the setting of complete carotid occlusion (Fig. 83.3). The differentiation of vasa vasorum from residual lumen (string) is extremely important, since in these cases the carotid artery cannot be salvaged. Any inadvertent attempt to perform angioplasty can result in catastrophic rupture of the fragile collaterals. The vasa vasorum are relatively well-marginated, tortuous vessels that do not correspond to the expected course of the ICA lumen, occupy an eccentric location, and may even be multiple.

### Teaching points

Contrast-enhanced MRA and CTA are the cross-sectional modalities of choice that help differentiate between string sign and complete carotid occlusion with high levels of accuracy. In cases of uncertainty, DSA will be definitive.

REFERENCES
1. North American Symptomatic Carotid Endarterectomy Trial Collaborators. Beneficial effect of carotid endarterectomy in symptomatic patients with high-grade carotid stenosis. *N Engl J Med* 1991; **325**: 445–53.

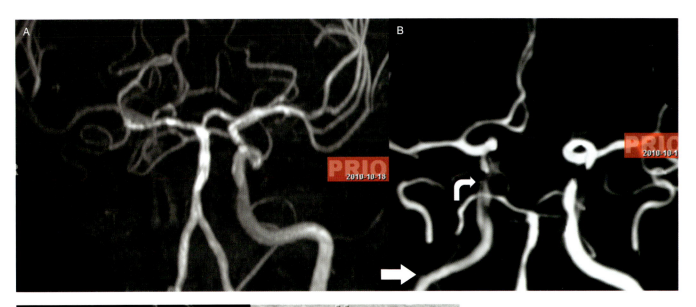

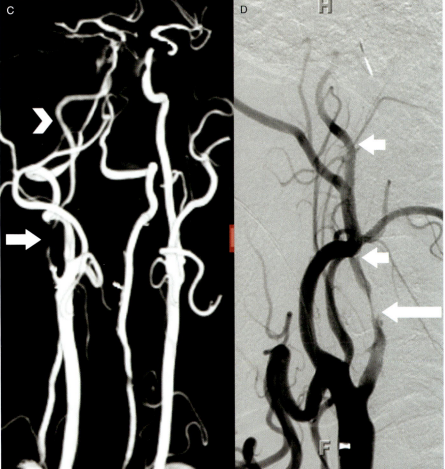

**Figure 83.1** (**A**) Time-of-flight (TOF) MRA in a patient with recurrent right hemispheric TIA events was suspicious for an occluded right internal carotid artery (ICA). No flow was noted in the cervical right ICA. (**B**) Contrast-enhanced MRA of circle of Willis demonstrates patency of right ICA (arrow) and a high-grade stenosis of cavernous ICA (curved arrow). (**C**) Although a flow gap is present in the proximal right ICA (large arrow), there is filling of cervical ICA (arrowhead) suggesting high-grade stenosis rather than occlusion on contrast MRA. (**D**) Flow is indeed confirmed on lateral DSA of the right common carotid artery. Note the string sign (arrow) and flow in the distal cervical ICA (small arrows).

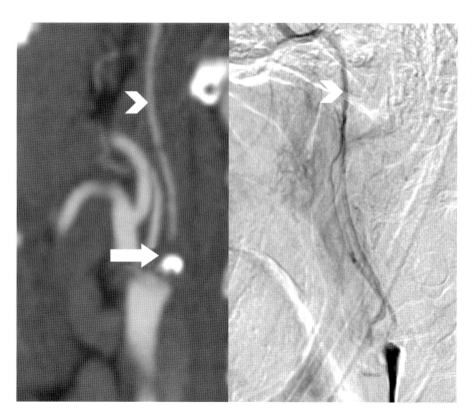

**Figure 83.2** String sign as evidenced on CTA and correlative DSA study. CTA shows a calcified plaque causing near-occlusive stenosis of ICA (arrow). The distal ICA is string-like and reduced in caliber on CTA and DSA (arrowhead).

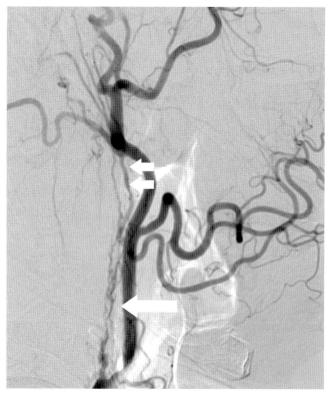

**Figure 83.3** Lateral view of carotid artery demonstrates tortuous, small vessels that are consistent with vasa vasorum (large arrow). These vessels reconstitute a small, distal cervical ICA (small arrows).

# **84** Carotid artery dissection

## Imaging description

CT angiography (CTA) is a highly sensitive and specific modality for large and medium vessel pathologies of the head and neck. Vessel wall thickening is often identified on CTA from a subintimal or intramural hematoma and frequently corresponds with "methemoglobin crescent sign" on MRA [1]. Dissecting aneurysms may be readily identified as focal outpouchings of the enhancing arterial lumen (Fig. 84.1), with or without associated thrombus, and often in an orientation parallel to the vessel. CTA is especially attractive in imaging patients with blunt or penetrating trauma, where imaging with MRI is difficult or sometimes contraindicated. Streak and beam hardening artifact from a patient's dental hardware may limit evaluation of the mid-cervical internal carotid artery (ICA), a commonly involved site for dissections.

MRI/MRA remains the initial screening modality of choice to evaluate patients with suspected non-traumatic cervical dissections. Fat-saturated axial T1- and T2-weighted sequences provide a sensitive technique to identify subtle dissections where no significant luminal narrowing may be appreciated on digital subtraction angiography (DSA). The periluminal (intramural) hematoma can be uniquely identified on MR imaging in the subacute stage (3–14 days). The classic finding is crescentic hyperintense signal peripheral to the flow void of an irregularly narrowed internal carotid artery. However, depending on the stage and composition of the hemorrhagic products, the signal on T1- and T2-weighted sequences may vary (Figs. 84.2, 84.3). In our experience, the presence of restricted diffusion on diffusion-weighted imaging (DWI) of the neck may also provide increased sensitivity for detection of intramural hematomas and detection of cervical dissections. Additionally, since both head and neck imaging are routinely performed, screening for ischemic intracranial complications can be simultaneously performed using DWI. 3D contrast-enhanced MRA of the neck has surpassed traditional time-of-flight (TOF) techniques, with higher spatial resolution and elimination of flow artifacts such as in-plane dephasing at arterial bends and signal loss due to slow or turbulent flow in carotid dissections [1].

DSA is now only needed as a problem-solving tool, or as a prelude to intervention. Detection of subtle intimal flap is best appreciated on DSA but seen in less than 10% of dissections.

The most common angiographic finding is a string sign, smooth tapered (or slightly irregular) luminal narrowing in approximately 65% of patients that may progress to an abrupt tapered, flame-like internal carotid artery occlusion.

## Importance

Early recognition of carotid artery dissection (CAD) helps with the institution of anticoagulant or antiplatelet therapy, which is highly effective in preventing the feared ischemic complications from CAD.

## Typical clinical scenario

Patients with cervical dissections may have a history of minor or major inciting events resulting in neck hyperextension or rotation, often with sudden transitional or decelerating movements. A classic clinical triad includes headache or neck pain, partial Horner's syndrome, and ischemic symptoms.

## Differential diagnosis

Carotid atherosclerotic disease can be distinguished from CAD on the basis of differing clinical presentations as well as imaging characteristics. Carotid atherosclerosis results in irregular narrowing of the proximal cervical ICA, commonly associated with involvement of the carotid bulb and the origin of the external carotid artery (Fig. 84.4). In contrast, the dissections tend to spare the proximal 2–3 cm of the cervical ICA. Calcifications, if present, favor atherosclerotic disease and are typically not encountered in CAD.

---

### Teaching points

It is important to remember that a classic sign of CAD, crescentic hyperintense signal from methemoglobin, is only present in the subacute stage and therefore cannot be relied upon in the acute stages of dissection. The diagnosis can be easily accomplished with MRA or CTA, and DSA is rarely needed.

---

REFERENCES

1. Ansari SA, Gemmete JG, Parmar H, Ibrahim M, Gandhi D. Cervical artery dissections: diagnosis, management and role of endovascular therapy. *Neuroimaging Clin N Am* 2009; **19**: 257–70.

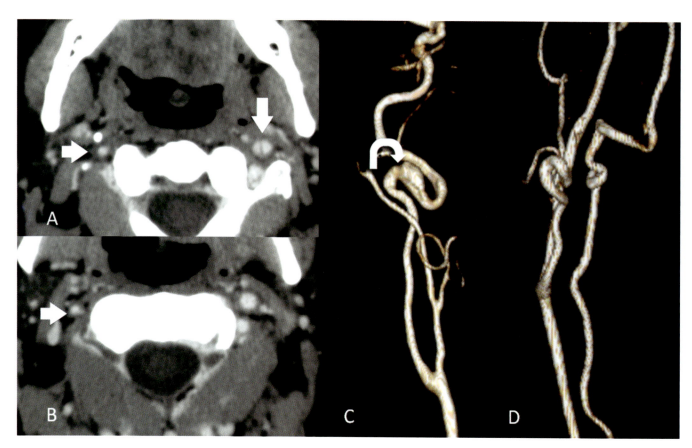

**Figure 84.1** (**A**, **B**) CTA of a patient with traumatic injury at presentation reveals bilateral CAD. An intimal flap is present in the left ICA (vertical arrow) and the right ICA is narrowed (horizontal arrow). (**C**, **D**) At 3-month follow-up, the patient has developed a dissecting aneurysm on the right (curved arrow) and the left ICA dissection has nearly healed.

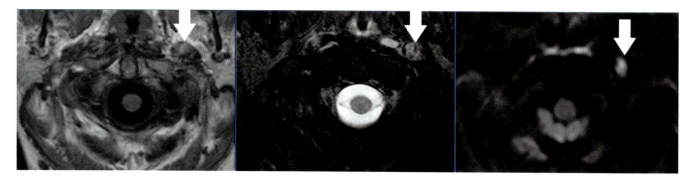

**Figure 84.2** Axial T1-weighted, T2-weighted, and DWI images are shown in succession in a patient with acute left ICA dissection on MRI. Note the acute hematoma in carotid wall on T1-weighted and T2-weighted images, but findings are even better appreciated on DWI images as an area of restricted diffusion.

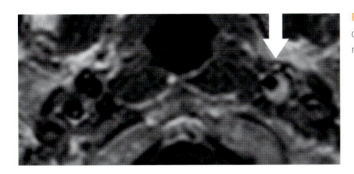

**Figure 84.3** The same patient as in Fig. 84.2, imaged a week later, demonstrates a typical, hyperintense, crescentric deposition of methemoglobin in the wall of the left ICA.

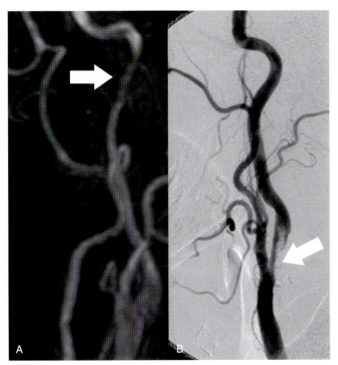

**Figure 84.4** Comparison of patients with (**A**) ICA dissection and (**B**) atherosclerotic disease. The ICA involvement in CAD is distal to the carotid bifurcation (horizontal arrow) but the atherosclerotic disease involves the carotid bifurcation and proximal ICA. There is a thrombus in the left ICA distal to stenosis (oblique arrow).

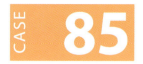

# Traumatic arterial injury

## Imaging description

Blunt and penetrating neck trauma can result in significant morbidity and mortality. While unstable patients, particularly those with penetrating injuries, are often directly taken for surgical exploration, relatively stable patients are evaluated with imaging for prompt diagnosis and treatment. Vascular injuries are significantly more frequent with penetrating injuries than with blunt neck trauma. Carotid artery is more frequently involved in penetrating injury. On the other hand, vertebral artery involvement is more common with blunt trauma.

The diagnosis of vascular injury can be made with either CTA or MRI/MRA, but CT is generally the technique of choice for initial evaluation of patients with neck and cervical spine injuries. This is especially relevant in patients with penetrating injuries, who may be suspected of having embedded metal fragments in the soft tissues (Fig. 85.1). Regardless of the mechanism of injury, similar imaging manifestations are seen on cross-sectional studies [1]. These include vascular dissections, dissecting aneurysms, arterial stenosis or occlusion, arteriovenous fistula, or frank extravasation (Figs. 85.1, 85.2, 85.3).

The imaging manifestations of dissections are discussed elsewhere (see Cases 4 and 84). Dissecting aneurysms (DAs) result from partial or complete disruption of arterial wall, resulting in collection of blood in the arterial wall or adjacent soft tissues. A DA is essentially the recanalized portion of this hematoma. On CTA or MRA, the DAs are eccentric to the lumen and communicate with it. The DAs are likely to be better defined and have a clearer margin, in contrast to areas of active extravasation of contrast, which will have a more irregular and heterogeneous appearance (Fig. 85.3). Occlusion of the artery is seen as lack of vessel enhancement on CTA or lack of signal in the vessel on time-of-flight (TOF) or contrast-enhanced MRA. Arteriovenous fistulas are the least common manifestations of neck injuries and more commonly seen with penetrating trauma, but may not be noted until days or sometimes months after initial trauma. The most common type of fistula in the neck is between the vertebral artery and perivertebral venous plexus (Fig. 85.4).

Cervico-cerebral angiography is generally not useful as a screening test but remains invaluable in evaluation of, and as a prelude to, endovascular repair of certain injuries (Figs. 85.2, 85.3, 85.4). It is also extremely useful for the diagnosis of a suspected injury if cross-sectional imaging techniques are degraded due to artifacts from metal fragments such as gunshot pellets or bullets.

## Importance

Injuries to the neck arteries carry a significant morbidity and mortality, especially so for injuries with penetrating mechanism, where mortality may be fairly high. The management of these lesions is multidisciplinary, with consideration often given to conservative therapy, anticoagulation or antiplatelet medications, surgical or endovascular repair. The factors that determine the treatment pathway include severity of vascular injury, presenting symptoms, and other associated injuries.

## Typical clinical scenario

Blunt trauma to the neck may occur from any mechanism that can result in sudden acceleration and deceleration, such as motor vehicle accidents, contact sports, and even chiropractic manipulation. The blunt neck trauma has a relatively low (<1%) rate of associated vascular injury. The majority of penetrating traumas are caused by gunshot and stab wounds, although these can result from any sharp objects.

## Differential diagnosis of traumatic injury

Subtle injuries may only result in thickening of vessel wall or a very small periluminal hematoma without vessel lumen alteration. In these cases, difficulty may arise in the detection of these changes, or in differentiating it from wall thickening related to atherosclerotic disease. In case of doubt, follow-up examination with a different cross-sectional modality, or in some cases angiography, is appropriate.

---

### Teaching points

Careful attention to the course of all the cervical vessels is essential in detecting vascular injuries. CT/CTA is becoming the technique of choice for initial screening, although angiography remains the gold standard for detection of subtle lesions and offers a possibility of endovascular repair in selected cases.

---

REFERENCES

1. Núñez DB, Torres-León M, Múnera F. Vascular injuries of the neck and thoracic inlet: helical CT-angiographic correlation. *Radiographics* 2004; **24**: 1087–100.

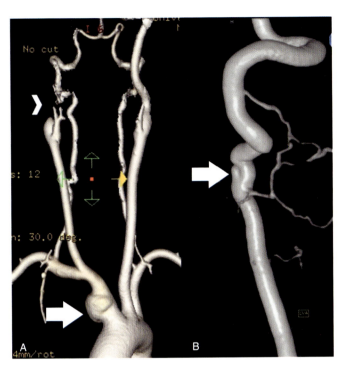

**Figure 85.1** CTA demonstrates several different post-traumatic lesions in a patient following a high-speed motor vehicle collision (MVC). (**A**) There is right ICA occlusion (arrowhead) and innominate artery dissecting aneurysm (arrow). (**B**) The left vertebral artery harbors a small dissecting aneurysm as well (arrow).

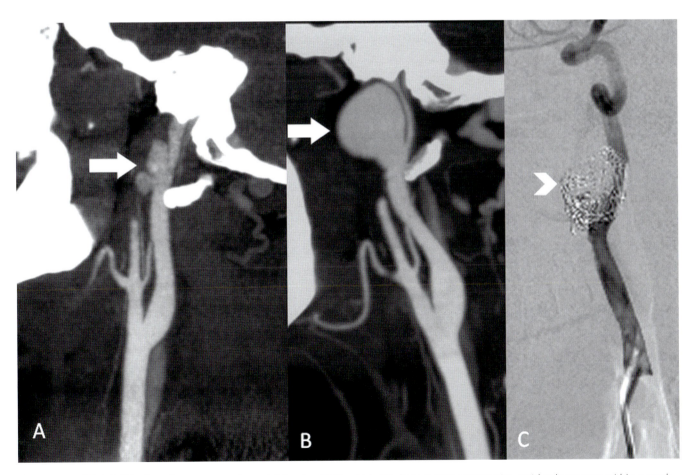

**Figure 85.2** (**A**) Left ICA dissecting aneurysm (arrow) following MVC, which (**B**) demonstrates progressive rapid enlargement within a week. (**C**) This was repaired endovascularly (arrowhead) with stent-assisted embolization.

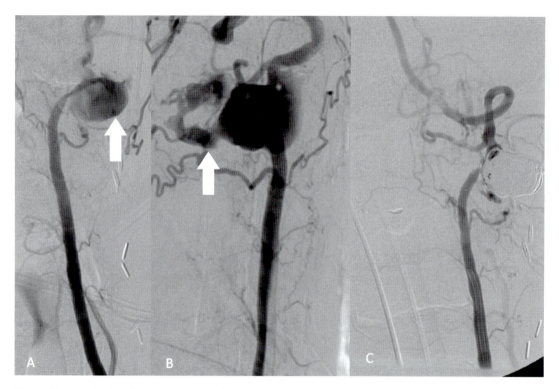

**Figure 85.3** (**A**, **B**) Rapidly expanding neck hematoma in a patient with ruptured left vertebral artery aneurysm following gunshot injury was studied with DSA. Note the irregular margins and contrast puddles, suggestive of active extravasation (arrows). (**C**) This was quickly controlled with embolization with stent assistance.

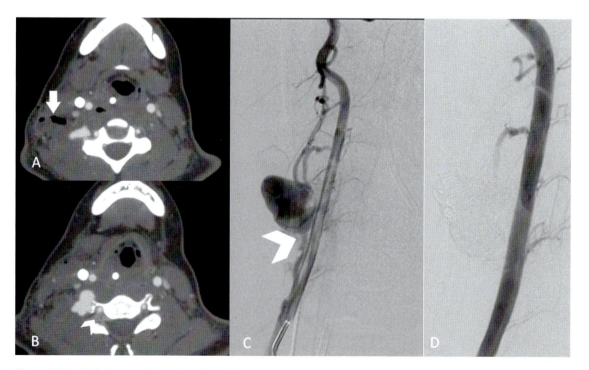

**Figure 85.4** (**A**) Stab wound (arrow) to the right neck resulting in right paravertebral and epidural AV fistula. (**B**) Note a large contrast collection in right paravertebral region, but there is additionally early filling of perivertebral venous plexus on this CTA (arrowhead). (**C**) Similar findings of a venous varix and early-filling veins are noted on right vertebral artery injection. (**D**) The varix and the fistula were obliterated with coils.

# CASE 86    Craniovertebral junction injuries

## Imaging description

Craniovertebral junction (CVJ) injuries are uncommon compared with other cervical spine traumatic injuries but they have a much higher rate of mortality and morbidity. When there is an associated fracture of the occipital condyles, clivus, or C1 vertebra, these injuries are easily identified on CT although plain radiograph diagnosis may be problematic. Some CVJ injuries, however, present with only ligamentous disruption and intact bones, making the diagnosis difficult for those who are not familiar with the normative measurements of the distances between the occiput and C1 (Fig. 86.1) [1].

Two of the CVJ injuries that can present with only ligamentous disruption are atlanto-occipital dissociations (AOD) and atlanto-axial dissociations (AAD) (Figs. 86.2, 86.3). AOD and AAD are extension–distraction type injuries that are associated with rupture of the tectorial membrane, alar ligaments, atlanto-occipital membrane, and the capsular ligaments of the occiput–C1 and C1–C2 joints. AOD and AAD are more common in pediatric populations, associated with high-speed motor vehicle accidents and injury to other body parts, particularly the CNS. The diagnosis is suspected by indirect CT signs and confirmed with MRI.

Many measurements of the CVJ have been utilized to make these diagnoses, but perhaps the most practical one is the distance between the inferior tip of the clivus (basion) and the superior tip of the odontoid process in midline (basion-odontoid interval, BOI). A BOI measurement on midsagittal CT that is greater than 10 mm should be highly suspicious for AOD [1–4]. BOI is not significantly dependent on age and sex, and the 10 mm cut-off has very high accuracy in identifying CVJ injury. In very young children with underdeveloped odontoid processes the specificity may be slightly less [4].

The Power's ratio is the ratio of the basion–posterior atlas arch interval to the opisthion–anterior atlas arch interval, and it is abnormal at values greater than 1. The Power's ratio is very specific but not as sensitive and cannot be used to exclude CVJ injury [2,3]. The distance between the occipital condyle and the superior surface of C1 at the midpoint of the atlanto-occipital joint should not be greater than 2 mm, and the joint gap between the lateral mass of C1 and the articular surface of

C2 at midpoint should not be greater than 3.5 mm. These last two measurements are dependent on the patient's age and not easily applicable to young children.

## Importance

Although they are relatively rare injuries, failure to identify and treat AOD and AAD can result in catastrophic neurologic deterioration.

## Typical clinical scenario

The mortality rate of AOD and ADD is high. Patients who survive can present with a variety of neurologic findings, including quadriparesis and isolated cranial nerve palsies. Associated brain injury and other injuries are common.

## Differential diagnosis

In the setting of acute trauma there is no differential diagnosis. Congenital anomalies of the CVJ can mimic some of the findings and alter some of the measurements described above.

---

### Teaching points

CVJ injuries can present without bone fractures. BOI measuring greater than 10 mm is almost always associated with AOD.

---

REFERENCES

1. Chaput CD, Walgama J, Torres E, *et al.* Defining and detecting missed ligamentous injuries of the occipitocervical complex. *Spine (Phila Pa 1976)* 2011; **36**: 709–14.
2. Dziurzynski D, Anderson PA, Bean DB, *et al.* A blinded assessment of radiographic criteria for atlanto-occipital dislocation. *Spine (Phila Pa 1976)* 2005; **30**: 1427–32.
3. Gonzalez LF, Fiorella D, Crawford NR, *et al.* Vertical atlantoaxial distraction injuries: radiological criteria and clinical implications. *J Neurosurg Spine* 2004; **1**: 273–80.
4. Chang W, Alexander MT, Mirvis SE. Diagnostic determinants of craniocervical distraction injury in adults. *AJR Am J Roentgenol* 2009; **192**: 52–8.

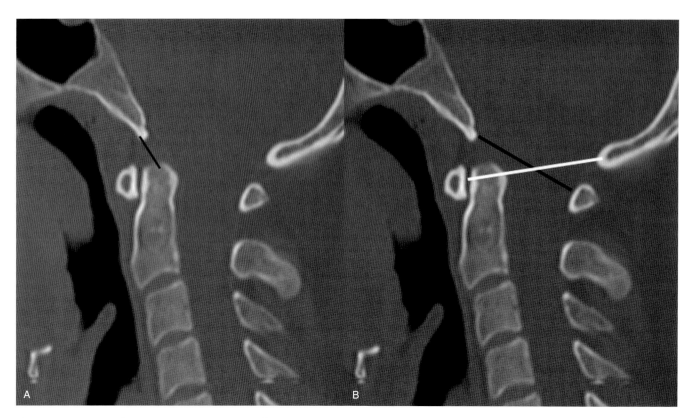

**Figure 86.1** (**A**) BOI: the distance between the tip of the clivus (basion) and odontoid (black line) should be less than 10 mm on CT. Up to 12 mm may be allowed in young children. (**B**) Power's ratio: the distance between the basion and the anterior aspect of the posterior arch of C1 (black line) divided by the distance between the opisthion (tip of the occiput) and the posterior cortex of the anterior arch of C1 (white line) should be less than 1.

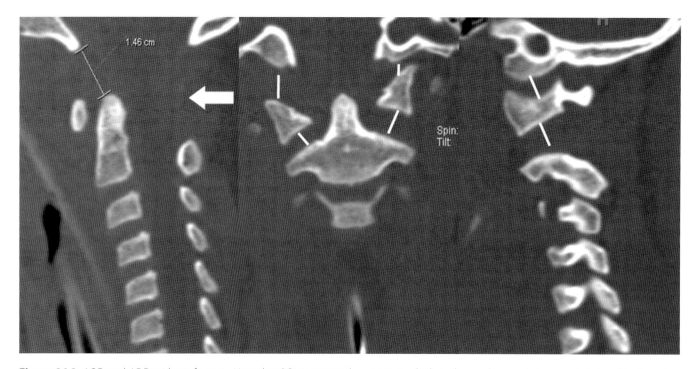

**Figure 86.2** AOD and ADD without fracture. Note that BOI is greater than 14 mm, which is always abnormal. Arrow points to widening of the distance between the opisthion and C1. Coronal and off-midline images reveal marked widening of the distances between the occipital condyles sand C1, as well as C1 and C2 (solid lines).

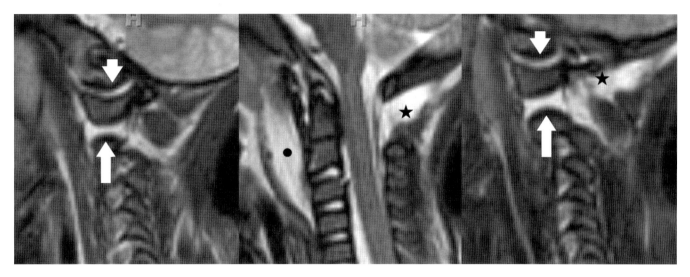

**Figure 86.3** ADD with minimal AOD on a different patient. Arrows point to the widened joint space between the lateral masses of C1 and C2. The atlanto-occipital joints are minimally widened (short arrows). Note prevertebral hematoma (black dot) and ruptured posterior atlanto-occipital membrane (black stars)

## Imaging description

C2, also known as axis, is one of the most complex and unusual vertebral bodies. It is crucial for weight-bearing as well as nodding and lateral movement of the head. Developmentally it has four ossification centers at birth, one each for a neural arch, one for the body, and one for the odontoid process. A secondary ossification center appears at the apex of the odontoid process (os terminale) between 3 and 6 years of age, and fuses to the odontoid process by the age of 12 years [1].

Classic imaging with radiography in case of a traumatic injury to C2 can exhibit linear lucency through the odontoid process or vertebral body. An open-mouth frontal-view radiograph can also show transverse or oblique fracture lines. However, it is increasingly being replaced by CT scan for possible traumatic injury to the cervical spine in the developed world [2]. CT is highly sensitive to detect lucent fracture lines and displacement of the fracture fragments, and for evaluation of the tip of the odontoid process or involvement of pedicles and foramen transversarium. In acute cases, soft tissue swelling anterior to C2 is visualized. Sagittal and coronal reconstructions increase the sensitivity of the CT scan, as sometimes axial imaging may be confusing. A 3 mm slice thickness is optimal, with no increasing advantage of having thinner sections [3]. Sagittal T1- and T2-weighted MRI exhibits high T2 signal bone marrow edema as well as soft tissue injury in the prevertebral compartment. The extent of possible cord compression is also well evaluated with MRI.

## Importance

The treatment options and further diagnostic work-up differ widely in different types of the odontoid C2 fractures. Type I fracture is considered as stable and does not require any surgery. Type II fracture is treated with primary fusion, as it is most likely to go on for non-union [1]. Type III fracture involves the C2 vertebral body and may involve the foramen transversarium. In that case, it is important to perform CTA or MRA of the neck to rule out possible dissection of vertebral arteries. These fractures also tend to be unstable and may need anterior fixation. Burst fracture is associated with retropulsion of posterior fragment and may need immediate decompression. Based on imaging findings and clinical status, it is important to explain the possible outcomes to the patient, including morbidity and side effects, along with the type of surgery [4].

## Typical clinical scenario

The most common symptom is neck pain, and the most common sign is that of myelopathy in case of cord injury. History of previous trauma is important. However, in elderly, osteoporotic patients, the trauma may be minor and not well recollected.

## Differential diagnosis

A secondary ossification center appears at the apex of the odontoid process between 3 and 6 years of age and fuses by the age of 12 years. Type I fracture (Fig. 87.1) is an avulsion of the tip of the odontoid process and is considered to be a stable fracture, treated only with immobilization. Type II fracture (Fig. 87.2) is a transverse fracture at the base of the odontoid process. It is the most common type of fracture of the odontoid process [1] and also the most likely to go on to non-union. Type III fracture (Fig. 87.3) extends into the body of C2 and may involve the foramen transversarium. A burst fracture (Fig. 87.4) is a comminuted fracture of the body of C2 with multiple fragments dislocated anteriorly and posteriorly. A hangman's fracture (Fig. 87.5) is a specific type of fracture affecting the C2 vertebral body; fractures of bilateral pedicles result in anterior subluxation of C2 vertebral body from its arch.

Congenital non-union of the tip of the odontoid process is known as os odontoideum. A well-corticated ossification center is seen above a truncated odontoid process (Fig. 87.6). There is no evidence for soft tissue swelling, history of trauma, or pain. Quite frequently, this is an incidental finding. Metastatic secondary deposit at the C2 vertebral body can result in pathologic fracture of the C2 odontoid process (Fig. 87.7). History of prior cancer and lack of history of trauma are frequently associated with this condition. Synovial proliferation in rheumatoid arthritis leads to erosion of the odontoid process, which can become thinned out and may result in C1–C2 subluxation (Fig. 87.8).

## Teaching points

Flexion/extension films are useful to assess stability. Source CT images may miss the fractures if the slice plane is parallel to the fracture line. It is very important to perform coronal and sagittal reconstructions. The body of the C2 vertebra fuses with the odontoid process between 3 and 6 years of age. Sclerotic margins of non-united odontoid process may indicate non-union of an old fracture. CTA should be performed, even in asymptomatic patients, if the fracture line extends to the foramen transversarium. MRI of the craniovertebral junction may be performed to assess the degree of cord compression. Marrow edema on T2-weighted imaging is able to differentiate between chronic non-union and acute fracture.

REFERENCES

1. Lustrin ES, Karakas SP, Ortiz AO, *et al.* Pediatric cervical spine: normal anatomy, variants and trauma. *Radiographics* 2003; **23**: 539–60.
2. Antevil JL, Sise MJ, Sack DI, *et al.* Spiral computed tomography for the initial evaluation of spine trauma: a new standard of care? *J Trauma* 2006; **61**: 382–7.

3. Phal PM, Riccelli LP, Wang P, Nesbit GM, Anderson JC. Fracture detection in the cervical spine with multidetector CT: 1-mm versus 3-mm axial images. *AJNR Am J Neuroradiol* 2008; **29**: 1446–9.

4. Lewkonia P, Dipaola C, Schouten R, *et al.* An evidence based medicine process to determine outcomes after cervical spine trauma: what surgeons should be selling their patients. *Spine (Phila Pa 1976)* 2012; **37**: E1140–7.

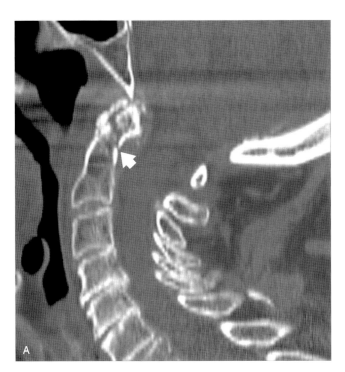
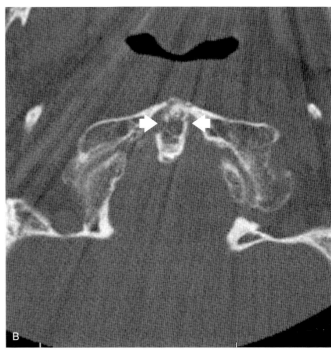

**Figure 87.1** Type I fracture. (**A**) Axial CT shows transverse lucency (arrow) into odontoid process, which could be confusing. (**B**) Sagittal reconstruction shows an oblique lucency (arrows) into odontoid process with mild posterior displacement of the tip of the odontoid process. Note the sclerotic transverse line of intact synchondrosis of odontoid process and C2 vertebral body.

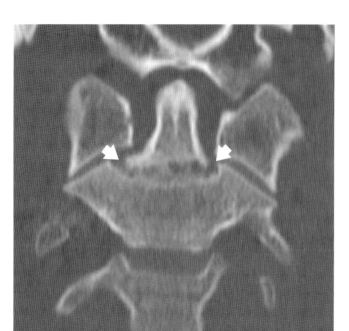

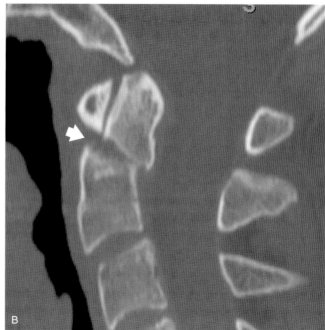

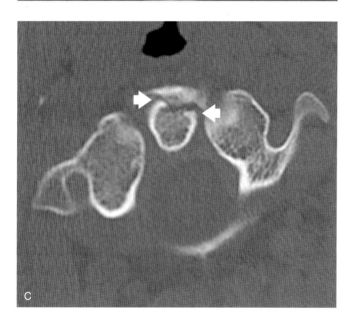

**Figure 87.2** Type II fracture. (**A**, **B**, **C**) Axial CT with sagittal and coronal reconstruction exhibits a fracture line along the embryonic fusion between the odontoid process and the C2 vertebral body (arrows).

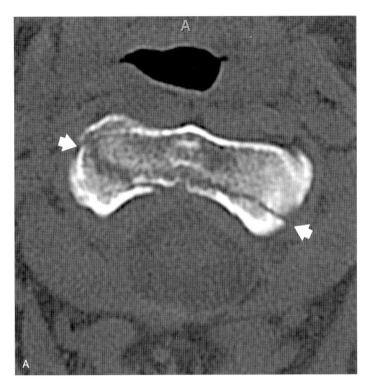

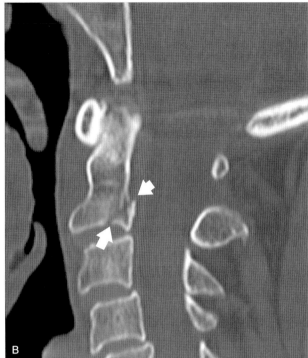

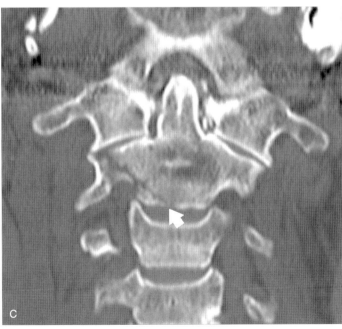

**Figure 87.3** Type III fracture. (**A**) Axial CT exhibits a transverse fracture line across the C2 vertebral body (arrows). (**B**) Sagittal CT reconstruction exhibits mild retropulsion of fracture fragment with oblique orientation of fracture line (arrows). (**C**) Coronal reconstruction exhibits the oblique fracture line extending from right lateral mass to inferior endplate of C2 vertebral body (arrow).

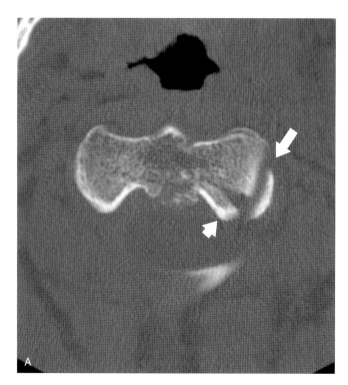
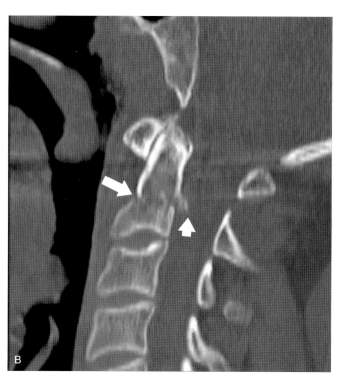

**Figure 87.4** Burst fracture. (**A**) Axial CT exhibits a comminuted fracture of C2 vertebral body with lateral (arrow) and posterior (short arrow) displacement of fracture fragments. (**B**) Sagittal CT reconstruction exhibits a fracture of C2 vertebral body (arrow) with characteristic posterior displacement (short arrow) of fracture fragment.

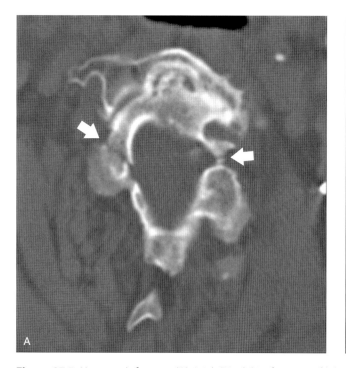
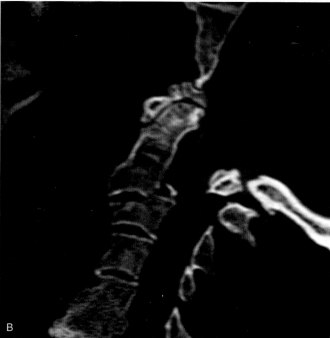

**Figure 87.5** Hangman's fracture. (**A**) Axial CT exhibits fractures of bilateral pedicles (arrows) of the C2 vertebral body. Due to abnormal angulation, the axial CT is mildly oblique. (**B**) Sagittal CTA reconstruction exhibits anterior displacement of skull base, C1 vertebra, and odontoid process with relation to the distal spinal column. An incomplete fracture line is also seen across the tip of the odontoid process.

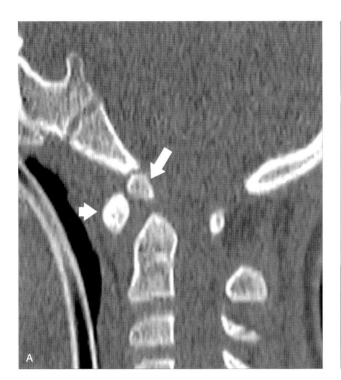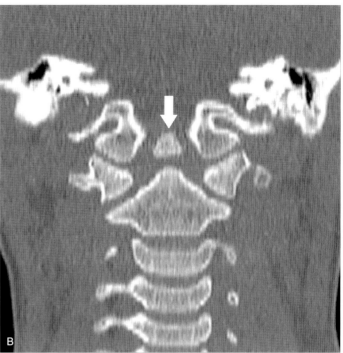

**Figure 87.6** Os odontoideum. (**A**) Sagittal CT reconstruction exhibits a rounded ossific fragment (arrow) in close proximity to basion with mild posterior subluxation of a truncated odontoid process with relation to the anterior tubercle of C1 (short arrow). Note the unfused synchondrosis of basioccipital and basisphenoid. (**B**) Coronal CT reconstruction exhibits a midline rounded ossific fragment (arrow) craniad to a smaller odontoid process.

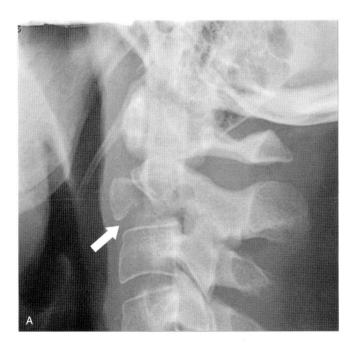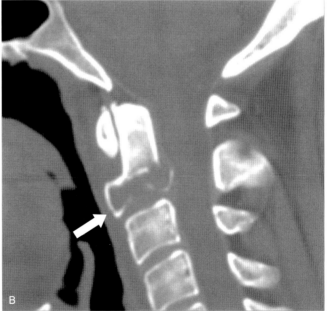

**Figure 87.7** Pathologic fracture with metastatic deposit from known renal cell carcinoma. (**A**) Lateral radiogram shows anterior displacement of a fractured C2 vertebral body (arrow). (**B**) Sagittal CT reconstruction exhibits a large expansile lytic lesion of C2 vertebral body, loss of height with mild anterior displacement of anterior cortical margin (arrow). (**C**) Coronal CT reconstruction exhibits an irregular lytic mass at C2 vertebral body (arrow). (**D**, **E**) Bone and soft tissue window of axial CT exhibits an expansile lytic soft tissue mass of C2 vertebral body extending into prevertebral spaces (arrow).

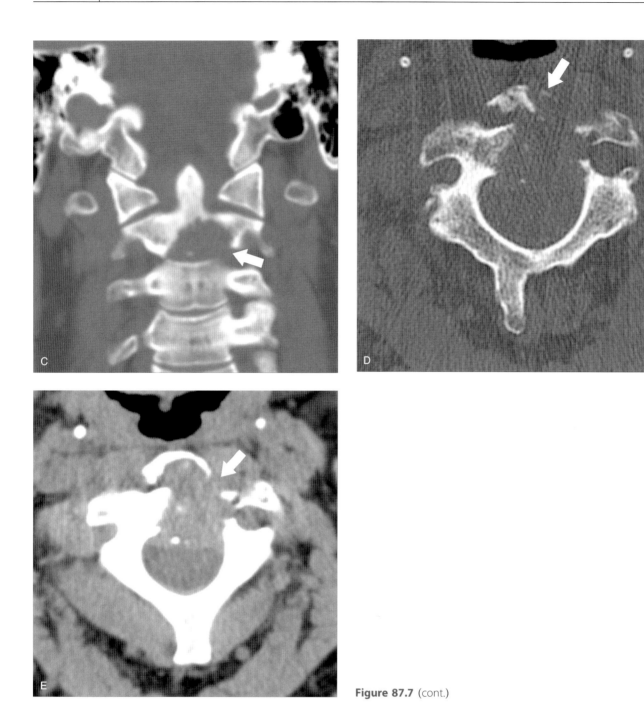

**Figure 87.7** (cont.)

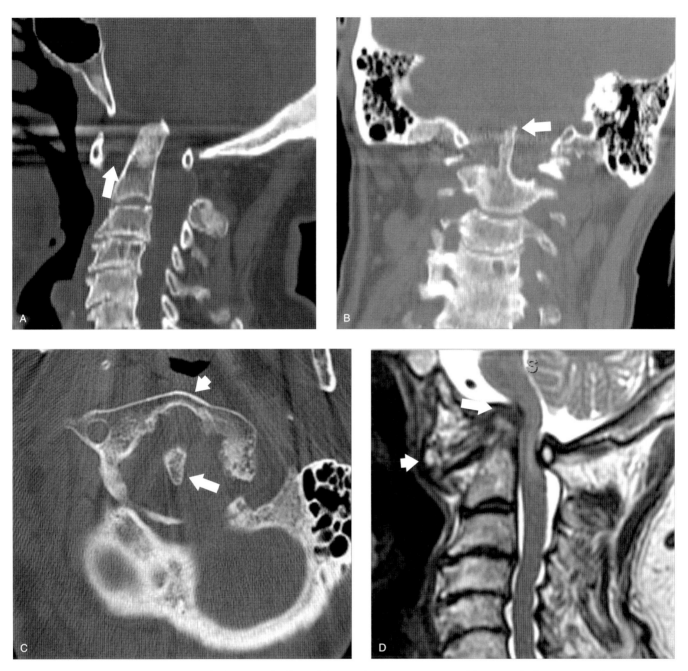

**Figure 87.8** Atlanto-axial subluxation with rheumatoid arthritis. (**A**) Sagittal CT reconstruction exhibits a marked posterior subluxation with superior displacement of odontoid process (arrow). (**B**) Coronal CT reconstruction exhibits characteristic marked thinning of odontoid process from the sides (arrow). (**C**) Axial CT exhibits marked posterior displacement of thinned-out elongated odontoid process (arrow) from anterior arch of C1 (short arrow). (**D**) T2-weighted sagittal MRI exhibits posterior displacement of odontoid process (arrow) with relation to anterior arch of C1 (short arrow) resulting in cord compression with intramedullary high T2 signal edema.

# Vertebral compression fractures

## Imaging description

Non-traumatic vertebral compression fractures (VCF) are common and often secondary to either osteoporosis or metastasis. Radiologists should try to determine the benign or malignant nature of the fracture each time they diagnose a VCF, as this has obvious implications for treatment and prognosis. MRI has the greatest accuracy among imaging modalities in this regard. Bone SPECT scan and FDG-PET are very sensitive but their specificity is markedly limited [1,2].

There are various signal changes, morphologic features and quantitative measurements that can help differentiate benign and malignant VCF [3]. Perhaps the most important signal characteristic is the T1 signal within the fractured vertebra: replacement of marrow fat by metastasis is almost always complete, whereas in osteoporotic VCF there are often areas of preserved marrow signal (Fig. 88.1). Identification of normal marrow signal on T1-weighted images, even in a small portion of the vertebral body, is a good indicator of a benign fracture. Abnormal marrow signal in the pedicles of vertebral bodies can be seen in both malignant and benign fractures, but abnormal signal within the posterior elements is more specific for malignant fracture. Linearly oriented band-like signal changes on either T1- or T2-weighted images favor benign fractures, as does fluid signal within the vertebral body (Fig. 88.1). The posterior border of the vertebral body provides important clues as to the nature of the fracture: a rounded bulge of the posterior border is suggestive of malignant fracture, whereas a triangular bulge is more consistent with benign fracture (Figs. 88.1, 88.2). Presence of paraspinal and/or epidural masses suggests metastasis, although benign fractures may have considerable hematoma when they are acute, which mimics soft tissue mass.

Metastatic VCF rarely occurs in the absence of other metastatic lesion in the spine. Identification of additional lesions in the spine, iliac bones, and ribs is highly suggestive of metastasis. On the other hand, benign-appearing old fractures at other levels suggest osteoporotic VCF. In the great majority of VCF, these features would allow correct identification of the cause.

The addition of DWI and/or opposed-phase chemical shift imaging to the conventional methods may increase accuracy. Metastatic VCF shows restricted diffusion on DWI and thus diminished apparent diffusion coefficient (ADC) values, and little signal loss on opposed-phase images due to replacement of fatty marrow by malignant cells [3,4].

One important caveat is multiple myeloma, which often mimics benign VCF (Fig. 88.3) [5]. Likewise, malignant melanoma metastases may have bright T1 signal secondary to melanin.

## Importance

Malignant fractures are treated differently.

## Typical clinical scenario

Back pain is the most common presenting symptom. Neurologic signs and symptoms may or may not be present, depending on the location of the VCF and the degree of canal compromise.

## Differential diagnosis

Trauma and infectious spondylodiscitis are two other causes of VCF. They can often be differentiated from spontaneous fractures based on history.

> ### Teaching points
>
> Benign VCFs have incomplete replacement of fatty marrow signal on T1-weighted images, triangular posterior border, and band-like signal changes in the vertebral body. Multiple myeloma fractures may mimic benign fractures.

REFERENCES

1. Cho WI, Chang UK. Comparison of MR imaging and FDG-PET/CT in the differential diagnosis of benign and malignant vertebral compression fractures. *J Neurosurg Spine* 2011; **14**: 177–83.
2. Tokuda O, Harada Y, Ueda T, Ohishi Y, Matsunaga N. Malignant versus benign vertebral compression fractures: can we use bone SPECT as a substitute for MR imaging? *Nucl Med Commun* 2011; **32**: 192–8.
3. Thawait SK, Marcus MA, Morrison WB, et al. Research synthesis: what is the diagnostic performance of MRI to discriminate benign from malignant vertebral compression fractures? Systematic review and meta-analysis. *Spine (Phila Pa 1976)* 2012; **37**: E736–44.
4. Régis-Arnaud A, Guiu B, Walker PM, et al. Bone marrow fat quantification of osteoporotic vertebral compression fractures: comparison of multi-voxel proton MR spectroscopy and chemical-shift gradient-echo MR imaging. *Acta Radiol* 2011; **52**: 1032–6.
5. Lecouvet FE, Vande Berg BC, Maldague BE, et al. Vertebral compression fractures in multiple myeloma. Part I. Distribution and appearance at MR imaging. *Radiology* 1997; **204**: 195–9.

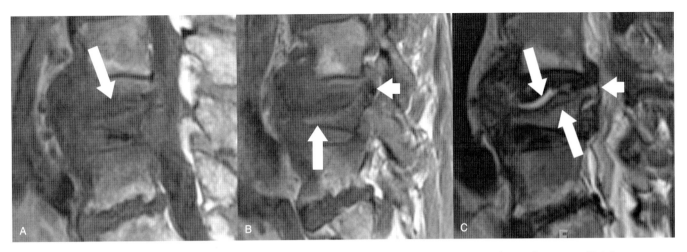

**Figure 88.1** Sagittal T1-weighted and T2-weighted images show L4 vertebral body fracture with complete replacement of bright marrow signal on (**A**) midsagittal T1-weighted image (arrow), but (**B**) an off-midline T1-weighted image shows some preservation of marrow signal (arrow), an important clue to the benign nature of this fracture. Also note the morphology of the fractured vertebra, with a pointy posterior wall of the vertebral body (short arrow). (**C**) T2-weighted image shows a linear band of hypointensity along the vertebral body (arrow), likely reflecting the fracture line below a band-like fluid signal (arrow), reliable signs of benign nature. A sizable disc herniation can be better separated from the fractured vertebra on T2-weighted image. Paraspinal soft tissue is more common with malignant fractures, although it can be present in acute benign fractures, as seen in this case.

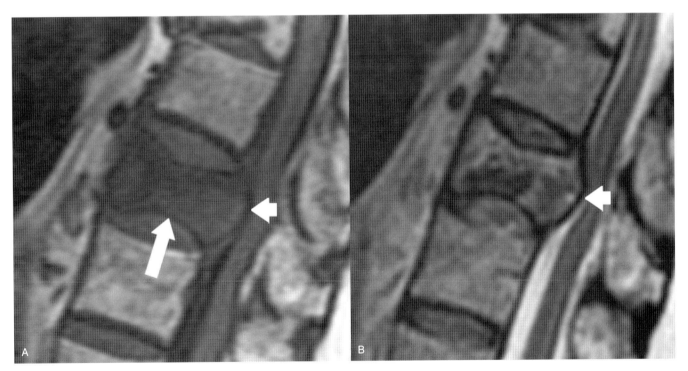

**Figure 88.2** Patient with history of colon cancer presented with acute-onset cauda equina syndrome due to a malignant compression fracture. (**A**) Note complete replacement of bright marrow signal on T1-weighted image (arrow), with rounded posterior bulge (short arrow). (**B**) T2-weighted image shows heterogeneous marrow signal without linear or band-like features. Also note lack of paraspinal soft tissue mass. No other metastasis was present in this patient's spine.

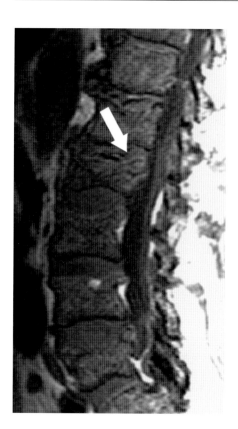

**Figure 88.3** Sagittal T1-weighted image of the lumbar spine of a patient with multiple myeloma (MM) showing fractures of the L2 and L4 vertebrae with some preservation of fat signal (arrow) within the vertebrae. Morphologically, MM fractures may mimic benign fractures, but heterogeneity of the marrow signal throughout the spine is a clue to the widespread involvement of the marrow.

# CASE 89 Sacral insufficiency fracture

## Imaging description

Insufficiency fractures occur when bone strength is not sufficient to withstand physiologic stress. The most common bones fractured are the thoracic and lumbar vertebral bodies. Sacral insufficiency fractures (SIF) are less common but they are commonly misdiagnosed [1]. The typical SIF is an H-shaped tri-part fracture with two vertical components through the sacral alae and a third horizontal component connecting them, usually through the upper sacral segments. Any permutation of these can be seen in a given patient, although isolated transverse component is rare.

Plain films are often non-diagnostic. CT is reliable, although in the acute phase findings may be very subtle secondary to decreased background bone density. MRI is very sensitive and shows the marrow edema associated with the fracture as increased signal on fluid-sensitive pulse sequences such as STIR and SE T2 and diminished signal on T1-weighted images in the bone surrounding the fracture (Figs. 89.1, 89.2). Contrast enhancement occurs in areas of edema. Bone scan is very sensitive but less specific than MRI and CT.

Despite the availability of very sensitive imaging tests, SIFs are frequently missed due to the non-specific nature of symptoms (lower back pain) usually leading to lumbar spine studies rather than dedicated sacral imaging, and common presence of degenerative changes in the lumbar spine which are presumed to account for the symptoms. It is difficult to see SIF on sagittal MRI (Fig. 89.3), and axial images may not even include the sacrum in routine lumbar MRI protocols. The coronal plane, which is the plane of choice for SIF detection, is not a part of back pain evaluation in many practices (Fig. 89.4).

## Importance

In women over 55 years of age the prevalence of SIF may be as high as 4% [2]. SIF is commonly missed in the setting of lower back pain. When appropriately diagnosed, SIF can be effectively treated with conservative measures or sacroplasty [3].

## Typical clinical scenario

Most patients are elderly women presenting with intractable lower back pain. Other associations include recent pregnancy, osteoporosis/osteomalacia, and prior radiation treatment.

## Differential diagnosis

Imaging findings on CT and MRI are often specific enough to make a definitive diagnosis, although in a patient with a history of cancer, sacral fractures may be misinterpreted as metastatic disease. Metastatic disease is only occasionally limited to the sacrum, however.

> ### Teaching points
>
> Sacral fractures are often missed because the radiologist is distracted by lumbar degenerative changes, coronal images of the sacrum are not obtained routinely, and axial images may not include the sacrum. Marrow edema in the sacrum on MRI and cortical discontinuity on CT should raise the possibility of SIF.

REFERENCES

1. Hatzl-Griesenhofer M, Pichler R, Huber H, Maschek W. [The insufficiency fracture of the sacrum: an often unrecognized cause of low back pain: results of bone scanning in a major hospital]. *Nuklearmedizin* 2001; **40**: 221–7.

2. Cho C, Mathis J, Kortman K. Sacroplasty. In Mathis JM, Golovac S, eds., *Image Guided Spine Interventions*, 2nd edn. New York, NY: Springer; 2010; pp. 355–74.

3. Frey ME, DePalma MJ, Cifu DX, *et al.* Percutaneous sacroplasty for osteoporotic sacral insufficiency fractures: a prospective, multicenter, observational pilot study. *Spine J* 2008; **8**: 367–73.

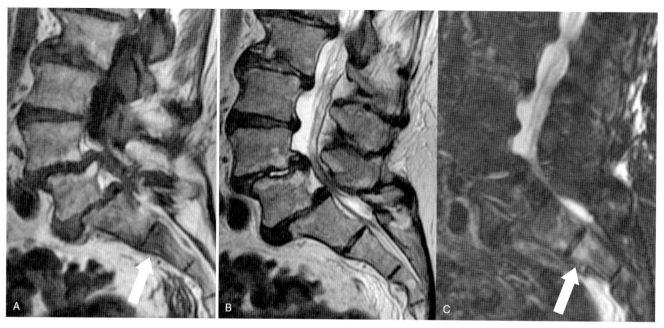

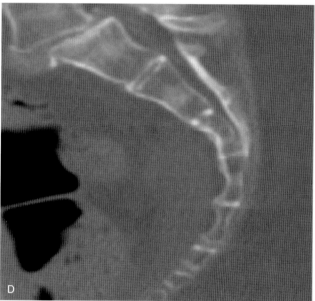

**Figure 89.1** Midsagittal (**A**) T1-weighted, (**B**) T2-weighted and (**C**) STIR MR images show extensive degenerative changes. Marrow edema seen in the S2 segment on T1-weighted and STIR images (arrow) is the only clue for a possible abnormality in the sacrum. (**D**) The midsagittal CT image does not show a fracture.

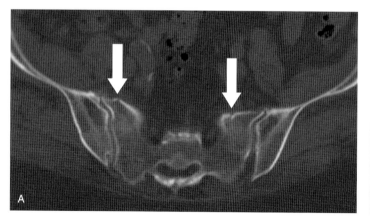

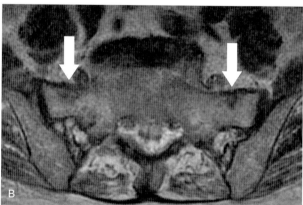

**Figure 89.2** (**A**) Axial CT image shows subtle cortical discontinuity on either side (arrows) compatible with SIF. (**B**) T2-weighted MR image of the same patient also shows the fractures (arrows) and associated subtle marrow edema.

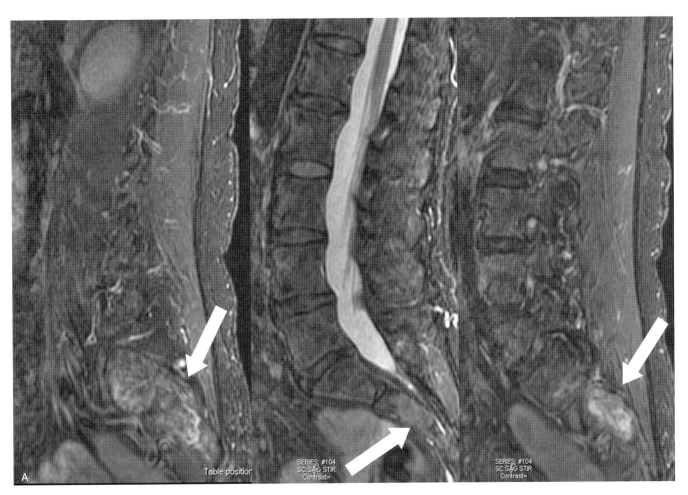

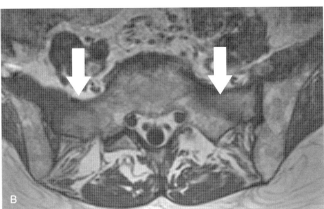

**Figure 89.3** (**A**) Sagittal STIR images show only minimal marrow edema in S2 in midline (middle) with marked marrow edema seen in only the very far lateral off-midline images (arrows) (right and left), compatible with SIF in the setting of severe back pain. (**B**) Axial T1-weighted image shows subtle decreased signal about the fracture lines on either side (arrows).

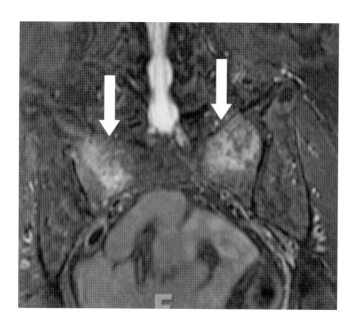

**Figure 89.4** Coronal STIR image of the same patient as in Fig. 89.2 shows the marrow edema (arrows) as a result of bilateral sacral vertical fractures.

# 90 Paget's disease of the spine

## Imaging description

Paget's disease of bone (PDB) is a chronic metabolic bone disorder characterized by bone thickening and deformity. The spine is the second most commonly affected site after the pelvis, with more than half of patients showing spinal involvement. The disease is usually polyostotic and involves multiple skeletal sites. In the spine, PDB can affect one or multiple segments. The most common site is the lumbar spine, with L4 and L5 being the most commonly involved segments.

PDB shows characteristic features on plain radiographs and CT of the spine that allow easy diagnosis [1]. These features include expansion of the vertebral body with increase in the anteroposterior and lateral vertebral dimensions and slightly decreased or unchanged vertebral height (Fig. 90.1). The vertebral body is almost always involved in a diffuse fashion, together with a variable portion of the neural arch. Loss of the concavity of the vertebral bodies anteriorly as well as posteriorly is a common feature. Trabecular hypertrophy paralleling the vertebral endplates, combined with thickening of the endplates and the cortex, results in an increased density in the vertebral periphery and a relatively lucent centre in the vertebral body, which is likened to a "picture frame" on radiographs and CT. The initial lytic phase of PDB does not occur in the spine. Progression of the sclerotic phase leads to the "ivory vertebra" appearance.

Although the MRI findings of PDB are often as characteristic as the plain radiograph and CT findings, radiologists tend to give a list of differential diagnoses for PDB rather than a single diagnosis in their MRI reports. All findings relating to vertebral expansion are easily recognizable on MRI (Figs. 90.2, 90.3). Areas that show sclerotic change on CT show decreased T1 and T2 signal on MRI (Fig. 90.4). In the early phases of PDB bone marrow edema may be present, manifesting as decreased T1 signal, increased T2 signal, and post-contrast enhancement. The marrow signal in the majority of cases is increased and more heterogeneous on T1-weighted images due to fatty replacement, and this allows exclusion of marrow-replacing and infiltrative processes such as metastases and lymphoma/leukemia.

## Importance

The prevalence of PDB in the general population is about 3%. The prevalence is higher in elderly populations, reaching 10% in individuals over the age of 80 years. Making the correct diagnosis of PDB prevents unnecessary work-up and anxiety.

## Typical clinical scenario

Back pain is the most common clinical symptom associated with Paget's disease of the spine, although not all patients are symptomatic. Back pain may be secondary to the primary bone disease or to expansion of the bone leading to spinal canal stenosis. Patients may present with compression fractures due to bone weakening and very rarely secondary to sarcomatous dedifferentiation.

## Differential diagnosis

The imaging appearance of PDB is characteristic and allows definitive diagnosis in the great majority of cases. In particular, expansion and squaring of the vertebral body with concomitant involvement of the posterior elements is the most important observation. In the "ivory vertebra" stage the differential diagnoses include metastases, osteosarcoma, carcinoid, and Hodgkin's lymphoma. In the very rare occurrence of the lytic phase of PDB in spine, other osteolytic processes should be considered.

### Teaching points

An expanded vertebral body and posterior element on MRI with heterogeneously increased marrow signal is characteristic for PDB.

REFERENCES

1. Dell'Atti C, Cassar-Pullicino VN, Lalam RK, Tins BJ, Tyrrell PN. The spine in Paget's disease. *Skeletal Radiol* 2007; **36**: 609–26.

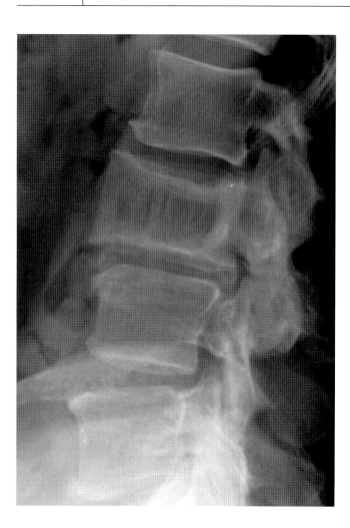

**Figure 90.1** Lateral plain radiograph of the lumbar spine shows the L3 vertebral body to have a slightly decreased height but increased width with flat anterior and posterior borders (loss of normal concavity), thickened trabeculae vertically as well as horizontally, with sclerotic borders of the vertebral body resembling a picture frame.

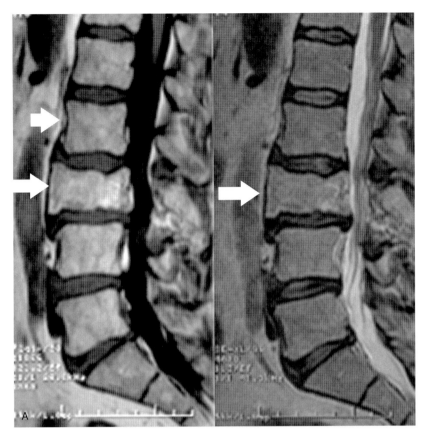

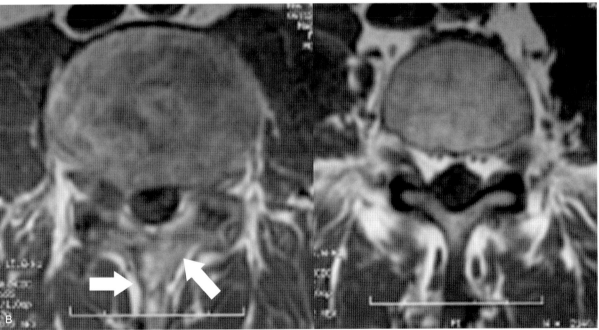

**Figure 90.2** (**A**) Sagittal T1-weighted (left) and T2-weighted (right) images of the lumbar spine show Paget's disease of the L3 vertebra, which is wider than the remaining lumbar vertebral bodies. Patchy increased T1 signal within the vertebral body is secondary to increased fat content. (**B**) Axial T1-weighted images of abnormal L3 (left) and normal L4 (right) vertebrae on the same scale reveal the marked relative enlargement of L3, with involvement of the laminae and spinous process (arrows).

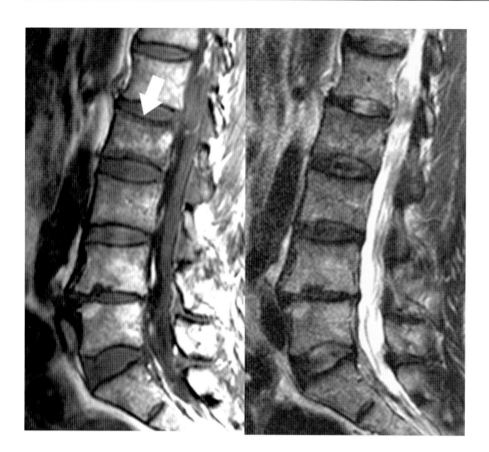

**Figure 90.3** Sagittal T1-weighted (left) and T2-weighted (right) images of the lumbar spine show hypointense borders of L2 (arrow) with a hyperintense vertebral body center and loss of concavity along the anterior border, compatible with Paget's disease.

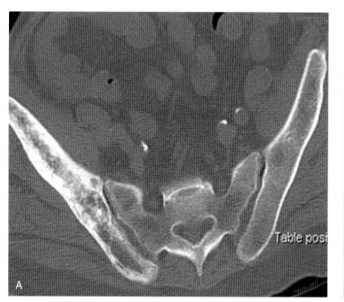
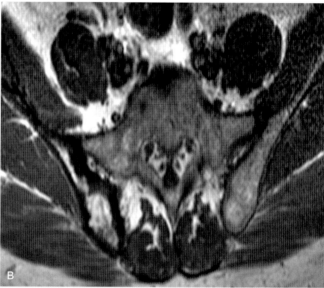

**Figure 90.4** Paget's disease of the pelvis. (**A**) Axial CT and (**B**) T1-weighted MR images through the pelvis show an expanded right iliac bone with marked thickening of the cortex and relatively increased fat in the center.

# 91 Renal osteodystrophy

## Imaging description

Renal osteodystrophy (ROD) is a general term for a variety of abnormalities of musculoskeletal system secondary to calcium and phosphate metabolic disorder in chronic end-stage renal disease. Hypocalcemia in chronic renal insufficiency leads to secondary hyperparathyroidism, which results in osteoclastic subperiosteal, subligamentous, subchondral, and trabecular bone resorption [1]. It also results in secondary osteomalacia and rickets due to aluminum intoxication, vitamin D deficiency, hypocalcemia, and acidosis. This can lead to complex bony changes. Osteosclerosis in renal osteodystrophy is related either to excessive osteoblastic bone production due to bone resorption or to increased production of mineralized osteoid. Reduced radiodensity in ROD reflects osteomalacia, osteitis fibrosa cystica, and osteoporosis [1].

When sclerotic changes occur in the spine, they do so parallel to the vertebral endplates, creating alternating bands of sclerosis along the endplates and a relative lucency in the middle, giving rise to radiographic findings of the "rugger jersey" spine, classically evaluated in the lateral radiographs [2]. In the spinal column, there is disappearance of transverse trabeculae with preservation of vertical trabeculae, resulting in characteristic vertical striations (Fig. 91.1). The prolonged T1 relaxation time on MRI seen in renal osteodystrophy is associated with increased marrow cellularity, thickened trabeculae, and peritrabecular fibrosis [3]. The overall result is decreased T1 signal of the vertebral bodies, which may be mistaken for lymphoma/leukemia involvement or diffuse metastasis. Secondary hyperparathyroidism may also result in soft tissue calcifications (Fig. 91.2)

## Importance

With increased availability of hemodialysis treatment, patients with end-stage renal disease survive longer, but continue to suffer from secondary complications, including ROD. Osteoporosis and osteomalacia associated with ROD put the patient at increased risk of pathologic fractures and can also cause cord compression due to bone expansion [4]. The diagnoses of ROD can result in additional dietary supplements of vitamin D analogs and phosphate binders to reduce the risk of fractures and complications. Spine surgery in patients with ROD also presents a unique set of challenges with increased hardware failure, necessitating alternative techniques [2].

## Typical clinical scenario

ROD takes place against a background of chronic end-stage renal disease. A history of chronic hemodialysis is very common. There is an increased risk of pathologic fractures, and focal back pain and neurological symptoms secondary to possible cord compression or nerve root impingement may also be present.

## Differential diagnosis

Paget's disease is a chronic metabolic disorder of abnormal bone remodeling in the adult skeleton. The commonest location in the spine is L4 and L5, but it can be seen at multiple levels. Trabecular coarsening and cortical thickening with areas of central osteopenia are seen (Fig. 91.3). Also known as marble bone disease, osteopetrosis is a congenital hereditary osteoclastic disorder resulting in diffuse increase in bone density with thickened bone cortex and bone-within-bone appearance (Fig. 91.4). Rickets is osteomalacia in the pediatric population due to impaired metabolism of vitamin D, phosphorus, calcium, or magnesium. There is blurring of normal trabeculae, as the normal osteoid bone is not laid down. There can be loss of distinction between cortex and medullary bone or bone-within-bone appearance of the vertebrae (Fig. 91.5). Lymphoreticular disease such as lymphoma can result in hypercellular bone marrow with loss of normal high T1 signal within the vertebral bodies and diffuse uniform post-contrast enhancement (Fig. 91.6).

## Teaching points

The "rugger jersey" pattern on lateral radiographs and CT scan of the spine is highly characteristic of renal osteodystrophy, but marrow signal changes on MRI may be mistaken for diffuse metastasis or lymphoma involvement. The bones of the appendicular skeleton can also have typical findings related to renal osteodystrophy.

REFERENCES

1. Jevtic V. Imaging of renal osteodystrophy. *Eur J Radiol* 2003; **46**: 85–95.

2. Veeravagu A, Ponnusamy K, Jiang B, Bydon M, *et al.* Renal osteodystrophy: neurosurgical considerations and challenges. *World Neurosurg* 2012; **78**: 191.E23–33.

3. Ito M, Ito M, Hayashi K, *et al.* Evaluation of spinal bone changes in patients with chronic renal failure by CT and MR imaging with pathologic correlation. *Acta Radiol* 1994; **35**: 291–5.

4. Macfarlane JD, Minhas A, Han KS, Boekhout M. Spinal cord compression in renal osteodystrophy. *Eur Spine J* 1995; **4**: 362–5.

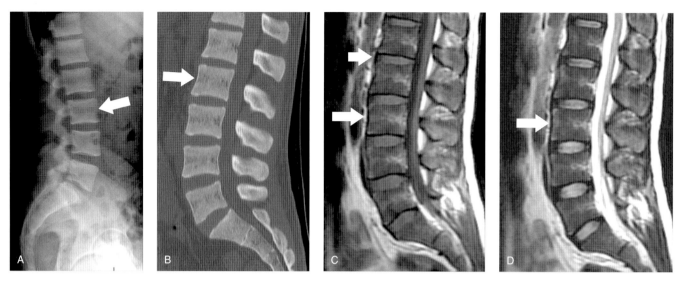

**Figure 91.1** Renal osteodystrophy. (**A**) Lateral radiogram exhibits sclerotic bands along the endplates of lumbar vertebrae with relative lucency in the middle (arrow), giving a typical "rugger jersey" appearance. (**B**) Sagittal reconstruction of overlapping helical axial CT of lumbar spine accentuates the "rugger jersey" appearance and exhibits vertical striations of compression trabeculae (arrow), signifying loss of transverse trabeculae. (**C**) Sagittal T1-weighted MR image exhibits loss of normal high T1 signal, especially along the sclerotic bone with residual high T1 signal that corresponds to lucency in the radiograph (arrow). Note relatively high T1 signal of intervertebral disc (short arrow). (**D**) Sagittal T2-weighted MR image exhibits similarly low T2 signal of lumbar vertebral bodies that is accentuated at sclerotic bands along the endplates with relatively normal bone marrow signal in the center (arrow).

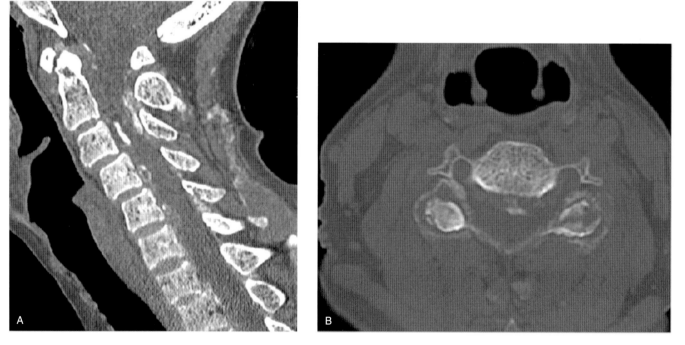

**Figure 91.2** (**A**, **B**) Sagittal and axial cervical spine CT images show diffuse sclerotic changes as well as calcifications in the periarticular tissues, posterior longitudinal ligament, and dura.

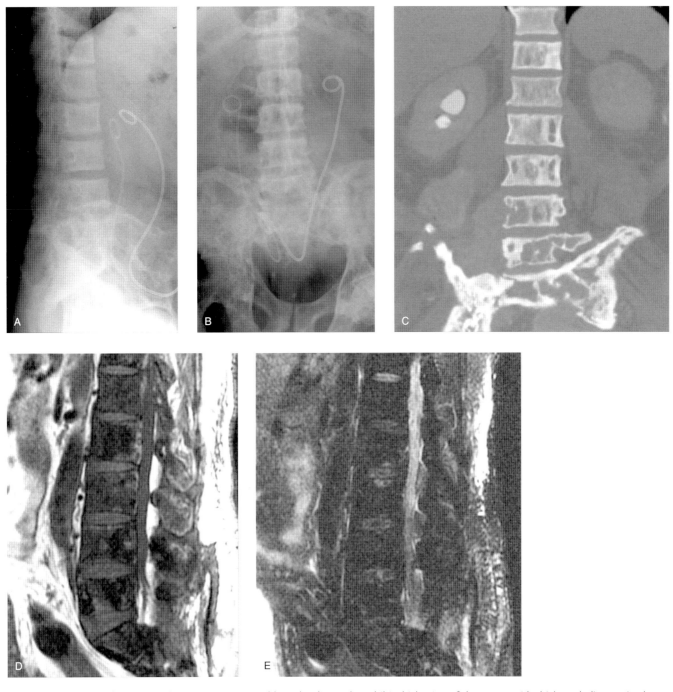

**Figure 91.3** Paget's disease. (**A**, **B**) Anteroposterior and lateral radiographs exhibit thickening of the cortex with thickened, disorganized trabeculae. Similar changes are seen at the visualized pelvic bones. (**C**) Coronal reconstruction of helical axial CT of lumbar spine exhibits better definition of coarsening of trabeculae with cortical thickening of the vertebral bodies and areas of central osteopenia. (**D**) Sagittal T1-weighted MR image exhibits heterogeneous but predominantly hypointense T1 signal. (**E**) Sagittal STIR MR imaging exhibits hypointense bone.

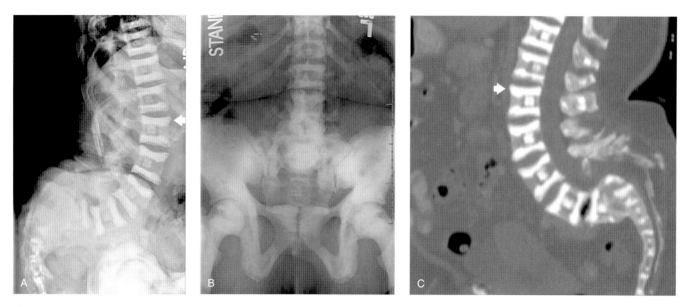

**Figure 91.4** Osteopetrosis. (**A**, **B**) Anteroposterior and lateral radiographs exhibit sharply demarcated sclerotic bands adjacent to the vertebral endplates (short arrow). Note the bone-within-bone appearance of the pelvic bones. (**C**) Sagittal reconstruction of helical axial CT exhibits sclerotic bands along the vertebral endplates (short arrow).

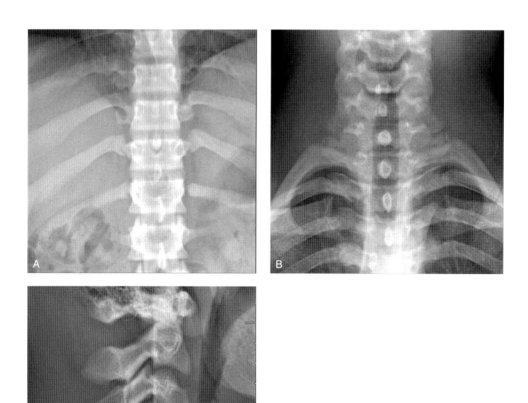

**Figure 91.5** Rickets. (**A**, **B**) Anteroposterior radiograms exhibit osteomalacia with blurring of trabeculae. (**C**) Lateral radiogram of cervical spine exhibits indistinct trabeculae with bone-within-bone appearance of vertebrae.

Renal osteodystrophy | CASE 91

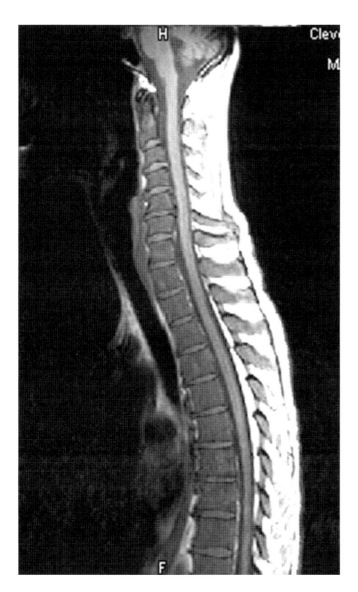

**Figure 91.6** Lymphoma. Sagittal T1-weighted MR image exhibits diffuse hypointense T1 signal. The intervertebral discs exhibit hyperintense T1 signal compared with the vertebral bodies.

## Imaging description

Calcific tendinitis of the longus colli muscle (CTLC) is an uncommon inflammatory process of the prevertebral and retropharyngeal soft tissues that manifests as retropharyngeal and prevertebral edema and a variable degree of calcification of the longus colli muscle tendon. The calcification of the tendon is characteristic of this entity in the proper clinical setting, while the accompanying retropharyngeal edema often leads to misdiagnosis and unnecessary surgical intervention [1,2]. Calcifications are variable in size and location but most commonly occur anterior to the C2 vertebra (Figs. 92.1, 92.2, 92.3).

## Importance

Making the diagnosis of calcific tendinitis by observing the characteristic calcification associated with the longus colli muscle tendon in the setting of acute neck pain and retropharyngeal edema eliminates the possibility of spinal or retropharyngeal infection, unnecessary antibiotic treatment, and aspiration or surgical drainage in some cases, and allows appropriate treatment with non-steroidal anti-inflammatory drugs (NSAIDs).

## Typical clinical scenario

Acute-onset neck pain and stiffness with or without dysphasia and odynophagia are the classic symptoms of CTLC. No sex predilection has been reported, and patients are usually middle-aged adults. A low-grade fever may occur. Mild elevation of erythrocyte sedimentation rate and leukocyte count can be seen.

## Differential diagnosis

Neck pain and retropharyngeal edema differential diagnosis is limited but includes entities such as retropharyngeal abscess and spinal infection that may require urgent surgical intervention (Table 92.1). The most common entity that would present with the same set of clinical and imaging findings is retropharyngeal cellulitis, which typically occurs in the setting of pharyngitis. Cellulitis (a.k.a. retropharyngeal edema or phlegmon) presents as diffuse swelling of the retropharyngeal soft tissue without an enhancing wall (Fig. 92.4). This does not require, nor does it respond to, surgical drainage and should be differentiated from retropharyngeal abscess, which manifests as a well-defined fluid collection in the retropharyngeal space with an enhancing wall and often associated marked mass effect on the surrounding structures. Infection

of the retropharyngeal nodes may lead to intranodal suppuration, which typically presents in children as a well-defined fluid collection with an enhancing wall in the lateral retropharyngeal space (Fig. 92.5). Although these features can be interpreted as abscess, these patients respond to conservative treatment well and rarely require surgical drainage. Spondylodiscitis may also present with neck pain and retropharyngeal edema and should be promptly diagnosed. In spondylodiscitis one can see inflammation in the prevertebral and epidural spaces as well as signal changes in the disc space and vertebral endplates (Fig. 92.6). Traumatic ligamentous injury may also generate retropharyngeal fluid collections, but the clinical context helps in differentiating this from other causes. Obstruction of the jugular vein can cause congestion of the retropharyngeal tissues as well as other structures in the neck.

**Table 92.1** Causes of retropharyngeal edema (cellulitis).

Pharyngitis
Retropharyngeal abscess
Nodal suppuration
Spondylodiscitis
Trauma
Venous obstruction
Recent anterior cervical spinal decompression surgery

## Teaching points

Calcification of the longus colli tendon in the setting of acute onset neck pain and retropharyngeal edema should provide the diagnosis of calcific tendinitis and eliminate unnecessary and potentially harmful work-up. These calcifications can be of variable size and appearance, are easily seen on CT but often very difficult to detect on MRI unless the radiologist is specifically searching for them.

REFERENCES
1. Offiah CE, Hall E. Acute calcific tendinitis of the longus colli muscle: spectrum of CT appearances and anatomical correlation. *Br J Radiol* 2009; **82**: e117–21.
2. Naqshabandi AM, Srinivasan J. Teaching neuroimages: acute calcific tendinitis of longus colli mimicking meningismus. *Neurology* 2011; **76**: e81.

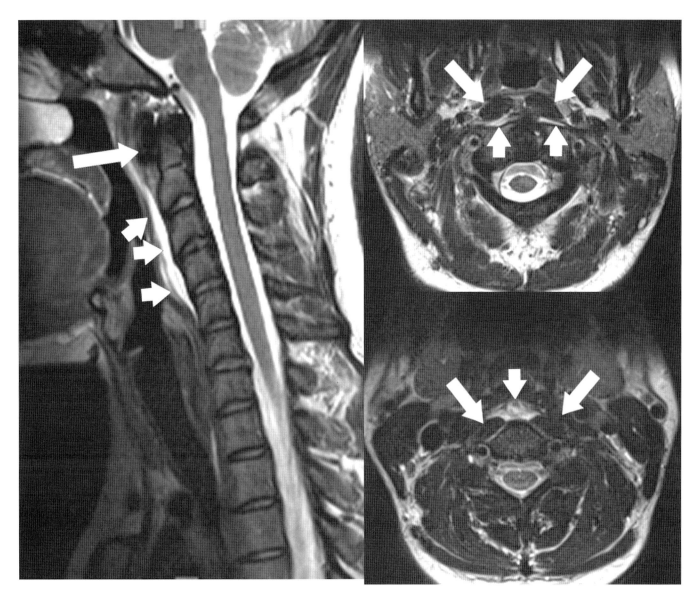

**Figure 92.1** Sagittal T2-weighted image shows hyperintense signal (short arrows) in the retropharyngeal region compatible with edema. Note the subtle hypointensity below the anterior arch of C1 (arrow), indicating calcification of the longus colli tendon. Arrows on the axial T2-weighted images point to the longus colli muscles. Only a small portion of the calcification is included in the upper right image. Note that fluid/edema (short arrows) is present both posterior (prevertebral space) and anterior (retropharyngeal space) to the longus colli muscles.

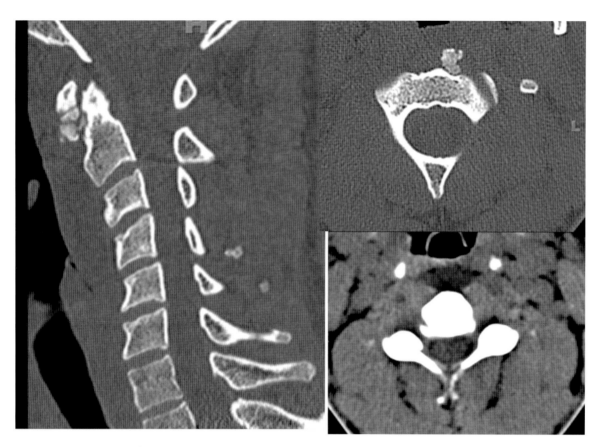

**Figure 92.2** CT images of the same patient as in Fig. 92.1 show the tendon calcification much more clearly. This is the most common location for tendon calcification.

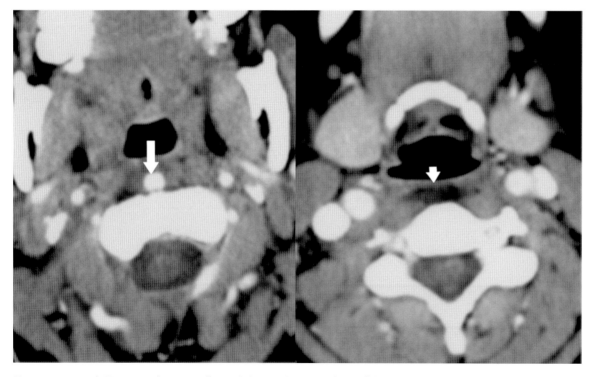

**Figure 92.3** Axial CT images show a midline calcification (arrow) in front of the C2 vertebral body with retropharyngeal edema (short arrow), compatible with CTLC.

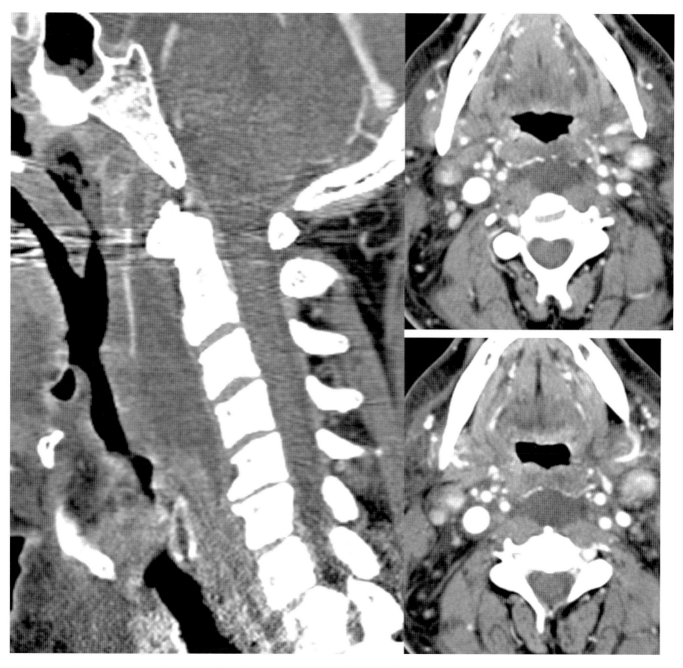

**Figure 92.4** Retropharyngeal phlegmon (cellulitis). Sagittal and axial CT images of the neck show a prominent swelling of the retropharyngeal soft tissues that bulges towards the pharyngeal airway. Positive mass effect and absence of tendon calcification separates this retropharyngeal cellulitis from CTLC. Retropharyngeal abscess would have an enhancing wall and demonstrate some asymmetry.

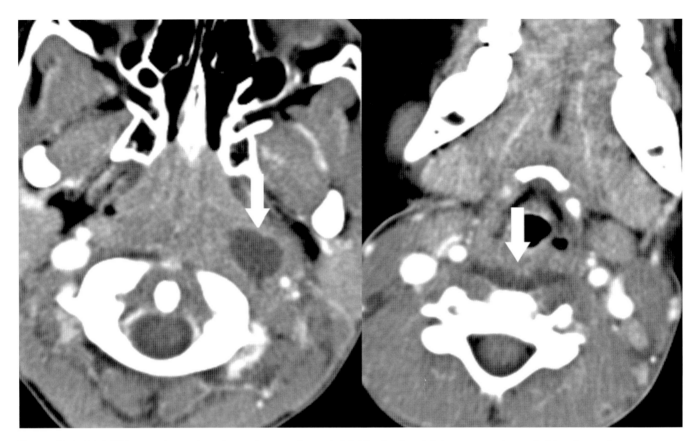

**Figure 92.5** Axial CT images show a lateral retropharyngeal rounded fluid collection (left image, arrow), a typical location and appearance for retropharyngeal lymph node suppuration. Mild retropharyngeal edema usually accompanies this (right image, arrow).

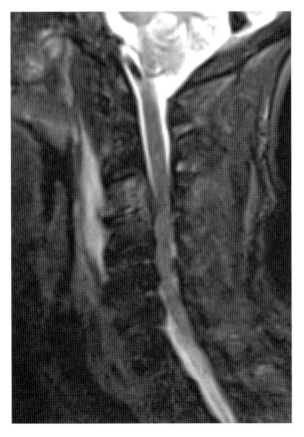

**Figure 92.6** Sagittal STIR image of the cervical spine shows retropharyngeal edema and abnormally increased signal within the C4–C5 disc space and adjacent endplates, indicating discitis and vertebral osteomyelitis.

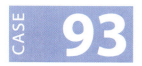

# 93 T2 hyperintense disc herniation

## Imaging description

Most disc herniations are hypointense on T2-weighted images, similar to the degenerated intervertebral disc they are associated with, which allows easy recognition and characterization of disc herniations on T2-weighted images thanks to increased contrast between the hypointense disc material and the hyperintense CSF and epidural fat. A small group of disc herniations are hyperintense on T2-weighted images with a diminished contrast between the disc material and CSF/epidural fat, leading to diagnostic errors (Fig. 93.1). In particular, relatively large T2 hyperintense fragments within the lateral recesses or foramina of the lumbar spine can go undetected because the thecal sac shows no significant contour deformity (Fig. 93.2). Yet disc herniations in the lateral recesses and foramina may potentially be more symptomatic, with more obvious radiculopathy due to compression of the descending or exiting nerve roots. In the cervical spine, T2 hyperintense disc herniations extending to the neural foramina can be missed because of high T2 signal of the epidural venous plexus, particularly on the gradient echo sequences. Foraminal disc herniations usually present with clear radiculopathy (Fig. 93.3). There is no clear understanding of why some disc herniations have increased T2 signal. There have been studies of acute traumatic disc herniations showing elevated T2 signal associated with disc herniations [1,2], but no systematic assessment of non-traumatic disc herniations with regards to T2 hyperintensity has been reported other than some anecdotes [3,4]. If contrast is given, T2 bright disc herniations usually show a rim enhancement.

## Importance

Compared to other sites of disc herniations, lateral recess herniations have a better correlation with the patient's symptoms.

## Typical clinical scenario

Relatively acute back pain and radiculopathy.

## Differential diagnosis

In the proper clinical setting with characteristic imaging findings, a definitive diagnosis is easily made once the lesion is visualized. To decrease the chance of missing these herniations, axial T1-weighted images may be very helpful, as the herniated disc looks very different than the epidural fat. If contrast material is given, some disc herniations show marked enhancement, to the extent that the lesion may mimic an extradural mass such as schwannoma or meningioma (Fig. 93.4). On close inspection there is always a portion of the disc material, albeit small, that does not enhance.

## Teaching points

Some disc herniations show increased T2 signal, making them difficult to diagnose on T2-weighted images, particularly when they are in the lateral recess of the lumbar spine or foramina of the cervical spine.

REFERENCES

1. Dai L, Jia L. Central cord injury complicating acute cervical disc herniation in trauma. *Spine (Phila Pa 1976)* 2000; **25**: 331–5.
2. Rizzolo SJ, Piazza MR, Cotler JM, *et al.* Intervertebral disc injury complicating cervical spine trauma. *Spine* 1991; **16**: S187–9.
3. Sadanand V, Kelly M, Varughese G, Fourney DR. Sudden quadriplegia after acute cervical disc herniation. *Can J Neurol Sci* 2005; **32**: 356–8.
4. Mahapatra AK, Gupta PK, Pawar SJ, Sharma RR. Sudden bilateral foot drop: an unusual presentation of lumbar disc prolapse. *Neurol India* 2003; **51**: 71–2.

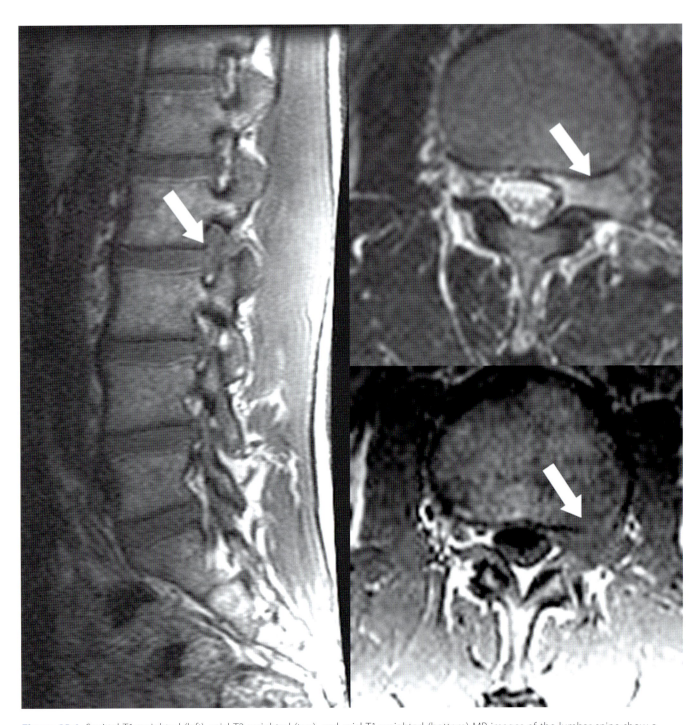

**Figure 93.1** Sagittal T1-weighted (left), axial T2-weighted (top), and axial T1-weighted (bottom) MR images of the lumbar spine show a large left foraminal disc herniation (arrows) which has a bright signal on T2-weighted images. Note absence of compression of the thecal sac. T1-weighted images show effacement of the epidural fat much more reliably. This patient had a severe left L2 radiculopathy.

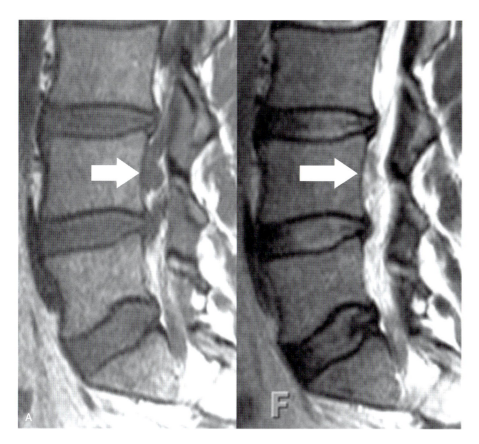

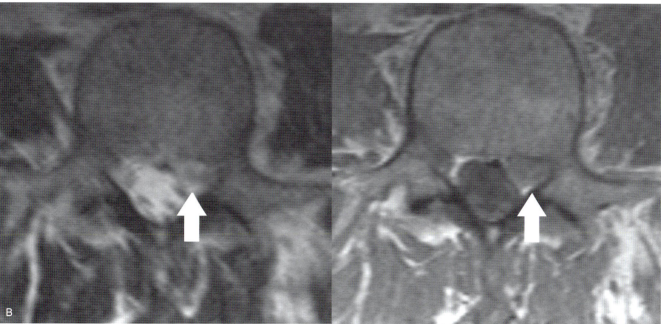

**Figure 93.2** (**A**) Sagittal T1-weighted and T2-weighted images show a T2 bright disc herniation in the lateral recess compressing the descending L4 nerve root. These are the only sagittal images that show the herniated disc. (**B**) Axial T1-weighted image reveals a large free disc fragment in the left lateral recess which is not reliably seen on the motion-degraded axial T2-weighted image due to its high T2 signal.

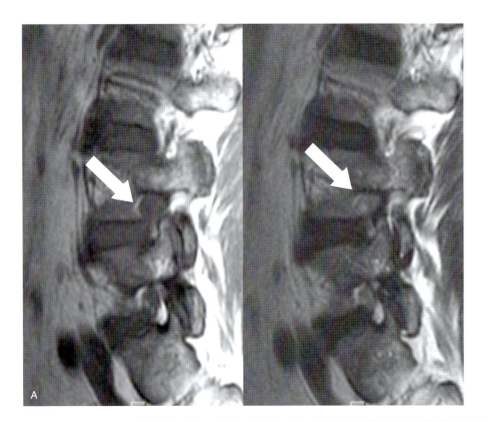

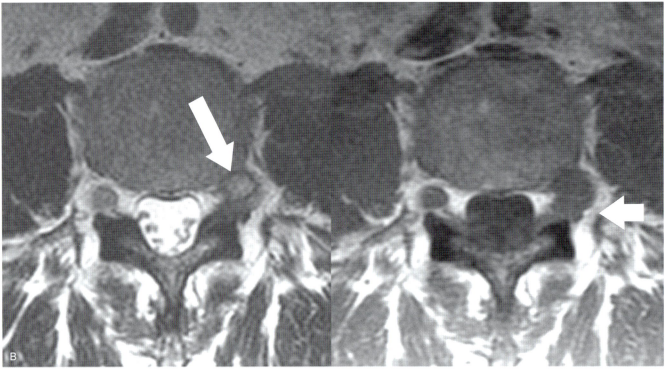

**Figure 93.3** (**A**) Sagittal and (**B**) axial T1-weighted and T2-weighted images show a left foraminal disc extrusion (arrows) which compresses the dorsal root ganglion (short arrow). Again note that it is easier to see the herniated disc on T1-weighted images.

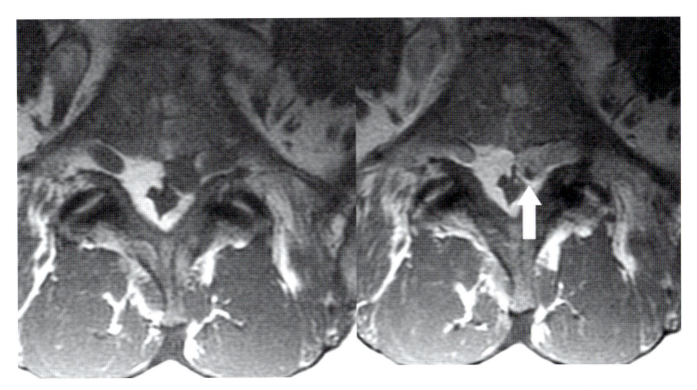

**Figure 93.4** Axial pre-contrast (left) and post-contrast (right) T1-weighted images show a large free disc fragment within the left lateral recess that shows marked enhancement. Note a small non-enhancing portion (arrow), which helps to differentiate this from an extradural mass lesion.

## Imaging description

Cervical myelopathy (CM) can result from extrinsic compression of the cord or cord inflammation, demyelination, ischemia, or infection. The most common reason for CM is spondylosis of the cervical spine. MRI is the modality of choice in the work-up of CM, and it can differentiate intrinsic cord lesions from extrinsic ones such as cervical spondylosis. In patients with CM secondary to cervical spondylotic changes, MRI shows narrowing of the spinal canal, complete effacement of the CSF spaces at the stenotic level(s), and deformity of the cord, although presence of these findings does not always predict clinically detectable CM. Although the primary mechanism of cervical spondylotic myelopathy is the compression of nervous tissue, there is some evidence that ischemia at the cellular level may be a contributing factor [1].

Increased T2 signal within the cord at the level of compression can be seen in some patients and heralds a worse outcome after surgical decompression compared to patients who do not have increased T2 signal in their cords [2]. Other factors that are associated with lack or diminished levels of improvement following surgery include old age, longer duration of symptoms, diminished T1 signal in the cord, and worse preoperative neurologic status [2–4].

Significant controversy still exists with regards to the surgical versus conservative management of patients with spondylotic myelopathy [1]. Interestingly, the value of contrast enhancement in the cord in predicting the outcome has not been investigated at all, perhaps because most of the studies performed are retrospective and routine cervical spine MRI protocols do not include contrast-enhanced sequences. When contrast is given, abnormal contrast enhancement can be seen within the cord in spondylotic CM, although the prevalence of this finding is not known (Figs. 94.1, 94.2). A contrast-enhancing cord lesion usually prompts a differential diagnosis (unnecessarily in the case of compressive myelopathy) that includes inflammatory and demyelinating disorders of the cord.

## Importance

Delaying treatment for compressive myelopathy for the work-up of an enhancing cord lesion may have a negative impact on outcome.

## Typical clinical scenario

Signs and symptoms of CM include gait disturbance, often with imbalance, lower extremity stiffness and jerking, upper and/or lower limb sensory loss and/or weakness, loss of hand dexterity, bowel and bladder dysfunction including urgency and incontinence, Lhermitte sign, and neck and/or unilateral or bilateral upper limb pain. Although it certainly can be present, the majority of patients do not report significant neck or upper limb pain [1].

## Differential diagnosis

Enhancing cord lesion differential diagnosis is broad and includes inflammatory, demyelinating, infectious, and toxic etiologies. When cord enhancement is associated with marked spinal canal stenosis secondary to spondylotic changes and T2 hyperintensity in the cord, the presumptive diagnosis should be spondylotic cervical myelopathy. Clinical and imaging follow-up to demonstrate resolution of abnormal enhancement is important and may take several months.

## Teaching points

Abnormal contrast enhancement seen in patients with cervical cord compression should not dissuade radiologists from considering the diagnosis of spondylotic myelopathy in the appropriate clinical setting.

REFERENCES

1. Tracy JA, Bartleson JD. Cervical spondylotic myelopathy. *Neurologist* 2010; **16**: 176–87.
2. Okada Y, Ikata T, Yamada H, Sakamoto R, Katoh S. Magnetic resonance imaging study on the results of surgery for cervical compression myelopathy. *Spine (Phila Pa 1976)* 1993; **18**: 2024–9.
3. Morio Y, Teshima R, Nagashima H, *et al.* Correlation between operative outcomes of cervical compression myelopathy and MRI of the spinal cord. *Spine (Phila Pa 1976)* 2001; **26**: 1238–45.
4. Yukawa Y, Kato F, Yoshihara H, Yanase M, Ito K. MR T2 image classification in cervical compression myelopathy: predictor of surgical outcomes. *Spine (Phila Pa 1976)* 2007; **32**: 1675–8.

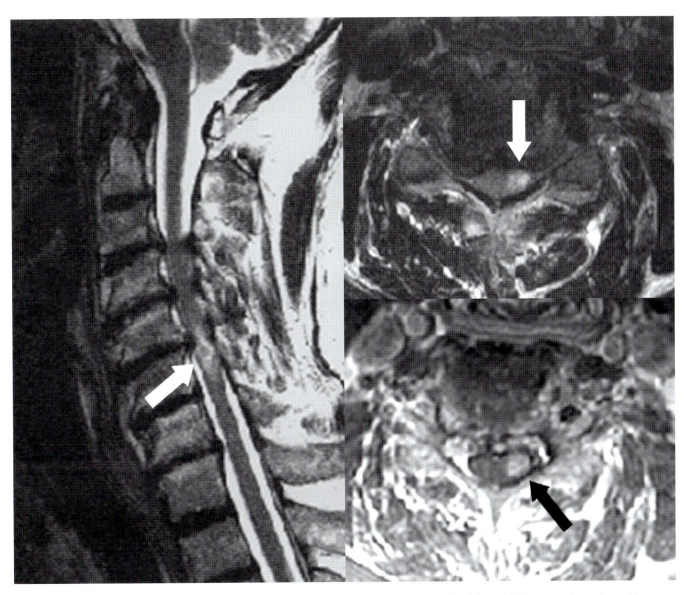

**Figure 94.1** Sagittal T2-weighted, axial T2-weighted (upper), and post-contrast axial T1-weighted (lower) MR images of a patient with acute CM and radiculopathy show a focal cord lesion displaying increased T2 signal and prominent contrast enhancement (arrows). A large disc herniation causes cord compression and marked canal compromise at this level. The patient underwent surgical decompression of the spine. Follow-up MRIs showed resolution of abnormal enhancement in 5 months.

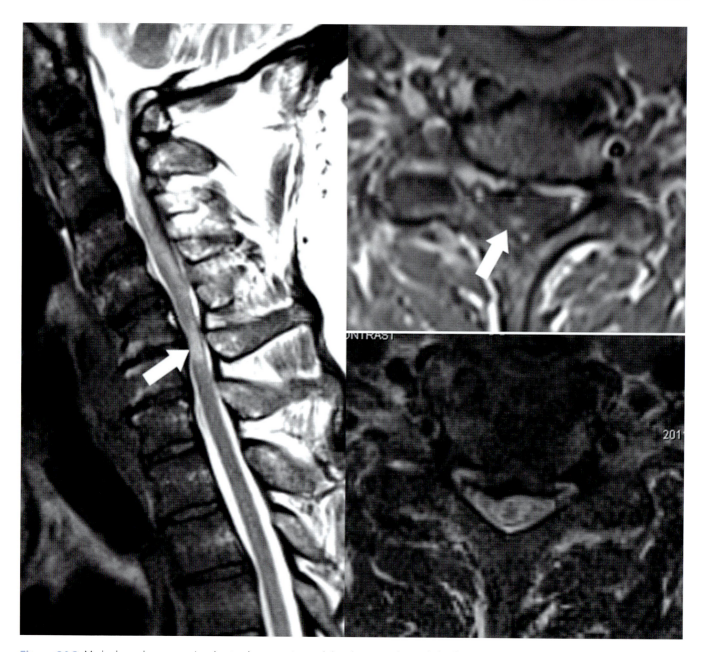

**Figure 94.2** Marked canal compromise due to degenerative endplate hypertrophy and disc herniation is noted at C5–C6 level with a T2 hyperintese cord lesion and a punctuate enhancement (arrows) seen. No evidence of underlying inflammatory or demyelinating disease was found in clinical work-up, and enhancement resolved.

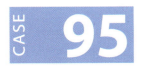
# Postoperative disc herniation versus postsurgical scarring

## Imaging description

MRI is the modality of choice for evaluation of the post-discectomy spine if there is a suspicion for recurrent disc herniation. Intravenous gadolinium should be routinely administered, as it helps in the differentiation of recurrent disc herniation from postoperative scarring. Moreover, it may assist with diagnosis of postoperative arachnoiditis and spinal infection. Sagittal as well as axial images should be routinely obtained in postoperative spine without and with intravenous gadolinium (Figs. 95.1, 95.2, 95.3)

Differentiation between recurrent disc herniation and scar is crucial in the management, but it is not an easy task. This is because of accompanying postsurgical alterations and edema, as well as frequent co-incidence of scar and herniated disc. Herniated disc is generally low in T1 signal and T2 signal. One may be able to identify a thin band of very low signal surrounding the disc, suggestive of fibers of annulus. However, the disc material may occasionally be bright on T2-weighted sequences. Recurrent disc herniation generally does not enhance with intravenous contrast other than at its periphery [1]. However, it is imperative that the imaging should begin promptly after contrast administration. The disc may enhance homogeneously on delayed enhanced images and may therefore be inseparable from scar.

Postsurgical scar is generally ill-defined, demonstrates low T1 as well as T2 signal, and enhances with contrast administration. The scar is infiltrative and does not exert mass effect on the nerve root of the thecal sac. However, scar often coexists with recurrent disc, and it may not always be possible to differentiate reliably between the two.

## Importance

Accurate differentiation of recurrent disc herniation from scar formation may allow improved treatment choices and proper selection of patients who may benefit from a second surgery.

## Typical clinical scenario

The most common setting for reimaging patients after a laminectomy and discectomy is for recurrent symptoms of back pain and/or radiculopathy.

## Differential diagnosis

Recurrent disc and scar demonstrate similar signal intensities on unenhanced T1-weighted sequence. The disc has a globular or polypoid appearance, and it is usually contiguous with the parent disc unless sequestrated. An overlying, peripheral rim of dark signal may outline the disc, enhancing after contrast administration. The disc substance itself generally does not enhance. Mass effect on the nerve or thecal sac points to the disc, whereas retraction of the thecal sac toward a soft tissue lesion is suggestive of scar.

---

### Teaching points

MRI is the examination of choice in postoperative pain following surgery for disc disease. An examination with gadolinium contrast allows the differentiation between postoperative scar and recurrent disc herniation with a very high accuracy. If postoperative scar is the predominant pathology, the issue of reoperation should be considered very carefully.

---

REFERENCES

1. Bundschuh CV, Modic MT, Ross JS, Masaryk TJ, Bohlman H. Epidural fibrosis and recurrent disk herniation in the lumbar spine: MR imaging assessment. *AJR Am J Roentgenol* 1988; **150**: 923–32.

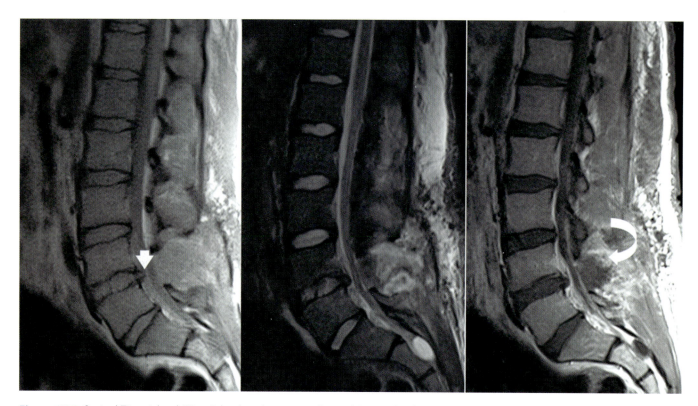

**Figure 95.1** Sagittal T1-weighted, T2-weighted, and contrast-enhanced T1-weighted images are shown in succession. This patient developed sudden left-sided pain following left L4–L5 microdiscectomy. Note a postoperative collection (curved arrow) and diffuse epidural soft tissue anterior to the thecal sac. There is a small recurrent disc herniation marked by the short arrow. The peripheral band of low intensity and maintained connection to the disc differentiate the disc from adjacent postoperative soft tissue thickening.

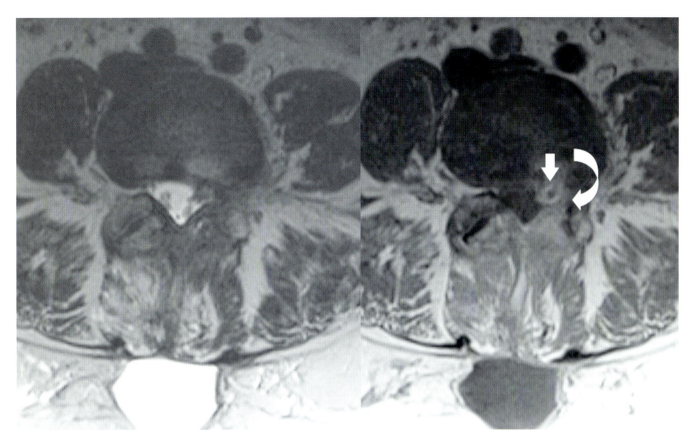

**Figure 95.2** Coexistent scar and recurrent left paracentral disc herniation at L3–L4 level. A small extruded disc fragment in the left lateral recess is marked with an arrow on enhanced T1-weighted axial image. Peripheral rim of enhancement and presence of mass effect on adjacent L4 nerve root on T2-weighted image differentiate this from the more extensive and laterally located scar (curved arrow).

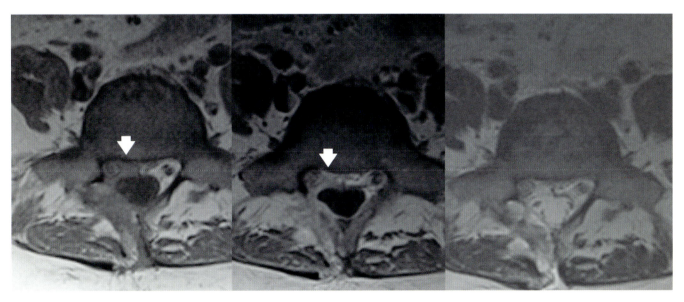

**Figure 95.3** Axial T1-weighted, contrast-enhanced T1-weighted, and T2-weighted images from L5–S1 level. Diffuse postoperative epidural fibrosis (scarring) in this patient exists along the right L5 laminectomy, lateral and anterior to the thecal sac on the right (arrow). Note the infiltrative nature of the scar surrounding the nerve root as well as the presence of enlargement and subtle high signal in the S1 nerve root.

# Degenerative endplate alterations

## Imaging description

Disc degeneration is accompanied by loss of hydration in the nucleus pulposus and declining structural integrity of the annulus fibrosus. The nucleus pulposus loses its high signal on T2-weighted images and there is a loss of disc height. Alterations in the adjacent vertebral endplates and vertebral marrow are commonly identified adjacent to the degenerated disc. These changes have been classified based on the pathologic changes in the vertebral endplate.

Modic type 1 marrow change signifies vascularized marrow, appearing hypointense on T1-weighted and hyperintense on T2-weighted sequences (Fig. 96.1). Type 2 changes occur with more chronic disc degeneration, with fatty changes in the adjacent marrow (Fig. 96.2). This type of degenerative change demonstrates high signal on T1-weighted and slightly high signal on T2-weighted images. Type 3 changes represent sclerosis and marrow fibrosis, resulting in dark signal on T1- and T2-weighted sequences [1]. The vertebral endplates in type 1 and type 2 change may enhance with contrast. There is relatively little evidence that the exact type of marrow changes harbor any clinical significance. However, it is imperative that radiologists be aware of the spectrum of signal abnormalities that can occur in the marrow and not confuse these with more sinister pathologies.

On radiographs and CT, the endplate changes appear as areas of sclerosis. The definition of endplate is sharp (Figs. 96.1, 96.2) and no erosive changes are identified.

## Importance

Marrow changes accompanying degenerative disc disease are commonly mistaken for discitis and osteomyelitis. Differentiation between these two processes may, however, occasionally prove to be quite difficult or even impossible.

## Typical clinical scenario

Degenerative endplate changes are mainly identified on studies performed for the evaluation of back pain or radiculopathy.

## Differential diagnosis

Endplate and degenerative marrow alterations are frequently confused with discitis and osteomyelitis. In the majority of cases these processes can be differentiated from each other, but it may occasionally be extremely difficult.

Discitis is an inflammatory process that is a result of infection that initially seeds in the vertebral endplate. As it progresses, it causes destruction of the endplate and spreads to the disc. With progressive destruction of the disc, fluid starts to accumulate and there is developing paravertebral and/or epidural inflammatory change (Fig. 96.3). Destruction and erosive changes of the endplate are a hallmark of discitis/osteomyelitis (Figs. 96.3, 96.4) and accompany the developing edema in the marrow, whereas the endplates are generally intact in degenerative changes. In discitis, the disc is hyperintense on T2-weighted studies and demonstrates enhancement, but in degenerative disease it is hypointense, although in rare cases there can be T2 hyperintensity within the disc space in the setting of degenerative disease. The enhancement is intense in discitis/osteomyelitis but fairly subtle in deneneratrive endplate change. Additionally, paraspinal inflammatory changes are a hallmark of discitis but not appreciated in degenerative disease. Also, acute-phase reactants such as erythrocyte sedimentation rate (ESR) and C-reactive protein (CRP) are almost always elevated in discitis. While these are non-specific, when they are negative they can be used to exclude discitis.

## Teaching points

Although extensive marrow alterations may accompany degenerative disc disease, these can be differentiated from discitis because of sparing of the endplate margins, lack of high T2 signal in the disc, and relatively modest enhancement with contrast. In the rare case of T2 hyperintensity in the disc in degenerative disease, correlation with clinical history and markers of inflammation (CRP and ESR) provide further help in this differential diagnosis. Short-term imaging follow-up may be important in difficult cases. Invasive tissue sampling should rarely be necessary.

REFERENCES

1. Modic MT, Steinberg PM, Ross JS, Masaryk TJ, Carter JR. Degenerative disk disease: assessment of changes in vertebral body marrow with MR imaging. *Radiology* 1988; **166**: 193–9.

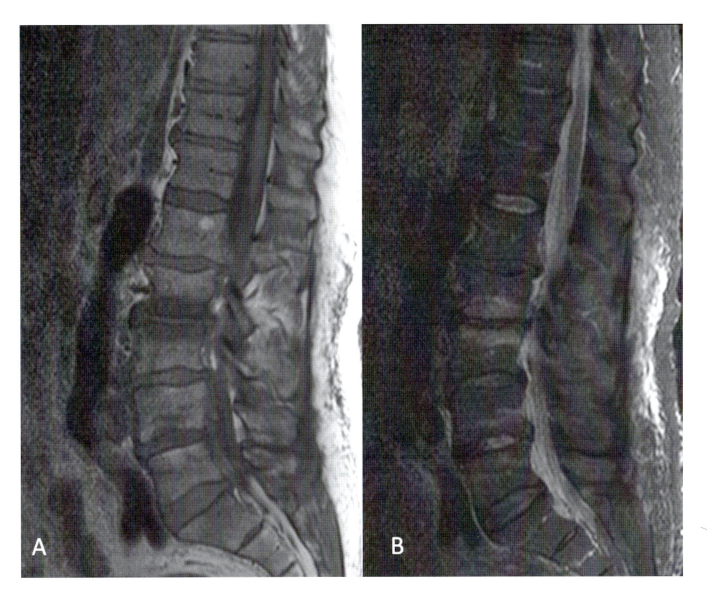

**Figure 96.1** Sagittal (A) T1-weighted and (B) fat-suppressed T2-weighted images demonstrate Modic type 1 changes at L2–L3 level. Note symmetric, low-intensity bands that demonstrate high signal edema on T2-weighted study. The endplates remain well defined and the disc has low T2 signal, suggesting degenerative process.

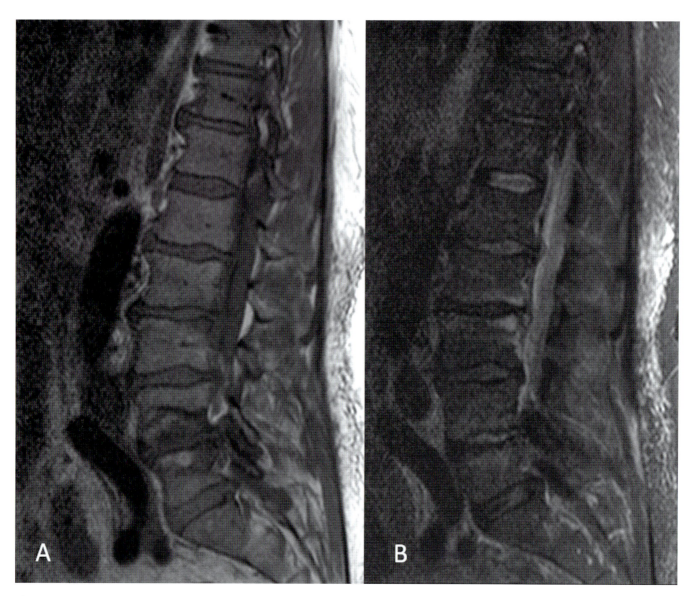

**Figure 96.2** Sagittal (**A**) T1-weighted and (**B**) fat-suppressed T2-weighted images reveal a combination of type 1 and type 2 marrow alterations at L4–L5 level. Again, note that the endplates are well corticated and there is no paravertebral of epidural edema.

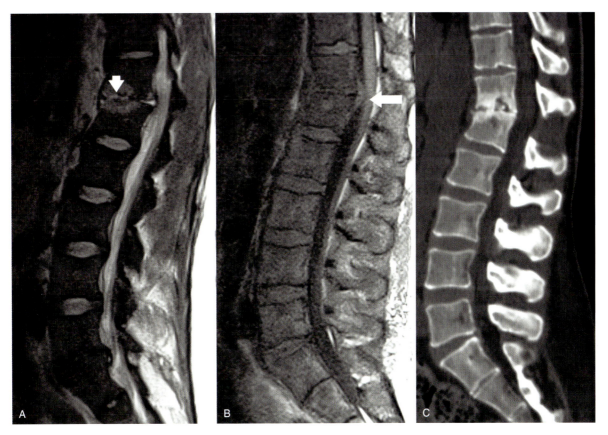

**Figure 96.3** Discitis/osteomyelitis at T12–L1 level is evident. (**A**) The features favoring the inflammatory process include asymmetric loss of disc space, high T2 signal in the disc, and loss of endplate margins (cortical line, short arrow). (**B**) Additionally, the presence of a small epidural inflammatory mass on sagittal T1-weighted image (horizontal arrow) is very suspicious for an inflammatory process. (**C**) The diagnosis is further supported on CT, which reveals irregular sclerosis and endplate destruction.

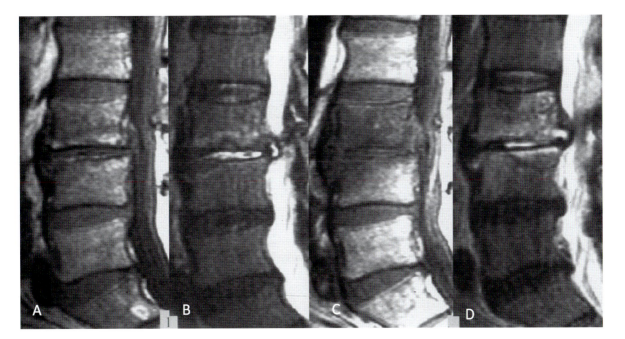

**Figure 96.4** Discitis/osteomyelitis (DO) may progress rapidly if undiagnosed. (**A, B**) In this patient with L3–L4 DO, the diagnosis was missed initially. (**C, D**) Note progressive abnormality of marrow signal on an MR image obtained 2 weeks later, reduction of disc space, and developing epidural phlegmon.

## Imaging description

Spina bifida properly refers to lack of fusion of the posterior bony element of the spinal canal. However, it is commonly confused with spinal dysraphisms, which are malformations of the spinal column and/or spinal cord across previous stages of development. The classification of spinal dysraphism takes into account the clinical, neuroradiological, and embryological features [1]. The neural placode is a segment of flattened, non-neurulated embryonic neural tissue [2]. It can be terminal or segmental, depending on its location with relation to the cord.

Clinically, spinal dysraphism can be categorized into open and closed varieties, depending on the location of the neural placode. In open spinal dysraphism (OSD), the placode is directly exposed to the environment and surrounded by partially epithelialized skin. In closed spinal dysraphism (CSD) the placode is covered with a full-thickness skin [3]. In 50% of patients with CSD, cutaneous birthmarks are also present. Therefore the term "occult spinal dysraphism" is not favored.

MRI offers a unique perspective on the relationship of the neural placode with the spinal cord and spinal column and makes an important contribution to the diagnosis and classification of spinal dysraphism.

## Importance

Gastrulation (week 2–3 of gestation), primary neurulation (week 3–4 of gestation), and secondary neurulation (week 5–6 of gestation) are the three basic embryonic stages leading to the development of mature spine. Abnormality of development at any of these stages can lead to spinal dysraphism. Clinical diagnosis of OSD is easier, given the exposure of the neural placode to the environment. It is important to assess for commonly associated conditions such as Chiari II malformation and hydrocephalus. CSDs are more diverse and may not to be clinically evident at birth unless associated with subcutaneous masses or cutaneous birthmarks [2]. When discovered in childhood or adulthood, it is important to look for associated abnormalities such as tethered cord, syringomyelia, dermal sinuses, vertebral anomalies, and intraspinal masses. A comprehensive classification of spinal dysraphism, based on embryogenesis, clinical findings, and radiological features, is summarized in Table 97.1.

## Typical clinical scenario

OSDs and most of the CSDs with subcutaneous mass are usually diagnosed at birth or in early infancy. They may also be detected by prenatal ultrasound or fetal MRI. In neonates,

**Table 97.1** Classification of spinal dysraphisms.

| Open spinal dysraphisms (OSD): without full skin cover |
| --- |
| • Myelomeningocele |
| • Myelocele |
| • Hemimyelocele Myelocele |
| • Hemimyelomeningocele |

| Closed spinal dysraphisms (CSD): with intact skin cover |
| --- |
| With a subcutaneous mass |
| • Meningocele |
| • Lipomyelomeningocele |
| • Lipomyelocele |
| • Myelocystocele |
| • Terminal myelocystocele |
| Without a subcutaneous mass<br>Simple dysraphic states |
| • Filum lipoma |
| • Intradural lipoma |
| • Tight filum terminale |
| • Persistent terminal ventricle |
| • Dermal sinus |
| Complex dysraphic states |
| • Diastematomyelia |
| • Caudal agenesis |
| • Segmental spinal dysgenesis |
| • Dorsal enteric fistula |
| • Neurenteric cyst |

screening with ultrasound to locate the position of conus medullaris and to investigate possible subcutaneous masses can also be performed [4]. However, many cases of CSD may be discovered in older children or adults, and these may be clinically occult. The presentation can be as subtle as a midline posterior dermal sinus, but may be associated with tethered cord syndrome (TCS) with progressive motor dysfunction, sensory deficits, foot drop, muscle atrophy, pain, or sphincter dysfunction.

## Differential diagnosis

A bifid spine may not be associated with spinal dysraphism. Conditions with OSD include myelomeningocele (Fig. 97.1), which accounts for about 98% of the cases, and myelocele (Fig. 97.2). In myelomeningocele, the neural placode protrudes above the cutaneous surface due to expansion of the underlying subarachnoid spaces. However, in myelocele, the placode is at the same level as the surface of the skin.

CSDs with subcutaneous masses include meningocele (Fig. 97.3), lipomyelomeningocele (Fig. 97.4), lipomyelocele (Fig. 97.5), myelocystocele, and terminal myelocystocele (Fig. 97.6). In lipomyelocele the placode–lipoma interface lies within the spinal canal, while in lipomyelomeningocele the placode–lipoma interface lies outside the spinal canal. In meningocele only CSF-filled cyst lined with dura protrudes posteriorly from the defect in spina bifida, but the spinal cord is generally tethered to the neck of the fluid-filled sac. In a terminal myelocystocele the terminal syrinx cavity, including terminal portion of the cord, herniates within a meningocele.

Simple CSDs without subcutaneous mass include lipoma of filum terminale (Fig. 97.7), intradural lipoma (Fig. 97.8), tight filum terminale (Fig. 97.9), persistent terminal ventricle, and a dermal sinus with and without epidermoid. All posterior dermal sinuses above the natal crease should be suspected of occult spinal dysraphism and further evaluated. This is the most challenging category for a neuroradiologist.

Complex CSDs without subcutaneous mass include conditions such as diastematomyelia (Fig. 97.10), caudal agenesis (Fig. 97.11), segmental spinal dysgenesis (Fig. 97.12), neurenteric cyst, and dorsal enteric fistula. A tuft of hair high along the back is commonly associated with diastematomyelia. Caudal regression and agenesis may be associated with lower limb abnormalities or anorectal malformations.

## Teaching points

MR features of spinal dysraphism may appear complex and complicated, with the possibility of overlapping features. However, an approach based on clinical, embryological, and MR imaging features helps to arrive at proper diagnoses. With the increasing usage of prenatal ultrasound, fetal MRI, and neonatal ultrasound, an early diagnosis is possible.

REFERENCES

1. Tortori-Donati P, Rossi A, Cama A. Spinal dysraphism: a review of neuroradiological features with embryological correlations and proposal for a new classification. *Neuroradiology* 2000; **42**: 471–91.
2. Rossi A, Gandolfo C, Morana G, *et al.* Current classification and imaging of congenital spinal abnormalities. *Semin Roentgenol* 2006; **41**: 250–73.
3. Rufener S, Ibrahim M, Parmar HA. Imaging of congenital spine and spinal cord malformations. *Neuroimaging Clin N Am* 2011; **21**: 659–76.
4. Chern JJ, Aksut B, Kirkman JL, *et al.* The accuracy of abnormal lumbar sonography findings in detecting occult spinal dysraphism: a comparison with magnetic resonance imaging. *J Neurosurg Pediatr* 2012; **10**: 150–3.

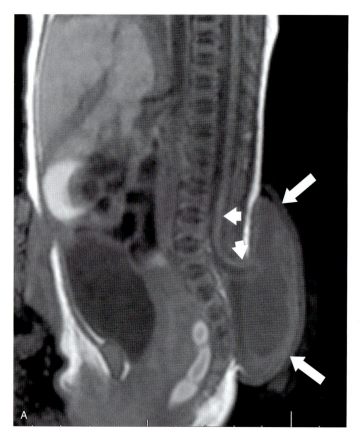

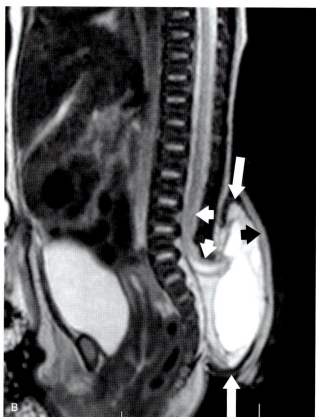

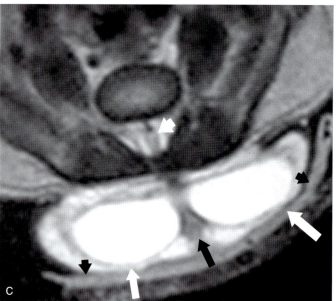

**Figure 97.1** Myelomeningocele. (**A**) T1-weighted sagittal MR image exhibits a meningeal outpouching through a large posterior defect in the lumbosacral spine (arrows). The low-lying spinal cord enters the outpouching (short arrows) and ends in the terminal placode. (**B**) T2-weighted sagittal MR imaging exhibits a fluid-filled cystic outpouching containing terminal spinal cord (short white arrows) and exposed to the environment (white arrows). It is covered externally by a piece of gauze (short black arrow). (**C**) T2-weighted axial MR image exhibits the cystic outpouching (arrow) containing the terminal placode (black arrow), covered by a piece of gauze (short black arrows). Note the terminal portion of the low-lying spinal cord within the spinal canal (short white arrow).

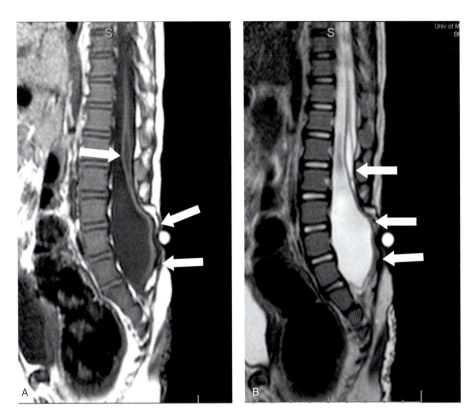

**Figure 97.2** Myelocele. (**A**) T1-weighted sagittal and (**B**) T2-weighted sagittal MR images exhibit the terminal neural placode protruding from the posterior bony defect, flush with the skin surface (arrows). Note the low-lying spinal cord with the terminal syrinx (arrow).

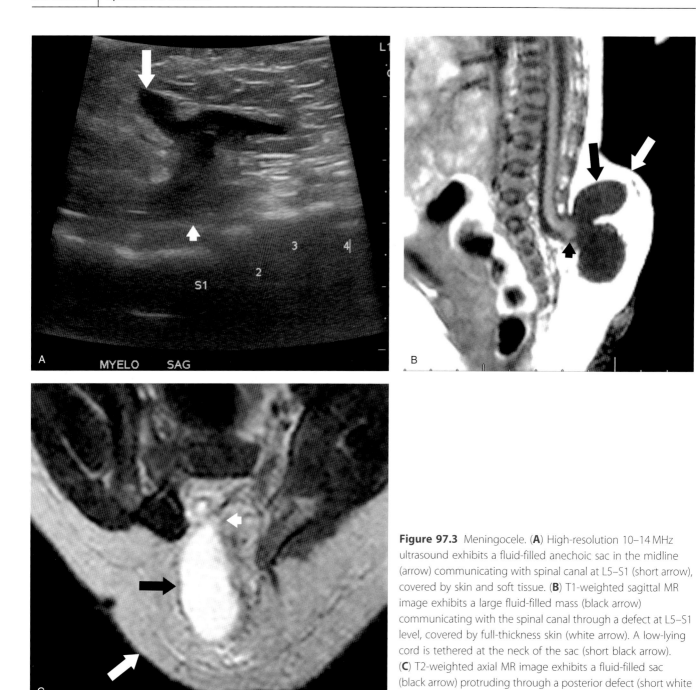

**Figure 97.3** Meningocele. (**A**) High-resolution 10–14 MHz ultrasound exhibits a fluid-filled anechoic sac in the midline (arrow) communicating with spinal canal at L5–S1 (short arrow), covered by skin and soft tissue. (**B**) T1-weighted sagittal MR image exhibits a large fluid-filled mass (black arrow) communicating with the spinal canal through a defect at L5–S1 level, covered by full-thickness skin (white arrow). A low-lying cord is tethered at the neck of the sac (short black arrow). (**C**) T2-weighted axial MR image exhibits a fluid-filled sac (black arrow) protruding through a posterior defect (short white arrow) and covered by full-thickness skin (white arrow).

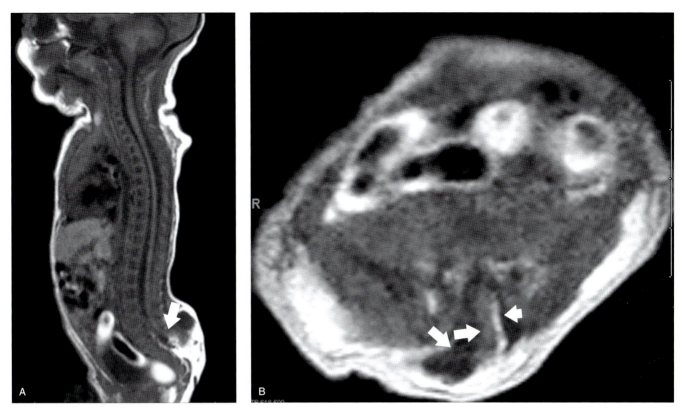

**Figure 97.4** Lipomyelomeningocele. (**A**) T1-weighted sagittal MR image exhibits a fluid-filled cavity protruding posteriorly and covered with full-thickness skin. Note the low-lying cord (arrow) entering the posterior outpouching. (**B**) T1-weighted axial MR image shows that the spinal cord projects out of the spinal canal and courses into the fluid-filled cavity. It attaches to a lipoma (short arrow) outside the anatomic boundary of the spinal canal.

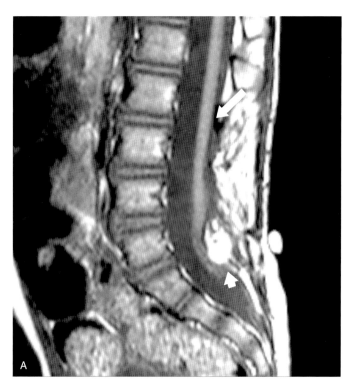

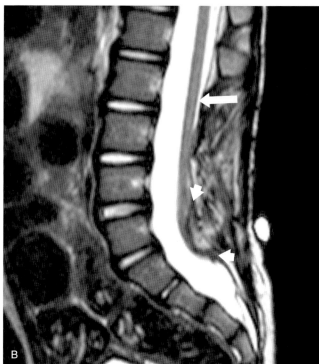

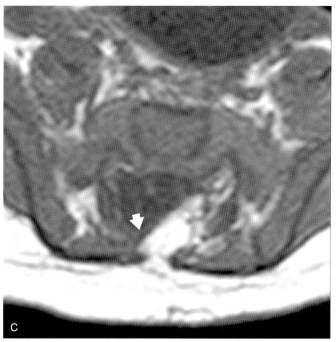

**Figure 97.5** Lipomyelocele. (**A**) T1-weighted and (**B**) T2-weighted sagittal MR images show a lipoma (short arrows) protruding posteriorly from a bony defect at L5–S1 level. Note the low-lying tethered spinal cord (arrow). (**C**) T1-weighted axial MR image shows the posterior defect with intraspinal lipoma communicating with subcutaneous lipoma. Note that the placode–lipoma interface (short arrow) is within the bony boundary of the spinal canal.

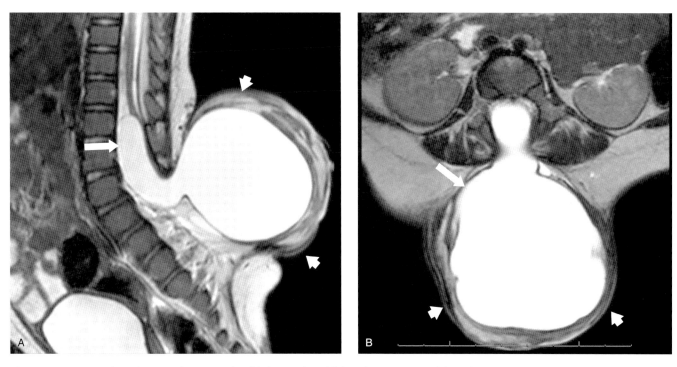

**Figure 97.6** Terminal myelocystocele. T2-weighted (**A**) sagittal and (**B**) axial MR images exhibit a large posteriorly protruding meningocele (short arrows) containing a terminal syrinx (arrow).

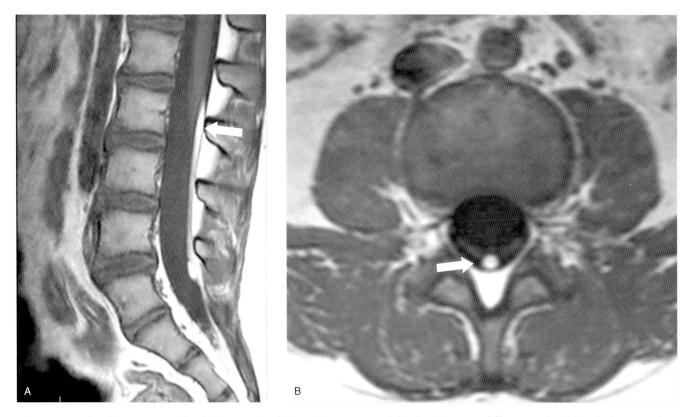

**Figure 97.7** Filum lipoma. T1-weighted (**A**) sagittal and (**B**) axial MR images exhibit that the terminal filum is replaced by a high T1 signal linear lipoma (arrow).

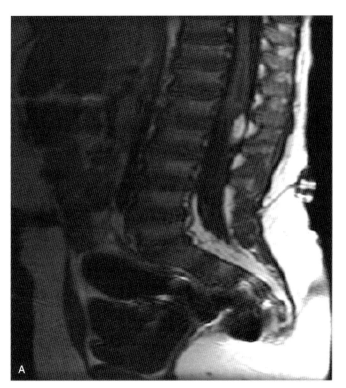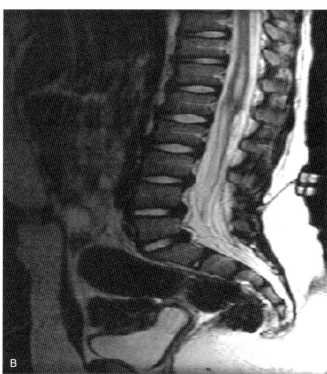

**Figure 97.8** Intradural lipoma and dorsal dermal sinus. (**A**) T1-weighted and (**B**) T2-weighted sagittal MR images exhibit a lipoma attached to the dorsal surface of the conus medullaris. Also note a dorsal dermal sinus tract at L4 level marked by a surface marker.

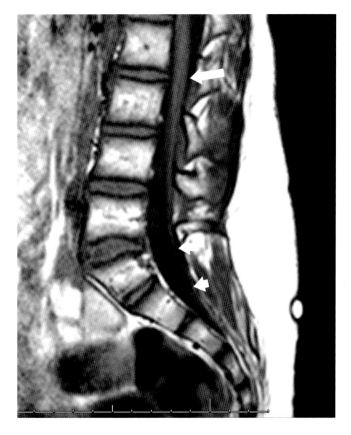

**Figure 97.9** Tight filum terminale. T1-weighted sagittal MR image exhibits a low-lying cord (arrow) with thickened filum terminale (short arrows).

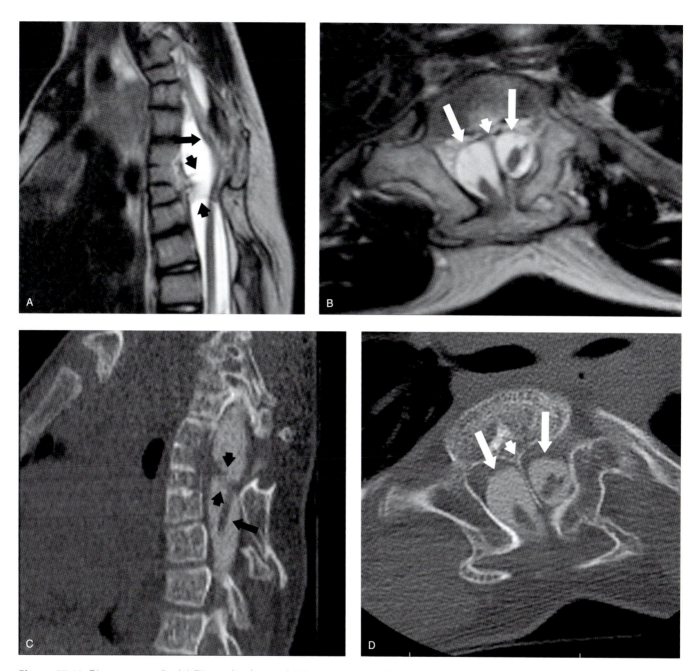

**Figure 97.10** Diastematomyelia. (**A**) T2-weighted sagittal MR image exhibits faint transverse septum (short black arrows) with posteriorly deviated hemicord (black arrow). (**B**) T2-weighted axial MR image exhibits a fibro-osseous midline septum (short arrow) with two separate dural sacs (arrows) containing hemicords. (**C**) Sagittal reconstruction of CT myelogram exhibits transverse septum (short black arrows) with hemicord (black arrow). (**D**) Axial CT myelogram exhibits a fibro-osseous midline septum (short arrow) with two separate dural sacs (arrows) containing hemicords.

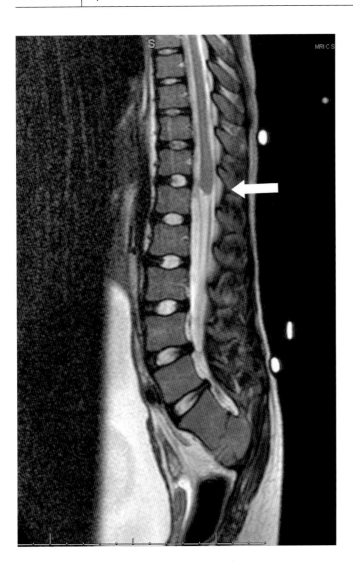

**Figure 97.11** Caudal regression. T2-weighted sagittal MR image exhibits abrupt termination of a wedge-shaped conus medullaris (arrow) with tapering of dural sac that ends high. Note the subtotal sacrococcygeal agenesis. There is "double bundle" configuration of the nerve roots of cauda equina.

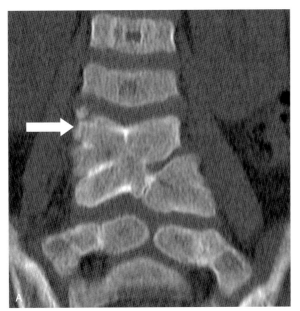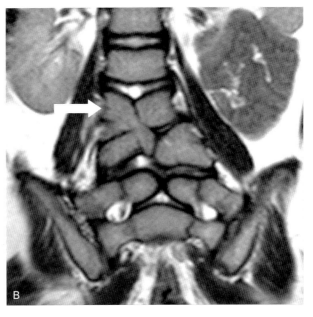

**Figure 97.12** Segmentation fusion anomaly. (**A**) Coronal reconstruction of CT scan of lumbar spine and (**B**) T2-weighted coronal MR image exhibit complex segmental anomaly (arrow) including butterfly vertebra, hemivertebra, and partial sagittal partition.

## Imaging description

In a radiological study, termination of conus medullaris below L2 vertebral level is considered tethering of the cord. However, tethered cord syndrome (TCS) is the constellation of symptoms and signs of motor and sensory dysfunction that are caused by excessive traction and tension on the spinal cord [1]. A majority of cases with TCS are associated with anomalies in nervous system development and are related to spinal dysraphism. Completely intradural processes such as lipoma of filum terminale (Fig. 98.1), abnormal fibrous adhesions, and shortened filum terminale are also associated with tethered cord. They are sometimes known as primary TCS, with terms like tight filum, fatty filum, and filum terminale syndrome [1]. Closed spinal dysraphisms such as lipomyelomeningocele, diastematomyelia, neurenteric cyst, lumbosacral lipoma (Fig. 98.2), dermal sinus, and thickened filum terminale are increasingly associated with tethered cord [2]. Almost all children born with open spinal dysraphisms such as spinal meningoceles (Fig. 98.3), myelomeningocele (Fig. 98.4), and myeloschisis have tethered cord [3]. More recently, TCS has been broadened to include patients with tethering of cervical or thoracic cord, and also patients with increased tension on the lower cord, in spite of having a normal position of conus [1]. TCS is also been associated with diverse conditions including trauma, infection, and neoplasm.

With increasing tension on the spinal cord, the blood flow and oxidative metabolism become impaired, with resultant ischemic injury and diminished conduction in both motor and sensory nerve fibers. In 24–30% of patients with TCS, there is an association with terminal syringomyelia (Fig. 98.4B), which is different from that caused by Chiari formation or arachnoiditis [4]. The epicenter of syringomyelia associated with tethered cord is very close to the tethering site or dysraphism [5]. It is also well established that TCS is a cause of scoliosis [6].

MRI is the modality of choice to evaluate patients with suspected tethered cord and scoliosis. Apart from low-lying conus medullaris terminating below L2 level, a thickened filum measuring more than 2 mm at L5–S1 level or a small lipoma of filum terminale are seen. Ultrasound can be used for determining the conus level in the newborn, but the sonographic window disappears at 2 months of age.

## Importance

There are conflicting opinions regarding surgical management of patients with tethered cord. A few studies indicate that reversal of upper motor neuron function is poor even after surgery if there is onset of neurologic deficit. Based on these observations, prophylactic release of tethered cord is advocated [2]. However, not all the patients with tethered cord actually developed TCS, with lesser degrees of tethering remaining subclinical. It is suggested that the surgical release of tethered cord should be performed on appearance of an upper motor neuron sign. The technical goal of untethering surgery is to remove the tension from the spinal cord, while the therapeutic goal is to stabilize symptomatology and cord function [1]. Depending on the cause of tethering, a wide variety of surgeries are performed. A large majority of children with repaired myelomeningocele has a tethered spinal cord, although only 10–30% develop a symptomatic TCS [6]. As early untethering for secondary TCS is essential [7], it is important to critically evaluate postsurgical MR images.

## Typical clinical scenario

The clinical presentation of tethered spinal cord depends on the age group and etiology. Cutaneous stigmata in neonates, such as presence of nevi, posterior midline lipomas, tufts of hair, hemangiomas, and dermal sinuses may be the only sign. There is a high association with a presence of anorectal malformations, scoliosis, and orthopedic lower limb deformity. In childhood and adolescence, gait difficulty, progressive motor dysfunction, sensory deficits, progression of scoliosis, foot drop, pain, and sphincter dysfunction are seen.

## Differential diagnosis

Low-lying conus as a normal variant. In a small minority of patients, it is possible to have a low-lying conus medullaris without evidence for filum lipoma or thickening of terminal filum on axial imaging. There is absence of any of the neurological symptomatology associated with TCS.

The low position of the conus in the postoperative setting causes difficulties in interpretation. After repair of spinal dysraphism and untethering of the cord, there is a high incidence of retethering. However, radiologic low position of conus medullaris in the postoperative setting cannot be used to diagnose retethering. Correlation with clinical symptoms is essential. Measuring spinal cord motion using phase-contrast MRI may be helpful in this setting, although experience with this method is limited.

---

### Teaching points

The classic imaging appearance is conus medullaris terminating below the inferior endplate of L2 vertebra, a tight filum terminale with associated tethering mass. It is seen in a majority of cases with open or closed spinal dysraphism, but can also be seen in completely intradural conditions, scar tissue from prior surgery, trauma, infection, and neoplasm. Terminal syringomyelia can be seen in up to a third of patients with tethered cord. The high incidence of retethering following surgery for spinal dysraphism demands critical evaluation of the postsurgical spine.

REFERENCES

1. Lew SM, Kothbauer KF. Tethered cord syndrome: an updated review. *Pediatr Neurosurg* 2007; **43**: 236–48.

2. Cornette L, Verpoorten C, Lagae L, *et al.* Tethered cord syndrome in occult spinal dysraphism: timing and outcome of surgical release. *Neurology* 1998; **50**: 1761–5.

3. Bowman RM, Mohan A, Ito J, *et al.* Tethered cord release: a long-term study in 114 patients. *J Neurosurg Pediatr* 2009; **3**: 181–7.

4. Beaumont A, Muszynski CA, Kaufman BA. Clinical significance of terminal syringomyelia in association with pediatric tethered cord syndrome. *Pediatr Neurosurg* 2007; **43**: 216–21.

5. Lee JY, Phi JH, Cheon JE, *et al.* Preuntethering and postuntethering courses of syringomyelia associated with tethered spinal cord. *Neurosurgery* 2012; **71**: 23–9.

6. Hudgins RJ, Gilreath CL. Tethered spinal cord following repair of myelomeningocele. *Neurosurg Focus* 2004; **16**: E7.

7. Ohe N, Futamura A, Kawada R, *et al.* Secondary tethered cord syndrome in spinal dysraphism. *Childs Nerv Syst* 2000; **16**: 457–61.

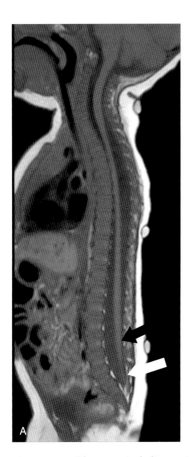
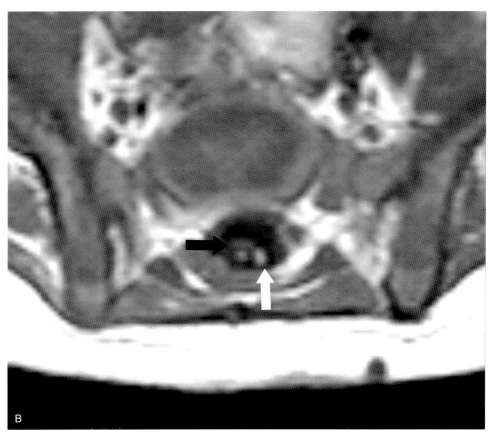

**Figure 98.1** Filum terminale lipoma in anorectal malformation with sacral dysgenesis. (**A**) T1-weighted sagittal image exhibits truncated sacral column. The tethered spinal cord is low-lying (black arrow) with presence of a lipoma of filum terminale (white arrow). (**B**) T1-weighted axial image exhibits a thickened filum terminale (black arrow) at L5–S1 level with small lipoma of filum terminale (white arrow).

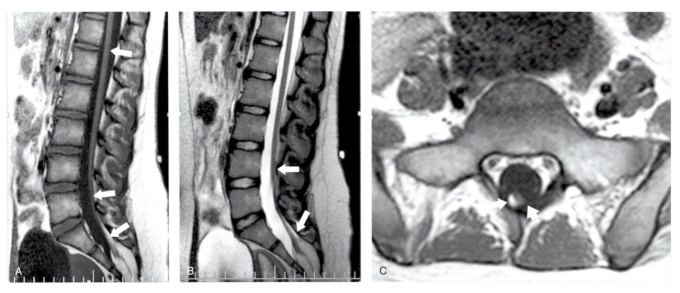

**Figure 98.2** Intradural lipoma. (**A**) T1-weighted sagittal image exhibits presence of large lobulated high T1 signal intradural lipoma within the sacral canal, contiguous with a lipoma of filum terminale with tethering of the cord (arrows). (**B**) T2-weighted sagittal image exhibits high T2 signal intradural lipoma with a tethered cord (arrows) that does not exhibit normal definition of conus medullaris. (**C**) T1-weighted axial image exhibits a thickened filum terminale at the level of L5–S1 (short arrow), with lipoma of filum terminale (arrow).

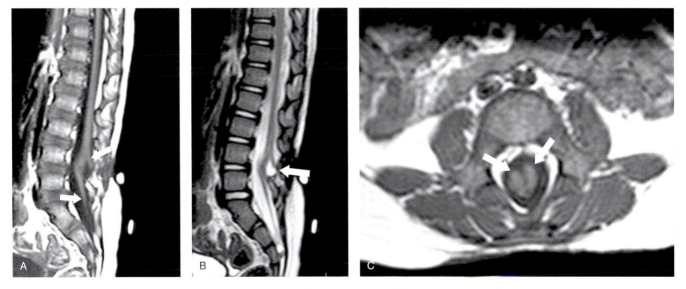

**Figure 98.3** Split cord in meningocele repair. (**A**) T1-weighted sagittal image exhibits low-lying spinal cord, splitting at L4 level with one hemicord adherent to posterior margin of dura, at previous meningocele repair (arrow) and another extending inferiorly into the sacral canal (arrow). (**B**) T2-weighted sagittal image exhibits a hemicord adherent to a posterior defect at the site of previous meningocele repair. (**C**) T1-weighted axial image exhibits split cords (arrows) at L4 level.

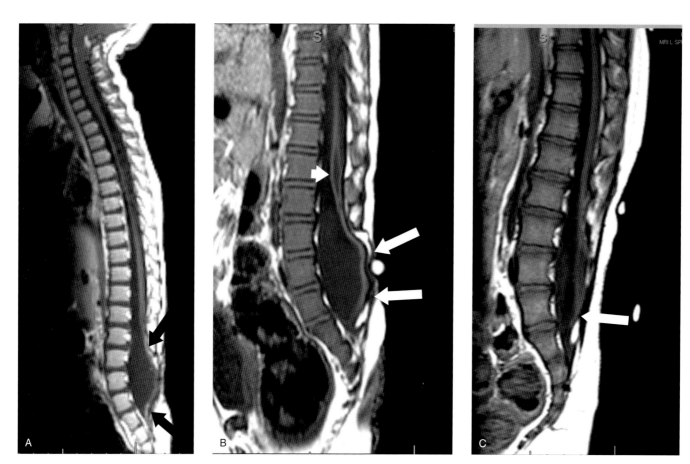

**Figure 98.4** Myelocele progressing into terminal syringomyelia with postsurgical retethering. (**A**) Post-contrast T1-weighted sagittal image in a newborn exhibits spina bifida aperta from L3 to S1 levels with myelocele (black arrows) showing a neural placode flush with skin and tethering of the cord. (**B**) T1-weighted sagittal image at the age of 2 years exhibits myelocele (arrows) with tethered cord. There is interval development of terminal syrinx (short arrow). (**C**) T1-weighted sagittal image at the age of 3 years exhibits repaired myelocele with the tethering of the cord (arrow) but without recurrence of syrinx.

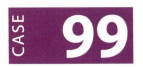

## Imaging description

Hans Chiari described Chiari malformations as a congenital condition in the late nineteenth century [1]. Inferior descent of at least one cerebellar tonsil more than 5 mm below the inferior margin of the foramen magnum is considered diagnostic (Fig. 99.1) [2]. There is a slight female preponderance. With the advent of MRI, it is seen with increasing frequency, in up to 1% of people undergoing imaging [3]. However, more than 50% of the individuals who are diagnosed with Chiari I malformation are asymptomatic. Apart from cerebellar descent, peg-like configuration of cerebellar tonsils with somewhat oblique orientation of the vertical sulci and elongated fourth ventricle with normal location are important imaging features (Fig. 99.2A). As a result of abnormal flow of CSF at the foramen magnum, Chiari malformation type I can lead to spinal cord syrinx formation (Fig. 99.3A) [4]. Factors associated with syrinx formation include increased tonsillar descent of more than 10 mm, basilar invagination, retroverted odontoid process (Fig. 99.3B), and hydrocephalus [5]. While cervical spine is more frequently affected (Fig. 99.3C), syrinx formation can also take place only in the lower segments [6]. Hence total spine imaging should be considered in a patient with Chiari I malformation. Phase-contrast magnetic resonance imaging is increasingly utilized to evaluate the effect of tonsillar ectopia on CSF flow. Reduced flow in posterior subarachnoid space (Figs. 99.1B, 99.3B) is generally considered a sign of an abnormal CSF flow, with increasing correlation between symptomatic Chiari I malformation and asymptomatic tonsillar ectopia [7]. Abnormal tonsillar pulsations are also associated with a pegged tonsillar morphology [5].

## Importance

With an incidence as high as 1% of total brain imaging patients, 5 mm inferior descent characterizing Chiari I malformation may easily be overlooked or overinterpreted. It is important to correlate with symptoms specific to Chiari I malformation and utilize CSF flow analysis for clinical significance. Further investigations of total spine with MRI should be performed in patients suspected of syringomyelia.

## Typical clinical scenario

Up to 50% of the patients are asymptomatic. A typical "Chiari I spell" includes headaches with coughing and syncope with sneezing. A typical headache, symptomatic for Chiari I malformation, should have a tussive component, a short duration, and lack of migrainous features [5]. When associated with syringomyelia, atypical scoliosis, unsteadiness of gait, and dissociated sensory loss with neuropathy are often encountered. In rare cases with brainstem compression, neck pain, torticollis, ataxia, lower cranial nerve palsies, or hypersomnolence can be seen.

## Differential diagnosis

Acquired tonsillar herniation, also known as acquired Chiari I malformation, is associated with conditions that result in small posterior fossa, such as retroverted odontoid process (Fig. 99.3B), basilar invagination, achondroplasia, craniosynostosis, and Paget's disease. Increased intracranial pressure and intracranial masses (Fig. 99.5A) also cause inferior descent of cerebellar tonsils. Benign intracranial hypotension secondary to CSF leak (Fig. 99.6A) or LP shunt that results in tonsillar descent is associated with thickening and enhancement of dura and sagging of brainstem.

## Teaching points

Inferior position of cerebellar tonsils for more than 5 mm below foramen magnum with peg-like configuration is diagnostic of Chiari I malformation, although this finding should not be overemphasized when seen incidentally, as more than 50% of individuals with this condition never develop symptoms. In young asymptomatic children less than 4 years old, follow-up studies may exhibit improvement. Increasing degrees of tonsillar descent and abnormal tonsillar pulsation on cine phase-contrast CSF flow MR imaging are associated with presence of syringohydromyelia of the cord. Associated findings such as retroverted odontoid process and basilar invagination have a higher incidence of syringohydromyelia.

REFERENCES

1. Chiari H. Über Veränderungen des Kleinhirns infolge von Hydrocephalie des Grosshirns. *Dtsch Med Wochenschr* 1891; **17**: 1172–5.
2. Barkovich AJ, Wippold FJ, Sherman JL, Citrin CM. Significance of cerebellar tonsillar position on MR. *AJNR Am J Neuroradiol* 1986; **7**: 795–9.
3. Aitken LA, Lindan CE, Sidney S, *et al.* Chiari type I malformation in a pediatric population. *Pediatr Neurol* 2009; **40**: 449–54.
4. Lipson AC, Ellenbogen RG, Avellino AM. Radiographic formation and progression of cervical syringomyelia in a child with untreated Chiari I malformation. *Pediatr Neurosurg* 2008; **44**: 221–3.
5. Strahle J, Muraszko KM, Kapurch J, *et al.* Chiari malformation type I and syrinx in children undergoing magnetic resonance imaging. *J Neurosurg Pediatr* 2011; **8**: 205–13.
6. Greitz D. Unraveling the riddle of syringomyelia. *Neurosurg Rev* 2006; **29**: 251–64.
7. Hofkes SK, Iskandar BJ, Turski PA, *et al.* Differentiation between symptomatic Chiari I malformation and asymptomatic tonsilar ectopia by using cerebrospinal fluid flow imaging: initial estimate of imaging accuracy. *Radiology* 2007; **245**: 532–40.

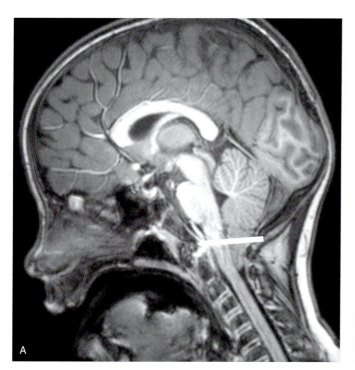
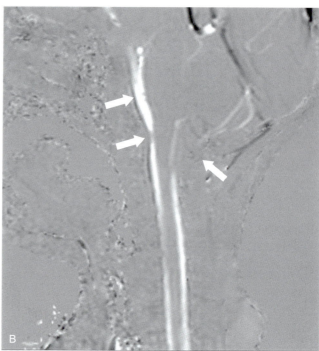

**Figure 99.1** Congenital Chiari I malformation in a 6-year-old with night-time headaches. (**A**) T1-weighted sagittal imaging. A line from basion to opisthion corresponds to inferior margin of foramen magnum. There is 16 mm inferior herniation of bilateral cerebellar tonsils with peg-like configuration. (**B**) Cine phase-contrast MR imaging in the sagittal plane exhibits lack of trans-foramen magnum CSF flow posteriorly, with patent flow anterior to cervical medullary neuraxis (arrows).

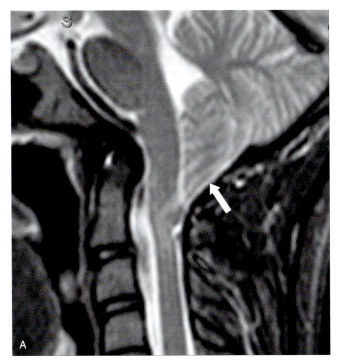

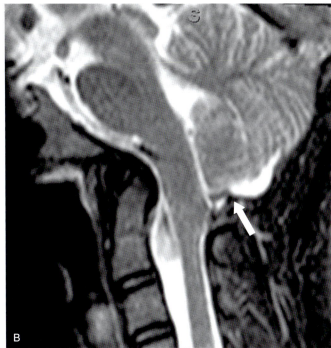

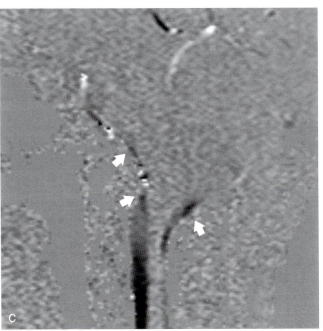

**Figure 99.2** Congenital Chiari I malformation in a 13-year-old with facial nerve weakness and tongue paresthesias. (**A**) T2-weighted sagittal image exhibits 9 mm inferior descent of cerebellar tonsils reaching up to posterior tubercle of C1. Note the oblique tonsillar folia with "sergeant's stripes" configuration (arrow). There is elongation of fourth ventricle with mildly retroflexed odontoid process without basilar invagination. (**B**) T2-weighted sagittal image following suboccipital craniotomy, C1 laminectomy, and duraplasty for decompression exhibits adequate CSF around tonsils (arrow). (**C**) Phase-contrast CSF flow MR imaging in the sagittal plane exhibits presence of CSF flow at anterior and posterior foramen magnum (arrowheads).

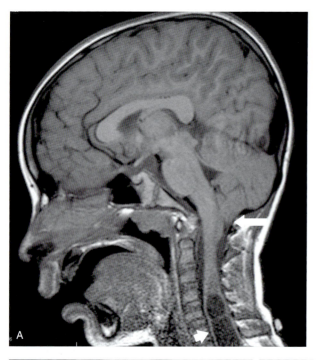
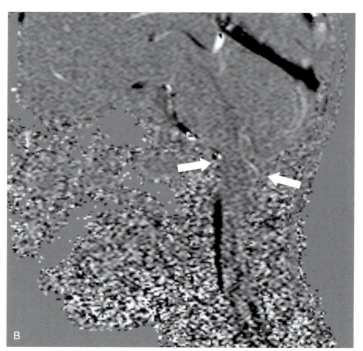
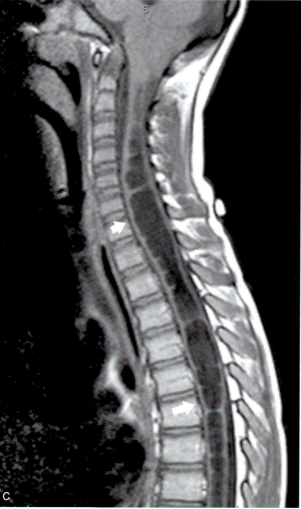

**Figure 99.3** Congenital Chiari I malformation with syringohydromyelia in a 5-year-old with footdrop and wide-based gait. (**A**) T1-weighted sagittal image exhibits inferior herniation of cerebellar tonsils (arrow) with peg-like configuration, reaching up to posterior tubercle of C1 vertebra. There is syringomyelia of cervical cord (short arrow). (**B**) Phase-contrast CSF flow imaging in the sagittal plane exhibits lack of normal CSF flow at the anterior or posterior margin of foramen magnum (arrows). Retroverted odontoid process is apparent. (**C**) T1-weighted sagittal image exhibits syringohydromyelia of spinal cord from cervical region to conus medullaris (short arrows). (**D**) T1-weighted sagittal image following suboccipital craniotomy (arrow), C1 laminectomy, and duraplasty exhibits decompression with improvement in the severity of cervical syrinx (short arrow). (**E**) Phase-contrast CSF flow MR imaging in the sagittal plane exhibits patent CSF flow at the anterior and posterior margins of foramen magnum (arrows).

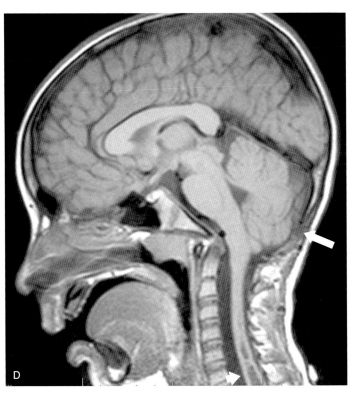

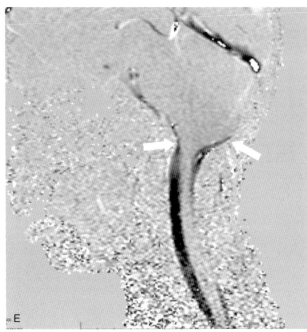

**Figure 99.3** (cont.)

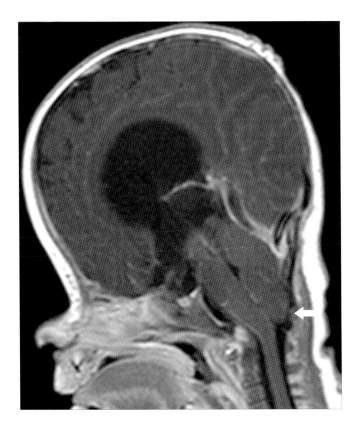

**Figure 99.4** Congenital Chiari I malformation in 2-month-old with Alpert syndrome. Post-contrast T1-weighted sagittal image exhibits inferior herniation of bilateral cerebellar tonsils with rounded inferior margins, reaching up to posterior tubercle of C1 vertebra (arrow). The rest of the images revealed multiple sutural synostosis, narrow cranial base, hydrocephalus, and venous flow abnormalities.

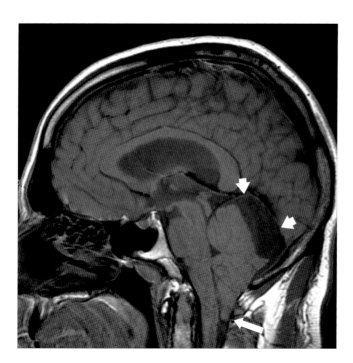

**Figure 99.5** Cerebellar tonsillar herniation in a 49-year-old with superior cerebellar arachnoid cyst. T1-weighted sagittal image exhibits inferior herniation of cerebellar tonsils, reaching below the posterior tubercle of C1 vertebra (arrow), secondary to mass effect from an arachnoid cyst superior to cerebellum (short arrows).

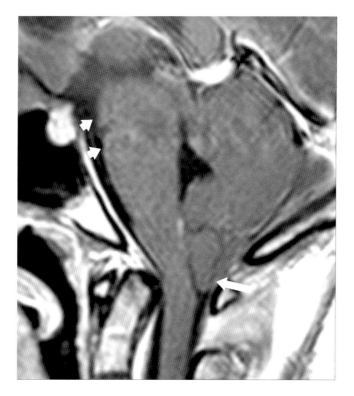

**Figure 99.6** Cerebellar tonsillar herniation in a 17-year-old with benign intracranial hypotension secondary to spontaneous CSF leak at thoracic spine. Post-contrast T1-weighted sagittal image exhibits inferior herniation of cerebellar tonsils reaching up to posterior tubercle of C1 with mildly rounded inferior margin (arrow). There is sagging of brainstem structures with mild patchy enhancement of the ventral surface (short arrows).

## Imaging description

Spinal vascular malformations (SVMs) are a rare and hetero-geneous group of entities with various subsets that present with differing clinical and imaging appearances. There are multiple proposed classifications and there is considerable overlap in entities within the reported literature. Two of the most commonly encountered SVMs, dural arteriovenous fis-tulas (DAVF) and spinal cord arteriovenous malformations (AVM), constitute a large majority of these lesions.

DAVFs are acquired shunts that are located within the dura, most commonly in the nerve root sheath. It is supplied by the meningeal branch of a radicular artery and the drainage is into a dilated vein coursing intradurally and eventually into peri-medullary venous plexus (Fig. 100.1). The imaging manifest-ations are simply a result of dilated perimedullary veins, venous hypertension, and its effect on the spinal cord. Enlarged venous structures can result in perimedullary flow voids that are best demonstrated on T2-weighted sequences (Fig. 100.2). Long-standing venous hypertension can result in cord edema and expansion. There may be faint enhancement of the cord on contrast administration. The perimedullary venous system may also demonstrate enhancement after con-trast administration (Fig. 100.3).

Although spinal digital subtraction angiography (DSA) is always needed to confirm the findings and as a prelude to endovascular repair, it can be more focused with the help of non-invasive assessments such as contrast-enhanced MRA or CTA. DSA allows depiction of precise anatomy of the shunt, study of shunt dynamics, and detection of spinal medullary vessels (anterior or posterior spinal arter-ies). Precise treatment is based on the anatomy of the shunt and cord blood supply. However, endovascular treatment is often attempted first, given its high success rate and low rate of complications [1].

Spinal cord AVMs are intradural shunting lesions that can be perimedullary (on the surface of the cord) or intramedul-lary. These lesions receive supply from radiculo-medullary arteries that follow the ventral (anterior spinal artery) or dorsal (posterior spinal artery) nerve roots. MRI can reveal areas of low signal intensity within the cord substance that may indicate a nidus, with or without surrounding signal changes in the cord (Fig. 100.4). The adjacent spinal cord may harbor intranidal aneurysms, edema, hemorrhage, or syrinx [1]. Because of presence of a shunt, the perimedullary venous system may be engorged and display areas of flow voids on T2-weighted sequence. DSA is imperative in the characterization of these lesions and helps identify the arterial feeders, aneurysms, or pseudoaneurysms as well as the status of the venous system.

## Importance

Spinal vascular malformations are frequently missed on imaging studies despite their pathognomonic imaging characteristics. It is not uncommon for the patients with DAVF to experience significant clinical deterioration before diagnosis. A lag between onset of symptoms and diagnosis is common, on average 10.5 months in one series.

## Typical clinical scenario

Spinal DAVFs are the most frequent SVMs in older adults, usually presenting after the fourth or fifth decade of life with a strong male predominance (5:1). Classic symptoms at presen-tation include progressive motor and sensory disturbance, with spasticity, paresthesias, pain, bladder and bowel disturb-ances, and sexual dysfunction. Hemorrhage is an extremely rare presentation of DAVFs.

In contrast, spinal cord AVMs usually present in younger patients, typically in the third decade of life, but they can be diagnosed in children and teenagers [1]. Within the pediatric population, a male predominance is present, but no sexual predominance is found in the adult population. Hemorrhage is the most common presentation, occurring in approximately half of all patients with spinal cord AVMs. In these cases, there is onset of sudden, new neurological deficits.

## Differential diagnosis

The imaging signs of spinal DAVFs and AVMs are character-istic and pathognomonic. What is missing generally is aware-ness of these entities and potential consideration of these lesions in a patient with progressive neurologic deterioration. Cord expansion and enhancement in DAVF cases can be mistaken for tumors. However, the enhancement in the DAVFs is typically faint and ill-defined, and therefore distinct from the enhancement pattern of tumors.

---

### Teaching points

Spinal DAVFs constitute a majority of SVMs and present in older, predominantly male patients. Diagnosis can be made on MRI with recognition of perimedullary vessels, cord edema and expansion. Hemorrhage is very uncommon in DAVFs but is the most common presenting feature of true cord AVMs.

---

REFERENCES

1. da Costa L, Dehdashti AR, terBrugge KG. Spinal cord vascular shunts: spinal cord vascular malformations and dural arteriovenous fistulas. *Neurosurg Focus* 2009; **26**: E6.

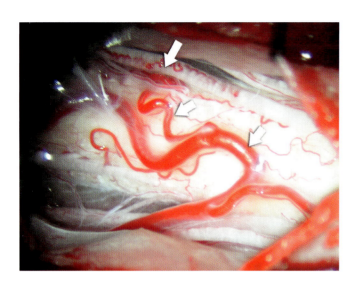

**Figure 100.1** An intraoperative image of DAVF illustrates the typical anatomy and pathophysiology. Note the fistula on the nerve sleeve (arrow), draining into a tortuous and arterialized coronal venous plexus (short arrows). Image courtesy of Paul Park MD.

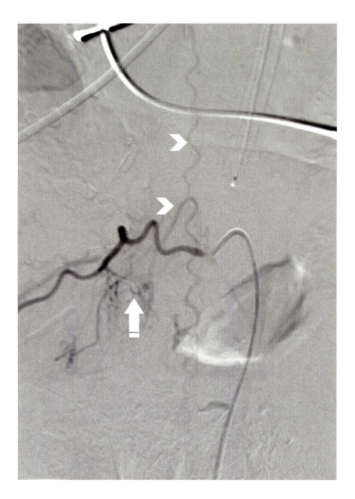

**Figure 100.2** DSA image of a DAVF demonstrates a right T11 nerve root fistula (arrow) supplied by the right T11 radicular artery. The dilated and superiorly draining vein is marked with arrowheads.

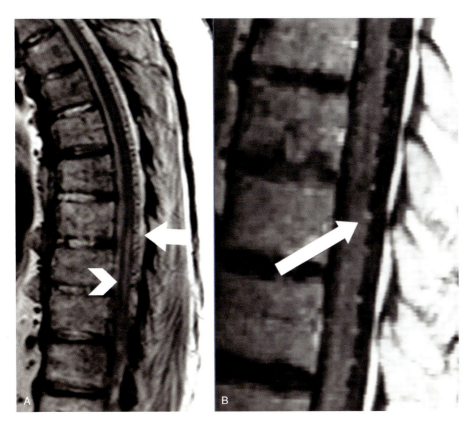

**Figure 100.3** Typical MR findings in a DAVF. (**A**) Sagittal T2-weighted study reveals typical engorged vessels seen as flow voids in subarachnoid space (arrow) as well as cord expansion and edema (arrowhead). (**B**) Sagittal T1-weighted enhanced image (of another patient) demonstrates the enhancement of perimedullary veins (arrow).

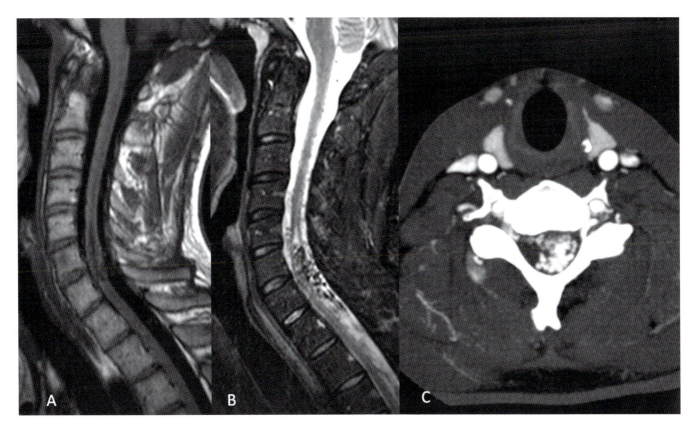

**Figure 100.4** Sagittal (**A**) T1-weighted and (**B**) T2-weighted images of a cervical AVM. Note the flow voids within the cord substance as well as subarachnoid space on T2-weighted sequence and a cord syrinx. (**C**) CTA confirms intramedullary enhancing nidus suggestive of an AVM.

# CASE 101 Cord compression

## Imaging description

Compression of the spinal cord by an extrinsic mass such as tumor or abscess often constitutes a medical emergency [1]. One of the common causes for spinal cord compression is metastatic epidural spinal cord compression (MESCC), first described by Spiller in 1925 [2]. It requires rapid diagnosis and treatment to avoid permanent progressive pain, diminished quality of life, and paralysis culminating in death [1,3]. MESCC is discovered in 5–10% of cancer patients, with lung carcinoma (Fig. 101.1), prostate cancer, and breast carcinoma the most common causes, followed by non-Hodgkin's lymphoma (Fig. 101.2), renal cell cancer, multiple myeloma (Fig. 101.3), and plasmacytoma (Fig. 101.4) [1,3,4]. In more than 85% of the patients, the cord compression is due to epidural growth of metastasis to vertebral bodies by hematogenous spread (Figs. 101.1D, 101.3D). The gradual compression can be precipitated in acute process by collapse of vertebral body (Fig. 101.4). In about 15% of patients, paravertebral tumor can grow directly into the spinal canal through an intervertebral foramen (Fig. 101.2D), leading to cord compression. This is more commonly seen in lymphomas (Fig. 101.2) and neuroblastomas [3].

MRI is the method of choice for diagnosis of MESCC, with a sensitivity of 93%, specificity of 97%, and accuracy of 95%, and it is often the first and only technique in making the diagnosis. It influences treatment planning and is able to differentiate benign vertebral body collapses from metastasis in patients with cancer [5].

The most common treatment options includes steroids, radiation therapy, and surgery and the combinations thereof, taking into account the severity of spinal cord compression, the radiosensitivity or resistance of the primary tumor, the mechanical instability of the spine, and systemic conditions [1,3].

## Importance

MESCC causes damage to the cord by compression and vascular compromise. Direct compression can cause demyelination and axonal damage. Vascular damage by early cord compression results in occlusion of epidural venous plexus, resulting in vasogenic edema and associated neurological dysfunction that can be reversed by corticosteroids. However, in the terminal stages of compression, the arterial blood flow to the spinal cord is compromised, resulting in cord ischemia and infarction leading to irreversible neurological damage [3]. It is very important to make early diagnosis of cord compression, with immediate and effective communication to the caretaking team.

## Typical clinical scenario

Apart from backache, commonly present for about 2 months in more than 95% of patients at diagnosis [3], lower extremity weakness is present in about 35–75% of patients. Other symptoms include sensory loss, motor deficits, pain, ataxia, and altered bowel and bladder function [1].

## Differential diagnosis

Apart from metastatic secondary deposits, spontaneous epidural hemorrhage, sometimes associated with AVM and rarely with cavernous hemangioma (Fig. 101.5), can also give rise to severe compromise of the spinal canal [6]. Infectious conditions such as pyogenic spondylitis or epidural abscess (Fig. 101.6) can also cause severe compression of the spinal cord [7] and acute neurologic deterioration. Benign neoplastic conditions such as meningioma and schwannomas can result in significant cord compression, although the symptoms are usually more subacute or chronic. Spinal meningeal cyst in the extradural compartment, especially type I cyst (Fig. 101.7), is a relatively rare condition but can result in significant cord compression. Epidural lipomatosis, frequently seen in chronic steroid users (Fig. 101.8), can also result in compression of the spinal cord [8].

## Teaching points

Cord compression is a medical emergency that requires prompt diagnosis, effective communication, and immediate management. Metastatic deposits, epidural abscesses, and hematomas are among the most common reasons for acute cord compression. In a patient with known malignancy, new-onset back pain with or without weakness and other clinical symptoms should raise suspicion for epidural deposits and the possibility of cord compression. As multiple sites of spinal cord compression may be present in epidural abscesses and metastases, imaging of the entire spine is advisable.

REFERENCES

1. Ribas ES, Schiff D. Spinal cord compression. *Curr Treat Options Neurol* 2012; **14**: 391–401.

2. Spiller WG. Rapidly progressive paralysis associated with carcinoma. *Arch Neurol Psychiatry* 1925; **13**: 471.

3. Cole JS, Patchell RA. Metastatic epidural spinal cord compression. *Lancet Neurol* 2008; **7**: 459–66.

4. Jung JM, Yoon SH, Hyun SJ, *et al.* Extraosseous multiple myeloma mimicking spinal epidural metastasis. *J Clin Neurosci* 2012; **19**: 1448–50.

5. Colletti PM, Siegal HJ, Woo MY, *et al.* The impact on treatment planning of MRI of the spine in patients suspected of vertebral metastasis: an efficacy study. *Comput Med Imaging Graph* 1996; **20**: 159–62.

6. Saracen A, Kotwica Z. Thoracic spinal epidural cavernous haemangioma with an acute onset: case report and the review of the literature. *Clin Neurol Neurosurg* 2013; **115**: 799–801.

7. Reihsaus E, Waldbaur H, Seeling W. Spinal epidural abscess: a meta-analysis of 915 patients. *Neurosurg Rev* 2000; **23**: 175–204.

8. Alvarez A, Induru R, Lagman R. Considering symptomatic spinal epidural lipomatosis in the differential diagnosis. *Am J Hosp Palliat Care* 2012; doi: 10.1177/1049909112457012.

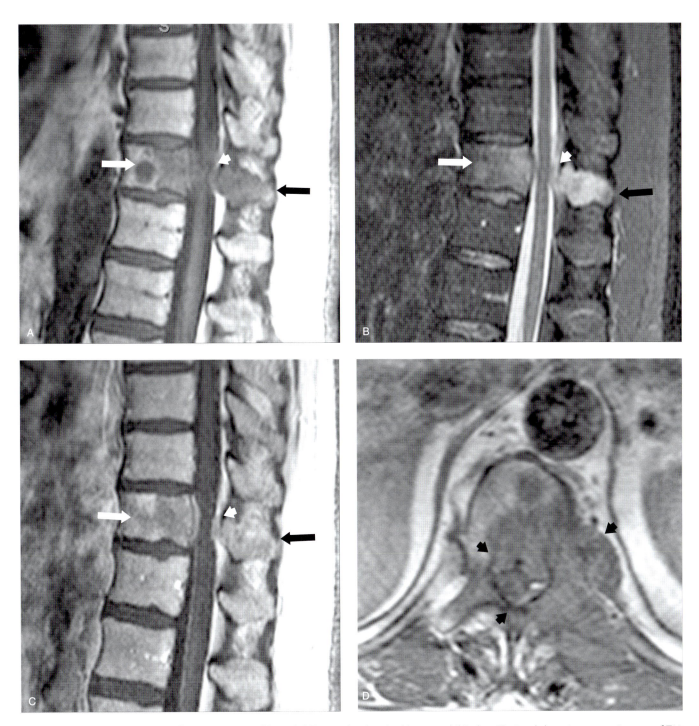

**Figure 101.1** Metastatic disease from carcinoma of lung. (**A**) T1-weighted sagittal image exhibits low T1 signal deposit at posterior part of T11 thoracic vertebra (white arrow), also involving the spinous process (black arrow) with epidural intraspinal extension (short white arrow). (**B**) T2-weighted sagittal image shows high T2 signal lesion within the vertebral body (white arrow) and spinous process (black arrow), extending into epidural spaces (short white arrow) resulting in spinal canal stenosis. (**C**) Post-contrast T1-weighted sagittal image exhibits patchy enhancement of the metastatic lesion within the vertebral body (white arrow) and spinous process (black arrow) as well as the epidural component (short white arrow). (**D**) T1-weighted axial image exhibits expansile low T1 signal lesions involving the anterior end of left-sided rib (short black arrow), posterior part of the vertebral body (short black arrow), extending into both the pedicles, involving the posterior elements (short black arrow), with anterior and posterior epidural extension resulting in compression of lower thoracic cord.

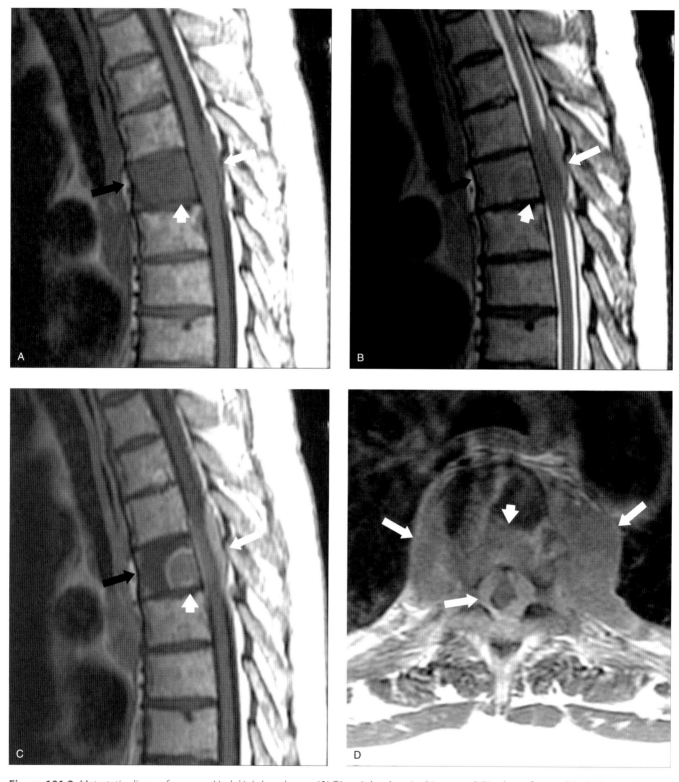

**Figure 101.2** Metastatic disease from non-Hodgkin's lymphoma. (**A**) T1-weighted sagittal image exhibits loss of normal high T1 signal in the T5 vertebral body (black arrow) with presence of a posteriorly situated focus (short white arrow) which is not apparent on non-contrast T1-weighted image. Note the epidural extension of the mass (white arrow). (**B**) T2-weighted sagittal image exhibits a low T2 signal of T5 vertebra (black arrow); a rim of high T2 signal outlines the posteriorly situated lesion (short white arrow). The epidural mass exhibits a low T2 signal (white arrow) with lack of normal CSF surrounding the thoracic cord. (**C**) Post-contrast T1-weighted sagittal image shows patchy post-contrast enhancement of the posteriorly situated focus (short white arrow) as well as the epidural mass (white arrow). The rest of the bone marrow continues to exhibit low T1 signal. (**D**) Post-contrast T1-weighted axial image shows patchily enhancing, large bilateral paraspinal soft tissue masses (arrows on either side), extending into epidural spaces (middle arrow) through intervertebral foramina and resulting into cord compression. Patchy enhancement of the posterior vertebral lesion is also seen (short arrow).

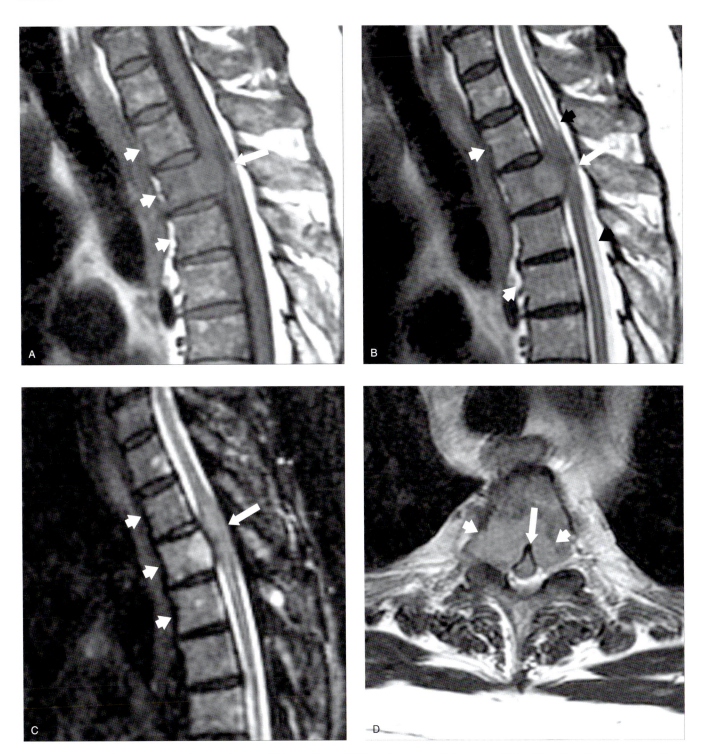

**Figure 101.3** Epidural metastatic deposits from multiple myeloma. (**A**) T1-weighted sagittal image exhibits diffuse low T1 signal of spinal column (short arrows) with an expansile epidural extension at T3 vertebral body (arrow). (**B**) T2-weighted sagittal image exhibits patchy high T2 signal of posterior vertebral deposit at T3 level and diffuse low T2 signal of the spinal column (short white arrows). The epidural deposits also exhibit low T2 signal with effacement of CSF surrounding the cord (white arrow). Note the posterior dural margin (short black arrows). (**C**) STIR sagittal image exhibits low signal at vertebral bodies (short arrows) with high signal at posterior vertebral deposit. The epidural deposits also exhibit low signal with effacement of CSF (arrow). (**D**) Post-contrast T1-weighted axial image exhibits patchily enhancing posterior vertebral lesion with epidural extension (short arrows) resulting in cord compression (arrow).

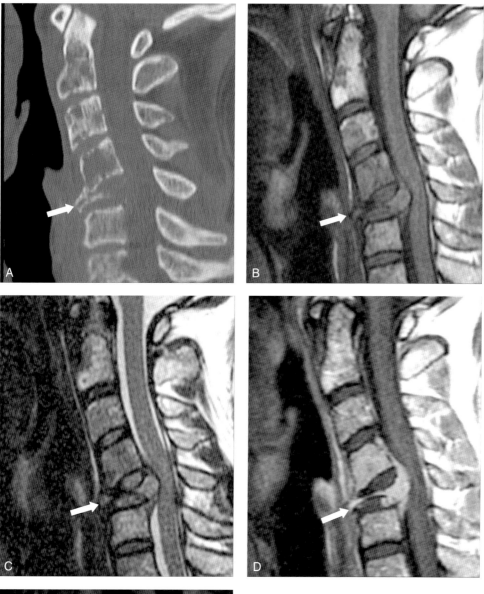

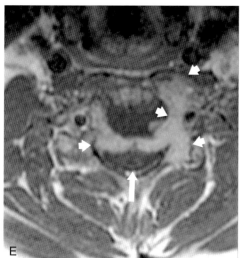

**Figure 101.4** Plasmocytoma metastatic deposit. (**A**) Sagittal reconstruction of CT scan of cervical spine exhibits a C5 vertebra plana with more than 90% loss of height (arrow). There is extensive bone destruction at other visualized cervical vertebrae. (**B**) T1-weighted sagittal image exhibits patchy low T1 signal corresponding to areas of bone destruction. There is a C5 vertebra plana with anterior epidural extension of expansile soft tissue (arrow). (**C**) T2-weighted sagittal image exhibits patchy low T2 signal of the spinal column with effacement of CSF surrounding the cervical cord at C5 level (arrow) and resultant cord compression. (**D**) Post-contrast T1-weighted sagittal image exhibits patchy post-contrast enhancement of spinal deposits including the collapsed C5 vertebra (arrow) and epidural component. (**E**) Post-contrast T1-weighted axial image exhibits patchy post-contrast enhancement of the epidural mass (short arrows), which also extends into intervertebral foramina to involve the left prevertebral space (short arrow). There is marked cord compression (arrow).

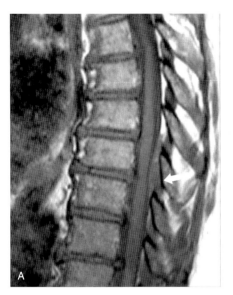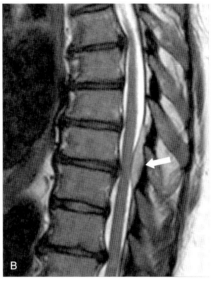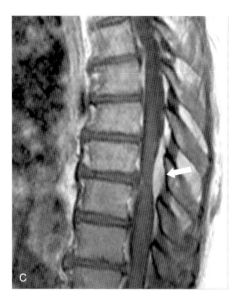

**Figure 101.5** Epidural cavernous hemangioma. (**A**) T1-weighted sagittal image shows a low T1 signal posterior epidural mass at T8–T9 level (arrow). (**B**) T2-weighted sagittal image exhibits mildly high T2 signal of the posterior epidural mass (arrow) with effacement of CSF surrounding the cord. (**C**) Post-contrast T1-weighted sagittal image shows intense post-contrast enhancement (arrow) of posterior epidural mass.

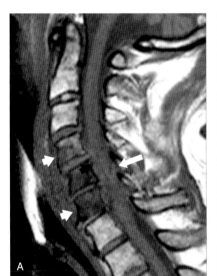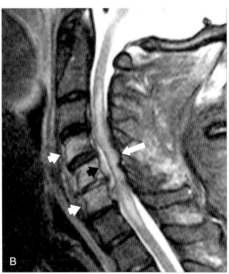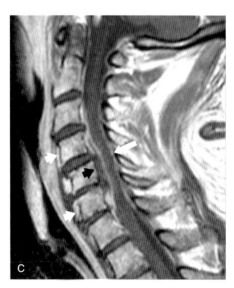

**Figure 101.6** Epidural abscess. (**A**) T1-weighted sagittal image exhibits low T1 signal of contiguous C4–C6 vertebrae (short white arrows). An anterior epidural component (short black arrow) resulting in cord compression (white arrow) is not readily apparent on T1-weighted images. (**B**) T2-weighted sagittal image exhibits a patchy high T2 signal from C4–C6 vertebrae (short white arrows) and at C5–C6 intervertebral disc. Anterior epidural abscess (short black arrow) results in compression with edema of cervical cord (white arrow). (**C**) Post-contrast T1-weighted sagittal image exhibits patchy post-contrast enhancement of C4–C6 vertebrae (short white arrows) and C5–C6 intervertebral disc. There is intense peripheral enhancement of anterior epidural abscess (short black arrow) and the surface of the cervical cord (white arrow).

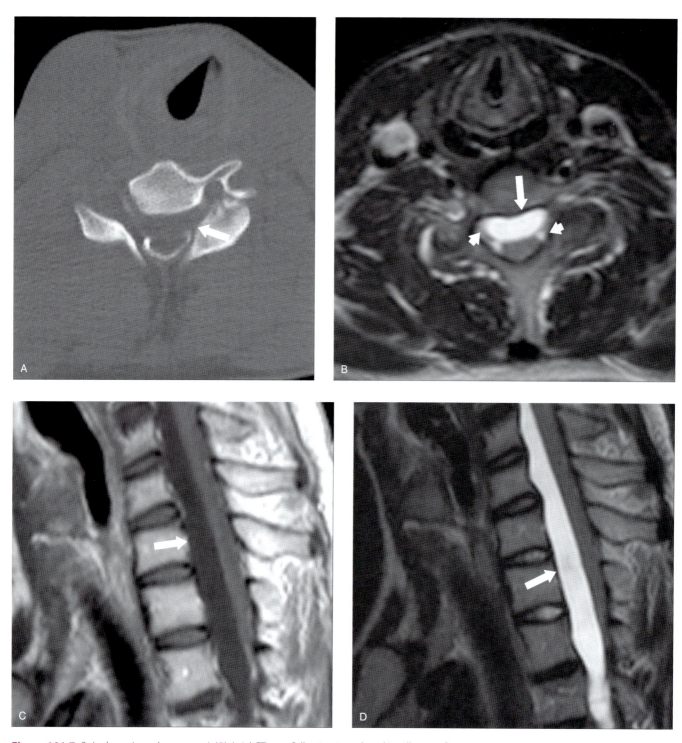

**Figure 101.7** Spinal meningeal cyst, type I. (**A**) Axial CT scan following intrathecal instillation of non-ionic adequate contrast exhibits effacement of contrast column anterior to posteriorly displaced cervical cord at C6 level, concerning for an epidural mass (arrow). There is no evidence for bone destruction. (**B**) T2-weighted axial image exhibits a CSF intensity anterior epidural lesion (arrow) with posterior displacement of cervical cord and stretching of spinal nerve roots (short arrow). (**C**) T1-weighted sagittal image exhibits a long segment low T1 signal, CSF intensity lesion at anterior epidural spaces (arrow) with posterior displacement of the cord. (**D**) T2-weighted sagittal image exhibits high T2 signal long segment anterior epidural lesion (arrow).

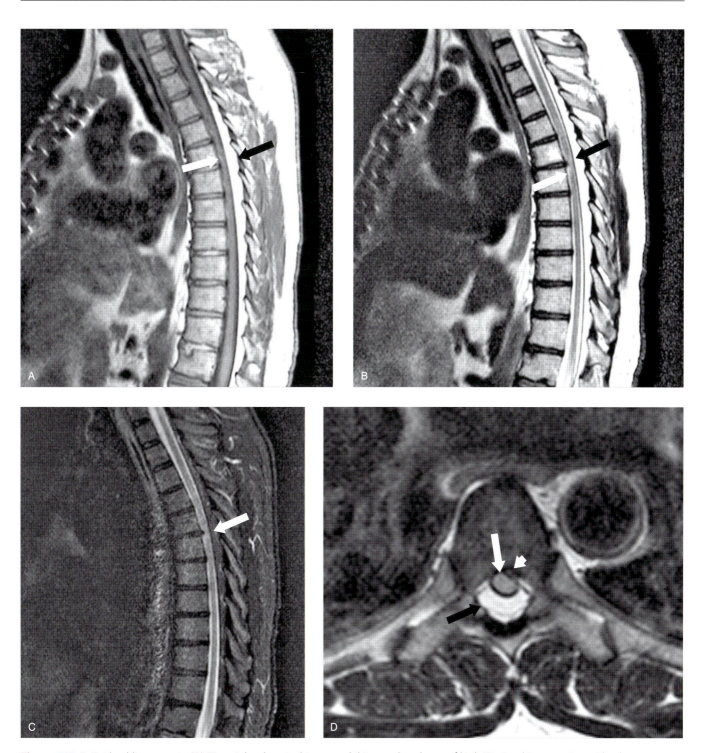

**Figure 101.8** Epidural lipomatosis. (**A**) T1-weighted sagittal image exhibits an abundance of high T1 signal in posterior epidural spaces (black arrow), compatible with epidural lipomatosis at thoracic spine resulting in cord compression at upper thoracic level (white arrow). (**B**) T2-weighted sagittal image exhibits a small posterior spur at T5–T6 level (short white arrow), exacerbating the spinal canal stenosis from high T2 signal epidural lipomatosis (black arrow), resulting in cord compression (white arrow). (**C**) STIR sagittal image exhibits low signal of epidural lipomatosis (arrow) with resultant cord compression. (**D**) T2-weighted axial image exhibits presence of left paracentral posterior spur (short white arrow) and an abundance of high T2 signal posterior epidural fat (black arrow) resulting in cord compression with high T2 intramedullary signal (white arrow).

# Demyelinating/inflammatory spinal cord lesion

## Imaging description

In a previously healthy adult patient presenting with an acute to subacute myelopathy, first a compressive lesion such as a large disc extrusion or mass associated with bone metastasis should be ruled out. MRI is uniquely suited for the evaluation of these patients with its ability to evaluate the spine as well as the cord and nerve roots. Once an extrinsic compression is excluded a demyelinating, inflammatory, or neoplastic intrinsic cord lesion is usually responsible for the symptoms. An enhancing cord mass with associated edema and focal expansion of the cord is usually attributed to primary or secondary neoplasms, although a demyelinating plaque can have very similar features (Fig. 102.1). In about 10–20% of multiple sclerosis (MS) patients the first presentation is related to a solitary spinal cord lesion, most frequently in the cervical cord [1]. While most of these patients will have a relatively typical plaque with a focal T2 hyperintense lesion involving no more than 50% of the surface area of the cord on axial images and no longer than two vertebral body height on sagittal images, some patients may have an enhancing "mass" with associated edema and cord expansion (Fig. 102.2). Neuromyelitis optica is a separate demyelinating process of the cord associated with optic neuritis, and may present with similar imaging features. Acute transverse myelopathy is an immune-mediated inflammatory disorder of the cord with variable etiology that can present with enhancing cord lesions (Fig. 102.3).

## Importance

Mistaking a demyelinating cord lesion for a tumor may lead to unnecessary and potentially dangerous procedures such as surgical biopsy and resection.

## Typical clinical scenario

The clinical presentation varies depending on the spinal cord segment affected and the degree of involvement. Paresthesia, spastic paresis, paraplegia, hyperreflexia, neurogenic bowel and bladder, and sexual dysfunction may be seen, and may progress in a few days.

## Differential diagnosis

It may be impossible to differentiate a demyelinating plaque from a spinal cord ependymoma or astrocytoma with imaging alone, and clinical features including CSF findings play a critical role in establishing the diagnosis. Tumefactive demyelinating plaques usually demonstrate homogeneous, nodular, or ring enhancement during the acute and subacute phase, which may last 2–8 weeks. Cysts and hemorrhage within or in the vicinity of the lesion and heterogeneous contrast enhancement support the diagnosis of neoplasm. Neuromyelitis optica, although different than MS in its pathogenesis, may present with enhancing mass-like demyelinating lesions that are identical to MS. In acute transverse myelitis, the cord usually shows more diffuse swelling and the enhancement is more heterogeneous. Sarcoidosis can rarely present with an enhancing intramedullary mass, but most frequently the enhancement is dural-based or leptomeningeal. Spinal arteriovenous fistula-related cord signal changes can rarely show enhancement, but this does not resemble a nodular mass. Imaging of the brain may be helpful in differentiating tumors from demyelinating/inflammatory processes, as multifocal involvement is common with the latter, in contrast to the primary cord tumors, which tend to be isolated.

## Teaching points

An enhancing nodular mass in the spinal cord may be the first presentation of multiple sclerosis or other demyelinating/inflammatory processes.

REFERENCES

1. Bot JC, Barkhof F. Spinal-cord MRI in multiple sclerosis: conventional and nonconventional MR techniques. *Neuroimaging Clin N Am* 2009; **19**: 81–99.

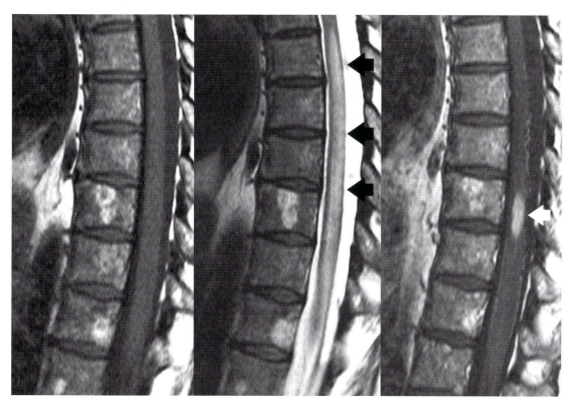

**Figure 102.1** Sagittal T1-weighted, T2-weighted, and post-contrast T1-weighted images of the thoracic spine show an enhancing nodular "mass" with marked surrounding edema which was later proven to be a demyelinating plaque. Incidentally noted are vertebral hemangiomas and some prominent veins.

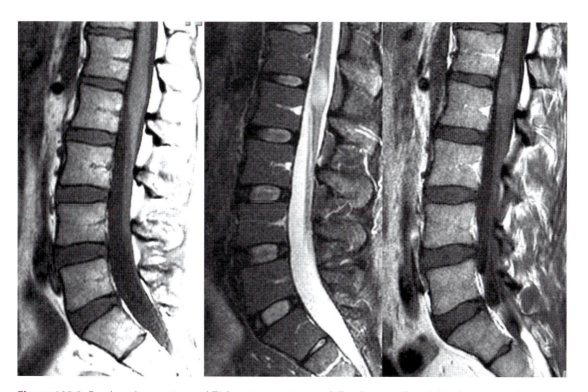

**Figure 102.2** Focal cord expansion and T2 hyperintense intramedullary lesion with peripheral contrast enhancement are seen on sagittal T1-weighted, STIR, and post-contrast T1-weighted images of a patient who presented with subacute myelopathy and unremarkable prior medical history. Clinical work-up revealed multiple sclerosis.

**467**

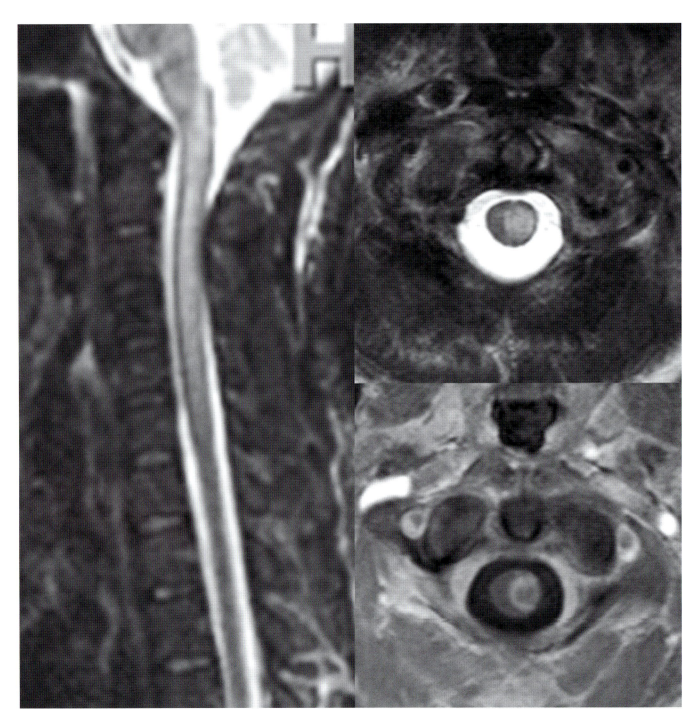

**Figure 102.3** Sagittal STIR, axial T2-weighted, and axial post-contrast T1-weighted images show an intramedullary mass-like lesion with enhancement. The patient received a diagnosis of neuroinflammatory disease, which could not be further specified.

# 103 Subacute combined degeneration

## Imaging description

Subacute combined degeneration (SCD) is characterized by dysesthesia, disturbance of position sense, and spastic paraparesis or tetraparesis that occurs as a result of demyelination of the white matter tracts in the dorsal and lateral columns of the cervical and upper thoracic cord secondary to vitamin $B_{12}$ deficiency. MRI shows symmetrical T2 hyperintensity in the posterior and lateral columns of the cord that usually extends in a continuous fashion throughout the cervical cord and sometimes the upper thoracic cord (Fig. 103.1) [1]. Involvement of anterior columns and enhancement on post-contrast sequences are rare. DWI shows restricted diffusion in the same distribution. MRI may be completely normal in some cases, however. Nitrous oxide inhalation, either as an anesthetic agent or as a recreational drug, can act on the vitamin $B_{12}$ metabolism and result in the same clinical presentation and MRI findings [2]. $N_2O$-provoked SCD may occur in patients who have normal levels of vitamin $B_{12}$. Copper deficiency is another less common reason for SCD [3].

## Importance

Early diagnosis is essential to prevent significant cord damage. After vitamin $B_{12}$ supplementation, patients show clinical and radiologic improvement. Early initiation of treatment is more likely to result in complete recovery.

## Typical clinical scenario

Dementia, cerebellar ataxia, optic atrophy, psychosis, and mood disorders are the most common neuropsychiatric manifestations of $B_{12}$ deficiency. Patients may have macrocytic anemia and history of vegetarian diet, gastric bypass surgery, or gastrointestinal malabsorption. SCD presents with symmetric dysesthesia, disturbance of positional sense, and spastic paraparesis.

## Differential diagnosis

Bilateral symmetric dorsal column hyperintensity can be seen in multiple sclerosis, but this usually does not extend more than two vertebral heights. $N_2O$ toxicity, copper deficiency, and AIDS-related vacuolar myelopathy can have very similar signal changes in the cord. Historically, syphilis cord involvement (tabes dorsalis) was the most common disease entity involving the dorsal cord.

## Teaching points

SCD presents with characteristic T2 hyperintensity in the dorsal columns of the cervical cord, and early initiation of vitamin $B_{12}$ supplementation is critical for good outcome.

REFERENCES

1. Vide AT, Marques AM, Costa JD. MRI findings in subacute combined degeneration of the spinal cord in a patient with restricted diet. *Neurol Sci* 2012; **33**: 711–13.
2. Guttormsen AB, Refsum H, Ueland PM. The interaction between nitrous oxide and cobalamin. Biochemical effects and clinical consequences. *Acta Anaesthesiol Scand* 1994; **38**: 753–6.
3. Jaiser SR, Winston GP. Copper deficiency myelopathy. *J Neurol* 2010; **257**: 869–81.

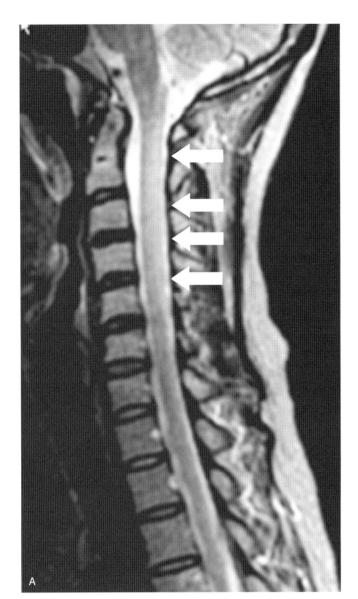
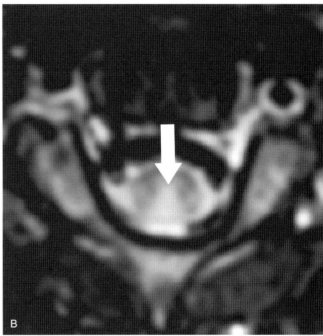

**Figure 103.1** (**A**) Sagittal and (**B**) axial T2-weighted images show an area of hyperintense signal in the posterior aspect of the spinal cord extending throughout most of the cervical cord (arrows). Axial image shows the bilateral posterior column involvement clearly (arrow) as a triangular hyperintense signal in the dorsal cord in midline. The posterior columns are also a favorite site for multiple sclerosis plaques, which are generally not as extensive in the craniocaudal direction.

## Imaging description

Apparent anterior displacement of the thoracic cord on sagittal T2-weighted MRI with expansion of the CSF space posterior to the cord in patients with myelopathy is a frequently missed finding (Fig. 104.1). Approximation of the entire thoracic cord to the ventral aspect of the canal is a common normal finding, particularly in patients with accentuated kyphosis. When this happens in a focal area with associated cord contour deformity, radiologists should suspect a CSF-signal space-occupying structure (i.e., intradural arachnoid cyst) that is pushing the cord (Fig. 104.2) or an anterior thoracic cord herniation that is pulling the cord (Fig. 104.3). Alternatively, intradural arachnoid bands can tether the cord and result in a similar appearance (Fig. 104.4). CT myelography is often diagnostic and can differentiate between these possibilities.

Intradural arachnoid cysts are congenital cysts and they are nearly always posterior to the cord [1]. Eighty percent of them are located in the thoracic spine. Most intradural arachnoid cysts are connected to the subarachnoid space and show gradual filling on myelography, with a minority presenting as a filling defect. Intradural cysts anterior to the spinal cord are unlikely to be congenital in origin and may develop on the basis of prior subarachnoid hemorrhage and archnoiditis [2].

Anterior thoracic cord herniation is a rare entity in which the spinal cord is displaced into a ventral dural defect, creating a marked focal cord deformity [3,4]. The dural defect is inferred on imaging and confirmed during surgical repair. The etiology of thoracic cord herniation is not clear but presumed to be related to disc herniations or osteophytic changes weakening the dura [5]. CT myelography or high-resolution heavily T2-weighted MRI is diagnostic.

In the absence of an intradural cyst or thoracic cord herniation, intradural arachnoid bands tethering the cord may be responsible from the MRI appearance and the patient's symptoms. Intradural bands are rare, and probably represent the sequela of arachnoiditis. These are difficult to directly visualize even on high-resolution CT myelography exams but may be inferred by subtle differences in contrast concentration in the CSF in the vicinity of the cord deformity.

## Importance

Surgical treatment of intradural cysts, bands, and thoracic cord herniation often results in improvement of the patient's myelopathy.

## Typical clinical scenario

Progressively worsening various neurologic deficits, depending on the level and degree of cord compromise.

## Differential diagnosis

Neuroenteric cyst can be considered in the differential diagnosis of intradural cysts; these are often complex, large cysts associated with vertebral anomalies and extension of the cyst into the mediastinum. Cystic schwannomas can mimic intradural cysts, although these usually have an avidly enhancing solid component, albeit small.

### Teaching points

Focal contour deformity of the cord on MRI without apparent mass in patients with myelopathy should be worked up with CT myelography for the possibility of intradural cysts, dural bands, and idiopathic cord herniation.

REFERENCES

1. Khosla A, Wippold FJ. CT myelography and MR imaging of extramedullary cysts of the spinal canal in adult and pediatric patients. *AJR Am J Roentgenol* 2002; **178**: 201–7.

2. Ginanneschi F, Palma L, Rossi A. Arachnoid cyst and arachnoiditis following idiopathic spinal subarachnoid haemorrhage. *Br J Neurosurg* 2008; **22**: 578–9.

3. Kumar R, Taha J, Greiner AL. Herniation of the spinal cord: case report. *J Neurosurg* 1995; **82**: 131–6.

4. Brugières P, Malapert D, Adle-Biassette H, *et al.* Idiopathic Spinal Cord Herniation: Value of MR Phase-Contrast Imaging. *AJNR Am J Neuroradiol* 1999; **20**: 935–9.

5. Brus-Ramer M, Dillon WP. Idiopathic thoracic spinal cord herniation: retrospective analysis supporting a mechanism of diskogenic dural injury and subsequent tamponade. *AJNR Am J Neuroradiol* 2012; **33**: 52–6.

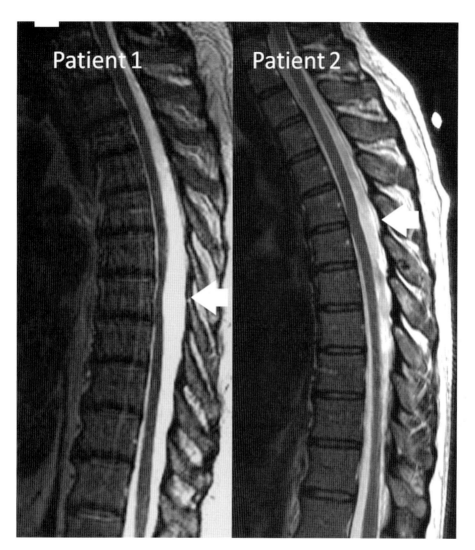

**Figure 104.1** Sagittal T2-weighted images of the thoracic spine in two different patients with myelopathy show apparent focal displacement of the cord anteriorly with relative expansion of the posterior subarachnoid space at these levels, which were initially missed.

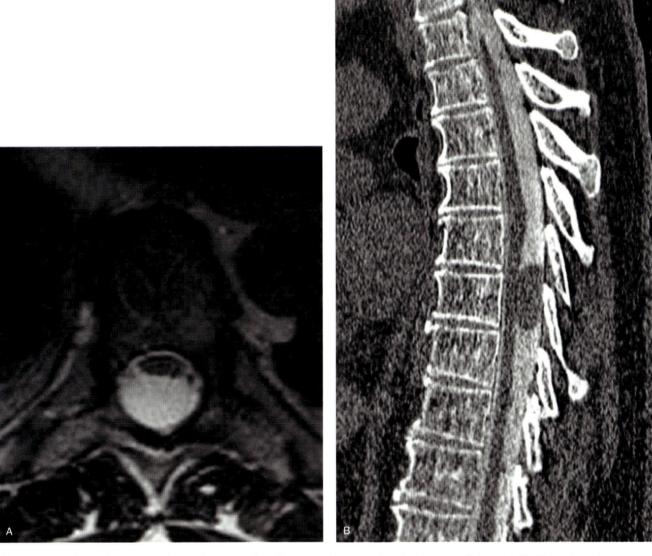

**Figure 104.2** (**A**) Axial T2-weighted MRI of patient 1 from Fig. 104.1 shows anterior displacement of the cord. (**B**) CT myelography revealed a large filling defect compatible with an arachnoid cyst, which was removed surgically.

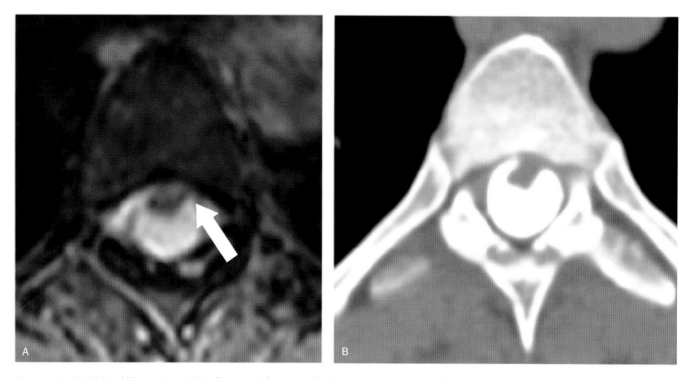

**Figure 104.3** (**A**) Axial T2-weighted MRI of patient 2 from Fig. 104.1 shows a focal cord deformity anteriorly (arrow). (**B**) The cord is small, deformed, and glued to the ventral surface of the thecal sac on CT myelogram. During surgery a ventral dural defect was found through which the cord was herniated and tethered.

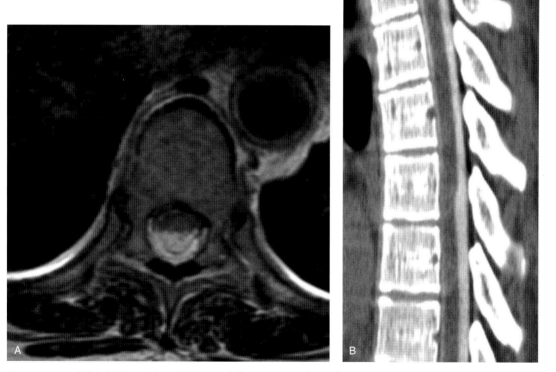

**Figure 104.4** (**A**) Axial T2-weighted MRI on a different patient shows flattening of the posterior surface of the cord, with (**B**) CT myelogram showing no filling defect or cord herniation. In surgery, an arachnoid band crossing the subarachnoid space and tethering the cord was found.

## Imaging description

CSF leaks in the spine are most commonly seen following iatrogenic or post-traumatic arachnoid and dural tears. However, spontaneous CSF leaks are increasingly identified as a cause of spontaneous intracranial hypotension (SIH).

The dural tear can result in formation of a pseudomeningocele or fistula at the site of traumatic or iatrogenic injury (spinal surgery, lumbar puncture). On MRI, focal disruption of the dural lining and the contour of the thecal sac can be identified (Figs. 105.1, 105.2), and, in case of large leaks, obvious collections of CSF may be present outside the dura (Fig. 105.3).

The localization of the precise site of CSF leak presents significant challenges in patients with SIH. Conventional CT myelography (CTM) is often very useful in demonstrating the site of leakage, and is considered the modality of choice. However, it may fail to demonstrate very small leaks and may not precisely localize the site in the presence of fast CSF leaks [1,2]. MR myelography with intrathecal gadolinium has been shown to be complementary when no demonstrable leak has been shown on CTM (Fig. 105.2). While its use remains off-label, several studies have shown safety of low-dose intrathecal gadolinium [1].

Fast CSF leaks may also not be reliably detected on conventional CTM. Dynamic CTM or digital subtraction myelography may be helpful and complementary in such patients (Fig. 105.3). It has also been suggested that the presence of extra-arachnoid collections on spinal MRI may be used as a predictive sign for rapid CSF leaks [2]. In such cases, conventional CTM may be omitted, and patients can undergo dynamic CTM directly.

## Importance

Precise localization of the site of CSF leakage is potentially helpful in directing therapeutic procedures. Targeted blood patch or fibrin glue injections can be useful for slow leaks, but surgical correction may be needed for fast, high-volume leaks.

## Typical clinical scenario

Patients typically present with orthostatic headaches, although a wide range of other manifestations may also be present depending on the severity and chronicity of leakage.

## Differential diagnosis

Collections of fluid adjacent to the dural sac may be observed in many patients after spinal surgery. The causes include postoperative seromas, hematomas, abscess, and CSF leaks. Therefore, especially in postoperative patients, careful correlation is necessary with the clinical presentation. Hematomas and abscess can be readily differentiated from CSF collections based on MR signal characteristics and peripheral enhancement (in the case of abscess). In some cases, percutaneous fluid aspiration may be necessary to distinguish seromas from CSF collections.

---

### Teaching points

The majority of CSF leaks in patients with SIH are located in the spine. Conventional CTM, MR with intrathecal gadolinium, and dynamic CTM are the techniques used to locate and characterize such leaks. The presence of extra-arachnoid CSF collections on MRI may predict rapid CSF leak.

---

REFERENCES

1. Akbar JJ, Luetmer PH, Schwartz KM, *et al.* The role of MR myelography with intrathecal gadolinium in localization of spinal CSF leaks in patients with spontaneous intracranial hypotension. *AJNR Am J Neuroradiol* 2012; **33**: 535–40.

2. Luetmer PH, Schwartz KM, Eckel LJ, *et al.* When should I do dynamic CT myelography? Predicting fast spinal CSF leaks in patients with spontaneous intracranial hypotension. *AJNR Am J Neuroradiol* 2012; **33**: 690–4.

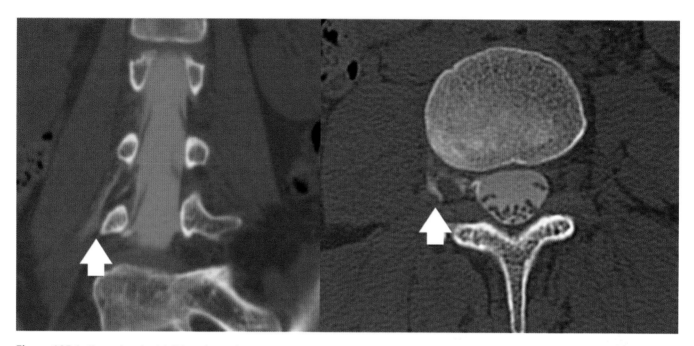

**Figure 105.1** Coronal and axial CT myelography images in a patient with SIH reveal a small contrast leak along the right L4 nerve root (arrows). Note the contrast extending outside the nerve root sleeve into paraspinal soft tissues.

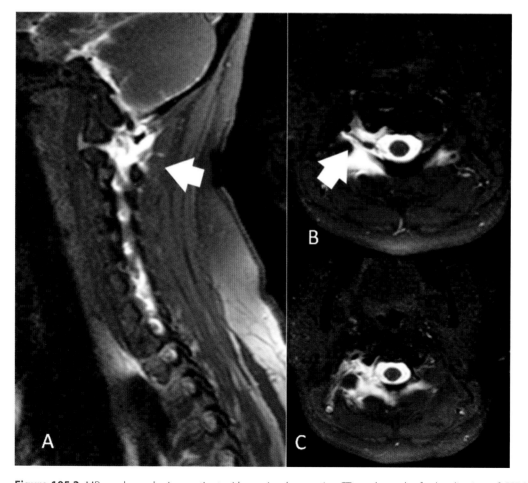

**Figure 105.2** MR myelography in a patient with previously negative CT myelography for localization of CSF leak. High-resolution fat-saturated (**A**) sagittal and (**B**, **C**) axial images of the cervical spine are obtained after intrathecal administration of gadolinium. The site of leakage is at C1–C2 level. Note the disruption of the dura and a large CSF collection (arrows).

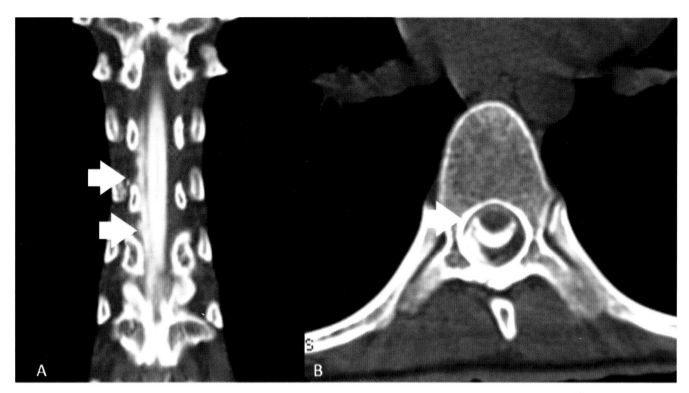

**Figure 105.3** Utility of dynamic CT myelography in localization of fast leaks. (**A**) Conventional CT myelography confirmed a CSF leak (arrows) in the lower thoracic region but failed to definitively localize the leak. (**B**) Dynamic CT myelography reveals a small defect in the dura at T8 level on the right (arrow).

## Imaging description

With the advent of modern chemotherapeutic medicine, sophisticated delivery of radiation, and efficient management of complex side effects and complications, cancer patients are living longer. There is also increasing incidence of leptomeningeal cranial and spinal metastasis due to the spread of malignant tumor cells through the subarachnoid space, which is typically seen in advanced cancer cases [1]. However, in 20% of patients it can present after a disease-free interval, and in 5–10% of cases it can be the first manifestation of cancer [1].

CSF analysis is one of the earliest investigations in patients presenting with myelopathy and polyradiculopathy. However, for positive analysis in a case of leptomeningeal metastatic disease, multiple CSF sampling may be necessary to get positive cytology [2]. Drop metastasis from primary CNS tumor is most commonly seen with medulloblastoma in children (Fig. 106.1). It can be seen in cases of intracranial ependymoma (Fig. 106.2), germinoma, or choroid plexus papilloma. In adults, it is more commonly seen in cases of anaplastic astrocytoma (Fig. 106.3), glioblastoma (Fig. 106.4), or ependymoma [3]. Disseminated hematogenous spread from an extracranial malignant neoplasm is commonly seen with adenocarcinomas, more commonly from breast (Fig. 106.5) or lung. It can also be seen from adenocarcinoma of the gastrointestinal tract, such as esophagus or stomach [4]. Sometimes drop metastasis from rare intracranial conditions such as primary leptomeningeal oligodendroglioma is also seen (Fig. 106.6). Other systemic conditions, including melanoma, leukemia, and non-Hodgkin's lymphoma, are also associated with an increasing incidence of leptomeningeal spinal metastasis.

Magnetic resonance imaging with gadolinium enhancement is the technique of choice to evaluate patients with suspected leptomeningeal metastasis. The leptomeningeal drop metastasis presents itself in various patterns. The most challenging pattern is presence of a solitary enhancing focus at the bottom of the thecal sac, which can look like intradural fat on post-contrast T1-weighted sagittal imaging (Fig. 106.1). Hence, a fat-saturated post-contrast T1 sagittal image is very helpful. Another challenging pattern is that of an intramedullary nodule communicating with the surface. Sometimes it can be difficult to distinguish it from hematogenous intramedullary cord metastasis (Fig. 106.2). However, sometimes a tail of enhancement along the surface of the cord can be seen, to recognize it as leptomeningeal metastases. Diffuse, thin surface enhancement of the cord with sheet-like smooth coating of the rootlets of the cauda equina can also be seen (Fig. 106.3). There is lack of nodularity, and sometimes the enhancement can be subtle. Conversely, multifocal discrete nodules can be seen along the rootlets of the cauda equina and also on the surface of the spinal cord (Fig. 106.4). There can be ropelike thickening of the cauda equina rootlets (Fig. 106.5), which can

be contiguous with sugarcoating of the surface of the cord (Fig. 106.6). Sometimes thick surface nodules do not exhibit any appreciable enhancement; however, a rind of soft tissue can be seen around the cord and along the cauda (Fig. 106.7).

## Importance

Leptomeningeal metastasis generally presents at a late stage in the disease and can be treated only with radiation or chemotherapy, preferably intrathecal. Even though the median survival is short despite therapy, in selected patients treatment can result in significant palliation. It is important to differentiate this condition from other inflammatory and infective conditions, which are treated with antibiotics and steroids.

## Typical clinical scenario

Leptomeningeal drop metastasis is generally seen in patients with known advanced cancer, and it is rarely a presenting symptom. It may be asymptomatic in the early stages but generally presents with severe pain and polyradiculopathy with relentless progression. Depending on the distribution, the patient may have nuchal rigidity and myelopathy. However, the element of radiculopathy dominates over the element of myelopathy.

## Differential diagnosis

Infectious conditions such as pyogenic meningitis and tuberculous meningitis can exhibit smooth and thick or thin sheet-like enhancement, which can be indistinguishable from leptomeningeal carcinomatosis. Small schwannomas or neurinomas along the cauda, as seen in neurofibromatosis, can also present as discretely enhancing nodules, without sheet- or rope-like enhancement (Fig. 106.8). Post-viral conditions such as Guillain–Barré syndrome can exhibit thick enhancement of the nerve roots of the cauda equina, but present with motor signs. Sarcoidosis, postoperative changes, and adhesions secondary to subarachnoid hemorrhages can also mimic leptomeningeal metastases.

---

### Teaching points

It is important to distinguish between leptomeningeal drop metastases and leptomeningeal enhancement from other causes such as previous surgery, Guillain–Barré syndrome, post-radiotherapeutic and chemotherapeutic polyradiculopathy, and infectious and inflammatory conditions such as pyogenic or tuberculous meningitis or sarcoidosis. Sometimes nodular, mass-like leptomeningeal metastases do not enhance avidly on post-contrast studies. Efforts should be made not to miss a small focus of enhancement at the bottom of the thecal sac when there is no simultaneous enhancement of cord or cauda.

REFERENCES

1. Chamberlain MC. Leptomeningeal metastasis. *Curr Opin Oncol* 2010; **22**: 627–35.

2. Ren S, Huang Y, Shah P, Manucha V. Metastatic squamous cell carcinoma in cerebrospinal fluid: why a rare diagnosis on cytology? *Acta Cytol* 2012; **56**: 209–13.

3. Shah A, Redhu R, Nadkarni T, Goel A. Supratentorial glioblastoma multiforme with spinal metastases. *J Craniovertebr Junction Spine* 2010; **1**: 126–9.

4. Emoto S, Ishigami H, Yamaguchi H, *et al.* Frequent development of leptomeningeal carcinomatosis in patients with peritoneal dissemination of gastric cancer. *Gastric Cancer* 2011; **14**: 390–5.

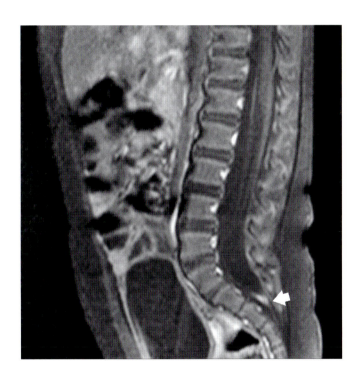

**Figure 106.1** Medulloblastoma drop metastasis. Fat-saturated post-contrast T1-weighted sagittal MR image exhibits a solitary focal mass at the bottom of the thecal sac (arrow) in routine surveillance MR scan in a patient treated for medulloblastoma.

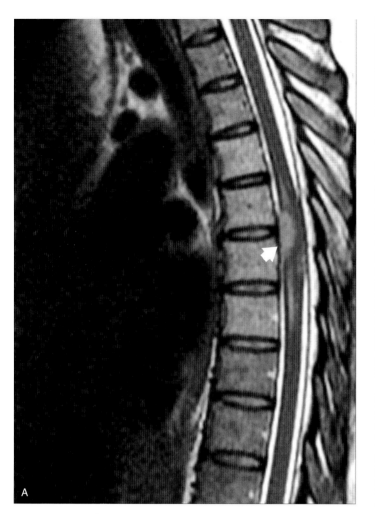

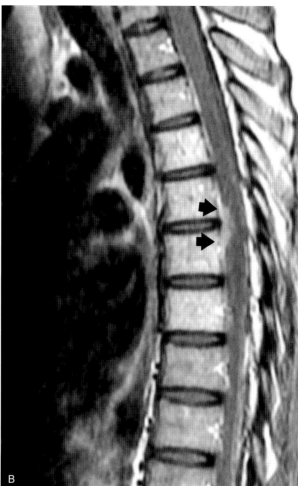

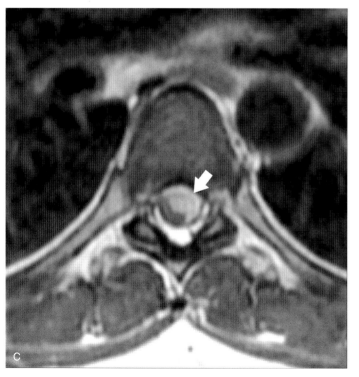

**Figure 106.2** Ependymoma drop metastasis. (**A**) T2-weighted sagittal MR image exhibits a faintly high T2 signal plaque-like mass on the ventral cord surface (short white arrow) in a patient with recently treated posterior fossa ependymoma. (**B**) Post-contrast T1-weighted sagittal MR imaging exhibits patchy post-contrast enhancement, reaching up to the cord surface with a faint tail of contrast enhancement along the ventral surface of the cord (short black arrows). (**C**) Post-contrast T1-weighted axial MRA image exhibits enhancing cord mass with surface enhancement (white arrow). Sometimes such nodules are difficult to distinguish from intramedullary cord metastasis due to hematogenous spread.

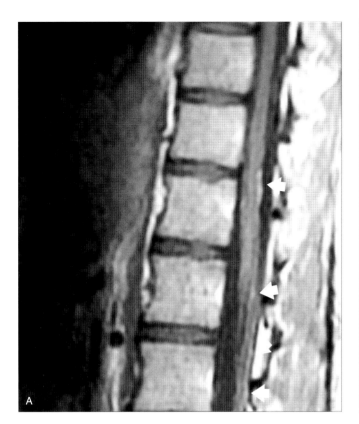
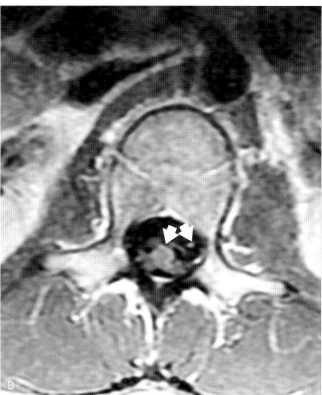

**Figure 106.3** Anaplastic astrocytoma drop metastasis. T1-weighted post-contrast (**A**) sagittal and (**B**) axial MR imaging exhibits diffuse thin surface enhancement of the dorsal surface of the cord (short white arrows) with sheet-like smooth coating, also seen along the conus and cauda equina rootlets (short white arrows), in a patient presenting with polyradiculopathy, 2 years after resection of intracranial anaplastic astrocytoma.

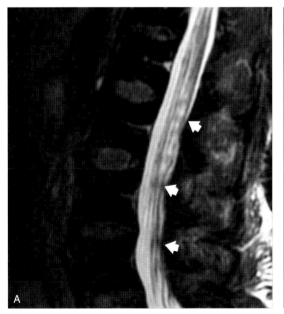
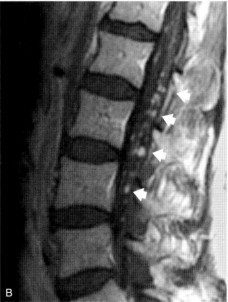

**Figure 106.4** GBM drop metastasis. (**A**) Fat-saturated T2-weighted sagittal MR imaging exhibits rope-like thickening of cauda equina with nodularity (short white arrows) on chemotherapy for GBM diagnosed 6 months back, in a patient complaining of low back and buttock pain. (**B**) Fat-saturated post-contrast T1-weighted sagittal MR imaging of the lumbar spine exhibits presence of multifocal discrete nodules along the rootlets of the cauda equina (short white arrows). (**C**) Fat-saturated post-contrast T1-weighted sagittal MR imaging of the thoracolumbar region exhibits multifocal discrete nodules with sugarcoating along the surface of the cord (short white arrows).

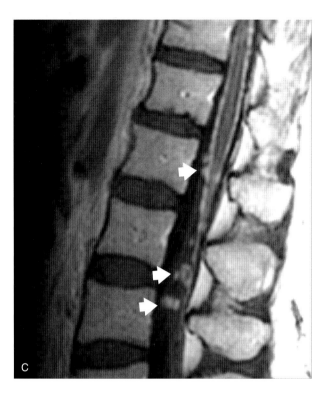

**Figure 106.4** (cont.)

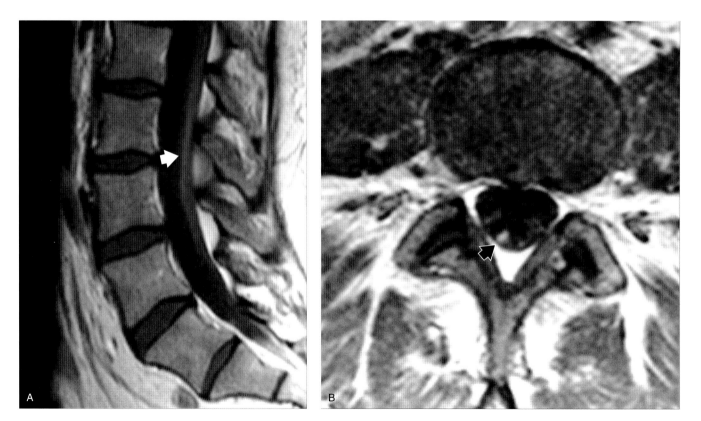

**Figure 106.5** Leptomeningeal carcinomatosis from breast cancer. Post-contrast T1-weighted (**A**) sagittal and (**B**) axial MR imaging exhibits rope-like thickening and enhancement of an isolated rootlet of cauda equina (short white and black arrows). The patient was surgically treated for carcinoma breast 6 years previously, had chemotherapy for lung metastasis 4 years back, and presented with lower extremity weakness.

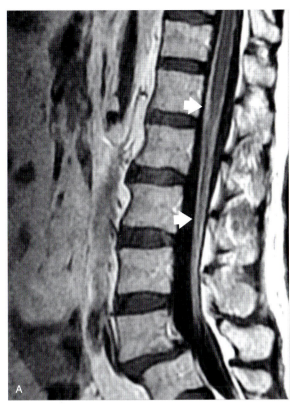

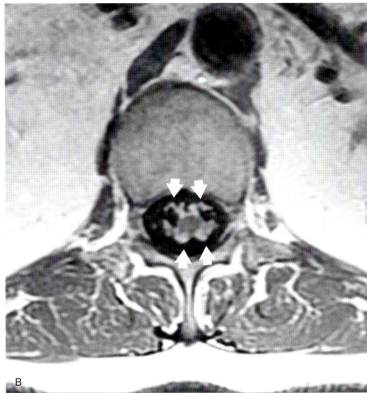

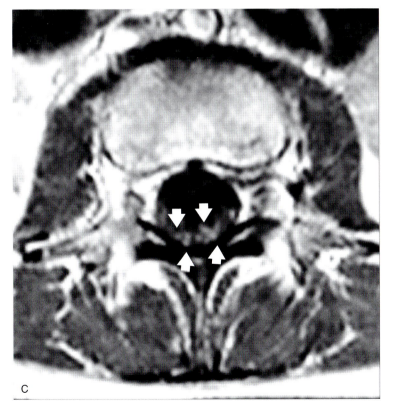

**Figure 106.6** Drop metastasis from leptomeningeal oligodendroglioma. (**A**) Post-contrast T1-weighted sagittal MR image exhibits sugarcoating of the cord surface (short white arrows) extending over the cauda equina, in a patient with known leptomeningeal oligodendroglioma, complaining of weakness of all four extremities. (**B**, **C**) Post-contrast T1-weighted axial MR imaging exhibits ropelike thickening and enhancement of the rootlets of cauda equina (short white arrows).

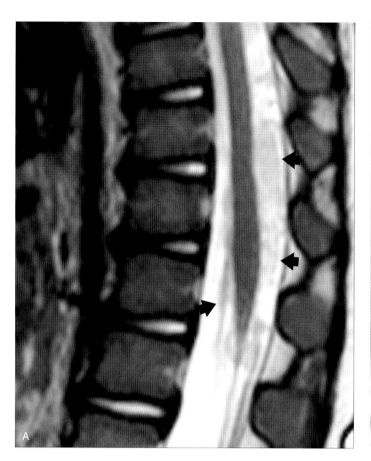

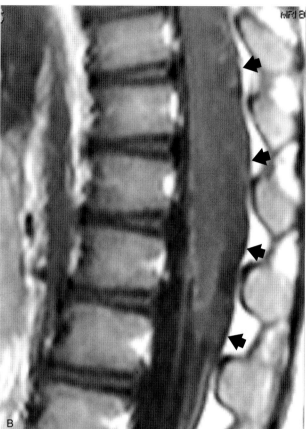

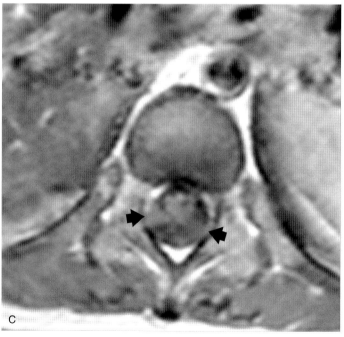

**Figure 106.7** Drop metastasis from atypical teratoid rhabdoid tumor (ATRT). (**A**) Fat-saturated T2-weighted sagittal MR imaging exhibits numerous coalescent low T2 signal nodules on the surface of distal spinal cord with mild thickening of rootlets of cauda equina (short black arrows) in a patient with known ATRT and recent-onset lower extremity weakness. (**B**) Post-contrast T1-weighted sagittal MR imaging exhibits multifocal coalescent nodule isointense to cord, predominantly on the dorsal surface and along the cauda (short black arrows) with only minimal enhancement. There is mild nodular enhancement of the ventral surface of the cord and cauda. (**C**) Post-contrast T1-weighted axial MR image exhibits isointense nodules along the cauda without significant enhancement (short black arrows).

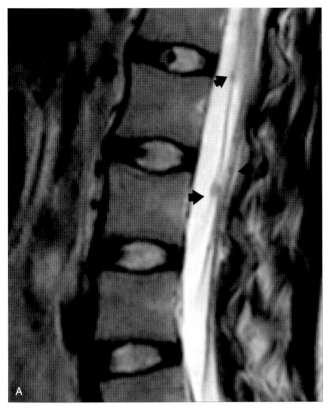

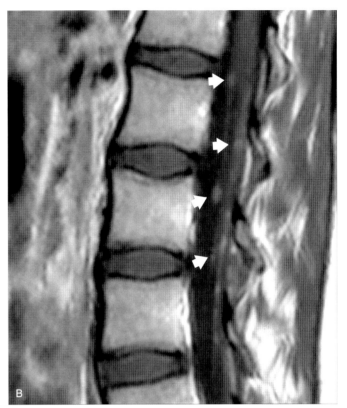

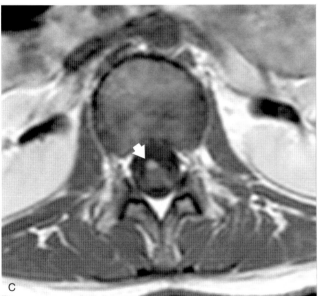

**Figure 106.8** Multifocal schwannomas of cauda equina in neurofibromatosis 2 (NF2). (**A**) Fat-saturated T2-weighted sagittal MR imaging exhibits isointense nodularity along the rootlets of cauda equina (short black arrows). (**B**) Post-contrast T1-weighted sagittal MR image exhibits uniform intense enhancement of the nodules (short white arrows) without surface enhancement of the cauda.
(**C**) Post contrast T1 weighted axial MR imaging exhibits enhancing schwannoma ventral to conus (short white arrow) without surface enhancement of cauda or conus.

# Index

abscesses
  brain *see* brain abscess
  neck 350, 353, 370–1
  peritonsillar 364, 368
  retropharyngeal 414
  spinal epidural 458, 464, 475
acute cerebral infarction 8–9
acute disseminated encephalomyelitis (ADEM)
      58–61
  diffuse infiltrating pontine glioma vs. 105, 108
  optic neuritis 336
  osmotic myelinolysis vs. 65, 71
adenoid cystic carcinoma, parotid gland 344, 347
adrenoleukodystrophy (ALD) 219–21
  neonatal (NALD) 219
adrenomyeloneuropathy (AMN) 219, 222–3
AIDS *see* HIV infection/AIDS
Alexander's disease 219
allergic fungal sinusitis 310–12
Alpert syndrome 453
amyloid angiopathy, cerebral (CAA) 26, 30–1
anaplastic astrocytoma
  low-grade glioma vs. 92, 100
  pediatric 80, 88
  spinal leptomeningeal drop metastases
      478, 481
anatomic variations 245–64
anesthesia, FLAIR sulcal hyperintensity secondary
      to 245–8
aneurysms, intracranial 21
  anterior clinoid process air cells vs. 264–5
  CT angiography pitfalls 260–3
  giant 23
  ruptured 17–18
  sellar or parasellar 181, 190
  *see also* dissecting aneurysms
anoxic-ischemic brain injury 4–7
anterior cerebral artery aneurysm 22
anterior clinoid process, asymmetric
      pneumatization 264–5
anterior communicating artery aneurysm 18
anterior thoracic cord herniation 471, 474
anti-vascular endothelial growth factor (VEGF)
      agents, glioblastoma pseudoresponse 112–13
aqueductal stenosis, adult onset 232
arachnoid bands, spinal intradural 471, 474
arachnoid cysts
  cerebellar tonsillar herniation with 454
  spinal intradural 471, 473
  suprasellar 240, 244
arachnoid granulations 255–6
arachnoid pits 324, 327
arterial injuries, traumatic 384–6
arteriovenous fistulas (AVFs)
  dural *see* dural arteriovenous fistulas
  neck injuries 384, 386
arteriovenous malformations (AVMs)
  cerebral
    developmental venous anomalies vs. 46, 48
    dural arteriovenous fistulas vs. 49
    hemorrhage from 26, 28

head and neck 360, 362
  spinal cord 455, 457
artery of Percheron territory infarction 213, 216
artifacts 245–64
*Aspergillus fumigatus* 316
astrocytomas
  anaplastic *see* anaplastic astrocytoma
  juvenile pilocytic *see* pilocytic astrocytoma,
      juvenile
  low-grade 92, 95, 98
  oligodendrogliomas vs. 114
  pineal 125, 138
  subependymal giant cell (SEGA) 153, 159
atlanto-axial dissociation (AAD) 387–9
atlanto-axial subluxation, rheumatoid arthritis
      390, 397
atlanto-occipital dissociation (AOD) 387–9
atypical teratoid rhabdoid tumor (ATRT)
      80, 86, 484

back pain 398, 401, 405, 419
basilar artery, acute thrombosis 1–2
basion-odontoid interval (BOI) 387–8
Battle sign 307
benign external hydrocephalus (BEH) 257–8
benign mixed tumor (BMT), salivary glands 344–6,
      364–5
bevacizumab, glioblastoma pseudoresponse 112–13
blood vessels, head and neck 381–4
bone erosion
  invasive fungal sinusitis 316–18
  malignant otitis externa 304, 306
brain abscess 191–2
  primary CNS lymphoma vs. 116, 123, 191
  tuberculosis vs. 191, 198, 204
  tuberculous 198
brain atrophy
  benign external hydrocephalus vs. 257–8
  moyamoya disease 40–1
brain death 4–5
brain metastases
  abscesses vs. 191, 206
  intraventricular 140, 146, 151
  lymphoma 116, 120–1
  neurosarcoidosis vs. 72
  pineal region 125, 137
  primary intraosseous meningioma vs. 161,
      168–70
  tuberculosis vs. 198, 205
brain sagging, intracranial hypotension
      234–5, 449
brain tumors 80–181
  acute disseminated encephalomyelitis vs. 58
  hemorrhagic
    amyloid angiopathy vs. 30, 32
    cavernous malformations vs. 52
    giant aneurysms vs. 23, 25
    intracerebral hematomas vs. 26, 29
    intraventricular (IVTs) 139
  metastatic *see* brain metastases
  pediatric posterior fossa 80

pineal region 125–6
  spinal leptomeningeal drop metastases 478
  tumefactive demyelinating lesion vs. 55
  *see also specific types*
brainstem gliomas 105
branchial anomalies
  first branchial cleft cysts 350–1
  second branchial cleft cysts 357
  third branchial apparatus anomaly 370
breast cancer
  brain metastases 198, 206
  leptomeningeal carcinomatosis 249, 478, 482
  metastatic epidural spinal cord compression
      458
  primary CNS lymphoma vs. 119
burst fractures, odontoid process 390, 394

calcific tendinitis of longus colli 414–16
calcifications
  arteriovenous malformations 26, 28
  cavernous malformations 52–3
  giant aneurysms 23–4
  neurocysticercosis 194, 197
  renal osteodystrophy 409–10
capillary malformations 360
caput medusa appearance 47
carbon monoxide poisoning 207, 209
carotid artery
  atherosclerotic disease 381, 383
  complete occlusion, with hypertrophied vasa
      vasora 378, 380
  dissection (CAD) 381–3
  near-occlusive stenosis 378–80
  traumatic injuries 384–5
cauda equina syndrome 399
caudal agenesis/regression 435, 444
cavernous hemangiomas
  intraventricular 140, 150
  primary intraosseous 161, 165
  spinal epidural 463
cavernous malformations (CMs) 52
  amyloid angiopathy vs. 30
  giant aneurysms vs. 23, 25
cavernous sinus
  internal carotid artery aneurysms 23
  pituitary macroadenoma invasion 180
  Tolosa-Hunt syndrome 331
cellulitis
  phlegmonous orbital 331
  retropharyngeal *see* retropharyngeal edema
central pontine osmotic myelinolysis 65–6
  diffuse infiltrating pontine glioma vs. 105
cephaloceles, sphenoid 324–6
cerebellar tonsillar herniation
  acquired 449, 454
  congenital *see* Chiari I malformation
cerebral amyloid angiopathy (CAA) 26, 30–1
cerebral blood volume, relative (rCBV)
  gliomas 114–15
  primary CNS lymphoma 116, 119
cerebral edema, cortical venous thrombosis 43–5

cerebral infarction
  acute 8–9
  acute disseminated encephalomyelitis vs. 58, 61
  lacunar 250, 253
  moyamoya disease 40–1
  multiple small infarcts 13, 16
  pontine 65, 68
  primary CNS vasculitis 34–5
  reversible cerebral vasoconstriction syndrome 37
  subacute 13
  see also stroke
cerebral vasoconstriction syndrome, reversible (RCVS) 37
cerebrospinal fluid (CSF) leaks
  intracranial hypotension 234, 449, 454
  spinal 475–7
  spontaneous 324, 326
cerebrovascular diseases 1–52
cervical myelopathy 424–6
cervical spine
  ligamentous craniovertebral junction injuries 387
  odontoid fractures 390
  spondylodiscitis 414, 418
  spondylosis 424–5
  T2 hyperintense disc herniations 419, 422
Chiari I malformation 449–53
  acquired 449, 454
  intracranial hypotension vs. 234–5
children see pediatric patients
cholesteatomas
  acquired 299
  attic 299, 301
  congenital 299
  pars flaccida 299–300
  pars tensa 299–301
  petrous apex 294, 297
cholesterol granulomas (CG)
  middle ear 299
  petrous apex 294–6
chondrosarcoma
  clivus 276, 281
  petrous apex 294, 298
  skull base 267
chordoid glioma of third ventricle 140
chordoma
  clivus 275–7
  sellar/suprasellar 181, 189
choroid plexus
  carcinoma 140, 143
  cysts 140, 149
  metastases 146
  papilloma 80, 89, 140, 143, 478
  tumors 140
clival lesions 276
coagulopathies, acute intracerebral hematoma 26, 28
cochlear dysplasia 285–8
cochlear implantation 285, 288–9
collaterals, puff of smoke 40, 42
colloid cysts 153–8
computed tomography angiography (CTA) 260–3
  carotid artery dissection 381–2
  dural arteriovenous fistulas 49
  intracranial aneurysms 21–2
  near-occlusive carotid stenosis 378, 380

subarachnoid hemorrhage 17
  traumatic arterial injuries 384–5
computed tomography myelography (CTM), CSF leaks 3, 476–7
computed tomography perfusion (CTP), acute cerebral infarction 8
concussion (mild traumatic brain injury) 224–6
conus medullaris, low-lying 445
copper deficiency 469
cord sign 43, 45
cortical venous thrombosis, isolated (ICVT) 43
cranial nerves
  clival lesions 276
  malignant otitis externa 304
  neurosarcoidosis 72
  perineural spread 282–3
craniopharyngiomas 140, 171, 176
  intrasellar 180, 188
  Rathke's cleft cysts vs. 240, 243
craniovertebral junction injuries 387
crescent sign, methemoglobin 381, 383
Creutzfeldt–Jakob disease disease (CJD) 207–8
  Wernicke's encephalopathy vs. 213, 216
cryptococcosis 250, 253
CSF see cerebrospinal fluid
cystic hygroma see lymphatic malformation
cystic nodal metastasis 357–9
cystic periventricular leukomalacia 250
cysticercosis see neurocysticercosis

demyelinating lesions
  brain 55–73
  spinal cord 466–8
  tumefactive (TDL) 55–7
dense basilar artery sign 1–2
dense middle cerebral artery (MCA) sign 1–2
dermal sinuses, dorsal 435, 442, 445
developmental venous anomalies (DVA) 46
  thrombosis 43, 45–6, 48
diabetes mellitus
  invasive fungal sinusitis 316
  malignant otitis externa 304
diastematomyelia 435, 443, 445
diffuse axonal injury (DAI) 224, 226
  amyloid angiopathy vs. 30, 33
diffuse infiltrating pontine glioma (DIPG) 105–6
diffusion-weighted imaging (DWI)
  acute cerebral infarction 8–9
  carotid artery dissection 381–2
  global anoxic brain injury 4–6
digital subtraction angiography (DSA)
  carotid artery dissection 381
  CNS vasculitis 34
  intracranial aneurysms 21, 23
  subarachnoid hemorrhage 17
  vascular malformations 49, 455–6
discectomy, postoperative complications 427–9
discitis-osteomyelitis 430, 433
dissecting aneurysms 384–5
  carotid artery 381–2
dorsal enteric fistula 435
DSA see digital subtraction angiography
dural arteriovenous fistulas (DAVFs)
  cerebral 49
    hemorrhage 26, 51
  spinal 455–7

dural sinus thrombosis 1
  intravascular clot 1, 3
dural venous thrombosis, cortical venous involvement 43
DWI see diffusion-weighted imaging

embolic infarcts, vertebral artery dissection 10
empty sella sign 238–9
eosinophilic granuloma 161, 167
ependymomas 80, 83
  intraventricular 140, 142
  spinal leptomeningeal drop metastases 478, 480
epidermoid tumors 240, 244
epidural abscess, spinal 458, 464, 475
epidural hematoma/hemorrhage, spinal 458, 463, 475
epidural lipomatosis, spinal 458, 465
external auditory canal (EAC)
  carcinoma 304
  first branchial cleft cyst 350
  malignant otitis externa 304, 306
extrapontine osmotic myelinolysis 65, 67

fibrillary low-grade astrocytoma 92, 95
fibrous dysplasia (FD)
  clivus 276, 278
  primary intraosseous meningioma vs. 161, 164
  skull base 267–9
  sphenoid bone 271, 274
filum terminale
  lipoma 435, 441, 445–7
  thickened 445–7
  tight 435, 442, 445
first branchial cleft cyst 350–1
FLAIR sulcal hyperintensity secondary to general anesthesia 245–8
fungal sinusitis
  allergic 310–12
  invasive 310, 316–19

ganglioglioma, third ventricular 148
gemistocytic low-grade astrocytoma 92, 98
general anesthesia, FLAIR sulcal hyperintensity secondary to 245–8
germ cell tumors (GCT), pineal region 125–6, 130, 132
germinomas
  leptomeningeal drop metastases 478
  pineal region 125–6, 130, 132
  suprasellar region 171, 178
ghosting artifacts, giant aneurysms 23
glioblastoma multiforme (GBM)
  brain abscess vs. 191, 193
  pediatric 80
  pineal 139
  primary CNS lymphoma vs. 116, 122
  pseudoprogression 109–11
  pseudoresponse to treatment 112–13
  spinal leptomeningeal drop metastases 478, 481
gliomas
  brainstem 105
  chordoid, of third ventricle 140
  classification 92
  diffuse infiltrating pontine 105–6
  low-grade (LGG) 92, 97
  optic nerve 336, 340
  pediatric 80, 92

gliomas (cont.)
  pineal 125, 138–9
  relative cerebral blood volume (rCBV) 114–15
  tectal 125, 138, 232–3
  tumefactive demyelinating lesion vs. 55
  see also astrocytomas; glioblastoma multiforme;
    oligodendroglioma
glioneural tumor of fourth ventricle, rosette
  forming 140
global anoxic brain injury 4–7
glomus tympanicum paraganglioma 299
glutaric aciduria type I 259
goiter, multinodular 374
granulation of middle ear, chronic 299, 303
granulomas
  cholesterol (CG) 294–6, 299
  CNS tuberculosis 198, 200–2
  neurosarcoidosis 72
granulomatous optic neuropathy 336, 339
Guillain–Barré syndrome (GBS) 478
Guillain–Mollaret triangle 217

hangman's fracture 390, 394
head and neck cancer
  cystic nodal metastasis 357
  perineural spread 282–4
  see also squamous cell carcinoma
head enlargement, benign external hydrocephalus
  257–8
hearing loss, sensorineural
  acquired 289
  congenital 285
hemangioblastoma 80, 91
hemangioma 360, 363
  see also cavernous hemangiomas
hematological malignancies
  progressive multifocal leukoencephalopathy 62
  see also lymphoma
herpes encephalitis 210–12
  low-grade glioma vs. 92, 103
HIV infection/AIDS
  cryptococcosis 253
  primary CNS lymphoma 116, 118
  progressive multifocal leukoencephalopathy
    62–4
  toxoplasmosis 193
  tuberculosis 198
HIV leukoencephalopathy 62
human papilloma virus (HPV)-related squamous
  cell carcinoma of neck 357
hydrocephalus
  adult onset, secondary to aqueductal stenosis
    232–3
  benign external (BEH) 257–8
  tumor-related 80, 125, 153
hyperparathyroidism, secondary 409
hypertension, intracerebral hemorrhage 26–7, 30
hypertrophic olivary degeneration (HOD) 217–18
hypertrophic pachymeningitis, idiopathic 72

idiopathic hypertrophic pachymeningitis 72
idiopathic intracranial hypertension (IIH) 238–9
  spontaneous CSF leaks 324, 327
immunocompromised patients
  invasive fungal sinusitis 316
  primary CNS lymphoma 116, 118

progressive multifocal leukoencephalopathy 62
  see also HIV infection/AIDS
infectious diseases 191–210
inflammatory diseases
  brain 55–73
  spinal cord 466, 468
infundibular dilatation, artery origins 17, 19,
  21–2
infundibular histiocytosis, neurosarcoidosis vs. 72
innominate artery dissecting aneurysm 385
insular ribbon sign 9
internal carotid artery (ICA)
  complete occlusion, with hypertrophied vasa
    vasora 378, 380
  dissection (CAD) 381–3
  giant aneurysms 23–4
  near-occlusive stenosis 378–80
  traumatic injuries 385
internal cerebral vein thrombosis 213, 215
intervertebral discs 419–30
  cervical spondylodiscitis 414, 418
  degenerative changes 430–2
  discitis 430, 433
  herniation and cord compression 424–6
  postoperative herniation vs. postsurgical scarring
    427–9
  T2 hyperintense herniations 419–23
intracerebral hematoma (ICH)
  acute 26
  amyloid angiopathy 26, 30–1
  cortical venous thrombosis 43, 45
  reversible cerebral vasoconstriction syndrome
    37–8
  subarachnoid hemorrhage 17–18
intracranial hemorrhage
  acute disseminated encephalomyelitis 58
  cavernous malformation-related 52, 54
  moyamoya disease 40
  see also intracerebral hematoma; subarachnoid
    hemorrhage
intracranial hypertension, idiopathic see idiopathic
    intracranial hypertension
intracranial hypotension 234–7
  cerebellar tonsillar descent 234–5, 449, 454
  spontaneous see spontaneous intracranial
    hypotension
intradural cysts, spinal 471
intraparotid lymph nodes (IPLN) 342–4
  first branchial cleft cyst vs. 350
intraventricular tumors (IVTs) 139
invasive fungal sinusitis 310, 316–19
inverted papilloma, paranasal sinus 310, 314
isolated cortical venous thrombosis (ICVT) 43
ivory vertebra 405
ivy sign 40–1

JC virus 62
jugular vein obstruction 414
juvenile nasal angiofibroma (JNA) 328–30
juvenile pilocytic astrocytoma see pilocytic
    astrocytoma, juvenile

labyrinthine aplasia (Michel's anomaly) 285, 289
labyrinthitis ossificans (LO) 289–91
lacrimal gland orbital pseudotumor 331, 333
lacunar infarcts 250, 253

Langerhans cell histiocytosis (LCH)
  intracranial 171, 179, 181, 189
  petrous apex 294
large vestibular aqueduct (LVA) 285
lateral medullary syndrome 10–11
Leigh's disease 207, 209
leptomeningeal drop metastases, spinal 478
leptomeningeal/meningeal carcinomatosis
  FLAIR sulcal hyperintensity 245, 249
  neurosarcoidosis vs. 72
leukodystrophies, inherited 219–20
limbic encephalitis 210, 212
lipoma
  filum terminale 435, 441, 445–7
  intradural 435, 442, 447
  lumbosacral 445
  pineal 125, 138
lipomatosis, spinal epidural 458, 465
lipomyelocele 435, 440
lipomyelomeningocele 435, 439, 445
longus colli, calcific tendinitis of 414–16
low-flow vascular malformations (LFVMs) 360
low-grade gliomas (LGGs) 92, 97
lumbar spine
  Paget's disease of bone 405–8
  T2 hyperintense disc herniations 419–21
lung carcinoma
  brain metastases 32, 198, 205, 212
  metastatic epidural spinal cord compression
    458–9
  spinal leptomeningeal drop metastases 478
lymph nodes
  acutely infected 357, 359
  cystic metastasis 357–8
  intraparotid (IPLN) 342–4, 350
  reactive, parathyroid adenoma vs. 372
  suppurative retropharyngeal 414, 418
lymphatic malformation (cystic hygroma) 360, 362
  cystic nodal metastasis vs. 357
  first branchial cleft cyst vs. 350, 352
lymphoma
  clival lesions 276
  cranial intraosseous metastases 161, 168
  metastatic epidural spinal cord compression
    458, 460
  orbital 331, 334
  primary CNS see primary CNS lymphoma
  secondary CNS 116, 120–1, 151
  spine 409, 413
  tumefactive demyelinating lesion vs. 55

macrocephaly, benign external hydrocephalus
  257–8
magnetic resonance angiography (MRA)
  carotid artery dissection 381
  dural arteriovenous fistulas 49
  intracranial aneurysms 21–3
  near-occlusive carotid stenosis 378–9
  traumatic arterial injuries 384
magnetic resonance (MR) myelography, CSF leaks
  475–6
magnetic resonance venography (MRV), idiopathic
  intracranial hypertension 238–9
malignant otitis externa (MOE) 304–6
marble bone disease 409, 412
McCune–Albright syndrome 267

medulla, infarction 217
medulloblastoma (MB) 80–1
    spinal leptomeningeal drop metastases
        478–9
melanoma
    parotid gland 342
    sinonasal 316, 322
    vertebral compression fractures 398
meningeal carcinomatosis see leptomeningeal/
        meningeal carcinomatosis
meningeal cysts, spinal 458, 463
meningeal enhancement, intracranial hypotension
        234
meningiomas
    en plaque, with hyperostosis 161, 165
    intracranial aneurysms vs. 263
    intraventricular 140, 145
    neurosarcoidosis vs. 72, 78
    optic nerve 336, 341
    parasellar 180, 187
    pineal 125, 135
    primary intraosseous (PIM) 161–3
    skull base intraosseous 267
    spinal cord compression 458
    suprasellar 171–4
meningitis
    acute pyogenic 198, 202
    FLAIR sulcal hyperintensity 245, 249
    neurosarcoidosis vs. 72
    sensorineural hearing loss 289, 291
    spinal leptomeningeal metastases vs. 478
    tuberculous see tuberculous meningitis
meningoceles
    Meckel's cave region 294, 298
    spinal 435, 438, 445, 447
metabolic disorders 213–20
metachromatic leukodystrophy 219
metastases
    brain see brain metastases
    clivus 276
    cystic nodal 357–9
    odontoid fractures 390, 395
    parotid gland 342–3
    petrous apex 294
    spinal intramedullary 478
    spinal leptomeningeal drop 478
    vertebral compression fractures 398–400
metastatic epidural spinal cord compression
        (MESCC) 458–62
methemoglobin crescent sign 381, 383
MGMT promoter methylation 109
Michel's anomaly 285, 289
middle cerebral artery (MCA)
    acute occlusion 1, 8–9
    aneurysm 18
    dense sign 1–2, 9
middle ear, chronic granulation 299, 303
mild traumatic brain injury (mTBI) 224–6
Mondini's malformation 285, 287, 288
moyamoya disease (and syndrome) 40
mucocele, paranasal sinus 310, 313
mucoepidermoid carcinoma
    parapharyngeal space 364
    parotid gland 344, 348
mucopolysaccharidosis 250, 254
mucormycosis 316

mucous retention cysts, nasopharynx 354
multiple sclerosis (MS)
    acute disseminated encephalomyelitis vs. 58
    optic neuritis 336
    osmotic myelinolysis vs. 65, 70
    primary CNS lymphoma vs. 116
    progressive multifocal leukoencephalopathy
        62
    spinal cord lesions 466–7
multiple small cerebral infarcts 13, 16
myelocele 434, 437, 448
myelocystocele 435
myeloma, multiple
    spinal cord compression 458, 461
    vertebral compression fractures 398, 400
    see also plasmacytoma
myelomeningocele 434, 436, 445
myeloschisis 445

nasal angiofibroma, juvenile (JNA) 328–30
nasopharyngeal carcinoma
    clival invasion 276, 280
    juvenile nasal angiofibroma vs. 328
    parapharyngeal space 369
nasopharyngeal cysts 354
nasopharyngeal tonsillar crypt cysts 354, 356
neck 354–64
    abscesses 350, 353, 370–1
    calcific tendinitis of longus colli 414–16
    craniovertebral junction injuries 387
    cystic nodal metastasis 357–9
    ligamentous injuries 414
    low-flow vascular malformations 360
    odontoid fractures 390
    pain, acute 390, 414
    parapharyngeal masses 364
    traumatic arterial injuries 384–6
    vessels 381–4
    see also cervical spine
neonatal adrenoleukodystrophy (NALD) 219
neurenteric cysts 435, 445, 471
neurinomas, cauda equina 478
neuroblastoma 458
neurocysticercosis 194–7
    brain abscess vs. 191
    intraventricular 140
    Virchow–Robin spaces vs. 250, 254
neurocytoma, central 140, 144, 153, 160
neurodegenerative diseases 213–20
neurofibromatosis 1 (NF1)
    diffuse infiltrating pontine glioma vs. 105
    optic nerve glioma 336
neurogenic tumors, parapharyngeal space
        364, 366
neuromyelitis optica (NMO) 336, 466
neurosarcoidosis 72–8
    primary CNS lymphoma vs. 72, 116, 124
    third nerve enlargement 284
    tuberculosis vs. 198, 203
nitrous oxide inhalation 469
North American Symptomatic Carotid
        Endarterectomy Trial (NASCET) 378

odontoid process
    congenital nonunion 390, 395
    erosion, in rheumatoid arthritis 390, 397

fractures 390–3
    ossification centers 390
    pathological fractures 390, 395
oligoastrocytoma, third ventricular 146
oligodendroglioma (ODG) 115
    low-grade 114
    low-grade glioma vs. 92, 102
    spinal leptomeningeal drop metastases 478, 483
olivary degeneration, hypertrophic (HOD) 217–18
optic nerve
    glioma 336, 340
    meningioma 336, 341
optic neuritis (ON) 336–7
optic neuropathy
    chronic relapsing 336, 339
    granulomatous 336, 339
    ischemic 336
    radiation-induced 336, 338
orbital pseudotumor, idiopathic 331–3
orbits 331–7
    lymphoproliferative lesions 331, 334
    phlegmonous cellulitis 331
    sarcoidosis 331, 336, 339
os odontoideum 390, 395
osmotic myelinolysis (OM) 65–7
ossifying fibroma
    fibrous dysplasia vs. 267, 270
    paranasal sinus 310, 313
    sphenoid bone 271
osteomalacia 409, 412
osteomyelitis, vertebral 430, 433
osteopetrosis 409, 412
osteoporosis
    renal osteodystrophy 409
    sacral insufficiency fractures 401
    vertebral compression fractures 398–9
osteosarcoma, calvarial 161
otitis externa, malignant (MOE) 304–6
otitis media, chronic otomastoiditis with 303
otomastoiditis, chronic 303
oxygen inhalation-related FLAIR sulcal
        hyperintensity 245–8

Paget's disease of bone
    fibrous dysplasia vs. 267, 270
    pelvis 408
    spine 405–9, 411
papillary tumor of pineal region (PTPR) 125, 130
paraganglioma
    glomus tympanicum 299
    parapharyngeal space 364, 367
paranasal sinuses 310–28
    benign masses 310
    inverted papilloma 310, 314
    mucocele 310, 313
    ossifying fibroma 310, 313
paranasal sinusitis
    acute 310
    aggressive pyogenic 316–17
    allergic fungal 310–12
    chronic purulent 310, 316
    invasive fungal 310, 316–19
parapharyngeal masses 364
parapharyngeal space 364
parathyroid adenoma 372–3, 375, 377
Parinaud's syndrome 125

parotid glands
  abscess 350, 353
  benign mixed tumor 344–6, 364–5
  first branchial cleft cyst 350–1
  intraparotid lymph nodes 342, 344, 350
  malignant tumors 344, 347–8
  retention cysts 350, 352
pathological fractures
  odontoid process 390, 395
  renal osteodystrophy 409
  vertebral compression 398–400
pediatric patients
  benign external hydrocephalus 257
  diffuse infiltrating pontine glioma 105
  low-grade gliomas 92
  posterior fossa masses 80
  third branchial apparatus anomaly 370
pelvis, Paget's disease 408
perimesencephalic hemorrhage, benign 17, 19
perineural spread (PNS) 282–4
peritonsillar abscess 364, 368
periventricular leukomalacia, cystic 250
periventricular white matter disease,
    neurosarcoidosis vs. 72
peroxisomal disorders, early onset 219
persistent terminal ventricle 435
petechial hemorrhages
  cerebral amyloid angiopathy 30–1
  diffuse axonal injury 30, 33
petrous apex (PA)
  asymmetric pneumatization 264, 266, 294
  fluid entrapment in air cells 294–5
  surgical lesions 294
petrous apicitis 294
phleboliths 360
pilocytic astrocytoma, juvenile (JPA) 80, 84,
    92–3
  diffuse infiltrating pontine glioma vs.
    105, 107
  suprasellar 171, 177
pineal cyst 125–6, 133–4
pineal parenchymal tumor of intermediate
    differentiation (PPTID) 125, 128
pineal region tumors 125–6
pineoblastoma 125–6, 129
pineocytoma 125–7
piriform sinus, sinus tract from 370–1
Pittsburgh Compound B 30
pituitary apoplexy 180, 182, 186
pituitary hyperplasia 180, 187
pituitary macroadenomas 180–2, 184–5
  clival invasion 276, 278
  Rathke's cleft cysts vs. 240, 243
  suprasellar extension 171, 175, 180
  ventricular involvement 140, 152
plasmacytoma
  clivus 276, 279
  metastatic epidural spinal cord compression
    458, 462
  petrous apex 294
  skull 161
pleomorphic adenoma see benign mixed tumor
pneumatization
  arrested, of sphenoid bone 271–3
  asymmetric 264–6
polycystic kidney disease, intracranial aneurysm
    22

pons
  diffuse infiltrating glioma 105–6
  ischemic infarction 65, 68
  osmotic myelinolysis 65–6
popcorn appearance, cavernous malformations
    52–3
port-wine stains 360
post-concussion syndrome 224
posterior cerebral artery (PCA) territory infarcts
    13–14
posterior communicating artery, infundibular
    dilatation at origin 17, 19, 22
posterior fossa masses, children 80
posterior reversible encephalopathy syndrome
    (PRES) 229–31
  diffuse infiltrating pontine glioma vs. 105, 108
  osmotic myelinolysis vs. 65
Power's ratio 387–8
primary CNS lymphoma (PCNSL) 116–19
  brain abscess vs. 116, 123, 191
  intraventricular 140
  neurosarcoidosis vs. 72, 116, 124
primary CNS vasculitis (PCNSV, or primary
    angiitis of CNS, PACNS) 34, 37
primitive neuroectodermal tumor (PNET), pineal
    125, 136
progressive multifocal leukoencephalopathy (PML)
    62–4
prostate cancer, metastatic 161, 170, 458
pseudo-Chiari malformation 234–5
pseudotumor cerebri see idiopathic intracranial
    hypertension
pterygoid process, asymmetric pneumatization
    264, 266
puff-of-smoke collaterals 40, 42

radiation arteritis 36
radiation vasculopathy 44
radiotherapy
  glioblastoma pseudoprogression following
    109–11
  optic neuropathy complicating 336, 338
Rathke's cleft cyst 240–2
Refsum disease, infantile 219
renal cell carcinoma, metastatic 146, 395, 458
renal osteodystrophy 409–10
retention cysts
  nasopharynx 354
  parotid gland 350, 352
retropharyngeal abscess 414
retropharyngeal edema (cellulitis)
  calcific tendinitis of longus colli 414–15
  phlegmonous 414, 417
retropharyngeal lymph nodes, suppurative 414, 418
reversible cerebral vasoconstriction syndrome
    (RCVS) 37
rhabdomyosarcoma (RMS) 328, 330
rheumatoid arthritis, atlantoaxial subluxation
    390, 397
rhinosinusitis
  acute 316, 321
  chronic 310, 316
  see also paranasal sinusitis
rickets 409, 412
rosette-forming glioneural tumor of fourth
    ventricle 140
rugger jersey spine 409–10

sacral insufficiency fractures 401–4
salivary glands 342–50
  benign mixed tumor (BMT) 344–6, 364–5
  malignant tumors 344, 347–8
  see also parotid glands
sarcoidosis 72
  nervous system see neurosarcoidosis
  orbital 331, 336, 339
  spinal cord 72, 466
schwannomas
  cauda equina 478, 485
  parapharyngeal space 364, 366
  spinal cord compression 458
  third nerve 262
  trigeminal nerve 284
scoliosis, tethered cord and 445
second branchial cleft cysts 357
segmental spinal dysgenesis 435, 444
seromas, spinal epidural 475
sestamibi scintigraphy, Tc-99m 372–6
sinonasal melanoma 316, 322
sinonasal polyposis 310, 315
sinonasal squamous cell carcinoma 316, 320
sinovenous stenoses, idiopathic intracranial
    hypertension 238–9
sinovenous thrombosis (SVT) 238
sinusitis see paranasal sinusitis, rhinosinusitis
skull base 267–82
  asymmetric pneumatization 264–6
  clival lesions 276
  fibrous dysplasia 267–9
  perineural spread 282
  sphenoid bone pseudolesion 271
  spontaneous CSF leaks 324
sphenoid bone pseudolesion 271–3
sphenoid cephaloceles 324–6
spina bifida 434
spinal canal contents 434–79
spinal cord
  anterior thoracic herniation 471, 474
  apparent anterior displacement 471–2
  arteriovenous malformations (AVMs)
    455, 457
  demyelinating/inflammatory lesions 466–8
  intradural cysts 471
  intramedullary metastasis 478
  sarcoidosis 72, 79, 466
  subacute combined degeneration 469–70
  tumors 466
spinal cord compression 458
  disc herniation and 424–6
  metastatic epidural (MESCC) 458–62
  renal osteodystrophy 409
spinal dysgenesis, segmental 435, 444
spinal dysraphism 434–5
  classification 434
  closed (CSD) 434–5, 445
  occult 434
  open (OSD) 434, 445
spinal meningeal cysts 458, 463
spinal vascular malformations (SVMs) 455
spine 387–414
  CSF leaks 475–7
  intracranial hypotension and 234, 236
  leptomeningeal drop metastases 478
  lymphoma 409, 413
  Paget's disease of bone 405–9, 411

renal osteodystrophy 409–10
rugger jersey 409–10
see also cervical spine; intervertebral discs; lumbar spine; vertebrae
spondylitis, pyogenic, cord compression 458
spondylodiscitis, cervical 414, 418
spontaneous intracranial hypotension (SIH) 234, 237
spinal CSF leaks 475–6
spot sign, intracerebral hematoma 26–7
squamous cell carcinoma (SCC)
cystic nodal metastasis 357–8
human papilloma virus (HPV)-related 357
parotid metastases 342–3
sinonasal 316, 320
straight sinus thrombosis 3
string sign
carotid artery dissection 381
near-occlusive carotid stenosis 378–80
stroke
acute intracerebral hematoma 26
acute ischemic 8–9
dense artery sign 1–2
moyamoya disease 40
near-occlusive carotid stenosis 378
subacute 13
vertebral artery dissection 10
see also cerebral infarction
subacute cerebral infarction 13
subacute combined degeneration 469–70
subarachnoid hemorrhage (SAH) 17
associated vasospasm 37, 39
FLAIR sulcal hyperintensity 245, 249
reversible cerebral vasoconstriction syndrome-associated 37–8
vertebral artery dissection 10, 12
subdural fluid collections
benign external hydrocephalus vs. 257–8
intracranial hypotension 234–5
subdural hematomas
benign external hydrocephalus vs. 257, 259
intracranial hypotension 234
isodense 227–8
subependymal giant cell astrocytoma (SEGA) 153, 159
subependymoma 140
suboccipital rind sign 10
sulcal hyperintensity secondary to general anesthesia, FLAIR 245–8
superior sagittal sinus thrombosis, FLAIR sulcal hyperintensity 248
superior semicircular canal dehiscence (SSCD) 292–3
syringomyelia
Chiari I malformation and 449, 452
terminal 445, 448

temozolomide, glioblastoma pseudoprogression following 109–11
temporal bone
fractures 307–9
imaging 285–308
teratomas, pineal region 125
terminal myelocystocele 435, 441
tethered spinal cord 434, 438, 445
thiamine deficiency 213
thickened cortex sign 227–8
third branchial apparatus anomaly 370
thoracic cord herniation, anterior 471, 474
thrombolytic therapy, patient selection 8–9
thrombosis, acute 1–3
thyroglossal duct cysts 357
thyroid adenoma 372, 376
thyroid cancer nodal metastases 357, 359, 371
thyroid gland, hypermetabolic, sestamibi uptake 372, 374
thyroid ophthalmopathy 331, 334
thyroid/perithyroid abscesses 370
tissue plasminogen activator (tPA) therapy, patient selection 8
Tolosa–Hunt syndrome 331
tonsillar crypt cysts 354, 356
Tornwaldt's cysts 354–5
toxoplasmosis 191, 193
transverse myelopathy/myelitis, acute 466
transverse sinus thrombosis 3
trauma 224–7
acute intracerebral hematoma 26
arterial injuries to neck 384–6
craniovertebral junction injuries 387
isodense subdural hematoma 227–8
ligamentous neck injuries 414
mild traumatic brain injury 224–6
odontoid fractures 390
temporal bone fractures 307–8
traumatic brain injury, mild (mTBI) 224–6
tuberculosis
brain abscess vs. 191, 198, 204
CNS 198–202
tuberculous meningitis (TBM) 198–9
spinal leptomeningeal metastases vs. 478
spontaneous intracranial hypotension vs. 237
tuberous sclerosis 153, 159
Tullio's phenomenon 292
tumefactive demyelinating lesion (TDL) 55–7
tumefactive lesions, acute disseminated encephalomyelitis 58
tumors
brain see brain tumors
perineural spread 282–4

salivary glands 344
secondary see metastases
spinal cord 466

varicella vasculitis 36
vasa vasora, hypertrophied, with complete carotid occlusion 378, 380
vascular injuries, traumatic 384
vascular malformations
classification 360
low-flow (LFVMs), head and neck 360
spinal 455
vasculitis (angiitis), primary CNS (PCNSV) 34, 37
vasospasm, subarachnoid hemorrhage-associated 37, 39
vein of Galen thrombosis 3
venolymphatic malformations, parapharyngeal space 364, 368
venous angiomas, cerebral see developmental venous anomalies
venous malformations (VMs), head and neck 360–1
venous structures
CT angiography 260
intracranial aneurysms vs. 17, 20–1
venous thrombosis
internal cerebral veins 213, 215
intravascular clot 1, 3
isolated cortical (ICVT) 43
ventricle, persistent terminal 435
vertebrae
compression fractures 398–400
cord compression due to collapsed 458
degenerative end-plate changes 430–2
ivory 405
osteomyelitis 430, 433
Paget's disease 405–9, 411
renal osteodystrophy 409–10
vertebral artery
dissection (VAD) 10
traumatic injuries 384, 386
vertebrobasilar artery, giant aneurysm 25
Virchow–Robin spaces (VRS) 250–2
vitamin $B_{12}$ deficiency 469
von Hippel–Lindau syndrome 80

Wallenberg (lateral medullary) syndrome 10–11
Warthin's tumor 342, 344, 349
watershed ischemic lesions 229, 231
Wegener's granulomatosis 316, 321, 331, 335
Wernicke's encephalopathy 213–15

Zellweger syndrome 219